Concussions in Athletics

Semyon M. Slobounov • Wayne J. Sebastianelli
Editors

Concussions in Athletics

From Brain to Behavior

Springer

Editors
Semyon M. Slobounov
Professor of Kinesiology & Neurosurgery
Director of Center for Sports Concussion
  Research and Services
Penn State - Department of Kinesiology &
  Hershey Medical College
University Park, PA, USA

Wayne J. Sebastianelli
Kalenak Professor in Orthopaedics
Director of Athletic Medicine
Penn State - Hershey Medical College
University Park, PA, USA

ISBN 978-1-4939-0294-1   ISBN 978-1-4939-0295-8 (eBook)
DOI 10.1007/978-1-4939-0295-8
Springer New York Heidelberg Dordrecht London

Library of Congress Control Number: 2014931771

Printed on acid-free paper

Springer is part of Springer Science+Business Media (www.springer.com)

Foreword

I recently saw a 16-year-old cheerleader who had suffered five concussions. She has dropped from an A student to a C student who needs special help. Another patient, a 12-year-old former cheerleader, after two concussions had to drop back to the first grade level in school.

Concussion in sport is a big deal. It is a common problem with consequences. There is the short-term issue of a period when the athlete cannot continue to play. But then there are longer term issues of post-concussive symptoms including increased sensitivity for subsequent concussions (second impact syndrome). And, even though there is no obvious damage to the brain on routine neuroimaging, there may well be brain damage leading to reduction in cognitive abilities or even, in severe cases, posttraumatic encephalopathy. It's a big deal for another reason; it is a problem with children and young adults, and concussion can change their lives forever. Of course, concussion can also occur with auto accidents and with war injuries, as well as everyday life, and similar issues emerge. Studies of athletes can well be generalized to other situations.

With an acute injury, it is important to recognize that a concussion has occurred and determine its severity. There can be a variety of symptoms including difficulty in thinking, concentrating or remembering, headache, nausea, dizziness, and imbalance. Clinical assessment can include drowsiness, disorientation, slow reaction time, memory loss, difficulty with balance and coordination, and emotional lability. In the post-concussion syndrome all these symptoms and signs can persist for variable periods of time.

There are approximately 300,000 sports-related concussions annually in the USA. It is interesting to consider in what sports they occur. A nice paper by Marar et al. [1] looked in detail at the epidemiology of concussions in high school athletes. They reported on 1,936 concussions in 7,778,064 athletic exposures. Boys' football gives the largest number of concussion with more exposures and with the highest rate overall. After that in numbers of concussions are girls' soccer, boys' wrestling, girls' basketball, and boys' soccer. After boys' football, the next highest rate is boys' ice hockey, then boys' lacrosse.

So we are dealing with a common problem. But we certainly don't understand it well enough. What is happening in the acute and chronic states? Why does sensitivity increase for subsequent concussions? There are clinical issues all along. What is the best way to recognize and grade the severity of concussion? When is it relatively safe to return to the sport? Is clinical assessment enough? Can laboratory testing help? Are there ways to prevent concussion? How should it be treated? All these topics and more are dealt with in this nice book edited by Drs. Slobounov and Sebastianelli. They have enormous experience themselves at Penn State and have put together a distinguished group of authors to speak to the important issues.

This book should be of value to anyone dealing with persons with concussion—and that is almost everyone.

Bethesda, MD, USA   Mark Hallett

Reference

1. Marar M, McIlvain NM, Fields SK, Comstock RD. Epidemiology of concussions among United States high school athletes in 20 sports. Am J Sports Med. 2012;40(4):747–55. doi:10.1177/0363546511435626. Epub 2012 Jan 27.

Preface

Concussion in athletics, commonly known as mild traumatic brain injury (mTBI), is a growing public health concern with increased attention being focused on treatment and management of this frustrating epidemic. A critical decision confronting healthcare practitioners is to determine the appropriate time frame with respect to returning an injured athlete back to full participation. Premature return to play after a concussion increases an athlete's risk for recurrent brain injury and potentially increases the severity of injury. At present there is no definitive diagnostic tool prognosticating the brain's true return to normal. The common symptoms of concussion may be caused by abnormalities anywhere in the brain. Therefore, a multidisciplinary approach to understanding the true pathology and associated residual behavioral, psychosocial, neuropsychological, and neurological consequences of concussion injuries in athletes is necessary. The purpose of this book is to condense our current understanding of concussion, *From Brain to Behavior*, including the neuromechanisms, predispositions, and the latest developments in evaluation and management of concussive injuries.

This book is the partial product of a conference: "Concussion in Athletics: From Brain to Behavior" held at Pennsylvania State University in October 5–6, 2012. This conference received the generous support of The College of Health and Human Development, Penn State Hershey College of Medicine, the Departments of Kinesiology, Psychology, The Social Science Research Institute, and Springer. Due to this support, we were able to invite world known experts in the field supplementing the host Pennsylvania State University faculty. This conference experienced great success, evidenced by 180 attendees not only from the USA, but also from Canada, Israel, and Russia. It should be noted that the conference was not able to cover all aspects of concussion. A limited emphasis was given to the treatment and management of sports-related concussions. A limited discussion was developed in the area of rehabilitation and recovery of diminished neurocognitive and behavioral consequences of traumatic brain injury. We are very pleased with the fact that several chapters of this book provided by contributing authors address these less studied but still very important aspects of sports-related concussions. We are indebted to all authors for their great contribution to this book. We would also like to acknowledge the presentation of Dr. Albert King at this conference. Unfortunately, we are unable to include his presentation into the content of this book due to copyright issues.

Caring for athletes at any level is a distinct pleasure and privilege. We would like to thank the thousands of students and recreational athletes that we have cared for over the last several decades. They have allowed us to become part of their lives. This book represents a continuum of interest and concern for athletes with mTBIs, aka concussion. Although we have learned a tremendous amount since our research initially started, one can see from the excellent chapters in this textbook that more remains to be understood. To the trainers, coaches, and athletic administrative support personnel, our sincere thanks for helping us pursue a solution to this challenging problem. To our office staff, support staff, and partners, our sincere appreciation for giving us the time to pursue this endeavor. A special thanks to Katie Finelli for her dedication to our research and tremendous contribution to this book. It is with great pleasure we extend our thanks to our publishers and particularly to Richard Lansing and Barbara Lopez-Lucio for their efforts to make this book happen.

University Park, PA, USA   Semyon M. Slobounov
                                                                Wayne J. Sebastianelli

Contents

Contributors

Peter A. Arnett, Ph.D. Department of Psychology, Pennsylvania State University, University Park, PA, USA

Patrick S.F. Bellgowan, Ph.D. Laureate Institute for Brain Research, Tulsa, OK, USA

Erin D. Bigler, Ph.D. Department of Psychology and Neuroscience Center, Brigham Young University, Provo, UT, USA

Department of Psychiatry, University of Utah, Salt Lake City, UT, USA

Steven P. Broglio, Ph.D., A.T.C. NeuroSport Research Laboratory, School of Kinesiology, University of Michigan, Ann Arbor, MI, USA

Thomas A. Buckley, Ed.D. Department of Health and Kinesiology, Georgia Southern University, Statesboro, GA, USA

Robert C. Cantu, M.A., M.D., F.A.C.S., F.A.A.N.S., F.A.C.S.M. Emerson Hospital, Concord, MA, USA

Jonathon Cooke, M.D. Department of Neurological Surgery, Penn State Milton S. Hershey Medical Center, Hershey, PA, USA

Rimma Danov, Ph.D. Dr. Danov Neuropsychologist PC, Brooklyn, NY, USA

Stefan M. Duma, Ph.D. School of Biomedical Engineering and Sciences, Virginia Tech, Blacksburg, VA, USA

Michael R. Gay, Ph.D., A.T.C. Pennsylvania State Intercollegiate Athletics, Pennsylvania State University, University Park, PA, USA

Kevin M. Guskiewicz, Ph.D., A.T.C. College of Arts and Sciences, University of North Carolina at Chapel Hill, Chapel Hill, NC, USA

E. Mark Haacke, Ph.D. Department of Radiology, Wayne State University, Detroit, MI, USA

David A. Hovda, Ph.D. Departments of Neurosurgery and Molecular and Medical Pharmacology, David Geffen School of Medicine at UCLA, Los Angeles, CA, USA

Brian D. Johnson, Ph.D., M.S., R.T.(MR)(N) Department of Kinesiology, Pennsylvania State University, University Park, PA, USA

Zhifeng Kou, Ph.D. Departments of Biomedical Engineering and Radiology, Wayne State University, Detroit, MI, USA

Giuseppe Lazzarino, Ph.D. Department of Biology, Geology and Environmental Sciences, Division of Biochemistry and Molecular Biology, University of Catania, Catania, Italy

Mark R. Lovell, Ph.D. Department of Neurological Surgery, University of Pittsburgh, Pittsburgh, PA, USA

Andrew R. Mayer, Ph.D. Department of Cognitive Neuroscience, The Mind Research Network, Albuquerque, NM, USA

Andrew S. McIntosh, Ph.D., M.Biomed.E, B.App.Sci. (P.T.) Centre for Healthy and Safe Sports, The University of Ballarat, Ballarat, VIC, Australia

Victoria C. Merritt, M.S. Department of Psychology, Pennsylvania State University, University Park, PA, USA

Jessica Meyer, B.S. Department of Psychology, Pennsylvania State University, University Park, PA, USA

Karl M. Newell, Ph.D. Department of Kinesiology, Pennsylvania State University, University Park, PA, USA

Linda Papa, M.D., C.M., M.Sc. Department of Emergency Medicine, Orlando Regional Medical Center, Orlando, FL, USA

Amanda R. Rabinowitz, Ph.D. Department of Neurosurgery, University of Pennsylvania School of Medicine, Philadelphia, PA, USA

William J. Ray, Ph.D. Department of Psychology, Pennsylvania State University, University Park, PA, USA

Scott L. Rosenthal, B.S. Department of Kinesiology, Pennsylvania State University, University Park, PA, USA

Steven Rowson, Ph.D. School of Biomedical Engineering and Sciences, Virginia Tech, Blacksburg, VA, USA

Wayne J. Sebastianelli, M.D. Pennsylvania State University, University Park, PA, USA

Departments of Orthopaedics and Sports Medicine, Penn State Hershey, Bone and Joint Institute, State College, PA, USA

Stefano Signoretti, M.D., Ph.D. Department of Neurosciences—Head and Neck Surgery, Division of Neurosurgery, San Camillo Hospital, Rome, Italy

Semyon M. Slobounov, Ph.D. Professor of Kinesiology & Neurosurgery, Director of Center for Sports Concussion Research and Services, Penn State - Department of Kinesiology & Hershey Medical College, University Park, PA, USA

Barbara Tavazzi, Ph.D. Institute of Biochemistry and Clinical Biochemistry, Catholic University of Rome, Rome, Italy

Elizabeth F. Teel, M.S. Department of Kinesiology, Pennsylvania State University, University Park, PA, USA

Kirtley E. Thornton, Ph.D. The Brain Foundation, Lake Wylie, SC, USA

Dede M. Ukueberuwa, M.S. Department of Psychology, Pennsylvania State University, University Park, PA, USA

Roberto Vagnozzi, M.D., Ph.D. Department of Biomedicine and Prevention, Section of Neurosurgery, University of Rome Tor Vergata, Rome, Italy

Gray A. Vargas, M.S. Department of Psychology, Pennsylvania State University, University Park, PA, USA

Keith Owen Yeates, Ph.D. Section of Pediatric Psychology and Neuropsychology, Nationwide Children's Hospital, Columbus, OH, USA

Department of Pediatrics, The Ohio State University, Columbus, OH, USA

J. Christopher Zacko, M.S., M.D. Penn State Hershey Medical Center, Hershey, PA, USA

Chapter 1
Introduction

Semyon M. Slobounov and Wayne J. Sebastianelli

Abstract Concussion in athletics is a growing public health concern with increased attention being focused on treatment and management of this puzzling epidemic. A critical decision confronting health care practitioners is to determine the proper and safest time frame when clearing athletes to resume participation, as premature return-to-play after concussion may put injured athletes at high risk for recurrent and more severe brain injuries. Despite the increasing occurrence and prevalence of concussions in athletics, there is no universally accepted definition or "gold standard" for its assessment. Conventional brain imaging techniques lack the sensitivity to detect the subtle structural changes. Clinical management of sports-induced concussions has not changed much over the past decade. Advances in neuroimaging that include electroencephalography, functional magnetic resonance imaging, diffusion tensor imaging, and magnetic resonance spectroscopy offer the opportunity in developing research leading to a better understanding of the complexities and nuances of concussions. This may ultimately influence the clinical management of the injury and provide more accurate guidelines for return to sport participation. In this introductory chapter the authors review the major findings from advanced neuroimaging methods along with current controversy within the field of concussion research.

S.M. Slobounov, Ph.D. (✉)
Professor of Kinesiology & Neurosurgery, Director of Center for Sports Concussion Research and Services, Penn State - Department of Kinesiology & Hershey Medical College
University Park, PA, USA
e-mail: sms18@psu.edu

W.J. Sebastianelli, M.D.
Pennsylvania State University, University Park, PA, USA

Departments of Orthopaedics and Sports Medicine, Penn State Hershey,
Bone and Joint Institute, State College, PA 16803, USA
e-mail: wsebastianelli@hmc.psu.edu

S.M. Slobounov and W.J. Sebastianelli (eds.), *Concussions in Athletics:
From Brain to Behavior*, DOI 10.1007/978-1-4939-0295-8_1,
© Springer Science+Business Media New York 2014

Keywords Concussion • Return-to-play • Brain imaging • EEG • fMRI • DTI • MRS • Virtual reality

Clinical Research of Sports-Related Concussion

Each year, thousands of first responders, athletic trainers, coaches, and clinicians face a critical question: What is the time frame for safe return-to-sports participation after concussion? According to the current best practice established by the Concussion in Sports Group (CISG), an athlete must be completely asymptomatic at rest, with cognitive exertion and with activities of daily living prior to the initiation of a step-wise "Return-to-Play" protocol. An athlete is defined as "asymptomatic" once he/she has returned to baseline levels on self-reported symptom scales and clinical examination, including balance and neurocognitive function measures. While the current clinical standard of neuropsychological testing, postural control measures and symptoms checklists have been reported to be highly sensitive, there is no indication that resolution of these indices corresponds to recovery of the complex pathophysiology induced by concussion.

Mild traumatic brain injury (mTBI), commonly known as concussion, is gaining significant attention within the clinical and basic brain research communities. With some researchers reporting 1.6–3.8 million concussions occurring in sports [1], mTBI accounts for 80 % of all reported traumatic brain injuries [2]. The annual rate of diagnosed concussions over the past 10 years in high school sports demonstrated an increase of 16.5 % annually [3]. With such high rates of sports-related brain injury occurring during adolescence and young adulthood an emphasis has to be placed on fully understanding the short and long term consequences of this complex and still most puzzling neurological disorder [4].

The main goal of this introductory chapter is to provide a cursory review and empirical evidence from neuroimaging and clinical studies that go against the conventional wisdom that *typical* recovery following a sport-related concussion is rapid and full with no residual deficits. There is growing evidence that *atypical evolution* of mTBI may be more prevalent due to the fact that physical, neurocognitive, emotional symptoms and underlying neural alterations persist months or even years post-injury. Specifically, the findings of recent brain imaging studies challenge the conventional wisdom based upon neurocognitive assessment of concussion.

Allied health professionals treating concussed young people have been using the same approach to treatment for nearly two decades. Initially, focused on classification systems, clinicians would choose a system based on their general preference. With 41 different and most often controversial classification systems [5] and a return to play protocol based on a clinical construct [6], practitioners have been held to management and return to play standards that were based less on well researched physiologic data but more on clinical intuition and consensus statements from leaders in the field of neuropsychology [7]. Serial testing of patients' cognitive status was first recommended in the early 1980s as a mechanism to help the clinician determine when an athlete could safely return to athletic participation [8]. Contributing to the early treatment approach was the formation of neuropsychological assessment batteries [9, 10], which are still in clinical use today as the cornerstone of clinical management for sports-related concussion [11, 12]. These testing batteries primarily measure a patient's cognitive status. Initially performed with paper and pencil, cognitive test batteries designed for managing athletes recovering from sports-related concussion have now almost fully evolved to computer-based online batteries of tests which can be interpreted by many health care professionals [13].

Even with increased awareness of concussion and an increased presence of trained allied health professionals like athletic trainers monitoring high schools and college sports, concussion is still commonly misunderstood by some clinicians and can be over simplified in terms of its diagnosis and recovery [14, 15]. Athletes typically present clinically with a variety of physical and cognitive symptoms which can be reasonably detected with a thorough clinical evaluation both on the field and in the clinic or athletic training room [12]. One common tool that has been endorsed for sideline assessment or clinical use is the Sport Concussion Assessment Tool (SCAT-2) [12]. This clinical assessment tool has been endorsed in one form or another in the proceedings and consensus statements of the second and third International Conference on concussion for use on athletes recovering from mTBI. The use of which mandates the inclusion of a baseline measure taken when the athlete is asymptomatic. The SCAT-2 is designed to evaluate the patient using a composite score generated from: the Self-Reported Symptoms Score; Physical Signs Score; the Glasgow Coma Scale; Sideline Assessment—Maddock's Score; Cognitive Assessment (SAC); and Coordination Examination Scores. The athlete's overall score is recorded and then compared to the athlete's premorbid level of function on their pre-season baseline measure. This basic clinical assessment tool score along with other clinical findings on exam are used to determine when an athlete may be ready to progress back into exercise and athletic participation.

There is still a lack in belief among neuropsychological and clinical researchers that concussion results in long lasting structural injury to the neuron. This idea is reflected in the sentiment of nearly every consensus statement on concussion [7, 11, 12] and is frequently repeated in these statements. The authors of these statements frequently repeat that; "Concussion may result in neuropathologic changes, but the clinical symptoms largely reflect a functional disturbance rather than a structural injury." This clinical sentiment is repeated and re-examined in clinical research in which neuropsychologists and other clinical concussion researchers continue to promote the idea of cognitive functional recovery being representative of clinical recovery [11]. Objectively, this basic statement represents a construct flaw in their hypothesis. *All of the supportive data are mainly based on the restoration of cognitive functioning measured by neuropsychological testing and not based on the healing of the microstructural lesion.*

The above controversy is exaggerated even more by the fact that conventional MRI and CT scans are often negative due to the absence of macrostructural alterations. Over the past 10 years, animal studies and physiological reviews have demonstrated a complex series of neurometabolic cascades, neurovascular compromise and neurophysiologic impairment [16–19] stemming from the mechanical forces of sport-related concussion. The mechanical stretch of axons produces injury to the cytoarchitecture of the axon [20, 21] and surface architecture of the axon [22] which significantly impairs normal neurologic function [23] and leaves the neuron vulnerable to more significant insult repeatedly [22]. These forces are also capable of inducing short term and lasting vascular changes [24–26]. These are findings that the neurobiological research community and neuroimaging community have paid particular attention to in recent years, but have been identified for decades [27]. However, these findings are largely overlooked and underappreciated in the clinical management of sports-related concussion. *Inclusion of these findings, upon validation, into the clinical management of concussion must be considered, combining advanced neuroimaging techniques with data driven neuropsychological and neurological assessments.*

EEG Research in Concussion

Considering the high temporal resolution of electroencephalography (EEG) signal, EEG is highly suitable for examining neurophysiological correlates of fast sensory-motor and cognitive functions [28–30], susceptible to concussive impacts. Historically EEG was the first monitoring assessment tool to demonstrate the alteration of brain functions in subjects suffering from TBI [29–33]. Since then, considerable empirical evidence was accumulated indicating both (a) clinical value of EEG in terms of the accuracy of assessment of mTBI, and (b) conceptual significance of EEG in enabling the examination of neural substrates underlying neurological, behavioral and neuropsychological alterations in mTBI [31, 34–37].

Early EEG research in 300 patients clearly demonstrated the slowing of major frequency bands and focal abnormalities within 48 h post-injury [34]. A study by McClelland et al. has shown that EEG recordings performed during the immediate post-concussion period demonstrated a large amount of "diffusely distributed slow-wave potentials," which were markedly reduced when recordings were performed 6 weeks after injury [33]. A shift in the mean frequency in the alpha (8–10 Hz) band toward lower power and an overall decrease of beta (14–18 Hz) power in patients suffering from mTBI was observed by Tebano et al. [34]. The reduction of theta power [39] accompanying a transient increase of alpha-theta ratios [40, 41] was identified as residual symptoms in mTBI patients.

The most comprehensive EEG study using a database of 608 mTBI subjects up to 8 years post-injury revealed: (a) increased coherence in frontal–temporal regions; (b) decreased power differences between anterior and posterior cortical regions; and (c) reduced alpha power in the posterior cortical region, which was attributed to mechanical head injury [38]. A study by Thornton has shown a similar data trend in addition to demonstrating the attenuation of EEG within the high frequency gamma cluster (32–64 Hz) in mTBI patients [39]. Also, the usefulness and high sensitivity of EEG in the assessment of concussion have been demonstrated [40–44].

There is also a line of recent research indicating the efficacy of EEG-based ERP (event-related potentials) in detecting subtle and pervasive alterations of cognition-related waveforms in athletes suffering from mTBI, including multiple concussions [40, 41]. It appeared that the athletes with the history of previous mTBI exhibited significantly attenuated amplitude of posterior contralateral negativity (SPCN) compared to normal volunteers in the absence of working memory (WM) abnormalities [41]. Similarly, Broglio et al. reported significant decrement in the N2 and P3b amplitude of the stimulus-locked ERP in athletes with a history of concussion on average of 3.4 years post-injury [42]. Most importantly, no significant alterations were observed based on commonly used ImPACT tests. *Overall, these findings strongly support the notion that sport-related mTBI can no longer be considered as a transient injury.*

A number of reports from our research group clearly indicate that advanced use of EEG feature extraction may indeed detect subtle brain functional abnormalities in the absence of any clinical mTBI symptoms. Specifically, we applied advanced *EEG-wavelet entropy* measures to detect brain functional deficits in mTBI subjects. These EEG measures were significantly reduced primarily after the first and especially after the second mTBI far beyond 7 days post-injury. Most importantly, the rate of recovery of EEG entropy measures was significantly slower after the second mTBI compared to those after the first concussion [45]. In fact, we have recently reported the alteration of EEG signals in mTBI subjects detected by a novel measure of nonstationarity, named Shannon entropy of the peak frequency shifting [46]. These findings are complementary to our previously published concussion report indicating the presence of residual deficits in mTBI subjects detected by the multi-channel EEG signals classifier using a support vector machine [47].

Our research group also conducted an EEG resting state study and reported the alteration of cortical functional connectivity in mTBI subjects revealed by graph theory, independent component analysis (ICA) and low resolution brain electro-magnetic tomography analyses (LORETA). Overall, a clear departure from *small world like network* was observed in mTBI subjects [48]. We observed a reduction of the clustering coefficient (C_p) as an index of local structure and enhancement of path length (L_p) as an index of graph integration as a result of concussion. These results seem to be in agreement with "network randomization" hypothesis, as a general framework of abnormal brain functions commonly observed in neurological subjects, including those suffering from low-grade tumor and/or epilepsy.

Recently Arciniegas outlined the major limiting factors contributing to the limited capacity of EEG measures in clinical assessment of mTBI. These include: (a) the lack of control for subjects' homogeneity, (b) lack of research when EEG assessment was performed immediately after and serially over the first year of injury; (c) poor experimental designs when EEG data are collected independently from performance-based assessment of patients' functional status; (d) different time frame since injury when EEG measures were obtained [31]. Our research team partially addressed these limitations by obtaining further EEG evidence of a residual disturbance of the neuronal network that is involved in execution of postural movement in mTBI subjects. This was done by incorporating EEG and Virtual Reality

(VR) induced measures [49–52]. We designed an EEG study using a virtual reality (VR) graphics system aimed to examine the brain activation patterns preceding the loss of postural stability induced by a "Moving Room" experimental paradigm ([56], see special VR chapter by Dr. Slobounov et al. (Chap. 4)).

Similar to *typical* course of clinical recovery after mTBI, abnormalities on conventional EEG recording tend to resolve during the first several months post-injury [53]. EEG assessment could contribute to the development and refinement of differential diagnostic information among subjects with atypical clinical recovery following mTBI. That said, it is important to note that the differences in EEG profiles in subjects showing the *typical* and *atypical* functional recovery after mTBI may serve as a starting point from which to begin more fully investigating the neural substrates for differential recovery after traumatic brain injury [54]. With this in mind our research group combined EEG (alpha power difference during sitting versus standing upright postures) and balance measures (standing still with eyes open and closed) in subjects prior to injury (baseline testing, $n = 380$) and serially over 1 year post-injury ($n = 49$) to further examine the neural substrates of cerebral brain dysfunctions in mTBI subjects as injury evolves over time [54].

The major findings in our study are the following: (a) Percent alpha power suppression from sitting to standing postural conditions significantly increased in mTBI subjects shortly after the injury ($p < 0.01$); (b) Percent alpha power suppression significantly correlated with increased area of COP during standing posture with eye closed ($r^2 = 0.53$, $p < 0.01$); (c) The magnitude of alpha power suppression predicted the rate of recovery of this measure in subacute and chronic phases of injury ($r^2 = 0.609$, $p < 0.01$); Finally, 85 % of mTBI subjects who showed more than 20 % of alpha power suppression in the acute phase of injury did not return to pre-injury status up to 12 months post-injury [54].

Overall, the efficacy of serially implemented EEG measures in conjunction with balance assessment over the course of mTBI evolution to document residual cerebral dysfunction was clearly demonstrated. Specifically, alteration of EEG alpha power dynamics in conjunction with balance data in the acute phase of injury with respect to baseline measures may predict the rate of recovery from a single concussive blow. *As such, EEG measures (if properly executed in conjunction with other behavioral variables) are excellent tools to assess the status and prognosis of patients with concussion.*

Functional Magnetic Resonance Imaging and Concussion

Blood oxygen level-dependent (BOLD) MR: One of the more recent and popular advancements in neuroimaging, fMRI, has become a widely used research tool in probing the complexities of the brain [55]. Functional MRI uses the principal of BOLD contrast as an index of neuronal activity [56]. The BOLD signal in fMRI is sensitive to blood-based properties, specifically the local magnetic susceptibility produced by deoxyhemoglobin which cause a reduction in signal.

The assumption in BOLD fMRI is that an increase in neuronal activity within a brain region results in an increase in local blood flow, leading to reduced concentrations of deoxyhemoglobin in nearby vessels [57]. Therefore, the higher concentrations of oxyhemoglobin associated with neuronal activity results in higher signal intensities due to a reduction in local field inhomogeneities and signal dephasing caused by deoxyhemoglobin. For a more detailed review of MR physics or fMRI methodological and conceptual pitfalls see Horowitz [58] and Hillary et al. [59] respectively. The currently accepted notion is that BOLD fMRI most likely detects secondary effects of neuronal firing due to the *hemodynamic response*, allowing *indirect* assessment of the neuronal responses to cognitive and/or sensory-motor task demands [60].

There is hope that advanced brain imaging techniques like fMRI will be a valuable tool in the assessment of mTBI due to the limited ability of conventional brain imaging and current neuropsychological tests [61]. Recent brain imaging research, particularly fMRI, revealed alteration of the BOLD signal in concussed individuals while performing working memory, attention, sensory-motor and other neurocognitive tasks. Empirical findings have suggested that task-related fMRI studies may be a robust and more sensitive tool for assessment of residual functional motor and cognitive deficits, especially in the subacute phase of mTBI [62]. However, there is still debate in the literature regarding the values of advanced brain imaging data (e.g., fMRI, diffusion tensor imaging [DTI], magnetic resonance spectroscopy [MRS]) in a clinical assessment of concussion, at least as it pertains to athletics [12].

Since working memory (WM) deficits are nearly universal following most of the neurological disruption (including mTBI), the functional imaging clinical literature has focused on examining these deficits with respect to basic information processing. In functional imaging studies of mTBI, there have been more or less similarities in the findings, with most results [62–64] pointing to increased neural activity in several brain regions, but most consistently in the prefrontal cortex (PFC), and especially the dorsolateral prefrontal cortex (DLPFC). For example, McAllister et al. [64] have shown enhanced and more widespread BOLD signal in concussed subjects performing a series of cognitive tasks. In these fMRI studies, mTBI subjects within 1 month post-injury and age-matched normal controls performed the "*n*-back" working memory task. Significant differences between the two groups' brain activation patterns were shown in response to increasing working memory processing loads. The primary finding from McAllister's team was an increased activation in DLPFC in concussed subjects who successfully performed the "*n*-back" working memory task. Another interesting finding of this research group is that mTBI patients showed disproportionately increased activation during the moderate processing load condition [64]. Similarly, Jantzen et al. showed increased activation in the parietal, lateral frontal, and cerebellar regions in concussed subjects when compared with pre-injury in the absence of changes in cognitive performance [65]. The hyper-activation of PFC and possibly other regions of interest (ROIs) in mTBI may represent a "neural inefficiency" concept that has been linked to neurological patients' diminished performance of cognitive tasks [66, 68, 69].

It should be noted however that Chen et al. reported opposite findings suggesting a reduction (hypo-activation) of fMRI BOLD in the mid-DLPFC in symptomatic concussed subjects in conjunction with poorer performance on the WM tasks [67]. Later on, this group reported additional activation in concussed subjects in the posterior brain regions including the left temporal lobe that were not present in the normal controls [70]. Most recently, Chen et al. reported reduced activation in DLPFC and striatum in concussed athletes with depression who have no performance difference compared to patients without depression and healthy controls [71]. In a more recent Mayer et al. study, mTBI individuals also reported hypo-activation within several cortical and subcortical areas along with poor performance of auditory orientation and attention inhibition tasks [72]. Another study of mTBI patients within 6 weeks post-injury reported no significant difference in the brain activation patterns compared to normal volunteers, but there was an inverse correlation between medial temporal lobe activation and injury severity [73]. Clearly, whether research methodology pitfalls (i.e., differential time of scanning since injury, susceptibility artifact, SNR especially when dealing with group analysis), conceptual biases (e.g., selecting primarily frontal and anterior temporal ROIs as the common site for the brain damage after TBI) or inhomogeneity of the mTBI subjects (differential severity of acute brain injury and/or lack of control for the history of multiple concussive and sub-concussive blows) may cause controversial fMRI finding obtained in different research laboratories and requires further analysis. See also Slobounov et al. for further details [74].

Resting-State Functional Connectivity from fMRI

There has been recent focus in studies using BOLD fMRI to approximate brain activation patterns, specifically to incorporate baseline or "resting state" measurement of the BOLD signal. Conceptually, the human brain has two contradictory properties: (1) "segregation," which means localization of specific functions; and (2) "integration," which means combining all the information and functions at a global level within the conceptual framework of a "global integrated network" [75, 76]. Consistent with this conceptual framework, Biswal et al. were the first to document the spontaneous fluctuations within the motor system and high potential for functional connectivity in resting state fMRI (rs-fMRI) using intrinsic activity correlations [77]. Since this discovery of coherent spontaneous fluctuations, many studies have shown that several brain regions engaged during various cognitive tasks also form coherent large-scale brain networks that can be identified using rs-fMRI [78].

The recent advances in brain imaging technologies offer promise for improving clinical applicability of fMRI examining spontaneous modulations in the BOLD signal that occur during resting state [79]. In contrast to the traditional task-related approach, rs-fMRI has thus provided unique information about the behavior of networks in the absence of direct task and/or stimulation. In this approach, subjects generally are asked to lie quietly with eyes closed or while fixating on a crosshair. One of the reasons to use resting state functional connectivity for clinical applications is that the task-related increases in neuronal metabolism are usually small (5 %) when compared to the larger resting energy consumption (20 % of the body's energy, most of which supports ongoing neuronal signaling) [80] and eliminates differences based upon performance. Overall, ongoing spontaneous activity provides a window into the neural processing that appears to consume the vast majority of the brain resources, which might provide a more accurate and richer source of disease-related BOLD signal change [81].

Recent fMRI reports have indicated alterations of resting state functional connectivity in neurological populations, including mTBI and have brought new insight into better understanding the pathophysiology of these disorders. Nakamura et al. examined neural network properties at separate time points during recovery from TBI [82]. They reported that the strength but not the number of network connections diminished during the acute phase of TBI indicating the disruption of the neural system. Marguez de la Plata also reported a deficit in the functional connectivity of the hippocampus and frontal lobe circuits 6 months after traumatic diffuse axonal injury (DAI) [83]. In our own recent study, we focused on alterations of several interhemispheric brain functional networks at rest and in response to the YMCA physical stress test in subjects suffering from sports-related mTBI [84]. We found that interhemispheric connectivity was significantly reduced in the primary visual cortex, hippocampal, and DLPFC networks in mTBI subjects. Considering the fact that all mTBI subjects were clinically asymptomatic at the time of scanning, *our findings clearly indicate that functional brain alterations in the acute phase of injury are overlooked when conventional clinical, and neuropsychological examinations are used.*

Default Mode Network

The existence of a "default mode network" in the brain during the resting state was reported by Greicius et al. [85]. Both functional and structural connectivity between brain regions were examined to detect whether there are orderly sets of regions that have particularly high local connections (forming families of clusters) as well as limited number of regions that serve as relay stations or hubs [86]. It was suggested that the neural network of the brain has a small-world structure, namely high-cluster coefficients and low average path length allowing optimization of information processing [87]. Overall, network analysis is necessary to explore the integration phenomena observed in both resting states and in response to high-level information processing in the brain induced by cognitive and/or motor tasks.

As one of the resting state networks (RSN) of the brain, the default mode network (DMN) includes the precuneus/posterior cingulate cortex (PCC), medial prefrontal cortex (MPFC), and medial, lateral, and inferior parietal cortex [88]. Although the DMN is active during rest it is not actively involved in attention or goal-oriented tasks [89]. Despite the fact that the DMN is deactivated during specific tasks, the presence of the DMN during rs-fMRI has been reported and validated in several studies [89–91].

Presently, there are few reports focusing on alteration of DMN in mTBI. Mayer et al. [92] investigated the resting state DMN of subacute mTBI and showed that these subjects displayed decreased BOLD connectivity within the DMN and hyperconnectivity between the right prefrontal and posterior parietal cortices involved in the frontoparietal task-related network (TRN). However, inhomogeneities such as: (a) differential diagnosis of mTBI including the presence or absence of loss of consciousness (LOC); (b) time since injury; and (c) detailed subject's medical history that includes information on past head injuries influences fMRI data. In our own study, we examined DMN in mTBI athletes using rs-fMRI with specific focus on recruiting a homogeneous subject population and controlling for the number of previous concussions [98]. We have reported the major findings that there were disruptions in the connections that make up the DMN in mTBI subjects [93].

In our most recent rs-fMRI study, we focused on the functional integrity and strength of the brain functional connections that make up the DMN in subacutely concussed individuals [94]. Our expectation that DMN may be jeopardized as a result of mTBI was not confirmed. In fact, the functional integrity within the DMN (PCC, LLP, RLP, and DLPFC) lateral parietal ROI remained resilient to a single episode of concussive blow. The major ROIs constituting the DMN and the connectivity within these four ROIs were similar between NVs and mTBI subjects. However, the YMCA Bike Test disrupted the DMN, significantly reducing magnitude of connection between PCC and left lateral parietal ROI, PCC and right lateral parietal ROI, as well as between PCC and MPFC in mTBI subjects. Thus, while the DMN remained resilient to a single mTBI without exertion at 10 days post-injury, it was altered in response to the light intensity of physical stress [94].

Diffusion Tensor Imaging and Concussion

DTI is an advanced imaging technique that exploits the molecular diffusion or Brownian motion of water due to thermal energy. Due to this random diffusion, the displacement and motion of molecules can be used to gain information on microscopic tissue structures and characteristics that are beyond the basic resolution of MRI [95]. Brownian motion is random and this free diffusion is described as being isotropic yet the direction and mobility of water molecules can be restricted by certain tissue characteristics and structures that result in anisotropy [96]. In the white matter of the brain, this diffusion anisotropy becomes ever apparent as myelinated axonal fibers organized into bundles and tracts allow for quicker diffusion along axonal fibers as compared to diffusion oriented perpendicular to the fiber [97]. As the name implies a tensor model is fitted in order to obtain certain indices, λ_1, λ_2, and λ_3 that allow for a quantitative description of this anisotropic diffusion, where λ_1 is the axial diffusivity, and λ_2 and λ_3 are combined together to form the radial diffusivity [98]. Another important scalar measure reported in the literature is the fractional anisotropy (FA). The FA value is between 0 and 1, with 0 representing free diffusion in all directions and 1 representing diffusion confined to only one direction. More precisely the FA value is the ratio of the direction of maximal diffusion to the diffusion that is perpendicular to that main direction [99]. Further metrics include the apparent diffusion coefficient (ADC) which tries to correct image contrasts due to relaxation effects or diffusion, and the mean diffusivity (MD) which is an averaged value of diffusion.

Clearly, feasibility of DTI in isolation [100] and in conjunction with volumetric analysis [99] to monitor the evolution of moderate-to-severe TBI has been recently documented both in adult and pediatric patients. DTI studies are also gaining popularity in mTBI research. A recent review of the literature by Sharp and Ham have reported that DTI studies in the subacute and chronic stages display a decrease in FA and an increase in MD or both but opposite findings during an acute phase of injury [97]. As the injury and subsequent recovery from mTBI evolves, many cellular processes are taking place and changing the diffusion properties measured by DTI. These results suggest that even though DTI is sensitive to detect changes in the diffusion patterns, especially in the white matter, work still needs to be done to optimize the effectiveness and use of DTI. Also adding to the confusion in the literature is the lack of uniformity in DTI protocols and the ability to standardize the data, with multiple parameters that can be adjusted along with the number of different vendor platforms on which DTI is performed [101–103].

There are a few mTBI studies that use DTI and direct their focus on the pediatric to young adult population [104–109] with a majority falling into either adolescent or collegiate age groups. Similar to the DTI studies in adults during the acute phase of injury, studies report an increase in FA values and a reduction in ADC and radial diffusivity. An acute study by Wilde et al. took ten adolescents aging from 14 to 17 years old and performed DTI scans 1–6 days after mTBI [103]. Statistical analysis found a significant increase in FA as well as a decrease in ADC and radial diffusivity in the corpus callosum. Although in another study that recruited 18 collegiate male football players (mean age 22.08) who had suffered a concussion performed DTI scans within 5 days of injury and then follow-up scans at 6 months post-injury [112] there were contradictory results found in the chronic phase of injury. FA values were elevated in the 6-month scan from both the control group and the acute scan. It seems that time from injury is an important element when utilizing DTI. As scanning takes place further away from the initial insult, the majority of studies have shown some inconsistent results. In a subacute study of collegiate athletes (mean age 21.3) scanned at 30 days post-injury by Zhang et al. [105], no differences in FA values between the mTBI group and controls were observed with both voxel- and ROI-based analysis methods.

A recent voxel-based analysis of DTI study of high school athletes by Bazarian et al. performed DTI within a 3-month interval pre- and postseason [102]. Despite the small sample size, one athlete received a concussion during the season and had the largest number of affected voxels in the white matter. Specifically, this athlete showed significant changes of FA values in 3.19 % and mean diffusivity in 3.44 %

of white matter voxels from the preseason to postseason scan with an overall increase in FA and decrease in mean diffusivity values. Another investigation into collegiate concussion took ten concussed athletes (mean age 19.7) and scanned them with DTI at least 1 month post-injury [106]. Again a voxel based analysis was implemented and revealed significant increases in mean diffusivity only in the left hemisphere. It is also important to note that in this study a majority of subjects had a prior history of concussion. This highlights the importance in taking into consideration when analyzing data the history of previous mTBI or concussion. Another concern when using DTI in younger patients is the fact that there are differences between pediatric and adult brains. As the brain develops there are many changes seen in the grey and white matter that are associated with the changing microstructures of the tissues that coincide with process of myelination, synaptogenesis, and dendritic arborization [109]. Consequently ADC values are higher in pediatric populations and decrease with age and are associated with changes in brain water content [109] and FA has been shown to increase sharply from childhood to adolescence and a continued increase at a slower rate from adolescence to adult [109]. Overall, DTI offers valuable structural and molecular information and insight into the brain and as it becomes more commonplace in neuroimaging studies, work needs to be done to optimize its effectiveness.

Magnetic Resonance Spectroscopy and Concussion

MRS is a useful tool that allows for identification and quantification of cellular metabolites in vivo [110]. As with many MRI applications, there are a number of different parameters and pulse sequences that can be used in order to acquire MRS data, all of which have their advantages and disadvantages and can make comparisons between studies difficult. The metabolites in the brain that are most often studied are N-acetylaspartate (NAA), choline (Cho), and creatine-phosphocreatine (Cr) [111–113]. NAA is used as an indicator of neuronal and axonal integrity as decreased levels are seen after injury and associated with neuronal loss, metabolic dysfunction, or myelin repair [114].

The second most common MRS finding after head trauma behind decreases in NAA are increases in Cho levels [115, 116] which are a marker of cell membrane turnover [115]. The Cr peak, which is a combination of the two creatine-containing compounds (creatine and creatine phosphate), is an accepted indicator of cell energy metabolism [117, 118]. Despite the information MRS can yield about the metabolic response of the brain to injury, there are limited numbers of studies that utilize it to evaluate sports-related mTBI [119].

A recent study of collegiate athletes recovering from mTBI used MRS to assess the subacute phase of injury [119]. All subjects were clinically asymptomatic at the time MRS evaluation was performed and analysis was focused on the genu and splenium of the corpus callosum. The main finding was a reduction in NAA/Cr and NNA/Cho levels in both ROIs as compared to controls. The general findings in

MRS studies of mTBI have been a reduction in NAA and an increase in Cho with Cr remaining stable. However, recent studies by Gasparovic et al. imply that Cr may not be as stable as once thought and the sheer lack of numbers of MRS studies focused directly on the pediatric to young adult population makes interpretation of the results difficult [114]. More details about feasibility of recent sports-related MRS studies can be found in the special chapter by Dr. Lazzarino et al. (Chap. 6).

Concluding Statement

We understand that at present, advanced imaging studies are often not easily accessible, and the full implication of them is not yet established. Continuing research should indicate what will be cost-effective in determining safe return-to-play after brain injuries. However, it becomes clear that the proposed solution for existing controversies in sports concussion research needs to result in a combination of multiple modalities that will be able to concurrently record performance (functional) variables as well as structural/functional brain imaging (fMRI, DTI, MRS, EEG) variables. Clinicians should be interested not only in the restoration of successful functional performance (memory, attention, balance, executive functions) but also the structural (neural) network responsible for maximum performance. Numerous multimodal findings obtained in many research laboratories are indicative of the types of results to which clinicians should be attentive. These studies seek to find a behavioral and structural resolution. Is there ever ultimate restoration of a normal structural components and functional integrity, or permanent "brain reorganization?" With combined modality longitudinal studies, we can come closer to answering that question.

And the final thought: We believe that if concussion indeed, is a *complex pathophysiological process affecting the brain*, proper (physiological, brain imaging, etc.) diagnostic tools have to be validated and implemented in clinical practice. While we do not currently understand the true pathophysiology of concussion and/or contributing factors for permanent versus transitory physiological damage, the graded symptoms checklist or other subjective reports over serial evaluations will never bridge the knowledge gaps at the junction between neuroscience and clinical management of sports-related concussions.

References

1. Langlois JA, Rutland-Brown W, Wald MM. The epidemiology and impact of traumatic brain injury, a brief overview. J Head Trauma Rehabil. 2006;21:375–8.
2. Ruff RM. Mild traumatic brain injury and neural recovery, rethinking the debate. Neurorehabilitation. 2011;28:167–80.
3. Lincoln AE, Caswell SV, Almquist JL, Dunn RE, Norris JB, Hinton RY. Trends in concussion incidence in high school sports, a prospective 11-year study. Am J Sports Med. 2011;39:958–63.

4. Cantu RC, Aubry M, Dvorak J, Graf-Baumann T, Johnston K, Kelly J, et al. Overview of concussion consensus statements since 2000. Neurosurg Focus. 2006;21:E3.
5. Anderson T, Heitger M, Macleod AD. Concussion and mild head injury. Pract Neurol. 2006;6:342–57.
6. Canadian Academy of Sport Medicine Concussion Committee (CAoSMC C). CASM guidelines for assessment and management of sport-related concussion. Clin J Sport Med. 2000;10:209–11.
7. Aubry M, Cantu R, Dvorak J, Graf-Baumann T, Johnston K, Kelly J, et al. Summary and agreement statement of the 1st international conference on concussion in sport, Vienna 2001. Recommendations for the improvement of safety and health of athletes who may suffer concussive injuries. Br J Sports Med. 2002;36:6–10.
8. Hugenholtz H, Richard MT. Return to athletic competition following concussion. Can Med Assoc J. 1982;127:827–9.
9. Alves WM, Rimel RW, Nelson WE. University of Virginia prospective study of football induced minor head injury—status report. Clin Sports Med. 1987;6:211–8.
10. Barth J, Alves W, Ryan T, Macciocchi S, Rimel R, Jane J, et al. Mild head injury in sport, neuropsychological sequelae and recovery of function. In: Levin H, Eisenberg H, Benton A, editors. Mild head injury. New York: Oxford Press; 1989.
11. Moser RS, Iverson GL, Echemendia RJ, Lovell MR, Schatz P, Webbe FM, et al. Neuropsychological evaluation in the diagnosis and management of sports-related concussion. Arch Clin Neuropsychol. 2007;22:909–91.
12. McCrory P, Meeuwisse W, Johnston K, Dvorak J, Aubry M, Molloy M, et al. Consensus statement on concussion in sport 3rd international conference on concussion in sport held in Zurich, November 2008. Clin J Sport Med. 2008;19:185–200.
13. Bazarian JJ, Veenema T, Brayer AF, Lee E. Knowledge of concussion guidelines among practitioners caring for children. Clin Pediatr. 2001;40:207–12.
14. Chrisman SP, Schiff MA, Rivara FP. Physician concussion knowledge and the effect of mailing the CDC's "heads up" toolkit. Clin Pediatr. 2011;50:1031–9.
15. McCrea M, Prichep L, Powell MR, Chabot R, Barr WB. Acute effects and recovery after sport-related concussion, a neurocognitive and quantitative brain electrical activity study. J Head Trauma Rehabil. 2010;25:283–92.
16. Giza CC, Hovda DA. The neurometabolic cascade of concussion. J Athl Train. 2001;36:228–35.
17. Barkhoudarian G, Hovda DA, Giza CC. The molecular pathophysiology of concussive brain injury. Clin Sports Med. 2011;30:33–48.
18. Kan EM, Ling EA, Lu J. Microenvironment changes in mild traumatic brain injury. Brain Res Bull. 2012;87:359–72.
19. Goetz P, Blamire A, Rajagopalan B, Cadoux-Hudson T, Young D, Styles P. Increase in apparent diffusion coefficient in normal appearing white matter following human traumatic brain injury correlates with injury severity. J Neurotrauma. 2004;21:645–54.
20. Browne KD, Chen XH, Meaney DF, Smith DH. Mild traumatic brain injury and diffuse axonal injury in swine. J Neurotrauma. 2011;28:1747–55.
21. Yuen TJ, Browne KD, Iwata A, Smith DH. Sodium channelopathy induced by mild axonal trauma worsens outcome after a repeat injury. J Neurosci Res. 2009;87:3620–5.
22. Flamm ES, Ommaya AK, Coe J, Krueger TP, Faas FH. Cardiovascular effects of experimental head injury in the monkey. Surg Forum. 1966;17:414–6.
23. Grundl PD, Biagas KV, Kochanek PM, Schiding JK, Barmada MA, Nemoto EM. Early cerebrovascular response to head injury in immature and mature rats. J Neurotrauma. 1994;11:135–48.
24. Lewine JD, Davis JT, Bigler ED, Thoma R, Hill D, Funke M, et al. Objective documentation of traumatic brain injury subsequent to mild head trauma, multimodal brain imaging with MEG, SPECT, and MRI. J Head Trauma Rehabil. 2007;22:141–55.
25. Chason JL, Hardy WG, Webster JE, Gurdjian ES. Alterations in cell structure of the brain associated with experimental concussion. J Neurosurg. 1958;15:135–9.

26. Nevin NC. Neuropathological changes in the white matter following head injury. J Neuropathol Exp Neurol. 1967;26:77–84.
27. Faas FH, Ommaya AK. Brain tissue electrolytes and water content in experimental concussion in the monkey. J Neurosurg. 1968;28:137–44.
28. Glaser MA, Sjaardema H. The value of the electroencephalograph in cranio-cerebral injuries. West Surg. 1940;48:6989–96.
29. Jasper HH, Kershman J, Elvidge AR. Electroencephalographic study in clinical cases of injury of the head. Arch Neurol Psychiatry. 1940;44:328–50.
30. Williams D. The electro-encephalogram in acute head injury. J Neurol Psychiatry. 1941;4:107–30.
31. Arciniegas DB. Clinical electrophysiologic assessments and mild traumatic brain injury: state-of-the-science and implications for clinical practice. Int J Psychophysiol. 2011;82:41–52.
32. Geets W, Louette N. Early EEG in 300 cerebral concussions. Rev Electroencephalogr Neurophysiol Clin. 1985;14:333–8.
33. McClelland RJ, Fenton GW, Rutherford W. The postconcussional-syndrome revisited. J R Soc Med. 1994;87:508–10.
34. Tebano MT, Cameroni M, Gallozzi G, Loizzo A, Palazzino G, Pezzini G, et al. EEG spectral-analysis after minor head-injury in man. Electroencephalogr Clin Neurophysiol. 1988;70:185–9.
35. Montgomery EA, Fenton GW, McClelland RJ, Macflynn G, Rutherford WH. The psychobiology of minor head-injury. Psychol Med. 1991;21:375–84.
36. Pratapchand R, Sinniah M, Salem FA. Cognitive evoked-potential P300—a metric for cerebral concussion. Acta Neurol Scand. 1988;78:185–9.
37. Watson MR, Fenton GW, McClelland RJ, Lumsden J, Headley M, Rutherford WH. The postconcussional state—neurophysiological aspects. Br J Psychiatry. 1995;167:514–21.
38. Thatcher RW, Walker RA, Gerson I, Geisler FH. EEG discriminant analyses of mild head trauma. Electroencephalogr Clin Neurophysiol. 1989;73:94–106.
39. Thornton KE. Exploratory investigation into mild brain injury and discriminant analysis with high frequency bands (32–64 Hz). Brain Inj. 1999;13:477–88.
40. Duff J. The usefulness of quantitative EEG (QEEG) and neurotherapy in the assessment and treatment of post-concussion syndrome. Clin EEG Neurosci. 2004;35:198–209.
41. Gosselin N, Theriault M, Leclerc S, Montplaisir J, Lassonde M. Neurophysiological anomalies in symptomatic and asymptomatic concussed athletes. Neurosurgery. 2006;58:1151–60.
42. Broglio SP, Pontifex MB, O'Connor P, Hillman CH. The persistent effects of concussion on neuroelectric indices of attention. J Neurotrauma. 2009;26:1463–70.
43. Davis GA, Iverson GL, Guskiewicz KM, Ptito A, Johnston KM. Contributions of neuroimaging, balance testing, electrophysiology and blood markers to the assessment of sport-related concussion. Br J Sports Med. 2009;43(1):136–45.
44. Theriault M, De Beaumont L, Gosselin N, Filipinni M, Lassonde M. Electrophysiological abnormalities in well functioning multiple concussed athletes. Brain Inj. 2009;23:899–906.
45. Slobounov S, Cao C, Sebastianelli W. Differential effect of first versus second concussive episodes on wavelet information quality of EEG. Clin Neurophysiol. 2009;120:862–7.
46. Cao C, Slobounov S. Application of a novel measure of EEG non-stationarity as 'Shannon—entropy of the peak frequency shifting' for detecting residual abnormalities in concussed individuals. Clin Neurophysiol. 2011;122:1314–21.
47. Cao C, Tutwiler RL, Slobounov S. Automatic classification of athletes with residual functional deficits following concussion by means of EEG signal using support vector machine. IEEE Trans Neural Syst Rehabil Eng. 2008;16:327–35.
48. Cao C, Slobounov S. Alteration of cortical functional connectivity as a result of traumatic brain injury revealed by graph theory, ICA, and sLORETA analyses of EEG signals. IEEE Trans Neural Syst Rehabil Eng. 2010;18:11–9.
49. Slobounov S, Sebastianelli W, Moss R. Alteration of posture-related cortical potentials in mild traumatic brain injury. Neurosci Lett. 2005;383:251–5.

50. Slobounov S, Sebastianelli W, Newell KM. Incorporating virtual reality graphics with brain imaging for assessment of sport-related concussions. Conf Proc IEEE Eng Med Biol Soc. 2011;2011:1383–6.
51. Slobounov S, Slobounov E, Newell K. Application of virtual reality graphics in assessment of concussion. Cyberpsychol Behav. 2006;9:188–91.
52. Slobounov S, Tutwiler R, Sebastianelli W, Slobounov E. Alteration of postural responses to visual field motion in mild traumatic brain injury. Neurosurgery. 2006;59:134–9.
53. Nuwer MR, Hovda DA, Schrader LM, Vespa PM. Routine and quantitative EEG in mild traumatic brain injury. Clin Neurophysiol. 2005;116:2001–25.
54. Slobounov S, Sebastianelli W, Hallett M. Residual brain dysfunction observed one year post-mild traumatic brain injury, combined EEG and balance study. Clin Neurophysiol. 2012;123(9):1755–61.
55. Logothetis NK. What we can do and what we cannot do with fMRI. Nature. 2008;453(7197):869–78.
56. Ogawa S, Lee TM, Kay AR, Tank DW. Brain magnetic resonance imaging with contrast dependent on blood oxygenation. Proc Natl Acad Sci U S A. 1990;87:9868–72.
57. Ogawa S, Menon RS, Tank DW, Kim SG, Merkle H, Ellermann JM, et al. Functional brain mapping by blood oxygenation level-dependent contrast magnetic resonance imaging. A comparison of signal characteristics with a biophysical model. Biophys J. 1993;64(3):803–12.
58. Horowitz AL. MRI physics for radiologist, a visual approach. 3rd ed. New York: Springer; 1995.
59. Hillary FG, Steffener J, Biswal BB, Lange G, DeLuca J, Ashburner J. Functional magnetic resonance imaging technology and traumatic brain injury rehabilitation, guidelines for methodological and conceptual pitfalls. J Head Trauma Rehabil. 2002;17:411–30.
60. Jueptner M, Weiller C. Does measurement of regional cerebral blood flow reflect synaptic activity?—implications for PET and fMRI. Neuroimage. 1995;2:148–56.
61. Ptito A, Chen JK, Johnston KM. Contributions of functional magnetic resonance imaging (fMRI) to support concussion evaluation. Neurorehabilitation. 2007;22:217–27.
62. McAllister TW, Saykin AJ, Flashman LA, Sparling MB, Johnson SC, Guerin SJ, et al. Brain activation during working memory 1 month after mild traumatic brain injury, a functional MRI study. Neurology. 1999;53:1300–8.
63. McAllister TW, Sparling MB, Flashman LA, Guerin SJ, Mamourian AC, Saykin AJ. Differential working memory load effects after mild traumatic brain injury. Neuroimage. 2001;14:1004–12.
64. McAllister TW, Flashman LA, McDonald BC, Saykin AJ. Mechanisms of working memory dysfunction after mild and moderate TBI, evidence from functional MRI and neurogenetics. J Neurotrauma. 2006;23:1450–67.
65. Jantzen KJ. Functional magnetic resonance imaging of mild traumatic brain injury. J Head Trauma Rehabil. 2010;25:256–66.
66. Hillary FG, Schultheis MT, Challis BH, Millis SR, Carnevale GJ, Galshi T, et al. Spacing of repetitions improves learning and memory after moderate and severe TBI. J Clin Exp Neuropsychol. 2003;25:49–58.
67. Chen JK, Johnston KM, Frey S, Petrides M, Worsley K, Ptito A. Functional abnormalities in symptomatic concussed athletes, an fMRI study. Neuroimage. 2004;22:68–82.
68. Perlstein WM, Cole MA, Demery JA, Seignourel PJ, Dixit NK, Larson MJ, et al. Parametric manipulation of working memory load in traumatic brain injury, behavioral and neural correlates. J Int Neuropsychol Soc. 2004;10:724–41.
69. Chiaravalloti N, Hillary F, Ricker J, Christodoulou C, Kalnin A, Liu WC, Steffener J, DeLuca J. Cerebral activation patterns during working memory performance in multiple sclerosis using fMRI. J Clin Exp Neuropsychol. 2005;27:33–54.
70. Chen JK, Johnston KM, Collie A, McCrory P, Ptito A. A validation of the post concussion symptom scale in the assessment of complex concussion using cognitive testing and functional MRI. J Neurol Neurosurg Psychiatry. 2007;78:1231–8.

71. Chen JK, Johnston KM, Petrides M, Ptito A. Neural substrates of symptoms of depression following concussion in male athletes with persisting postconcussion symptoms. Arch Gen Psychiatry. 2008;65:81–9.
72. Mayer AR, Mannell MV, Ling J, Elgie R, Gasparovic C, Phillips JP, et al. Auditory orienting and inhibition of return in mild traumatic brain injury, a FMRI study. Hum Brain Mapp. 2009;30:4152–66.
73. Stulemeijer M, Vos PE, van der Werf S, van Dijk G, Rijpkema M, Fernandez G. How mild traumatic brain injury may affect declarative memory performance in the post-acute stage. J Neurotrauma. 2010;27:1585–95.
74. Slobounov S, Zhang K, Pennell D, Ray W, Johnson B, Sebastianelli W. Functional abnormalities in normally appearing athletes following mild traumatic brain injury, a functional MRI study. Exp Brain Res. 2010;202:341–54.
75. Varela F, Lachaux JP, Rodriguez E, Martinerie J. The brainweb, phase synchronization and large-scale integration. Nat Rev Neurosci. 2001;2:229–39.
76. Reijneveld JC, Ponten SC, Berendse HW, Stam CJ. The application of graph theoretical analysis to complex networks in the brain. Clin Neurophysiol. 2007;118:2317–31.
77. Biswal B, Yetkin FZ, Haughton VM, Hyde JS. Functional connectivity in the motor cortex of resting human brain using echo-planar MRI. Magn Reson Med. 1995;34:537–41.
78. Smith SM, Fox PT, Miller KL, Glahn DC, Fox PM, Mackay CE, et al. Correspondence of the brain's functional architecture during activation and rest. Proc Natl Acad Sci U S A. 2009;106:13040–5.
79. Fox MD, Raichle ME. Spontaneous fluctuations in brain activity observed with functional magnetic resonance imaging. Nat Rev Neurosci. 2007;8:700–11.
80. Raichle ME, Mintun MA. Brain work and brain imaging. Annu Rev Neurosci. 2006;29:449–76.
81. Fox MD, Greicius M. Clinical applications of resting state functional connectivity. Front Syst Neurosci. 2010;4:19.
82. Nakamura T, Hillary FG, Biswal BB. Resting network plasticity following brain injury. PLoS One. 2009;4(12):e8220.
83. de la Plata CDM, Garces J, Kojori ES, Grinnan J, Krishnan K, Pidikiti R, Spence J, Devous MD, Moore C, McColl R, Madden C, Diaz-Arrastia R. Deficits in functional connectivity of hippocampal and frontal lobe circuits after traumatic axonal injury. Arch Neurol. 2011;68:74–84.
84. Slobounov S, Gay M, Zhang K, Johnson B, Pennell D, Sebastianelli W, et al. Alteration of brain functional network at rest and in response to YMCA physical stress test in concussed athletes, RsFMRI study. Neuroimage. 2011;55:1716–27.
85. Greicius MD, Krasnow B, Reiss AL, Menon V. Functional connectivity in the resting brain, a network analysis of the default mode hypothesis. Proc Natl Acad Sci U S A. 2003;100:253–8.
86. Sporns O, Honey CJ, Kotter R. Identification and classification of hubs in brain networks. PLoS One. 2007;2:e1049.
87. Broyd SJ, Demanuele C, Debener S, Helps SK, James CJ, Sonuga-Barke EJ. Default-mode brain dysfunction in mental disorders, a systematic review. Neurosci Biobehav Rev. 2009; 33:279–96.
88. Raichle ME, MacLeod AM, Snyder AZ, Powers WJ, Gusnard DA, Shulman GL. A default mode of brain function. Proc Natl Acad Sci U S A. 2001;98:676–82.
89. Beckmann CF, DeLuca M, Devlin JT, Smith SM. Investigations into resting-state connectivity using independent component analysis. Philos Trans R Soc Lond B Biol Sci. 2005;360:1001–13.
90. Damoiseaux JS, Rombouts SA, Barkhof F, Scheltens P, Stam CJ, Smith SM, et al. Consistent resting-state networks across healthy subjects. Proc Natl Acad Sci U S A. 2006;103: 13848–53.
91. De Luca M, Beckmann CF, De Stefano N, Matthews PM, Smith SM. fMRI resting state networks define distinct modes of long-distance interactions in the human brain. Neuroimage. 2006;29:1359–67.

 92. Mayer AR, Mannell MV, Ling J, Gasparovic C, Yeo RA. Functional connectivity in mild traumatic brain injury. Hum Brain Mapp. 2011;32:1825–35.
 93. Johnson B, Zhang K, Gay M, Horovitz S, Hallett M, Sebastianelli W, et al. Alteration of brain default network in subacute phase of injury in concussed individuals, resting-state fMRI study. Neuroimage. 2012;59:511–8.
 94. Zhang K, Johnson B, Gay M, Horovitz SG, Hallett M, Sebastianelli W, et al. Default mode network in concussed individuals in response to the YMCA physical stress test. J Neurotrauma. 2012;29:756–65.
 95. Le Bihan D. Diffusion tensor imaging, concepts and applications. J Magn Reson Imaging. 2001;13:534–46.
 96. Snook L. Diffusion tensor imaging of neurodevelopment in children and young adults. Neuroimage. 2005;26:1164.
 97. Sharp DJ, Ham TE. Investigating white matter injury after mild traumatic brain injury. Curr Opin Neurol. 2011;24(6):558–63.
 98. Wilde EA, Merkley TL, Bigler ED, Max JE, Schmidt AT, Ayoub KW, et al. Longitudinal changes in cortical thickness in children after traumatic brain injury and their relation to behavioral regulation and emotional control. Int J Dev Neurosci. 2012;30:267–76.
 99. Shah S, Yallampalli R, Merkley TL, McCauley SR, Bigler ED, Macleod M, et al. Diffusion tensor imaging and volumetric analysis of the ventral striatum in adults with traumatic brain injury. Brain Inj. 2012;26:201–10.
100. Zhu T, Hu R, Qiu X, Taylor M, Tso Y, Yiannoutsos C, et al. Quantification of accuracy and precision of multi-center DTI measurements, a diffusion phantom and human brain study. Neuroimage. 2011;56:1398–411.
101. Bazarian JJ, Zhong J, Blyth B, Zhu T, Kavcic V, Peterson D. Diffusion tensor imaging detects clinically important axonal damage after mild traumatic brain injury, a pilot study. J Neurotrauma. 2007;24:1447–59.
102. Bazarian JJ, Zhu T, Blyth B, Borrino A, Zhong J. Subject-specific changes in brain white matter on diffusion tensor imaging after sports-related concussion. Magn Reson Imaging. 2012;30:171–80.
103. Wilde EA, McCauley SR, Hunter JV, Bigler ED, Chu Z, Wang ZJ, et al. Diffusion tensor imaging of acute mild traumatic brain injury in adolescents. Neurology. 2008;70:948–55.
104. Chu Z, Wilde EA, Hunter JV, McCauley SR, Bigler ED, Troyanskaya M, Yallampalli R, Chia JM, Levin HS. Voxel-based analysis of diffusion tensor imaging in mild traumatic brain injury in adolescents. AJNR Am J Neuroradiol. 2009;31:340–6.
105. Zhang K, Johnson B, Pennell D, Ray W, Sebastianelli W, Slobounov S. Are functional deficits in concussed individuals consistent with white matter structural alterations, combined FMRI & DTI study. Exp Brain Res. 2010;204:57–70.
106. Cubon VA, Putukian M, Boyer C, Dettwiler A. A diffusion tensor imaging study on the white matter skeleton in individuals with sports-related concussion. J Neurotrauma. 2011;28:189–201.
107. Henry LC, Tremblay J, Tremblay S, Lepore N, Theoret H, Ellemberg D, et al. Acute and chronic changes in diffusivity measures after sports concussion. J Neurotrauma. 2011; 28(10):2049–59.
108. Maugans TA, Farley C, Altaye M, Leach J, Cecil KM. Pediatric sports-related concussion produces cerebral blood flow alterations. Pediatrics. 2012;129:28–37.
109. Neil J, Miller J, Mukherjee P, Hüppi PS. Diffusion tensor imaging of normal and injured developing human brain—a technical review. NMR Biomed. 2002;15:543–52.
110. Shekdar K. Role of magnetic resonance spectroscopy in evaluation of congenital/developmental brain abnormalities. Semin Ultrasound CT MR. 2011;32:510–38.
111. Cecil KM. Proton magnetic resonance spectroscopy for detection of axonal injury in the splenium of the corpus callosum of brain-injured patients. J Neurosurg. 1998;88:795–801.
112. Belanger HG. Recent neuroimaging techniques in mild traumatic brain injury. J Neuropsychiatry Clin Neurosci. 2007;19:5–20.

113. Govind V. Whole-brain proton MR spectroscopic imaging of mild-to moderate traumatic brain injury and correlation with neuropsychological deficits. J Neurotrauma. 2010;27:483–96.
114. Gasparovic C, Yeo R, Mannell M, Ling J, Elgie R, Phillips J, et al. Neurometabolite concentrations in gray and white matter in mild traumatic brain injury, a 1H-magnetic resonance spectroscopy study. J Neurotrauma. 2009;26(10):1635–43.
115. Ross BD. 1H MRS in acute traumatic brain injury. J Magn Reson Imaging. 1998;8:829–40.
116. Signoretti S, Pietro V, Vagnozzi R, Lazzarino G, Amorini AM, Belli A, et al. Transient alterations of creatine, creatine phosphate, N-acetylaspartate and high-energy phosphates after mild traumatic brain injury in the rat. Mol Cell Biochem. 2009;333:269–77.
117. Vagnozzi R, Signoretti S, Cristofori L, Alessandrini F, Floris R, Isgro E, et al. Assessment of metabolic brain damage and recovery following mild traumatic brain injury, a multicentre, proton magnetic resonance spectroscopic study in concussed patients. Brain. 2010; 133:3232–42.
118. Walz NC. Late proton magnetic resonance spectroscopy following traumatic brain injury during early childhood, relationship with neurobehavioral outcomes. J Neurotrauma. 2008;25:94–103.
119. Johnson B, Zhang K, Gay M, Horovitz S, Hallett M, Sebastianelli W, et al. Metabolic alterations in corpus callosum may compromise brain functional connectivity in MTBI patients, an 1H-MRS study. Neurosci Lett. 2012;509:5–8.

Part I
Evaluation of Concussions—Current Development

Chapter 2
Consequences of Ignorance and Arrogance for Mismanagement of Sports-Related Concussions: Short- and Long-Term Complications

Robert C. Cantu

Abstract The major objective of this chapter is to provide my insights on short, and most importantly long-term complications from mismanagement of sports-related concussions. There is an expanding data base accumulating in neuroscience and clinical practice indicating the danger of long-term brain dysfunctions grounded on metabolic and structural deficits in the concussed brain. Although the exact mechanisms of these brain disorders still remained to be elucidated, the medical professionals in charge of concussed individuals have to be knowledgeable about epidemiology, pathophysiology, and current developments regarding evaluation, diagnostic imaging, management principles, complications, and prevention strategies. Clearly, both short- and long-term consequences of a single episode or multiple sub-concussive blows should NOT be overlooked while assessing injured athletes. There are several myths about concussion that I will elucidate in my final statements of this chapter, emphasizing still existing controversies and discrepancies between basic brain science and clinical management of sports-related concussions.

Keywords Concussion • Myths about concussion • Second impact syndrome

Short-Term Risks of Concussion Mismanagement

It is fun to think about how history may have changed if we knew centuries ago what we now know. A number of drivers were praising, as I would too, Dale Earnhardt Jr. for bringing forward his concussion symptoms after the Talladega crash. He did this because he was aware himself, that he'd had a concussion a few weeks before in

R.C. Cantu, M.A., M.D., F.A.C.S., F.A.A.N.S., F.A.C.S.M. (✉)
Emerson Hospital, Concord, MA, USA
e-mail: rcantu@emersonhosp.org

S.M. Slobounov and W.J. Sebastianelli (eds.), *Concussions in Athletics: From Brain to Behavior*, DOI 10.1007/978-1-4939-0295-8_2, © Springer Science+Business Media New York 2014

Kansas, and had concerned about his health. Drivers that were commenting were saying that just wouldn't have happened 10 years ago and that's probably true. NASCAR drivers driving cars are similar to fighter pilots on wheels. Their reaction times and their vision needs to be 100 %. I am very glad to see that he brought concussion issues to doctors even though it cost his team a great deal of money.

So, What Are the Short-Term Risks of Mismanaging a Concussion?

The most common result of not imposing physical and cognitive rest after a is taking concussion symptoms, concussion is greatly exacerbating concussion symptoms and causing something that would have recovered in a matter of days into something that may now go on for months and become post-concussive syndrome. Also, a much less common risk is *second impact* syndrome (SIS), which Bob Harbaugh and Dick Saunders first described in a JAMA article in 1984. It is interesting to me to see how my own practice has greatly changed in recent years, because of the awareness of concussions and post-concussion syndrome. I am actually inundated with post-concussive syndrome patients, most of whom have months of symptoms before ever see them.

Approximately 2 years ago, one of my colleagues and I, along with one of his graduate students wrote a paper looking at a retrospective analysis of 215 consecutive post-concussion patients. Those that had post-concussive syndrome had a disproportionate amount of a history of multiple prior concussions, as opposed to this being their first injury. Many of them took a double hit, which means your first hit may be to the head, and then you fall to the turf and slam your head a second time.

Double hits do seem to be associated with symptoms that last longer than a single hit, and may actually involve rotational forces, which are in one direction, and then rebound in the other opposite direction. Some suggest we should be thinking of those rotational forces as being summated or added. I will leave that up to further research that the biomechanists are doing, but it is a very interesting theory and it does correlate with what we see. The most common occurrence with post-concussive syndrome is athletes who are playing while still symptomatic. We wrote a paper a few years ago not about post-concussive syndrome, but catastrophic injuries. It was found that 38 % of individuals were playing while still symptomatic from a previous head injury that was sustained that season. We are finding the same thing with post-concussive syndrome.

Two young children cracking heads is unacceptable, and what we are realizing today, and what we are measuring today are primarily linear forces. For several years we have associated concussion risk being much higher with linear forces 80–100 g. We have also seen from the work of Dr. Guskiewicz and others, that just because you have 100 g impact, it is not necessarily associated with a concussion. Conversely, concussions can occur with *g* forces that are well under 100 g.

We now realize that it is not just those higher hits that are important. Today we realize concussion occurence is multifactorial and there is no known threshold.

I will try to make the case, although this has not been shown in the laboratory yet by Dr. Hovda that the sub-concussive hits count as well. In terms of how many hits kids are taking over a season, you can see at the college level that while the mean isn't terribly high, the extremes that the individuals are taking can be very high. Certainly at the high school level, over 1,000 hits a season is not uncommon.

Evidence that is emerging that I think should give us all cause for concern [1]. This data that of course needs to be replicated by other investigators, but it is data that shows decreased brain performance from repetitive trauma, even without a recognized concussion. This is presumably from the accumulation of sub-concussive blows over the course of the season. The trauma in this data has mostly been garnered from accelerometers in football helmets.

It is not just metabolic MRS studies that have shown changes, but DTI has shown changes similarly with baseline tests versus end of the season tests with fiber tracks integrity decreasing over the course of the season. Presumably, this is due to sub-concussive blows. Some of the studies have also used computer-based neuropsychological testing, and found deterioration in the test scores over the course of the season when compared with baseline. By using neuropsychological, fiber tract, and metabolic data, there is a suggestion that it may be these sub-concussive blows that are producing deleterious effects on brains. It is an accumulation of this data that has led me to start a book 2 years ago, and certainly the more controversial parts of the book are focusing on children in sports. I suggest taking tackle football away from youngsters *until the age of 14*, no body checking in ice-hockey until the age of 14 (which in the past 2 years has already almost happened with the age moving from 11 to 13), and no heading in soccer until the age 14. It does not make sense to me, that you have a very good batting helmet for baseball players, but then the helmet falls off of the player's head as they round the bases. This subjects them to epidural hematomas due to skull fractures from a thrown ball, when it would be so simple to put a chin strap that holds the helmet on the head.

Also, in sports that do not have helmets right now, but the mechanism of injury is a focal blow, meaning a stick to the head or face, like women's field hockey and lacrosse, I believe there should be helmets. Additionally, I feel very strongly and passionately that we are giving our officials a pass they do not deserve. They should either start calling sports appropriately, or they should be replaced. I think it is terrible that this is a problem that continues to go on. Pop Warner football was founded in 1929, although it was named in 1934 after Glenn Scooby Pop Warner. The organization has thrived, especially since the exposure that it has received on television.

With regard to neck strength, force equals mass times acceleration (*g*), or force divided by mass equals acceleration. Acceleration is what the brain is experiencing during a hit. If we look at it a different way, change of velocity over time, you have a much less change of velocity with a well-developed neck. Dom Comstock and I, as well as a few others have been working for a number of years on a study, testing neck strength with regard to concussion incidence. The data has correlated that the strongest necks have the lowest number of concussions, and the weakest necks have the highest number of concussions. Others have found the same theory, that neck strength reduces your risk of concussion. For example, the woodpecker has a large, strong neck, and it moves only in a linear straightforward manner—a woodpecker does not experience concussions, " ... never have headache." We are a strong believer in any athlete who is involved with a contact or collision sport should strengthen their neck muscles as well as their other core muscles as much as they can. Youngsters and females don't have testosterone and are not going to bulk up their neck muscles, so they aren't going to look any different, but they can strengthen them.

We do not know what the concussion threshold is today, but we do know that there are curves which suggest that the risk certainly goes up as the linear forces go up. Many of us feel that the rotational forces are more important than the linear, and that is really what should be researched further. This is especially true in sports where the head is swiveled on the neck from a hit like a helmeted football or lacrosse player. The reason that I believe that we do not yet have concussion thresholds despite a lot of good research is that we are not dealing with just biomechanical issues when we think about concussion. It is a complex situation. Yes, linear accelerations need to be known, rotational accelerations would be ideally known as well, duration of impact, location of impact, and tissue strain issues are all very relevant and in need of study.

However, there are also biological issues. There are rarely situations where the biological issues are matched up with the biomechanical situations to truly allow you to look at the whole picture when you talk about concussions. Some of the biological factors include history (how many concussions has somebody had, how severe were they, and what is the proximity of them), anticipation in terms of neck strength, age, gender (girls are more prone), hydration/volume (some science suggests that a dehydrated brain moves more inside the skull and is at greater risk of injury than a well-hydrated brain), as well as underreporting.

Concussions: Structural Versus Functional Brain Disorder

Dr. Ann McKee has found in some individuals that have died shortly after a concussion because of suicide, diffuse axonal swelling as well as axonal damage. In my opinion, concussion in part involves a neural metabolic cascade, a metabolic issue, but in part at least in some concussions, is *also a structural issue*. I believe that as we get better at MRI imaging, like DTI [2], we are going to be able to see those structural changes in concussion that we cannot currently see with routine MRIs. It is common knowledge that concussions are prevalent without loss of consciousness more than 90 % of the time, and that presents a problem. For those of us that have been on the sideline, and I was for a lot of years, it is not a great feeling knowing that we are probably missing multiple concussions for every one of which we are aware.

Subjects' Reports Versus Pure Evaluation

Theoretically by asking after the season, when there is no longer a feeling of possibly letting down their coaches of teammates, the athlete will be more likely to give honest answers. The incidence of concussion reported by individuals from these post-event studies is six to seven times what is known on the sideline. Some years ago we were a part of a Canadian study in which Paul Echlin was the lead author. This study looked at the incidence of concussion in junior "A" ice hockey that was reported from people on the bench, as opposed to physician observers in the stands. The physician observers in the stands had the responsibility of looking at people on the ice. When somebody got up slowly and seemed to have a problem but stayed in, they would go down between periods and examine them to determine if they had a concussion [3].

A seven times greater incidence of concussion was found from the physician observers, as compared with medical personnel on the bench. The national football league knows this is true as well, and that is why it now has athletic trainers up in a booth looking at the same television feeds that you and I get when we watch the game on television. The same feeds are now fed to the medical personnel on the sideline to be used as part of the concussion assessment. There have been multiple examples of individuals who were sent off the field and a body part was examined that was not the head, when it was a concussion that they had sustained. Colt McCoy is the most notable of them.

I am very pleased that Chris Nowinski, co-founder of the Sports Legacy Institute, and I held a meeting, dedicated to documenting the number of impacts occurring as well as potentially identifying what the threshold number should be for cumulative hits. We know that the numbers that youngsters are receiving are appreciable, we know from published data that roughly 60–70 % of those hits in the past have occurred during practice.

Coaching Preventive Strategies

If you change the way that practice occurs, you can dramatically reduce the number of hits individuals are taking to the head. The *winningest* college coach in this country is John Gagliardi from St. John University outside of Minneapolis St. Paul. He has over 800 victories, and during the season over the last 50 years he has never allowed tackling, only games are full contact. During practice the skill drills are all done and people tackling, but do not bring players to the ground—they just wrap people up. The NFL certainly gets that message too, because in the collective bargaining agreement during the 18-week long NFL season, players can only hit 14 times, less than once a week! Things are changing, and what we are doing is taking the trauma out of practice.

We protect little league pitcher's arms with good intentions, without question when we limit the number of pitches they can throw. However, medial collateral ulnar ligaments can be replaced and the arms can come back from high school to pitch in the big leagues. There are many examples of that including some big league players that are on their third Tommy John surgery operation, and still pitching in the big leagues. For a correctable condition, we have pitch counts for youngsters. We think there should be hit counts to the head because obviously the brain cannot be replaced.

We can modify how practices occur, and to their credit, Pop Warner football has reduced drastically the amount of hitting that they allow in practice. I think that we have an issue in soccer with regard to heading. We have studies that show structural changes in individuals' brains that have headed more than 1,300 times in a given season.

Second Impact Syndrome

SIS [4] is simply an individual that has sustained an initial brain injury, who while still symptomatic, sustains another brain injury that may be incredibly mild. What usually happens is that within minutes, there is a loss of autoregulation, which leads to massive blood flow inside the head, and increasing intracranial brain pressure. It is the capillary beds in our brain that have the ability to be dilated and hold extra blood, as do the arterials. In *SIS* this autoregulation, which keeps a constant flow of blood to our brain, is disrupted. In a normal situation, if your blood pressure goes up you find a constriction occurring in the arterial bed to keep a constant amount of blood flowing to the capillaries, and then to the tissue that needs it. On the other hand, the blood pressure returns to normal and the arterials go back to their normal size keeping the same amount of blood flow. When blood pressure goes down, we have dilation in that arterial bed to keep the same amount of blood in your capillaries.

What happens with an *SIS* is that the autoregulation is lost, and with blood pressures that are normal or even above normal because of adrenaline flowing from either pain or exertion, you find dilation in the arterial bed [4]. When that happens with normal or heightened blood pressure, you have a massive accumulation of blood in the capillaries of the brain. The brain inside the skull houses spinal fluid, brain, and blood. If you massively increase the amount of blood that is inside the blood vessels, you will massively increase intracranial pressure and cause brain herniation. Essentially, that is what we are seeing happen. *SIS* is usually bilateral and symmetrical, but it can occur unilaterally and it can occur with a small sliver of subdural hematoma [4]. The subdural is not causing much mass effect; however, it is this vascular engorgement of the brain that is causing the mass effect. This is not vasogenic edema, because there is grey and white matter differentiation. It is a massive increase of the volume of the brain due to blood.

Long-Term Risks of Mismanagement of Concussion

One of the long-term risks is prolonging your post-concussion syndrome, and the other is the issue of chronic traumatic encephalopathy (CTE). At Boston University we started out with four directors at the center for the study of traumatic encephalopathy [5]. Chris Nowinski, concussion advocate, a neuropsychologist Dr. Anne McKee, a famous for her work in CTE, and Bob Stern, who is a co-director. We established a brain donation registry, which now has over 500 people enrolled. We are hoping to register and study brains of asymptomatic individuals that live normal lives, and yet play contact sports. Right now we have over 130 brains, almost all of who have come from symptomatic people or those that have committed suicide. The symptomatic people you could have predicted would have had CTE by the emotional, behavioral, and cognitive symptoms they had.

What we do not have many of, are brains of individuals that were not symptomatic, but they will come from that registry. Bob Stern as P.I. I, along with Chris, Ann, myself and a crew of graduate students, are doing a longitudinal clinical research study on over a hundred NFL players compared to a group with no recognized brain trauma over the course of their lives. Structural issues using a variety of MRI modalities, magnetic spectroscopy, DTI, volume averaging MRI, and also biomarkers are being used to see whether or not we can have a profile that correlates highly enough to make a diagnosis of CTE in living people. The other part of the center is the brain bank with Dr. Ann McKee, which has gotten the majority of the exposure to date. Do you know who first described CTE? I asked this question recently at a conference, and immediately a hand went up and said Bennett Omalu. He did describe the first in National Football League players. Harrison Martlin described dementia pugilistica, he described the clinical syndrome, which is CTE but did not use those words. Well, I will give you the answer, because it was a graduate student that we are working with. He would call it mentoring, but I am not sure who is mentoring whom because he enlightened me to the answer of this. There is a British Medical Journal Article from 1957 by Macdonald Critchley, a renowned British neurologist, and I was aware of that article because a few years ago we did a book called Boxing in Medicine. In another book that was a tribute to Clovis Vincent that came out in 1949, a number of individuals were solicited to write chapters, and it was bound up in a volume and in the book there was one chapter written in English. In that volume the CTE of boxers was written by Macdonald Critchley (1949); therefore, it was the first time that was described. In NFL players Bennet Omalu was the first to recognize it, and he published the first case of it. Currently, CTE can only be diagnosed with certainty after death. You can actually have a very high clinical suspicion if the right clinical profile is there, but you cannot be 100 % certain.

Ann McKee's brain bank is the world's largest now in terms of CTE. Her first case was John Grimsley, which is an advanced case. The medial temporal lobe is just riddled with this staining identifying *hyperphosopholated tau protein*. Dave Duerson's brain was studied, and it was found that he had a moderately advanced case of CTE. Recently there was an article by Lahman and colleagues, who looked at death certificates of a number of NFL players who played over a 10-year period in the NFL, and they all had to play 5 years or more to be included in the study. When looking at the death certificates of these individuals, they found that the incidence of Alzheimer's disease and amyotrophic lateral sclerosis (omitting Parkinson's disease) was four times higher than what would have been predicted by the national average. We don't know from our work in Boston what the incidence of CTE is, and what the prevalence of it is in any population. It is unknown in the National Football League where we have the greatest number of brains. We know it occurs, and we know that it occurs in a very high percentage of those brains that we examine 45146, but we also know that those brains are an extremely skewed samples.

These brains were not studied, only the death certificates were looked at. These death certificates are filled out by a doctor which is never a happy task—and often a task that subsequently ends up being done as quickly as possible. This leads the information to not necessarily be as thorough as one would hope.

Furthermore, what is being described as Alzheimer's disease can possibly be chronic traumatic encephalopathy. These brains were not studied, so we will never know. The same is true for what is being described as amyotrophic lateral sclerosis, which is probably chronic traumatic encephalmyotrophy, which is a variant of CTE that Ann has described (along with the rest of her colleagues) in NFL players. CTE in most people is a progressive neurodegenerative disease believed to be caused by repetitive trauma to the brain which includes sub-concussive blows. This is NOT a prolonged post-concussive syndrome, nor is it solely the cumulative effects of concussions. Symptoms characteristically, although not always, begin decades after the individual has stopped sustaining brain trauma. The one sport with a fairly high incidence of CTE is boxing. It is fairly common that individuals in their 30s have already started to lose some foot speed, developed slurred speech, etc. We need to know about the risk factors for CTE, and we need to know how we can differentiate them from other situations. Suicide is associated with head trauma, including concussion. In terms of increased incidence, it is also associated with CTE; however, we do not yet fully understand all of the factors involved. It is certain that we do not know the prevalence or incidence of the disease, but we certainly know that we do not want to see anymore of our heroes having their brains examined because of suicide.

Concluding Statement: Myths About Concussion

Myth Number One: You Have To Be Hit in the Head to Have a Concussion

I think that most people now know this is not true. Just from whiplash you can have a concussion, from a blow to your back that snaps your head back or a blow to your chest which snaps it forward, or from a fall on your butt where the forces go up the spine. Of course, when we look at our blast victims, at least in our models, it isn't the pressure wave that is producing the concussion. It is the blast winds that are associated with it that are causing the head to shake violently and oscillate 10–14 times. This event can give somebody a lifetime of concussions from one blast.

Myth Number Two: You Have To Be Rendered Unconscious to Sustain a Concussion

More than 90 % of athletic concussions do not involve loss of consciousness.

Myth Number Three: Helmets Prevent Concussions

It is possible this could be true, if it were big enough, paired with enough energy attenuating materials maybe, but it is not practical. This would also be putting the neck at risk, so it is not going to happen. We are, however, getting better helmets all the time, and I personally am a strong advocate of going in that direction and not going in the direction of less protection. It is amazing how topics such as this have made their way into the media, because they are things that society in general needs to think about and know.

Myth Number Four: Mouth Guards Prevent Concussions

No, it is not only mouth guards that claim to prevent concussions. I am not against any of it but I am just against claims that cannot be substantiated.

Myth Number Five: You Can Always See a Concussion

You can always see if somebody is unconscious or if they cannot stand up, but you are not going to see most concussions. Most concussions are subtle, and it takes time, especially with mild concussions, to sort out whether somebody has had one or not.

Myth Number Six: Your Next Concussion Will Be Worse Than Your Last

Wrong. A Bruin's player scared for had his first concussion that consisted of four and a half months of symptoms, causing him to lose a season. With his second concussion, he experienced 2 weeks of symptoms, lost a month of playing, and was back playing the rest of that season. With his third concussion, he had 4 days of symptoms, and was back in 2 weeks. That was an exception, and it is not usually what we see, but it demonstrate that every concussion is unique. You cannot predict what the next one is going to be, unless somebody is on a trajectory that they are more easily concussed and each concussion is lasting longer.

Myth Number Seven: Three Concussions and You're Out

This myth really frustrates me because it is essentially saying in a very naive way that all concussions are created equally, but when they are not. Concussions are not created equally and each one needs to be handled on an individual basis. I strongly believe that you need to record in verbiage how long the symptoms lasted with each concussion. This way in the future, others working on managing an individual's concussion can have an idea about how severe their previous concussions were. If symptoms lasted months, that is not the same injury as symptoms that lasted hours or only a day.

Myth Number Eight: Signs and Symptoms Occur Immediately

Incorrect. Some individuals have very little in the way of symptoms immediately, and some are not aware that they have had a concussion immediately. How much of that is related to adrenaline and rationalization I'm not sure, but it is a reality that many people worsen hours after the incident. Some may not have symptoms really worsen until later that night or the next morning.

Myth Number Nine: Boys Suffer More Concussions Than Girls

The number of girls are now almost equal to boys in most sports. In ice hockey, basket ball, and soccer, in fact, girls have almost twice as many recognized concussions as boys. I stress "recognized" and I keep repeating it because we do not really know that they have twice as many concussions; but twice as many are recorded. It is possible that this is due to the fact that they are more honest in reporting their symptoms, or that is due to their weak necks. It could also be both, but only time will tell.

Myth Number Ten: Concussions Determine Risk of CTE

This has not shown to be true in the work we have done. Our work would suggest individuals that take the greatest amount of brain trauma are most likely to wind up with CTE, not the people that suffered spectacular concussions. If you play in a sport that takes a higher amount of brain trauma, arguably calling boxing a sport, you are going to have a greater chance for CTE than if you play a sport like football which has less head trauma. If you play football, the lineman are going to take a lot more hits to the head than the wide receivers or the quarterbacks, although the wide receivers and the quarterbacks may take a more spectacular hit. In a sport like ice hockey, you are going to take hits equal to or greater than a football player occasionally, but not as frequently. As we accumulate more and more cases going forward, we expect to see a similar trend—that boxing seems to have the greatest incidence and football is second. Sports like ice hockey, although it certainly has cases of CTE, now appear to have a lower risk for CTE.

References

1. Cantu RC. Role of diffusion tenser imaging MRI in detecting brain injury in asymptomatic contact athletes: World Neurosurgery; December 2013.
2. Bigler ED, Maxwell WL. Neuropathology of mild traumatic brain injury: relationship to neuroimaging findings. Brain Imaging Behav. 2012;6(2):108–36.
3. Cantu RC, Guskiewicz K, Register-Mihalik JK. A retrospective clinical analysis of moderate to severe athletic concussions. Am Acad Phys Med Rehabil. 2010;2:1088–93.
4. Cantu RC, Gean AD. Second-impact syndrome and a small subdural hematoma: an uncommon catastrophic result of repetitive head injury with a characteristic imaging appearance. J Neurotrauma. 2010;27:1557–64.
5. Baugh CM, Stamm JM, Riley DO, Gavett BE, Shenton ME, Lin A, Nowinski CJ, Cantu RC, McKee AC, Stern RA. Chronic traumatic encephalopathy: neurodegeneration following repetitive concussive and subconcussive brain trauma. Brain Imaging Behav. 2012;6(2):244–54.

Chapter 3
Neuropsychological Testing in Sports Concussion Management: An Evidence-Based Model when Baseline Is Unavailable

Peter A. Arnett, Amanda R. Rabinowitz, Gray A. Vargas, Dede M. Ukueberuwa, Victoria C. Merritt, and Jessica E. Meyer

Abstract Since Barth and colleagues' seminal study used baseline neuropsychological testing as a model for sports concussion management, many collegiate sports medicine programs have adopted variations of their approach. However, no evidence-based strategy has yet been clearly articulated for the use of neuropsychological tests in concussion management that involves consideration of cases in which no baseline testing has been conducted. In this chapter, we articulate an evidence-based model for neuropsychological sports concussion management in collegiate athletes for cases in which baseline data are not available. The model involves an algorithm that is based upon base rates of impairment in a typical neurocognitive sports concussion battery, with decision rules that differ slightly for males and females. Although we use our population of collegiate athletes and the tests we administer as a framework to provide concrete values to the proposed algorithm, our evidence-based model could easily be applied to other sports concussion populations and neurocognitive test batteries. Our proposed neuropsychological concussion management guidelines provide an evidence-based model, while at the same time remain consistent with trends in the literature, suggesting that increasingly individualistic clinical concussion management approaches are most prudent.

Keywords Concussion • Neuropsychology • Neurocognitive • Evidence-based • Return-to-play

P.A. Arnett, Ph.D. (✉) • G.A. Vargas • D.M. Ukueberuwa • V.C. Merritt • J. E. Meyer
Department of Psychology, Pennsylvania State University, 352 Moore Building,
University Park, PA 16802, USA
e-mail: Paa6@psu.edu

A.R. Rabinowitz
Department of Neurosurgery, University of Pennsylvania School of Medicine,
370 Stemmler Hall, Philadelphia, PA 19104, USA

S.M. Slobounov and W.J. Sebastianelli (eds.), *Concussions in Athletics:
From Brain to Behavior*, DOI 10.1007/978-1-4939-0295-8_3,
© Springer Science+Business Media New York 2014

Introduction

Barth and colleagues' [1] seminal study using baseline neuropsychological testing as a model for sports concussion management set a standard that continues to be influential today. Many school-based sports medicine programs have adopted variations of their approach, and a range of recommendations have been made for the use of neuropsychological testing within that framework. Although the literature is variable regarding how best to use neuropsychological testing, most investigators recommend the use of pre-injury baseline neuropsychological testing as the best practice for sports concussion management [1–7]. Still, baseline data is not always available and there is recognition that guidelines are needed for interpretation in such cases. In their "Consensus Statement on Concussion in Sport" article, McCrory and colleagues [6] suggested that an important area for future research was determining "best-practice" neuropsychological testing in cases where baseline data are not available. Also, in a position paper published under the aegis of the National Academy of Neuropsychology (NAN), Moser et al. [3] noted that neurocognitive tests can play a meaningful role in concussion management even in these cases. Nonetheless, neither article provides guidelines for how neuropsychological tests should be used when no baseline testing has been conducted.

The central goal of this chapter is to provide an evidence-based model for using neuropsychological testing in the management of sports-related concussion when no baseline is available. We will first summarize and evaluate existing approaches, focusing on the merits and limitations of baseline testing, the timing of testing post-concussion, and the "value-added" of neuropsychological tests in a sports concussion context. We then lay out the framework of our model. It is not our intent to suggest that the model presented in this article should replace the baseline model. Furthermore, a discussion of the case for or against the use of neurocognitive testing in a sports concussion framework goes well beyond the scope of this chapter and has been discussed at length by other investigators [8, 9]. However, we do touch upon the merits and limitations of such tests, as well as the pros and cons of conducting baseline testing.

Summary of Literature Recommendations for the Use of Neuropsychological Testing in Sports Concussion

Use of Baseline Testing

Although the literature is variable regarding how best to use neuropsychological testing, most investigators recommend the use of pre-injury baseline neuropsychological testing as best practice for sports concussion management [1–7]. As Guskiewicz et al. [2] and others [10] have articulated, the use of baseline testing for comparison with post-injury scores helps to control for idiosyncratic interindividual differences at baseline (e.g., ADHD, possible cumulative cognitive impact of prior concussions, cultural/linguistic differences, learning disorders, age, education, proneness to psychiatric issues). Controlling for such extraneous factors by using baseline testing should make neuropsychological tests more sensitive to the impact of concussions on specific individuals.

Still, the baseline paradigm for sports concussion is not without limitations. It has been criticized because there is no empirical evidence that the use of baseline testing improves diagnostic accuracy [8, 11], reduces risk of further injury [9], or predicts decline better than would be expected by chance alone [10].

Another significant limitation of the baseline model is the fact that most individual neuropsychological measures do not have well-established test–retest reliability for the types of intervals often used in sports concussion testing, when baseline and post-injury intervals can be years apart [9, 12–14]. As Mayers and Redick [13] note, a minimal standard for test–retest reliabilities for tests used to make clinical decisions is 0.70 and above. Test–retest reliability studies of the most commonly used computerized measure—the ImPACT—have been mixed. One study on the ImPACT [15] found generally acceptable levels of reliability (0.65–0.86 for the primary summary indices) when a group of healthy controls was tested 1–13 days apart. However, other investigators have found much lower test–retest reliability coefficients when using a longer interval between test administrations—between 0.23 and 0.38 for a 45-day test–retest interval [14], and between 0.30 and 0.60 for a 2-year test–retest interval [16], though the latter study reported somewhat higher values when intra-class correlations were used.

Test–retest reliabilities have generally been found to be acceptable for more traditional paper-and-pencil neuropsychological tests such as the Digit Span Test (0.80–0.91), Symbol Digit Modalities Test (SDMT) (0.72–0.80), Hopkins Verbal Learning Test-Revised (HVLT-R) (0.78), PASAT (0.80–0.90), and the COWAT (0.70–0.88) [12]. Despite these generally acceptable values, it is important to note that the time interval for establishing these reliabilities was considerably shorter than what typically occurs in the sports concussion framework.

Consideration of test–retest reliability coefficients such as these is critical because they are central to calculating the reliable change indices (RCIs) that are typically used to determine clinically significant change. If these reliability coefficients are low, then confidence intervals will be large and greater declines will be required post-concussion for change to be detected. Tests with low test–retest reliability coefficients, then, will be less sensitive to changes post-concussion than those with higher values.

An additional limitation of widespread baseline testing is logistical complexity and expense. Also, practice effects from prior test exposure can reduce neuropsychological tests' sensitivity post-concussion. Other limitations of the baseline model are outlined in Randolph et al.'s [9] recent critique. Overall, despite its utility in controlling for interindividual differences, the baseline model does have limitations. Given these considerations, using neuropsychological tests in the sports concussion framework when no baseline has been conducted should be considered.

Timing of Post-concussion Testing

There is no clear consensus on the timing of post-concussion neurocognitive testing. In Guskiewicz et al.'s [2] NATA Position Statement, the authors suggest that neurocognitive testing should ideally be conducted in the acute injury period to help determine the severity of the concussion, and then again when the athlete is symptom-free to help with return-to-play (RTP) decisions. However, they do not provide any clear indication of when during the acute injury period that testing might ideally occur.

In the ImPACT Test Technical Manual [17] on the "Best Practices" page from the ImPACT website (https://www.impacttest.com/pdf/improtocol.pdf), the authors recommend post-concussion ImPACT testing 24–72 h post-concussion to assess whether declines have occurred from baseline and to help with concussion management in general. They also recommend testing after this acute period once the athlete is symptom free both at rest and with cognitive exertion.

From the first consensus conference in sport [4], the participants recognized that the state of knowledge precluded any specific recommendations about timing of testing post-concussion, and they stated that clinical judgment should be applied on an individual basis. From the second consensus conference in sport, McCrory et al. [5] recommended that no neuropsychological testing be conducted until athletes were symptom free. They reasoned that there was nothing that such testing could contribute to RTP decisions, and that testing in the early post-concussion interval could contaminate future testing because of practice effects. They further noted that objective neurocognitive recovery could precede or follow self-reported symptom resolution.

The third consensus conference [6] maintained the recommendation that no neurocognitive testing be conducted until athletes were symptom free by their own self-report; however, these authors provided the caveat that some cases (especially children and adolescents) may warrant neurocognitive testing prior to symptom resolution. They reasoned that such testing could help with school and home management. A recent position statement published by the American Medical Society for Sports Medicine [18] was agnostic on this issue, asserting that the evidence was unclear regarding the optimal timing of post-concussion neuropsychological testing. In sum, the available literature indicates that there is no clear consensus on the timing of neuropsychological testing post-concussion.

The "Value-Added" of Neuropsychological Tests in a Sports Concussion Framework

Some investigators have argued that there is no "value added" to neuropsychological testing in the management of sports concussion, and that RTP decisions should strictly be based upon athletes' self-reported symptoms [8, 9]. However, research on this topic has revealed two important findings that counter such a recommendation: (1) A significant percentage of concussed athletes who report full symptom resolution still show objective neurocognitive deficits—either declines from baseline [19] or, when no baseline is available, worse neurocognitive performance than control subjects [20] and (2) neurocognitive tests can identify concussed athletes in the acute post-concussion period (within two days post-concussion) who deny any symptoms but show objective declines from baseline [7].

Although the "value-added" of neurocognitive tests to the concussion management process is controversial, beyond such considerations there are problems with relying exclusively on self-report of cognitive functioning in guiding RTP decisions. First, athletes have a high motivation to minimize symptoms following concussion because of their desire to return to play, a process articulated in Echemendia and Cantu's [21] "Dynamic Model for Return-to-Play Decision Making." Second, there is extensive literature demonstrating that self-reports of cognitive functioning are only weakly correlated with actual performance on objective cognitive tests, even in individuals who are motivated and who have not experienced any insult to the brain [22].

Harmon and colleagues [18] argue that there are at least three circumstances where post-concussion neurocognitive testing may be warranted: (1) In situations where athletes are presumed to be at high-risk because of prior concussions; (2) with athletes who are likely to minimize or deny symptoms so that they can return to play; and (3) to identify athletes with persistent deficits. Thus, these authors appear to recommend post-concussion neurocognitive testing under limited circumstances. One problem with only administering neurocognitive tests to athletes who are likely to minimize or deny symptoms is that such individuals can only be definitively identified if neurocognitive testing is conducted. Otherwise, how does one know? A limitation of only administering tests to identify athletes with persistent deficits is that, again, how does one know if athletes have "persistent deficits" if they are not actually tested? As indicated above, self-report of symptoms is suspect for a variety of well-established reasons, so relying on an athlete's self-report of symptoms is not going to be useful in identifying persistent deficits.

A Proposed Evidence-Based Model for Neurocognitive Concussion Management when no Baseline Is Available

Following Ellemberg and colleagues' [12] observation that the absence of scientifically validated algorithms for neuropsychological test interpretation has resulted in clinicians and researchers using idiosyncratic decision rules, as well as McCrory et al.'s [6] recommendation for "Best-Practice" guidelines, we articulate a model for the use of neuropsychological tests in a sports concussion framework when no baseline is available. We recognize that our model only represents a step in a process that should continue as new empirical knowledge about this topic accrues.

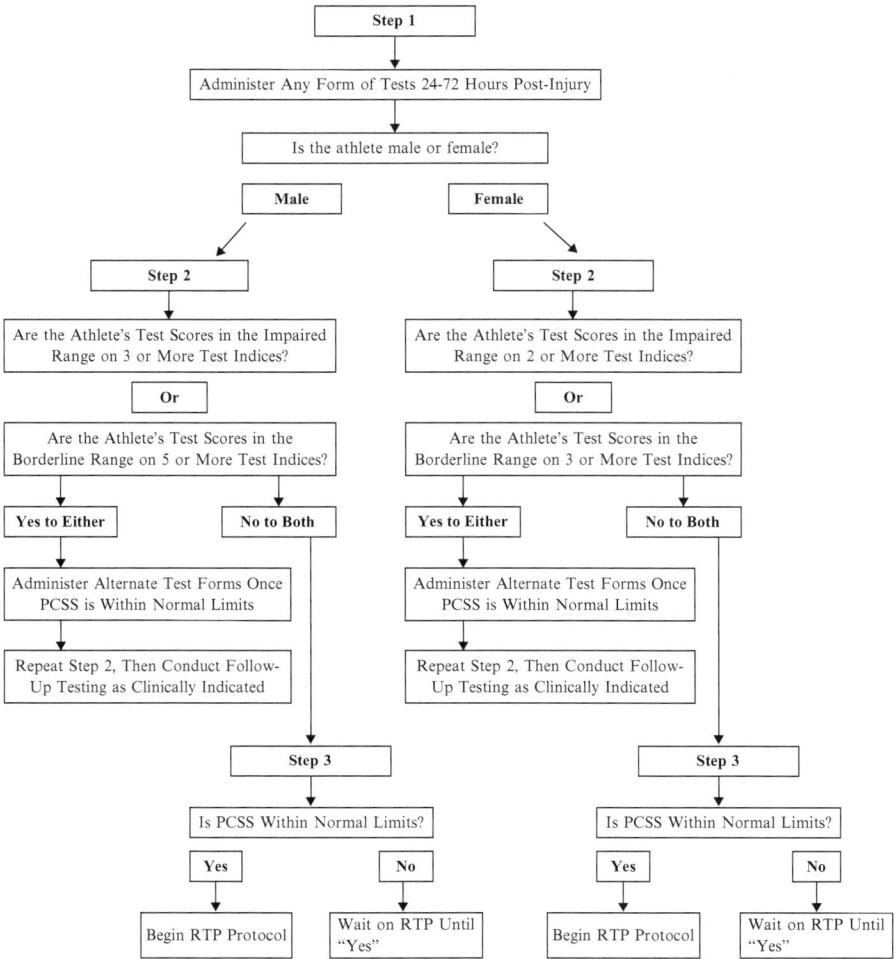

Fig. 3.1 Post-concussion neuropsychological testing algorithm when no baseline is available

Figure 3.1 illustrates our algorithm. Before discussing this in detail, we outline the tests in the battery on which the algorithm is based, which includes both computerized and paper-and-pencil tests. We then describe the evidence basis for each step of the algorithm. Note that there are separate decision rules for males and females. This is due to findings of gender differences in base rates of impairment using this same battery in Division I collegiate athletes [23]. Although there are factors that can influence the interpretation of neurocognitive test results including depression, number of prior concussions, and the presence of ADHD/learning disorders, we do not provide any systematic treatment of these issues, as they go beyond the scope of this chapter. Still, we acknowledge their potential importance in the interpretation of neurocognitive tests in the sports concussion context. Although the present article is not an empirical research paper, per se, the study on which we base some of the framework of the algorithm [23] was conducted in compliance with University Institutional Review Board requirements and American Psychological Association ethical guidelines.

Measures

The battery we use as the basis for our model includes both computerized and paper-and-pencil measures. Although the use of paper-and-pencil measures can be logistically more complex and expensive than using computerized tests alone because they require fact-to-face administration, including such tests is likely to increase the sensitivity of the battery. Also, if neuropsychological tests are only used post-concussion, then the cost of administration is considerably lower.

Computerized tests. Computerized tests include the ImPACT [24] and the Vigil Continuous Performance Test (CPT) [25]. The following summary indices from the ImPACT are included: verbal memory composite, visual memory composite, visuo-motor speed composite, and reaction time composite. Average delay (a reaction time index) is used for the Vigil CPT. Although more recent versions of the ImPACT are available, we based our algorithm on the 2.0 version because of the availability of data for our evidence-based model. This version appears to be highly correlated with more recent (including online) versions of the ImPACT.

Paper-and-pencil tests. These measures include the HVLT-R [26] (total correct immediate and delayed recall), the Brief Visuospatial Memory Test-Revised (BVMT-R) [27] (total correct immediate and delayed recall), the SDMT [28] (total correct within 90 s), a modified Digit Span Test [29] (total correct forward and backward sequences), the PSU Cancellation Task [30] (total correct within 90 s), Comprehensive Trail Making Test Trails 2 and 4 or 3 and 5 (CTMT) [31] (completion times for both parts), and the Stroop Color-Word Test (SCWT) [32] (time to completion for both color-naming and color-word conditions). Thus, across computerized and paper-and-pencil measures there are 17 test indices.

For most of the tests used, we suggest that alternate forms be used. The ImPACT has such alternate forms built into the program; alternate forms are available for all of the above paper-and-pencil tests with the exception of the modified Digit Span Test and SCWT.

Self-report. To measure post-concussion symptoms, we use the Post-Concussion Symptom Scale (PCSS). This measure includes a list of 22 common post-concussion symptoms. Examinees rate the extent to which they are currently experiencing each symptom on a scale from 0 to 6, with 0 indicating the absence of the symptom, and 6 being severe.

Algorithm of Decision Rules

As Fig. 3.1 shows, each step of the algorithm after the initial neuropsychological testing involves a question, and then an action depending on the answer to the question.

Step 1. The action at Step 1 is to administer the test battery at 24–72 h post-injury. The evidence basis for this stems from animal models showing that many elements of the neurochemical cascade in the brain following concussion peak at about 48 h post-injury, and the decrease in glucose metabolism that occurs at about 48 h post-injury is correlated with cognitive dysfunction in adult rats [33–35]. Also, neuro-cognitive research in humans has shown that the greatest cognitive impact post-concussion typically occurs within 24–72 h post-injury [1, 36–38], though there is considerable individual variability [38]. As such, testing athletes during this time interval should provide a likely estimate of the full impact of the concussion on the brain as manifested by neurocognitive test results. Also, if the athlete is free of neurocognitive impairment at this early stage (relative to base rates), then no further neurocognitive testing would necessarily need to be conducted post-concussion, and the RTP decision could be made based on other factors (e.g., self-reported symp-toms, vestibular signs). If the athlete does show signs of neurocognitive impairment at this point, then the objective neurocognitive data could be used to assist in getting temporary academic accommodations while symptomatic (e.g., deferral of exams and other assignments, testing in a room free from distraction, extra time on exams). A more detailed rationale for testing at this early time point post-concussion, and possibly before self-reported symptom resolution, is provided below in the section entitled, "Why Recommend Testing During the Acute Concussion Phase?"

Step 2. The algorithm has different Step 2s for males and females because the study on which these specific decision rules are based revealed slightly different base rates for males and females. In this study, we examined baseline performance in 495 col-legiate athletes on the same test battery outlined in this chapter [23], and impairment on a test was defined as performing 2 SDs or more below the mean of other athletes; borderline impairment was defined as 1.5 SD or greater below the mean. These criteria were used since currently there is no agreed upon definition of abnormally poor test performance on neuropsychological tests following concussion, and also to allow for some flexibility in decision making.

In this study, less than 10 % of males had five or more borderline scores, and less than 10 % of females had three or more borderline scores. Additionally, less than 10 % of males had three or more impaired scores, and less than 10 % of females had two or more impaired scores. We used these base rates as a foundation for the deci-sion rules in our model. In light of such data, male athletes who are tested post-concussion who show impairment on three or more tests and female athletes who show impairment on two or more tests evidence highly unusual performance that is likely to reflect the impact of their concussion (see Fig. 3.1). Similarly, male athletes who are tested post-concussion who show borderline scores on five or more tests and female athletes who show borderline scores on three or more tests display highly unusual performance that is likely to reflect the impact of their concussion. The application of these data in decision rules is shown at Step 2 in Fig. 3.1.

Ideally, concussion programs adopting this algorithm would be advised to use a base rate of impairment data collected from athletes participating in their specific programs. In this way, the data used are likely to be most valid for that group of athletes for a particular neurocognitive test battery. If such base rates differ from what we report, relevant values could simply replace what we report from our athletes in the algorithm. If base rates of impairment are not available, it should be noted that other studies using test batteries of comparable length have reported similar base rates of impairment using a similar number of test indices in healthy older adults [39, 40], as well as children and adolescents [41]. Thus, although the direct evidence basis for this recommendation concerning base rates relies only on our one study of collegiate athletes, findings from these other studies suggest that these data are likely representative of base rates of impairment more generally when individuals are tested on a neurocognitive battery similar in length to ours. Also, the data we rely on for concrete decision rules in the algorithm can be thought of as a vehicle for describing the model rather than something to be rigidly applied. Again, ideally, local base rate norms based upon whatever battery of tests is used, if different from what we report, would replace the specific values in the algorithm.

If male or female athletes receive a "yes" response at Step 2, for either the impaired or borderline criterion, then the action is to "Administer Alternate Test Forms Once PCSS is Within Normal Limits." The evidence basis for this stems from findings showing that even when athletes report that they are symptom free, many still show evidence for objective cognitive impairment [19]. Additionally, relying on self-report of cognitive functioning when determining when athletes can return to play is likely to be inaccurate given the consistently replicated low correlation found between objective neurocognitive test performance and self-reported neurocognitive functioning [22]. Thus, any athlete should have to perform within normal limits neurocognitively prior to returning to play, and such decisions should not be based on self-reported cognitive functioning alone. Following this recommendation after a "yes" response, the algorithm indicates, "Repeat Step 2, Then Conduct Follow-Up Testing as Clinically Indicated."

Step 3. If either male or female athletes have a "no" response at Step 2, then the algorithm moves to Step 3 to consider the following question: "Is PCSS Within Normal Limits?" The determination of "within normal limits" is made using normative data from our sample of collegiate athletes at baseline on the PCSS. Similar to our comment above concerning the ideal framework being the use of local norms to determine base rates, normative data from local samples would ideally be applied here to the PCSS. Scores falling within the broad average range (i.e., standard score of 80 or above) are considered "within normal limits." If the answer to this question is "yes," then the recommendation is to begin the RTP protocol. If the answer is "no," then the recommendation is to wait on starting the RTP until the PCSS is within normal limits.

One complicating issue involves cases where athletes have a "yes" response at Step 2 (meeting the below base rate impaired or a borderline criterion), yet report being within normal limits in terms of their symptom report. Given that the recommendation following such an outcome is to "Administer Alternate Test Forms Once PCSS is Within Normal Limits," how does one proceed? There are no clear evidence-based guidelines for how to proceed here in terms of the precise timing of the next post-concussion testing point. A broad guideline would be to recommend testing the athlete again between 5–10 days post-concussion, given that many studies show that most collegiate athletes show full cognitive recovery by that point [1, 30, 36, 37, 42–44]. With that said, other research shows that some collegiate athletes do not recover within that window and take longer than two weeks for their neurocognitive functioning to normalize [44, 45]. Thus, more research will clearly be needed to refine this broad guideline. Studies that examine the duration for normalization of brain functioning in athletes who report being normal in terms of symptom report but show impairments neurocognitively would be ideal. Given the current state of the literature, the most prudent approach would be to rely more on individualistic clinical concussion management strategies employed by skilled clinicians to determine temporal sequencing of testing in these cases [46]. Factors, such as the urgency with which an RTP decision needs to be made (e.g., if a crucial game is imminent vs. the athlete's sport not being "in season"), as well as other individualistic factors (e.g., prior concussion history, the presence of clinically significant depression), would need to be considered. Thus, the model allows for considerable flexibility at this stage not only due, in part, to the absence of clear research evidence to guide decision making, but also due to idiosyncratic factors that are nearly always going to be at play in the clinical management of concussion.

Why Recommend Testing During the Acute Concussion Phase?

One potentially controversial recommendation in our algorithm is to routinely test athletes in the acute stage more systematically post-concussion. Many athletes are likely to still be experiencing some symptoms at the 24–72 h post-concussion point, and some investigators and clinicians have asserted that such testing should be avoided on a number of grounds. First, given that athletes are still symptomatic, some posit that such testing cannot contribute anything to the RTP decision, because clinicians are typically not going to put athletes back to play who are still experiencing self-reported symptoms. Second, it has been suggested that such testing could exacerbate the athlete's symptoms. These are reasonable concerns; however, to our knowledge, there is no published study showing that recently concussed, still symptomatic adult athletes show more of an increase in symptoms following such neurocognitive testing than healthy controls. We assert that the value of such acute testing outweighs the potential minor risk (as yet empirically undemonstrated) of a temporary increase in symptoms. The caveat to this, of course, involves cases where symptoms are so severe that testing could be harmful in exacerbating already severe symptoms, or where the nature of such symptoms would likely substantially interfere with test performance (e.g., severe dizziness, nausea, or headache, among others). This is where individualistic concussion management again becomes important [46].

One benefit of such testing in the early acute phase is to help document the severity of the concussion. Athletes who show more normative impairments at this acute stage could be managed more conservatively once RTP procedures have begun than those who were back to their likely premorbid cognitive level, or nearly back to such a level. Another benefit, as noted earlier, is that early objective documentation of deficits could result in athletes quickly being able to secure needed academic accommodations during their recovery period. A third benefit of acute testing is that it may show that the athlete is in fact back to baseline neurocognitively, even at this early stage. If this is the case, then more rapid return to play could potentially occur. Although an athlete's medical well-being must always be the most important consideration of sports medicine professionals, athletes performing at a high level of sport (e.g., Division I college, the basis of our algorithm) could suffer significant harm in terms of their status on the team and ability to compete in important games and maintain their scholarships if they are held out of play for an unnecessarily long period of time.

A final benefit of conducting systematic testing during this acute period post-concussion and at other systematic time points is that the neurocognitive results following any future concussion could be compared with the results from the previous concussion to assess whether the range and severity of cognitive impairments increase. If athletes are tested at different points post-concussion, then such systematic comparisons would not be possible. Athletes who suffer multiple concussions and show an increased range and severity of cognitive impairments with each successive concussion can then be treated more conservatively.

Limitations

Our algorithm represents an initial attempt to develop systematic guidelines for decision-making post-concussion in cases where baseline data are not available. Although we provide systematic decision rules, there is much room for individualistic concussion management, and we spell out a number of examples where such factors come into play. The neuropsychological test battery we recommend is relatively lengthy and logistically complex; however, applying it in cases where baseline testing has not been conducted significantly reduces such complexity. Also, the algorithm can be adapted to different test (possibly shorter) batteries and different athlete groups when base rates of impairment data can be derived from such groups.

Future Directions

Future work should include studies to validate the algorithm in other samples independent of our lab group, particularly in test groups of collegiate athletes with and without concussions, followed by testing at the same time intervals as suggested by our model. Examining base rates of impairment on the test battery in individuals with ADHD and/or learning disorders would also be a valuable focus for future work.

More work is also needed concerning the objective impact of undergoing a neurocognitive concussion battery during the acute concussion phase in collegiate athletes. Measuring self-reported post-concussion symptoms prior to and after neuropsychological testing in concussed and non-concussed athletes would be one way of assessing this.

Our recommendations are necessarily tentative, given the limited evidence available for some aspects of the proposed algorithm (e.g., the ideal timing of post-concussion testing during the acute injury period, ideal temporal sequence of testing once athletes are normative symptomologically, but still impaired neurocognitively). However, we hope that our algorithm provides a template for improving neurocognitive concussion management in collegiate athletes.

Acknowledgement There are no conflicts of interest involved with this manuscript, and no sources of financial support.

References

1. Barth JT, Alves WM, Ryan TV, Macciocchi SN, Rimel RW, Jane JA, et al. Mild head injury in sports: neuropsychological sequelae and recovery of function. In: Levin HS, Eisenberg HM, Benton AL, editors. Mild Head Injury. New York: Oxford University Press; 1989. p. 257–75.
2. Guskiewicz KM, Bruce SL, Cantu RC, Ferrara MS, Kelly JP, McCrea M, et al. Recommendations on management of sport-related concussion: summary of the National Athletic Trainers' Association position statement. Neurosurgery. 2004;55:891–5.
3. Moser RS, Iverson GL, Echemendia RJ, Lovell MR, Schatz P, Webbe FM, et al. NAN position paper: neuropsychological evaluation in the diagnosis and management of sports-related concussion. Arch Clin Neuropsychol. 2007;22:909–16.
4. Aubry M, Cantu R, Dvorak J, Graf-Baumann T, Johnston K, Kelly J, et al. Summary and agreement statement of the first International Conference on Concussion in Sport, Vienna 2001. Br J Sports Med. 2002;36:3–7.
5. McCrory P, Johnston K, Meeuwisse W, Aubry M, Cantu R, Dvorak J, et al. Summary and agreement statement of the 2nd International Conference on Concussion in Sport, Prague 2004. Br J Sports Med. 2005;39:196–204.
6. McCrory P, Meeuwisse W, Johnston K, Dvorak J, Aubry M, Molloy M, et al. Consensus statement on concussion in sport—the 3rd International conference on concussion in sport held in Zurich, November 2008. Br J Sports Med. 2009;43(1):i76–90.
7. Van Kampen DA, Lovell MR, Pardini JE, Collins MW, Fu FH. The "value added" of neurocognitive testing after sports-related concussion. Am J Sports Med. 2006;30:1630–5.
8. Randolph C, McCrea M, Barr WB. Is neuropsychological testing useful in the management of sport-related concussion? J Athl Train. 2005;40:139–54.

9. Randolph C. Baseline neuropsychological testing in managing sport-related concussion: does it modify risk? Curr Sports Med Rep. 2011;10:21–6.
10. Echemendia RJ, Bruce JM, Bailey CM, Sanders JF, Arnett PA, Vargas G. The utility of post-concussion neuropsychological data in identifying cognitive change following sports-related MTBI in the absence of baseline data. Clin Neuropsychol. 2012;26:1077–91.
11. Randolph C, Kirkwood MW. What are the real risks of sport-related concussion, and are they modifiable? J Int Neuropsychol Soc. 2009;15:1–9.
12. Ellemberg D, Henry LC, Macciocchi SN, Guskiewicz KM, Broglio SP. Advances in sport concussion assessment: from behavioral to brain imaging measures. J Neurotrauma. 2009;26:2365–82.
13. Mayers LB, Redick TS. Clinical utility of ImPACT assessment for postconcussion return-to-play counseling: psychometric issues. J Clin Exp Neuropsychol. 2012;34:235–42.
14. Broglio SP, Ferrara MS, Macciocchi SN, Baumgartner TA, Elliott R. Test–retest reliability of computerized concussion assessment programs. J Athl Train. 2007;42:509–14.
15. Iverson GL, Lovell MR, Collins MW. Interpreting change on ImPACT following sport concussion. Clin Neuropsychol. 2003;17:460–7.
16. Schatz PS. Long-term test–retest reliability of baseline cognitive assessments using ImPACT. Am J Sports Med. 2010;38:47–53.
17. Lovell M. ImPACT version 2.0 clinical user's manual. Pittsburgh: ImPACT Applications Inc.; 2002.
18. Harmon KG, Drezner JA, Gammons M, Guskiewicz KM, Halstead M, Herring SA, et al. American Medical Society for Sports Medicine position statement: concussion in sport. Br J Sports Med. 2013;47:15–26.
19. Broglio SP, Macciocchi SN, Ferrara MS. Neurocognitive performance of concussed athletes when symptom free. J Athl Train. 2007;42:504–8.
20. Fazio VC, Lovell MR, Pardini JE, Collins MW. The relation between post concussion symptoms and neurocognitive performance in concussed athletes. NeuroRehabilitation. 2007;22:207–16.
21. Echemendia RJ, Cantu RC. Return to play following brain injury. In: Lovell MR, Echemendia RJ, Barth JT, Collins MW, editors. Traumatic brain injury in sports: an international neuropsychological perspective. Lisse: Swets & Zeitlinger B.V.; 2004.
22. Lezak MD, Howieson DB, Loring DW. Neuropsychological assessment. 4th ed. New York: Oxford University Press; 2004.
23. Barwick FH, Rabinowitz AR, Arnett PA. Base rates of impaired neuropsychological test performance among healthy collegiate athletes. In revision.
24. Lovell M, Collins M, Podell K, Powell J, Maroon J. ImPACT: immediate post-concussion assessment and cognitive testing. Pittsburgh: NeuroHealth Systems, LLC.; 2000.
25. Cegalis JA, Cegalis S. The Vigil/W Continuous Performance Test (manual). New York: ForThought; 1994.
26. Benedict RHB, Schretlen D, Groninger L, Brandt J. Hopkins Verbal Learning Test-Revised: normative data and analysis of inter-form and test-retest reliability. Clin Neuropsychol. 1998;12(1):43–55.
27. Benedict RHB. Brief Visuospatial Memory Test—revised: professional manual. Odessa: Psychological Assessment Resources; 1997.
28. Smith A. Symbol digit modalities test (SDMT) manual (revised). Los Angeles: Western Psychological Services; 1982.
29. Wechsler D. Wechsler Adult Intelligence Scale-III (WAIS-III). New York: Psychological Corporation; 1997.
30. Echemendia RJ, Putukian M, Mackin RS, Julian L, Shoss N. Neuropsychological test performance prior to and following sports-related mild traumatic brain injury. Clin J Sport Med. 2001;11:23–31.
31. Reynolds CR. Comprehensive trail making test (CTMT). Austin: Pro-Ed; 2002.
32. Trenerry MR, Crosson B, DeBoe J, Leber WR. Stroop neuropsychological screening test. Odessa: Psychological Assessment Resources; 1989.

33. Barkhoudarian G, Hovda DA, Giza CC. The molecular pathophysiology of concussive brain injury. Clin Sports Med. 2011;30:33–48.
34. Giza CC, DiFiori JP. Pathophysiology of sports-related concussion. Sports Health. 2011;3: 46–51.
35. Giza CC, Hovda DA. The neurometabolic cascade of concussion. J Athl Train. 2001; 36:228–35.
36. Rosenbaum AM, Arnett PA, Bailey CM, Echemendia RJ. Neuropsychological assessment of sports-related concussion: measuring clinically significant change. In: Slobounov S, Sebastianelli W, editors. Foundations of sport-related brain injuries. Norwell: Springer; 2006. p. 137–71.
37. Belanger HG, Vanderploeg RD. The neuropsychological impact of sports-related concussion: a meta-analysis. J Int Neuropsychol Soc. 2005;11:345–57.
38. Wilde EA, McCauley SR, Barnes A, Wu TC, Chu Z, Hunter JV, et al. Serial measurement of memory and diffusion tensor imaging changes within the first week following uncomplicated mild traumatic brain injury. Brain Imaging Behav. 2012;6:319–28.
39. Brooks BL, Iverson GL, White T. Substantial risk of 'accidental MCI' in healthy older adults: base rates of low memory scores in neuropsychological assessment. J Int Neuropsychol Soc. 2007;13:490–500.
40. Palmer BW, Boone KB, Lesser IM, Wohl MA. Base rates of "impaired" neuropsychological test performance among healthy older adults. Arch Clin Neuropsychol. 1998;13:503–11.
41. Brooks BL, Sherman EMS, Iverson GL. Healthy children get low scores too: prevalence of low scores on the NEPSY-II in preschoolers, children, and adolescents. Arch Clin Neuropsychol. 2010;25:182–90.
42. Covassin T, Schatz P, Swanik CB. Sex differences in neuropsychological function and post-concussion symptoms of concussed collegiate athletes. Neurosurgery. 2007;61:345–51.
43. Covassin T, Elbin R, Harris W, Parker T, Kontos A. The role of age and sex in symptoms, neurocognitive performance, and postural stability in athletes after concussion. Am J Sports Med. 2012;40:1303–12.
44. Echemendia RJ, Iverson GL, McCrea M, Broshek DK, Gioia GA, Sautter SW, et al. Role of neuropsychologists in the evaluation and management of sport-related concussion: an inter-organization position statement. Arch Clin Neuropsychol. 2012;27:119–22.
45. McClincy MP, Lovell MR, Pardini J, Collins MW, Spore MK. Recovery from sports concussion in high school and collegiate athletes. Brain Inj. 2006;20:33–9.
46. Lovell M. The management of sports-related concussion: current status and future trends. Clin J Sport Med. 2009;28:95–111.

Chapter 4
Feasibility of Virtual Reality for Assessment of Neurocognitive, Executive, and Motor Functions in Concussion

Semyon M. Slobounov, Wayne J. Sebastianelli, and Karl M. Newell

Abstract The purpose of the research presented in this chapter is to investigate if virtual reality (VR) neurocognitive, executive, and motor function assessment tools are susceptible to practice and fatigue effects similar to those currently used in a clinical practice. Fifteen athletically active and neurologically normal Penn State students participated in a VR "practice effect" study. Another 15 Penn State football players participated in an "effect of fatigue" study on neurocognitive, balance, and executive functions. Subjects performed VR tests on several occasions. The statistical analysis was conducted to examine the VR measures as a function of testing session (practice effect) and physical fatigue (prior to and after full contact practices). The number and type of the full contacts during the practices were assessed via a specially developed observational chart. There are several major findings of interest. First, all subjects reported the "sense of presence" and "significant mental effort" while performing the VR tests. Second, neither effect of testing day ($p > 0.05$) nor effect of VR testing modality ($p > 0.05$) was revealed by ANOVA. Third, physical fatigue did not influence the VR measures in the majority of football players under study ($p > 0.05$). However, there was a reduction in several VR performance measures in football players who sustained prior concussive injuries. The findings

S.M. Slobounov, Ph.D. (✉)
Professor of Kinesiology & Neurosurgery, Director of Center for Sports Concussion Research and Services, Penn State - Department of Kinesiology & Hershey Medical College, University Park, PA, USA
e-mail: sms18@psu.edu

W.J. Sebastianelli
Pennsylvania State University, University Park, PA, USA

Departments of Orthopaedics and Sports Medicine, Penn State Hershey, Bone and Joint Institute, State College, PA 16803, USA
e-mail: wsebastianelli@hmc.psu.edu

K.M. Newell
Department of Kinesiology, Pennsylvania State University, 267 Rec Building, University Park, State College, PA 16802, USA

S.M. Slobounov and W.J. Sebastianelli (eds.), *Concussions in Athletics: From Brain to Behavior*, DOI 10.1007/978-1-4939-0295-8_4,
© Springer Science+Business Media New York 2014

show that VR testing modalities implemented in this study and aimed to evaluate neurocognitive (spatial memory, attention), motor (balance), and executive functions may be used as a complementary tool in a clinical practice. VR testing modalities under laboratory conditions are easily transferable into field conditions, and can potentially be used as the side-line evaluation of subjects at risk for concussion.

Keywords Virtual reality (VR) • Practice effect • Fatigue effect • Concussion • Mild traumatic brain injury

Introduction

Mild traumatic brain injury (mTBI), the most common variant of what is known as concussion, has an annual reported incidence of 1.4 million cases in the United States alone [1, 2] and accounts for 80 % of all traumatic brain injuries (TBIs) [3, 4]. There are a number of immediate physical, cognitive, and emotional symptoms that arise from mTBI that include headache, dizziness, unsteady posture and gait, nausea, slurred speech, poor concentration, and short-term memory loss. For most sport-related concussions (80–90 %) the recovery is rapid, with spontaneous symptoms resolution within 10 days post-injury, thus referred to as *uncomplicated mTBI* [5, 6]. Yet when more challenging testing protocols are implemented [7] as many as 15–38 % of individuals suffering from mTBI have clinical symptoms that persist and may be detected for months or even years post-injury [8–10]. Prolonged clinical symptoms resolution exceeding 1 month post-injury associated with positive standard neuroimaging findings is referred to as *complicated mTBI* [11]. The definitional problems often are reflected in the lack of consistency and consensus among clinical practitioners and researchers dealing with mild TBI.

There is consensus among clinical practitioners dealing with sports-related concussions (mTBI) that neurocognitive, motor (predominantly whole body posture and balance), and executive functions (i.e., decision making and reaction time (RT)) are the most prominent deficits that concussed athletes experience at least within the acute phase of injury [8, 12, 13]. The Zurich Consensus Statement (2009) recommended that working memory, attention/vigilance, visual learning and memory, reasoning/problem solving, and speed of information processing are the most important neurocognitive functions that need to be accurately assessed to define the degree of brain damage induced by a concussive blow [5]. However, ecologically valid, sports-concussion-specific, and reliable assessment tools for detection of these neurocognitive functions have yet to be defined.

Several previous studies have identified a negative effect of mTBI on postural stability [14–16]. The use of postural stability testing for the management of sport-related concussion is gradually becoming more common among sport medicine clinicians. A growing body of controlled studies has demonstrated postural stability deficits, as measured by the Balance Error Scoring System (BESS), on post-injury day 1 [12, 17–23]. In the case of an *uncomplicated mTBI*, the recovery of balance occurred between day 1 and day 3 post-injury for most of the brain-injured subjects [22].

It appeared that the initial 2 days after an mTBI are the most problematic for subjects standing on the foam surfaces, which was attributed to a sensory interaction problem using visual, vestibular, and somatosensory systems [18, 23]. However, more recent studies by Cavanaugh et al. [24–26] have shown that advanced methods from nonlinear dynamics (i.e., approximate entropy, ApEn) may detect changes in postural control in athletes with *normal* postural stability measures based upon conventional balance testing, longer than 3–4 days after *uncomplicated* concussions. Our own recent study has also shown alteration of virtual-time-to-contact (VTC) measures in the absence of traditional measures of postural instability in concussed individuals [27]. Overall, there is an agreement that when more challenging testing modalities are introduced, balance deficiency in concussed athletes may be observed far beyond 7–10 days post-injury even after clinical symptoms resolution [10, 20, 27–37]. Specifically, application of nonlinear methods [24–26] and virtual reality tools [10, 27, 29–37] for assessment of postural data may reveal abnormal balance in the subacute phase of brain injury evolution even in *uncomplicated mTBI*.

Regardless of overall advances, both technological and conceptual, there is still no *gold standard* for accurate assessment of concussion in athletics. There are a few factors that exacerbate the problems with accurate assessment of mTBI. First, conventional neuropsychological (NP) tests are not designed to perform repeated measurements [38], and thus suffer from the so-called *practice effect*. Practice effects are particularly troublesome for post-injury cognitive impairment tracking, since they can confound interpretation [39]. Moreover, computerizing conventional neuropsychological tests that have validity for single assessments does not make them any more valid than the original paper and pencil versions for repeated testing, particularly at high frequency intervals. It provides administration, standardization, and data management advantages, but the tests are fundamentally the same as when given manually. Therefore it is not surprising that the results of follow-up tests in the acute phase of injury often appear to be better than those obtained from the initial baseline test.

Second, it should be noted that NP deficits persist in a significant minority (38 %) of concussed athletes even after they self-report that they are symptom-free [8]. Overall, currently used NP modalities, including computerized assessment of neurocognitive performance, cannot detect long-term cognitive decrement in majority of concussed individuals [8].

Third, most of the NP tests are lengthy and often boring which may induce mental and even physical fatigue. Several recent papers indicate that even normal volunteers may experience both self-reported and EEG-evidenced fatigue while taking NP tests [40]. This confounding factor may be exacerbated by the lack of control for subjects' efforts during administering NP tests (Iverson, personal communication 2010) that makes the interpretation of data at least questionable.

Finally, there is a growing concern regarding the lack of *ecological validity* and *transferability* of data obtained in a clinical setting to real-life situations. For example, a concussed subject may be *asymptomatic* based on traditional memory testing but cannot recall the coaches' instructions and immediate play actions required by coaches.

VR has the potential to overcome the aforementioned challenges and ultimately be used as a complementary tool for accurate assessment of the degree of damage induced by concussive blows. In fact, the Zurich Consensus Statement on concussion in sport [5] identified VR among the key areas of future research and possible clinical application.

VR is an interactive, computer-generated 3D environment that simulates the real world and provokes a sensation of immersion in the subjects. In fact, VR has recently emerged as a promising method in various domains of therapy, including brain damage rehabilitation, offering the potential to achieve significant successes in assessment, treatment, and improved outcome. Continuing advances in VR technologies along with cost reductions have stimulated both research and development of VR systems aimed at psychological, physical/behavioral, and emotional assessment/rehabilitation of brain-injured individuals. A growing number of diverse occupations that currently use the immersive and interactive properties of VR include athletes, drivers, parachutists, fire fighters, soldiers, divers, and surgeons. However, with respect to implication for clinical practice, it is still yet to be determined whether VR is *vulnerable* to practice and fatigue effects, similar to the modalities currently used in clinical practice. The overall objective of this chapter is to address these critical questions in two separate experiments.

Virtual Reality Applications, Methods, and Procedures

VR Visual Spatial Memory Test

The assessment of memory functions (i.e., spatial memory and its underlying distinct processes such as encoding, retention, and retrieval) was implemented via presentation of 3D simulation of a *virtual corridor*. TBI patients commonly experience memory problems, specifically in assessing their spatial location with respect to some external objects in the surrounding environment. For example, if the patient left the hospital room, he/she would have difficulty in finding his/her way back to the room, not remembering whether to turn *left* or *right*, move *forward* and/or *backward* in the hospital corridors.

The subjects (a) were shown the navigation route to encode (E) and then (b) requested to navigate purposefully with the goal of reaching specific target room location (active navigation, AN) using a high resolution joystick (www.magconcept.com). The subjects *moved* around using their right thumb to freely navigate in forward, backward, and side-to-side directions. The virtual corridor (see Fig. 4.1, including the floor plan of the *virtual corridor*) was generated by a VTC Open GL developing kit (HeadRehab, LLC, USA—www.HeadRehab.com) which provides a realistic VR environment and sense of presence (see also [51] for details). A total of three trials were allowed to successfully complete this test.

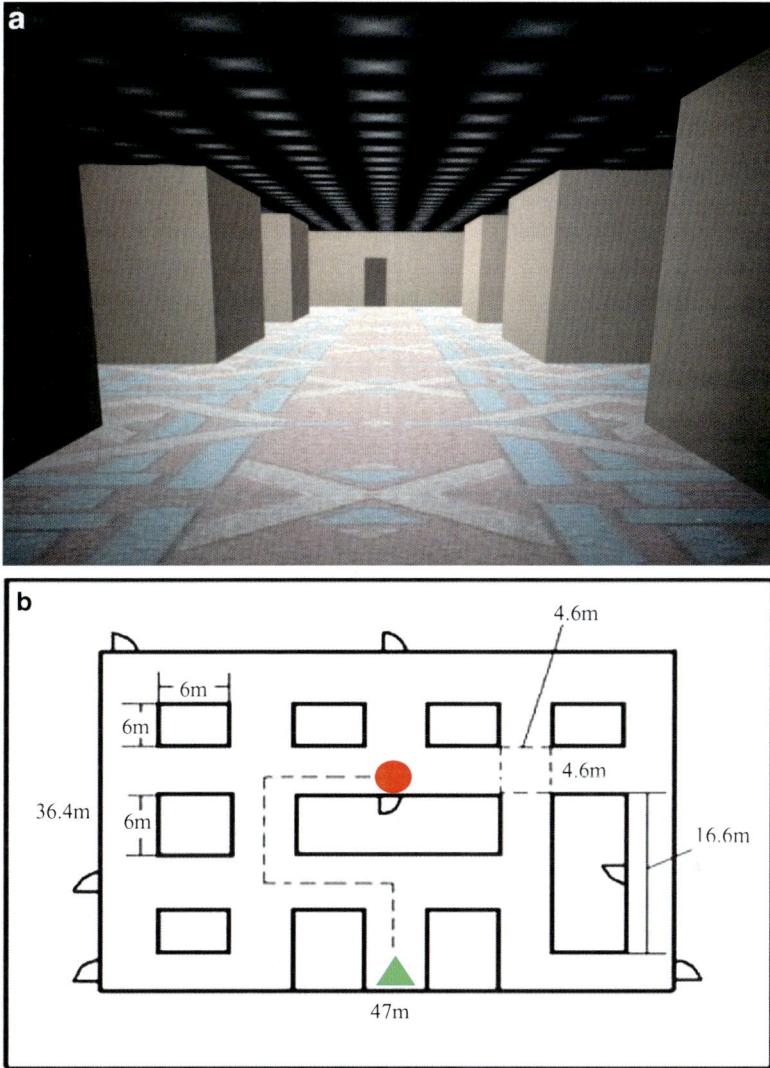

Fig. 4.1 (**a**) View of the virtual corridor used for navigation tasks under study; and (**b**) floor plan, and a sample of the route for one of the runs. The subjects were instructed to reproduce (e.g., retrieval) the previously shown routes (e.g., encoding) via navigating through virtual corridor by the joystick and to find the target location. It should be noted that starting position was the same for all runs

Assessment of "Sense of Presence" and Success Rate

All subjects were requested to report the illusion of forward self-motion and the sense of presence during VR navigation following the completion of this test similar to Jancke et al. [41]. It should be noted that sense of presence is understood to refer to the subjective feeling of being in a virtual environment while being unaware of one's real location and surroundings as well as the technology that delivers the stream of virtual input to the senses [42]. Subjects were instructed to rate the strength of *presence* on a scale ranged from 0 (no presence) to 10 (very strong presence), similar to Witmer and Singer [43].

The task performance success rate was assessed combining three variables: (1) accuracy of the task performance (find vs. not find presented route during encoding phase); (2) number of trials needed to successfully complete the test (total allowed $n = 3$); and (3) time needed to complete the test (30 s maximal allowed). These three data sets were used as an input for normalized reports of success rate ranges from 10 to 0 for each subject under study. It should be noted, we were able to detect spatial memory abnormalities in concussed individuals in subacute phase of injury, although diagnosed as *asymptomatic* based upon conventional neurocognitive assessment tools [44]. Current research is in progress to evaluate both convergent and discriminant validity of VR spatial memory module in the context of concussion evaluation that will be published elsewhere.

VR Recognition "A" Test

This test aimed to measure a subject's visual recognition performance in remembering and recognizing objects found within a virtual environment. This module can be used in conjunction with the recognition B test (see below). The subject's task is to passively navigate through the virtual corridor. Along his/her way there are seven objects that should be memorized. Both types and color of these objects are important to remember. Then, the subject is presented with a display panel of 14 different objects and given 120 s to select *only* the same seven objects previously seen in the virtual corridor. The number of correct/incorrect responses and time to perform the test are computed and converted into the scoring format from 10 to 0 (Fig. 4.2).

VR Recognition "B" Test

The subject is shown seven different objects slowly rotating for 60 s to memorize before passive navigation through the virtual corridor. Both the type and color of the objects are important memorizing properties. The subject is then passively navigated through the virtual corridor. If the subject recognizes an object from the seven objects previously shown in the display panel, he/she must press the trigger/button on the interactive device to select the recognized object. The total number of correct/incorrect responses is computed and converted into the scoring format from 10 to 0.

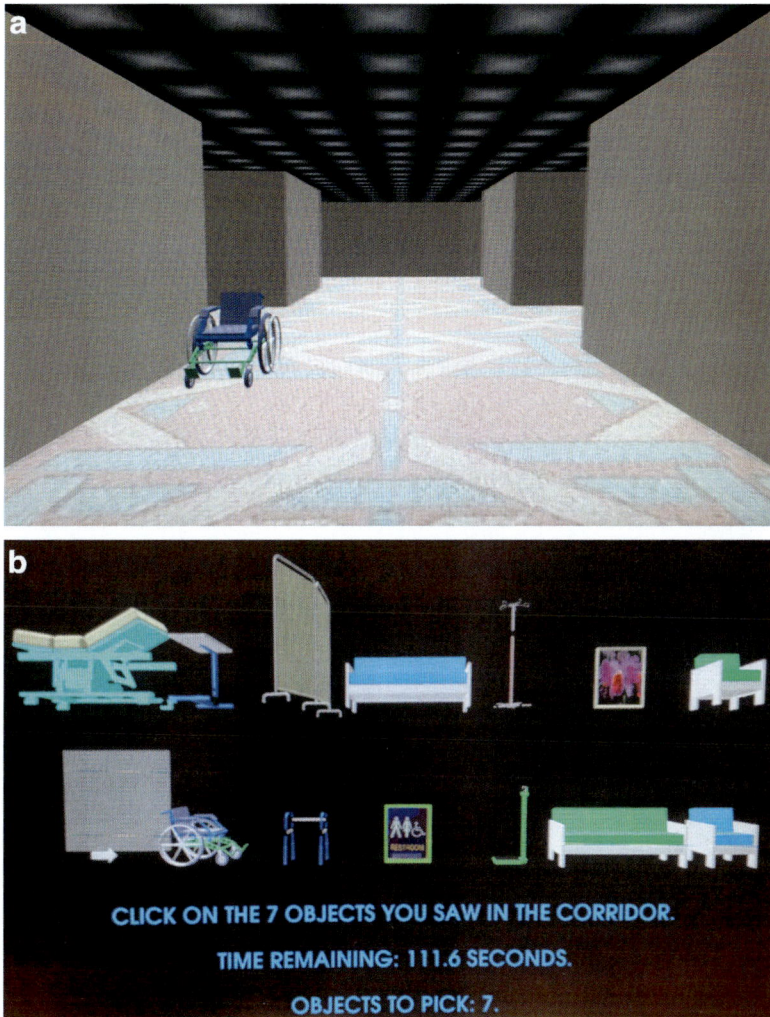

Fig. 4.2 (**a**) Different objects (total $n = 7$) are displayed to memorize while passively navigating via virtual corridor; (**b**) fourteen objects are displayed to recognize that were shown while navigating via virtual corridor

VR Assessment of Sustained Attention

Sohlberg and Matter in 1989 [45] proposed a clinical model of attention processes that outlined hierarchically organized levels of attention. Our personal experience in dealing with TBI patients on a daily basis is clearly in support of this clinical model of attention. Specifically, TBI patients, especially in acute stage of injury, most often are unable to sustain attention even for a short period of time. Their distractibility level increases significantly, affecting both everyday life and academic/learning activities.

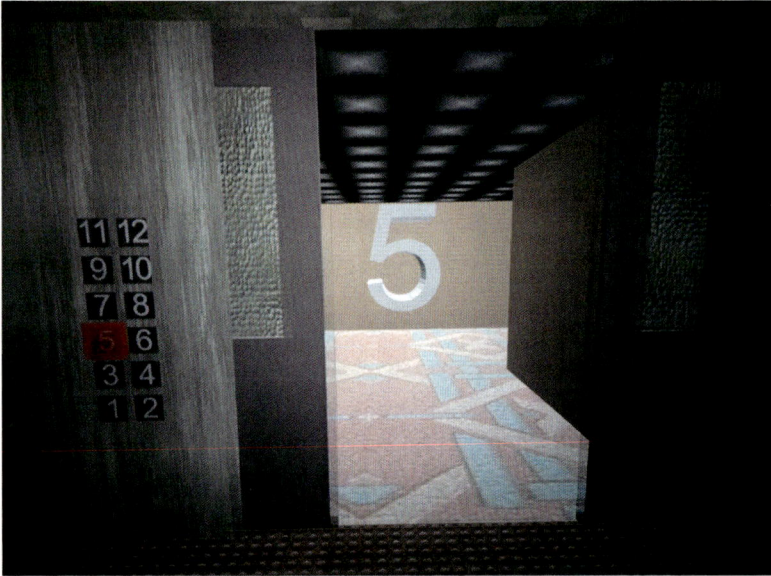

Fig. 4.3 The image of the Virtual Elevator module as perceived by the subject

The rate of recovery of this cognition function is influenced by numerous factors, such as the initial impact, degree of structural damage, and/or initial functional deficits, although not well documented in clinical research.

The attention deficit in TBI, specifically deficits in visual selective and sustained attention, is a prominent aspect of cognitive dysfunction after TBI. TBI patients frequently complain of distractibility and difficulty attending to more than one thing at a time. We designed the VR prototype of Everyday Attention [46] within the context of a *dual-task* paradigm to assess attention deficits in mild TBI. Our design of the VR attention module, *Virtual Elevator* (VE), was implemented by HeadRehab, LLC and is currently utilized in our laboratory for baseline and follow-up testing of concussed athletes (Fig. 4.3).

The VR advanced prototype of the Test of Everyday Attention (TEA) using the Virtual Elevator was implemented as the following:

- Sustained attention is being tested similar to the "Elevator Counting" test (1). The subjects are situated in the Virtual Elevator (VE) moving up (from floor 1 to floor 12) and down (from floor 12 to floor 1). There are visual separations that a subject should count in order to identify the *floor indicator* upon arrival (stop). There are numerous random trials that last for 10 min. The number of correct and incorrect counts assessed is used as an input to the comprehensive report.
- Elevator floor counting with distractions. Similar to (A) while additional sources of noise (external visual stimuli, i.e., adjacent buildings, windows, trees, people coming in and out, etc.) are being added.

- Dual-task version of VE is also elaborated to test the properties of "Divided Attention."

These data were used as an input for normalized reports of success rate ranges from 10 to 0 for each subject under study. It should be noted, we were able to detect attention deficits in concussed individuals in subacute phase of injury, although diagnosed as *asymptomatic* based upon conventional neurocognitive assessment tools, such as STROOP, SDMT, WMS-R Digit Span, Ruff 2 s and 7 s Selective Attention Test, and PASAT [44]. Current research is in progress to evaluate both convergent and discriminant validity of VR sustained attention module in the context of concussion evaluation that will be published elsewhere.

VR Assessment of Balance

Balance abnormalities specifically evident during visual-kinesthetic tasks are the most common symptoms in TBI patients suffering from sport-related concussions [18]. It should be noted that balance symptom resolution varies among mTBI patients and may last up to more than 1 year post-injury [10]. Our previous research has shown the presence of balance abnormalities and visual-kinesthetic disintegration, induced by VR visual field motion up to 30 days post-injury [29–31]. We have designed the VR moving room paradigm to examine postural stability via introducing the visual perturbation balance tasks [29]. The VR moving room appears to be an advanced tool allowing the detection of residual postural abnormalities as evidenced by impaired visual-kinesthetic integration [10].

The VR system that was used in this study includes: (a) VisMini portable stereo 3D projection system; (b) Draper Inc. 6 × 8 portable Cinefold surface screen; and (c) AMTI force plate for assessment of postural responses to visual field motion.

The field sequential stereo images were separated into right and left eye images using liquid crystal shutter glasses. An additional sensor was located on the subject's head to interact with the visual field motion. The visual field motion consists of a realistic looking moving room (see Fig. 4.4).

Preprogrammed manipulations of the VR moving room included the following: (1) viewing stationary VR room; (2) VR room forward–backward oscillatory translation within 18 cm displacement at 0.2 Hz; (3) VR room *Roll* around heading y-axis between 10 and 30° at 0.2 Hz; (4) VR room *Pitch* around interaural x-axis between 10 and 30° at 0.2 Hz; (5) VR room *Yaw* around vertical z-axis between 10 and 30° at 0.2Hz; and (6) VR room translation along x-axis within 18 cm displacement at 0.2 Hz. The subjects were instructed: (a) to acquire the Romberg stance and stand as still as possible on the force platform while viewing the computer-generated *moving room* visual scenes for 30 s trial duration (VR—balance 1 test); and (b) to produce whole body oscillations in synchrony with the motion of the VR room along x, y, and z axes (VR—balance 2 test).

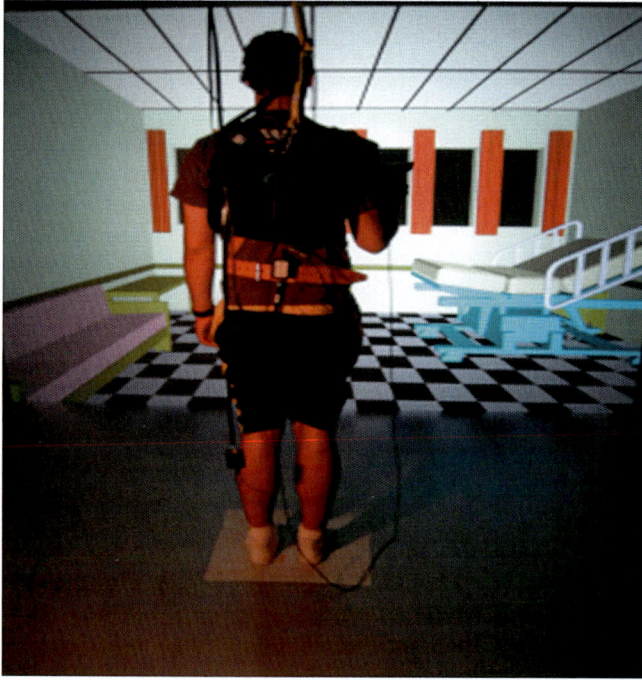

Fig. 4.4 AMTI force platform and 6° of freedoms ultrasound IS-900 micromotion tracking technology from "InterSense, Inc." was used to control the head and body kinematics and postural responses to visual manipulations of VR scenes

Normalized Assessment of Postural Stability

The area of the center of pressure (COP) was calculated from AMTI force platform data sampled at 100 Hz. A specially developed MATLAB program was used to estimate the subject response data obtained from the force platform similar to Slobounov et al. [36]. The COP area calculated from the data obtained for each individual subject (with respect to 450 records from normal age-matched volunteers) was used as an input for normalized reports of success rate (stable vs. unstable posture) ranges from 10 to 0 (loss of balance during the test).

Coherence values between quantities of moving room and subject responses were assessed using a specially developed MATLAB code. The auto-spectra for each signal were calculated by using Welsh's averaged periodogram method. Coherence was calculated based on the cross-spectra **fxy** and auto-spectra **fxx**, **fyy** with the spectra estimated from segments of data and the coherence **Rxy** estimated from the combined spectra:

$$\mathbf{Rxy}(\lambda)\,|\mathbf{2} = |\mathbf{fxy}(\lambda)|\,\mathbf{2}\,/\big(\mathbf{fxx}(\lambda)\,\mathbf{fyy}(\lambda)\big); \qquad (4.1)$$

The significance of coherence was also calculated. That is the confidence limit for zero coherence at the α %, and L, is the number of disjoint segments: sig $(\alpha) =$ $1-(1-\tilde{\alpha})1/(L-1)$. In addition, continuous wavelet transform (CWT) was performed to track the dynamics of coupling between subject body motion and visual scenes oscillation over the entire trial duration (30 s). The CWT is able to resolve both time and scale (frequency) events better than the short Fourier transform (STFT). In mathematics and signal processing, the CWT of a function f is defined by (1):

$$\gamma\left(\tau,s\right) = \int_{-\infty}^{+\infty} f\left(t\right) \frac{1}{\sqrt{|s|}} \overline{\psi\left(\frac{t-\tau}{s}\right)} \, \mathrm{d}t; \tag{4.2}$$

where τ represents translation, s represents scale which is related to frequency, and ψ is the mother wavelet. $\bar{z}$ is the complex conjugate of z. The mother wavelet is a complex Morlet wavelet, as it has both good time and frequency accuracy. The degree of coherence was converted to normalized score ranged from 10 (max dynamic balance) to 0 similar to Slobounov et al. [30, 36].

VR Assessment of Executive Function (Reaction Time)

Early and most recent research indicates that reaction time (RT), especially complex reaction time, significantly and reliably increased in mild TBI patients at least in acute phase of injury [13, 47–49]. Specifically, these finding have been replicated and confirmed in a number of studies [8, 50, 51]. Overall, it is widely accepted now that RT measures may serve as an index of the subject's integrity of executive functions, therefore may be used in clinical assessment of concussion [8, 13, 50] (Fig. 4.5).

We have designed a VR module of reaction time allowing the assessment of whole body response to unpredictable manipulation of optic flow. The subject was requested to oscillate forward and backward to follow the anterior–posterior (A–P) translation of the moving room at 0.2 Hz for 30 s trial duration.

Unpredictable change of moving room from A–P to medial–lateral (M–L) directions was randomized requiring the subject to respond via whole body motion and follow the motion of the moving room. The measured reaction time (ranged from 250 to 750 plus ms) and errors of anticipation (wrong direction of response) were calculated, interpolated, and converted into scoring system from 10 (best score, less than 250 ms compared to 450 samples from normal student-athletes volunteers) to 0 (more than 800 ms) and included in comprehensive reports. Current research is in progress to evaluate both convergent and discriminant validity of VR reaction time module with respect to RTclin and RTcomp derived from CogState-Sport [13] in the context of concussion evaluation that will be published elsewhere.

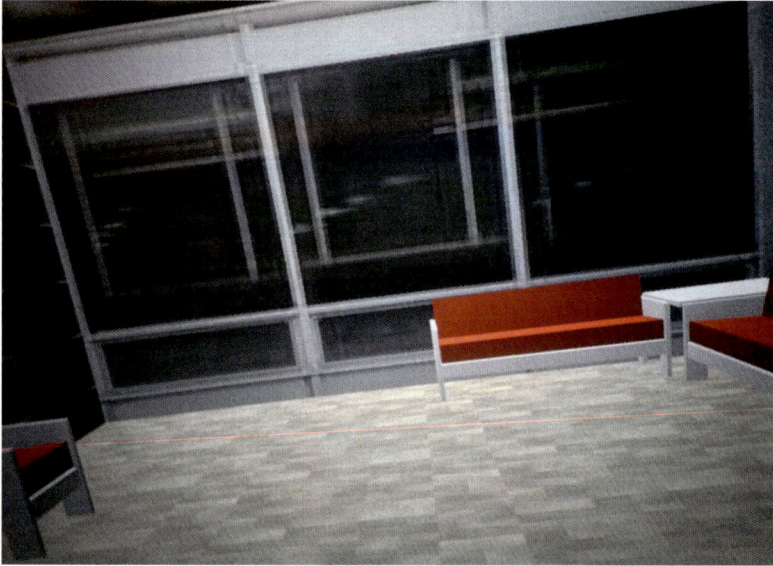

Fig. 4.5 Virtual room rolling to the left requiring subject to change direction of sway from AP to the left (ML) as fast as possible

Experimental Procedure: Effect of Practice

Subjects: Data were collected from 15 athletically active and neurologically normal undergraduate students recruited from the Pennsylvania State University. Average age was 21.4 years (SD = 1.3) and average estimated IQ, based upon Wechsler Test of Adult Reading (WTAR; The Psychological Corporation, 2001) test scores, was 108.9 (SD = 6.4). The sample was 70 % male and 30 % female. The reported racial/ethnic composition was 70 % Caucasian American, 10 % African American, 10 % Asian American, and 10 % mixed. Overall, subject percentages can be presented as 10 % multiples, given the usable sample consisted of 10 subjects. All participants had become involved in sports between ages 4 and 8 years old and had maintained their involvement, at either the recreational or collegiate level, as students at the university.

All participants were right-handed [52], and none were taking medications known to affect neurocognitive measurements. We ensured that participants were neurologically normal through a telephone screening questionnaire. Participants were excluded if they reported a prior history of (a) TBI, (b) learning disability or attention deficit hyperactivity disorder, (c) alcohol or drug abuse or dependence, (d) a neurological condition, or (e) a psychiatric disorder. Participants were also excluded if English was not their first language. All participants reported that they had slept 7–8 h the night before testing. Half of the subjects were tested between 10:00 am and noon, and the other half was tested between noon and 2:00 pm.

Subjects were requested to avoid taking any beverages containing caffeine at least 3 h prior to testing.

Procedures: Subjects were visiting our lab every other day for a total of three visits and performed sequence of (a) VR spatial memory navigation; (b) VR sustained attention; and (c) VR recognition, A and B; (d) VR balance tests; and (e) reaction time (RT). The order of testing modalities was randomized and necessary time between modalities was provided if needed to control for subjects' fatigue. The total time of testing was within 45 min.

Statistical analysis: Two-way within-subjects ANOVA was performed to assess the score differences between testing modalities ($n = 3$) as a function of testing day ($n = 3$). The threshold level of significance was set at $p < 0.05$.

Experimental Procedure: Effect of Fatigue Induced by Full Contact Football Practices

Subjects: Fifteen Penn State football players participated in this study. The subjects were males whose mean age was 20 ± 1.6 years. At the time of this study none of the subjects were injured and all were cleared for full contact sport participation by the team physician. Complete medical history of all players under study was available only to one of the authors (Dr. Sebastianelli). The other members of the research team did not have access to the subjects' medical records, thus were blind regarding the history of prior concussions until the completion of all results analysis.

VR assessment of spatial memory, balance, and executive functions (RT) was conducted prior to and within 30 min post-full contact practices. The number of blows during the practice was measured via reconstruction of impacts captured on video [53]. In addition, our research assistants registered the frequency and various types of impact experienced by the *targeted players* using a specially developed observation chart. The similar pre–post-full contact practice VR assessment was conducted 1 week later at the peak of preseason training load.

Results

Sense of Presence and Subjective Reports

All subject reports indicated that navigation via immersive VR environment induced a strong sense of presence. The scores for sense of presence for the spatial memory task were 6.8 ± 2.4, for the sustained attention task were 7.4 ± 1.7, and for the balance task were 9.2 ± 1.4. All subjects under study reported significant amounts of mental effort during the encoding phase of spatial memory task (8 ± 2) and during the retrieval phase (6 ± 2), that is consistent with our previous research [34, 54].

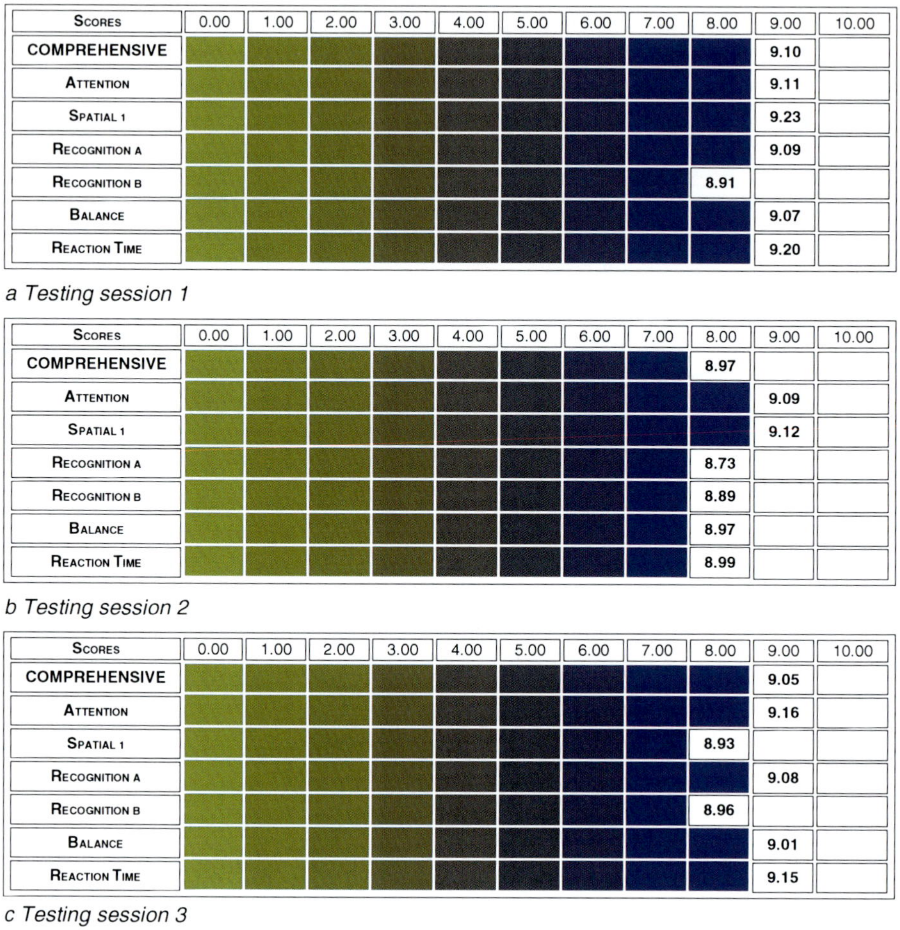

Scores	0.00	1.00	2.00	3.00	4.00	5.00	6.00	7.00	8.00	9.00	10.00
COMPREHENSIVE										9.10	
ATTENTION										9.11	
SPATIAL 1										9.23	
RECOGNITION A										9.09	
RECOGNITION B										8.91	
BALANCE										9.07	
REACTION TIME										9.20	

a Testing session 1

Scores	0.00	1.00	2.00	3.00	4.00	5.00	6.00	7.00	8.00	9.00	10.00
COMPREHENSIVE									8.97		
ATTENTION										9.09	
SPATIAL 1										9.12	
RECOGNITION A									8.73		
RECOGNITION B									8.89		
BALANCE									8.97		
REACTION TIME									8.99		

b Testing session 2

Scores	0.00	1.00	2.00	3.00	4.00	5.00	6.00	7.00	8.00	9.00	10.00
COMPREHENSIVE										9.05	
ATTENTION										9.16	
SPATIAL 1									8.93		
RECOGNITION A										9.08	
RECOGNITION B									8.96		
BALANCE										9.01	
REACTION TIME										9.15	

c Testing session 3

Fig. 4.6 Representative example from one subject on VR performance scores, including comprehensive, and those obtained from different testing modalities. Both visually and statistically there are no significant differences in performance scores as a function of testing day ($n = 3$)

Effect of Practice

Representative example of VR data obtained for three consequent testing sessions of one subject is shown in Fig. 4.6.

The overall VR results obtained from all 15 subjects on three testing sessions are shown in Fig. 4.7.

The ANOVA revealed neither main effect of testing day ($p > 0.05$) nor effect of VR testing modality ($p > 0.05$). In other words, no effect of practice was observed for either VR resting modalities.

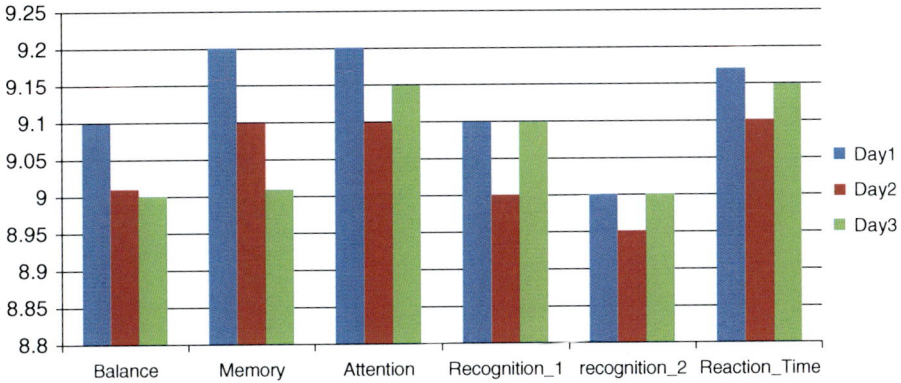

Fig. 4.7 Summary results of VR testing from all subjects under study ($n = 15$) as a function of testing day ($n = 3$). Both visually and statistically, no significant differences were observed within the testing modality and between tests indicating the lack of practice effect

Table 4.1 Subjects' performance on VR tests before and after full contact football practices inducing fatigue and the number of blows received

Players	Memory pre/post/post	Balance pre/post/post	RT pre/post/post	Impacts pr1/pr2
F001	8.3/8.7/8.4	8.6/9.1/8.8	9.4/9.1/8.3	46/38
F002	9.4/9.4/9.4	9.2/9.1/8.6	8.5/7.9/7.7	41/34
F003	7.5/7.9/8.1	9.3/9.0/9.1	8.6/8.9/8.0	37/42
F004	9.7/8.8/8.5	8.4/8.4/7.9	8.4/7.1/89	34/43
F005	6.9/8.3/8.1	7.4/7.9/6.8	8.5/7.2/8.3	36/38
F006	9.5/8.6/9.1	8.8/9.3/9.0	9.4/7.9/7.8	38/41
F007	8.1/8.6/5.4	9.3/7.8/5.6	7.7/5.5/4.2	37/43
F008	9.5/8.6/9.1	8.7/8.9/8.3	9.3/8.4/8.1	46/32
F009	8.4/8.9/9.3	8.3/8.1/7.6	7.9/8.1/8.3	41/39
F010	8.6/8.5/8/3	7.5/7.9/8.2	8.2/7.8/7.6	26/35
F011	8.6/8.5/5.3	7.8/5.6/5.1	9.2/8.8/4.9	29/35
F012	9.4/9.7/9.5	7.4/7.7/7.8	8.2/8.7/8.6	31/37
F013	7.4/6.7/5.2	8.6/8.1/6.1	9.5/6.7/4.2	34/31
F014	8.6/9.2/8.7	9.3/9.6/9/2	9.3/9.4/8.1	37/29
F015	9.3/9.6/9.0	7.8/8.5/8.1	8.4/7.8/8.4	35/41

The blow types included head-to-head, head-to-torso, blow to the back, blow to the torso, blow to the face, landing on the head, etc.

Effect of Fatigue

The results from effect of fatigue on VR assessment of memory, balance, and executive functions are summarized in Table 4.1. The subjects' fatigue was assessed via verbal responses that ranged from 0 (no fatigue) to 10 (extreme exhaustion). All subjects under study had reported fatigue scored $7 +/2.4$ after full contact practice.

As can be seen from Table 4.1, the fatigue did not influence the VR data for either of the testing dates obtained from 12 of the football players ($p > 0.05$). However, there was a negative effect of fatigue on three of the subjects, and upon further investigation it was found that of all of the 15 subjects tested they were the only ones to have a history of previously diagnosed concussions. It is important to note that players received approximately equal number of blows during both practices. The effect of multiple blows, in conjunction with fatigue, on performance measurement needs further investigation.

Discussion

There is a considerable debate in the literature regarding the best practices in treatment of athletes suffering from concussion. Up to date, there is still no "gold standard" and the absence of definite biomarkers for an accurate diagnosis or prognostication of sports-related concussions [55] continues. The lack of consent among clinical practitioners is also exacerbated even more by the fact that the majority of subjects with *uncomplicated mTBI* appeared to be *asymptomatic* based on anatomical MRI, CT, and/or conventional clinical and neuropsychological (NP) assessments shortly after the injury [56]. Therefore, the search for more accurate complementary concussion assessment tools is ongoing.

Here we tried to look at the effects of practice and fatigue on assessment of concussion and imply a VR-based assessment to see if it can overcome some of the downfalls of current clinical assessment tools. There are several major findings of interest that will be briefly discussed in the following text. *First*, VR induces a "sense of presence," an important feature of performance assessment tools that make it realistic and possibly transferrable to real-life situations. There are several reports indicating the differences in decision making processes and visual search behavior while performing visual-motor tasks in 2D vs. 3D sports-specific surrounding environment [57–59].

This research was grounded on previous empirical findings; for example, there are no differences in planned agility between expert and novice athletes, although a reactive agility test was able to discriminate skill between levels due to the inclusion of the sport-specific visual stimuli [60]. Indeed, human vision is 3D. Therefore, depth perception is critical for successful performance in various sports environments [61]. Most recent research has attempted to improve visual stimuli realism for examining visual-perceptual skill via 2D/3D video projections of *real-life* opponents to elicit reactive movement [62]. In our own research, we observed differential patterns of brain activation (fMRI BOLD) while performing the spatial navigation memory task in 2D vs. 3D virtual environment (unpublished study). Collectively, 3D realistic sports-specific virtual reality scenarios may enhance sensitivity of testing modalities used in a clinical setting. It is our ongoing line of research to examine the efficacy of 3D realistic sports-specific scenarios for assessment of performance indices in normal volunteers and student-athletes suffering the concussion.

Second, VR modules aimed to assess balance, neurocognitive, and executive functions appeared to be resilient to a *practice effect* and, thus, may be implemented in repeated fashion to track evolution of a measured function, for example, as result of recovery from brain injury. Clearly, every single existing NP (and/or other) tool currently used in a clinical practice may have a possible practice effect. Therefore, it should not be *overused* while evaluating the concussed individuals during follow-up testing [63]. The *practice effect* should be evaluated and considered while interpreting the evolution of repeated measures obtained during the follow-up testing. The reported findings regarding virtual reality testing modalities' resilience to practice effect may indicate the feasibility of VR modules for multiple uses in a clinical practice. That is being said, it is important to reiterate that the construct and discriminative validity as well as specificity of VR modules for assessment of concussion are yet to be determined.

Third, the VR modules implemented in this study appeared to be resilient to a *fatigue effect*, e.g., that may significantly confound evaluation of neurocognitive, balance, and executive functions as a sporting event is in progress. Clearly, comprehensive neuropsychological and behavioral evaluation of concussed individuals requires time and effort that may induce both physical and mental fatigue due to taking the tests [40]. Thus, dissociating fatigue symptoms due to concussion from those due to taking the tests is an important clinical issue. Moreover, it is also important to dissociate the athletes' performance level of neurocognitive, balance, and executive functions at different times during practices and/or games as a function of fatigue and/or concussion, if occurred. The resilience of VR modules to fatigue effect, but possible sensitivity to prior history of concussion, as reported in this study, may be considered as a valuable asset for side-line assessment of athletes in a clinical setting.

There are few limitations in this study. *First*, no objective measures of fatigue (e.g., biological and/or behavioral markers) were implemented in this study. *Second*, no clinically diagnosed acute concussed athletes participated in the *fatigue effect* study. The inclusion of clinically diagnosed concussed subjects in comparison with those with no history of concussion may contribute to understanding the sensitivity and discriminative values of the VR modalities. *Third*, for the noisy environment of a game's side-lines, VR applications in the present form may not be applicable unless noise protection procedures will be implemented.

Conclusion

These two separate experiments provide strong evidence that VR testing modalities upon clinical validation can be: (a) used repeatedly as testing measures since no evidence of *practice effect* was observed and documented; and (b) potentially used on the side-line of an athletic environment to estimate the neuropsychological, balance, and executive functions while ruling out the effect of possible *physical fatigues* as practice/game is in progress.

Acknowledgements This study was supported by NIH R01 grant: "Identification of Athletes at Risk for Traumatic Brain Injury." The authors would like to thank George Salvaterra, Katie Finelli, and Gregory Miskinis for their contribution to subjects' recruitment and data collection for this study.

References

1. Bazarian JJ, McClung J, Shan MN, Cheng YT, Flesher S, Schneider S. Emergency department management of mild traumatic brain injury. Acad Emerg Med. 2005;1(3):199–214.
2. Langlois JA, Rutland-Brown W, Wald MM. The epidemiology and impact of traumatic brain injury, a brief overview. J Head Trauma Rehabil. 2006;21:375–8.
3. Risdall JE, Menon DK. Traumatic brain injury. Philos Trans R Soc Lond B Biol Sci. 2011;366: 241–50.
4. Ruff RM. Mild traumatic brain injury and neural recovery: rethinking the debate. NeuroRehabilitation. 2011;28:167–80.
5. McCrory P, Meeuwisse W, Johnston K, Dvorak J, Aubry M, Molloy M, et al. Consensus statement on concussion in sport—the 3rd international conference on concussion in sport, held in Zurich, November 2008. J Clin Neurosci. 2009;16(6):755–63.
6. Makdissi M, Darby D, Maruff P, Ugoni A, Brukner P, McCrory PR. Natural history of concussion in sport: markers of severity and implication for management. Am J Sports Med. 2010;38(3):464–71.
7. Iverson GL, Brooks BL, Collins MW, Lovell MR. Tracking neuropsychological recovery following concussion in sport. Brain Inj. 2006;20:245–52.
8. Broglio SP, Ferrara MS, Macciocchi SN, Baumgartner TA, Elliott R. Test-retest reliability of computerized concussion assessment programs. J Athl Train. 2007;42(4):509–14.
9. Sedney CL, Orphanos J, Bailes JE. When to consider retiring an athlete after sports-related concussion. Clin Sports Med. 2011;30:189–200.
10. Slobounov S, Sebastianelli W, Hallett M. Residual brain dysfunction observed one year post-traumatic brain injury: combined EEG and balance study. Clin Neurophysiol. 2012;123(9): 1755–61.
11. Shenton ME, Hamoda HM, Schneiderman JS, Bouix S, Pasternak O, Rathi Y, et al. A review of magnetic resonance imaging and diffusion tensor imaging findings in mild traumatic brain injury. Brain Imaging Behav. 2012;6(2):108–37.
12. Guskiewicz KM, McCrea M, Marshall SW, Cantu RC, Randolph C, Barr W, et al. Cumulative effects associated with recurrent concussion in collegiate football players: the NCAA concussion study. JAMA. 2003;290:2604–5.
13. Eckner JT, Kutcher J, Richardson JK. Between-seasons test-retest reliability of clinically measured reaction time in national collegiate athletic association division I athletes. J Athl Train. 2011;46(4):409–14.
14. Lishman WA. Physiogenesis and psychogenesis in the post-concussional syndrome. Br J Psychiatry. 1988;153:460–9.
15. Ingelsoll CD, Armstrong CW. The effect of closed-head injury on postural sway. Med Sci Sports Exerc. 1992;24:739–43.
16. Wober C, Oder W, Kollegger H, Prayer L, Baumgartner C, Wober-Bingol C. Posturagraphic measurement of body sway in survivors of severe closed-head injury. Arch Phys Med Rehabil. 1993;74:1151–6.
17. Guskiewicz KM, Riemann BL, Perrin DH, Nashner LM. Alternative approaches to the assessment of mild head injury in athletes. Med Sci Sports Exerc. 1997;29(7):213–21.
18. Guskiewicz KM. Postural stability assessment following concussion: one piece of the puzzle. Clin J Sport Med. 2001;11:82–189.

19. Guskiewicz KM, Ross SE, Marshall SW. Postural stability and neuropsychological deficits after concussion in collegiate athletes. J Athl Train. 2001;36(3):263–73.
20. Guskiewicz K, Mihalik J. The biomechanics and pathomechanics of sport-related concussion: looking at history to build the future. In: Slobounov S, Sebastianelli W, editors. Foundations of sport-related brain injuries. NY. pp: Springer; 2006. p. 65–84.
21. Rieman B, Guskiewicz K. Effect of mild head injury on postural stability as measured through clinical balance testing. J Athl Train. 2002;35:19–25.
22. Peterson C, Ferrara M, Mrazik M, Piland S, Elliott R. Evaluation of neuropsychological domain scores and postural stability following cerebral concussion in sport. Clin J Sport Med. 2003;13(4):230–7.
23. Valovich T, Periin D, Gansneder B. Repeat administration elicits a practice effect with the balance error scoring system but not with the standardized assessment of concussion in high school athletes. J Athl Train. 2003;38(10):51–6.
24. Cavanaugh J, Guskiewicz K, Stergiou N. A nonlinear dynamic approach for evaluating postural control: new directions for the management of sport-related cerebral concussion. Sports Med. 2005;35(11):935–50.
25. Cavanaugh J, Guskiewicz K, Giuliani C, Marshall S, Mercer V, Stergiou N. Detecting altered postural control after cerebral concussion in athletes with normal postural stability. Br J Sports Med. 2005;39(11):805–11.
26. Cavanaugh JT, Guskiewicz KM, Giuliani C, Marshall S, Merser VS, Stergion N. Recovery of postural control after cerebral concussion: new insights using approximate entropy. J Athl Train. 2006;41(3):305–13.
27. Slobounov SM, Cao C, Sebastianelli W, Slobounov E, Newell K. Residual deficits from concussion as revealed by virtual time-to-contract measures of postural stability. Clin Neurophysiol. 2008;119:281–9.
28. Slobounov S, Sebastianelli W, Simon R. Neurophysiological and behavioral concomitants of mild brain injury in collegiate athletes. Clin Neurophysiol. 2002;113:185–93.
29. Slobounov S, Newell K, Slobounov E. Application of virtual reality graphics in assessment of concussion. Cyberpsychol Behav. 2006;9(2):188–91.
30. Slobounov S, Sebastianelli W, Tutwiler R, Slobounov E. Alteration of postural responses to visual field motion in mild traumatic brain injury. J Neurosurg. 2006;59(1):134–9.
31. Slobounov S, Sebastianelli W, Cao C, Slobounov E, Newell K. Differential rate of recovery in athletes after first versus and second concussion episodes. J Neurosurg. 2007;61(2):238–44.
32. Slobounov S, Sebastianelli W, Moss R. Alteration of posture-related cortical potentials in mild traumatic brain injury. Neurosci Lett. 2005;383:251–5.
33. Slobounov S, Cao C, Sebastianelli W. Differential effect of first versus second concussive episodes on wavelet information quality of EEG. Clin Neurophysiol. 2009;120:862–7.
34. Slobounov S, Zhang K, Pennell D, Ray W, Sebastianelli W. Functional abnormalities in asymptomatic concussed individuals: fMRI study. Exp Brain Res. 2010;202(2):341–54.
35. Slobounov S, Johnson B, Zhang K, Hallett M, Horovitz S, Sebastianelli W, et al. Alteration of brain functional network at rest and in response to YMCA physical stress test in concussed athletes: RsFMRI study. Neuroimage. 2011;55(4):1716–27.
36. Slobounov S, Sebastianelli W, Newell K. Incorporating virtual reality graphics with brain imaging for assessment of sport-related concussions. IEEE Engineering in Medicine and Biology Society. 33rd Annual International Conference, Boston, http://embc2011.embcs.org, 2011.
37. Slobounov S, Gay M, Johnson B, Zhang K. Concussion in athletes: ongoing clinical and brain imaging research controversies. Brain Imaging Behav. 2012;6(2):224–42.
38. Bartels C, Wegrzyn M, Wiedl A, Aukermann BV, Ehrenreich H. Practice effects in healthy adults: a longitudinal study on frequent repetitive cognitive testing. BMC Neurosci. 2010;11:118.
39. Schmidt JD, Register-Mihalik JK, Mihalik JP, Kerr ZY, Guskiewicz K. Identifying impairment after concussion: normative data versus individualized baselines. Med Sci Sports Exerc. 2012;44(9):1621–8.
40. Barwick F, Arnett P, Slobounov S. EEG correlates of fatigue during administering of a neuropsychological test battery. Clin Neurophysiol. 2011;123:278–84.

41. Jancke L, Cheetham M, Baumgartner T. Virtual reality on the role or prefrontal cortex in adults and children. Front Neurosci. 2009;3(1):52–9.
42. Wirth W, Hartmann T, Boecking S, Vorderer P, Klimmt C, Schramm H, et al. A process model of the formation of spatial presence experience. Media Psychol. 2007;9:493–525.
43. Witmer BG, Singer MJ. Measuring presence in virtual environments: a presence questionnaire. Presence Teleop Virtual Environ. 1998;7:225–40.
44. Gloyer K, Aukerman D, Sebastianelli W, Slobounov S. Application of virtual reality for assessment of concussion in sports. American Medical Society for Sports Medicine, AMSSM, 20th Annual Meeting, Salt Lake City, UT, 2011.
45. Sohlberg S, Mateer CA. Training use of compensatory memory books: a three stage behavioral approach. J Clin Exp Neuropsychol. 1989;11(6):871–91.
46. Andrew J, Bate JL, Mathias R, Crawford R. Performance on the test of everyday attention and standard tests of attention following severe traumatic brain Injury. Clin Neuropsychol. 2001;15(3):405–22.
47. MacFlynn G, Montgomery EA, Fenton DW, Rutherford W. Measurement of reaction time following minor head injury. J Neurol Neurosurg Psychiatry. 1984;47:1326–31.
48. Stuss DT, Stethem LL, Hugenholtz H, Picton T, Pivik J, Richard MT. Reaction time after head injury: fatigue, divided and focused attention, and consistency of performance reaction. J Neurol Neurosurg Psychiatry. 1989;52:742–8.
49. Warden DL, Bleiberg J, Cameron KL, Ecklund J, Walter J, Sparling MB, et al. Persistent prolongation of simple reaction time in sports concussion. Neurology. 2001;57(3):524–6.
50. Iverson GL, Lovell MR, Collins MW. Validity of ImPACT for measuring processing speed following sports-related concussion. J Clin Exp Neuropsychol. 2005;27(6):683–9.
51. Schatz P. Long-term test-retest reliability of baseline cognitive assessments using ImPACT. Am J Sports Med. 2010;38(1):47–53.
52. Chapman LJ, Chapman JP. The measurement of handedness. Brain Cogn. 1987;6:175–83.
53. Pellman EJ, Viano DC, Tucker AM, Casson IR, Waeckerle JE. Concussion in professional football: reconstruction of game impact and injuries. Neurosurgery. 2003;35:799–814.
54. Jaiswal N, Ray W, Slobounov S. Encoding required more cerebral resources than retrieval: combined EEG and virtual reality study. Brain Res. 2011;1347:80–9.
55. Bigler E, Bazarian J. Diffusion tensor imaging: a biomarker for mild traumatic brain injury? Neurology. 2010;74(8):626–7.
56. Bigler E, Maxwell W. Neuropathology of mild traumatic brain injury: relationship to neuroimaging findings. Brain Imaging Behav. 2012;6:108–36.
57. Vaeyens R, Lenoir M, Williams AM, Mazyn L, Philippaerts RM. The effects of task constraints on visual search behavior and decision-making skill in youth soccer players. J Sport Exerc Psychol. 2007;29(2):147–69.
58. Cochrane JL, Lloyd DG, Besier TF, Elliott BC, Doyle TLA, Ackland TR. Training affects knee kinematics and kinetics in cutting maneuvers in sport. Med Sci Sports Exerc. 2010;42(8):1535–44.
59. Lee MJ, Bourke P, Alderson JA, Lloyd DG, Lay B. Stereoscopic filming for investigating evasive sidestepping and anterior cruciate ligament injury risk. In: Stereoscopic Displays and Applications XXI. Paper presented at the SPIEIS & Electronic Imaging, 2010.
60. Farrow D, Young W, Bruce L. The development of a test of reactive agility for netball: a new methodology. J Sci Med Sport. 2005;8(1):52–60.
61. Vickers JN. Perception, cognition and decision training: the quiet eye in action. Champaign: Human Kinetics; 2007.
62. Lee MJC, Tidman S, Lay B, Bourke P, Lloyd D, Anderson J. Visual search differs but not reaction time when intercepting a 3D versus 2D videoed opponent. J Mot Behav. 2013;45(2):107–15.
63. Lovell M. Neuropsychological management of sport-related concussion. 2nd Penn State conference: Concussion in athletics: from brain to behavior, Oct 11–12, 2012.

Chapter 5
Feasibility of Electroencephalography for Direct Assessment of Concussion

William J. Ray, Elizabeth F. Teel, Michael R. Gay, and Semyon M. Slobounov

Abstract In this chapter, we will focus on sport-related concussions as studied through the use of electroencephalography. It should be noted that in this chapter the terms concussion and mild traumatic brain injury are used interchangeably.

Keywords Concussion • EEG • Power analysis • Coherence

W.J. Ray, Ph.D.
Penn State Center for Sports Concussion Research and Services,
Pennsylvania State University, University Park, PA 16802, USA

Department of Psychology, Pennsylvania State University,
University Park, PA 16802, USA
e-mail: wjr@psu.edu

E.F. Teel, M.S.
Department of Kinesiology, Pennsylvania State University,
University Park, PA 16802, USA
e-mail: eteel@live.unc.edu

M.R. Gay, Ph.D., A.T.C.
Pennsylvania State Intercollegiate Athletics, Pennsylvania State University,
University Park, PA 16802, USA
e-mail: mrg201@psu.edu

S.M. Slobounov, Ph.D. (✉)
Professor of Kinesiology & Neurosurgery, Director of Center for Sports Concussion Research and Services, Penn State - Department of Kinesiology & Hershey Medical College,
University Park, PA, USA
e-mail: sms18@psu.edu

S.M. Slobounov and W.J. Sebastianelli (eds.), *Concussions in Athletics:*
From Brain to Behavior, DOI 10.1007/978-1-4939-0295-8_5,
© Springer Science+Business Media New York 2014

Introduction

Worldwide, concussion is a critical public health problem that can lead to a variety of neurocognitive and psychological problems [1]. These problems can include loss of consciousness, cognitive deficits, depression, and, at a later period, the onset of dementia [2]. Concussion has been referred to as a "silent epidemic" and it is currently estimated that 1.6–3.8 million concussions occur each year in the United States, which may still be an underestimate [2]. Concussions can result from any event that causes the brain to make an impact with the skull. The most common examples are automobile accidents and contact sports.

Recent media presentations and scientific research have emphasized the role of concussion in athletics. The National Football League has supported studies of the long-term effects of concussion in professional athletes. Many universities have established centers for the study of concussion and several states have established laws related to concussion assessment and management in high school athletics as well as return to play guidelines. High school athletes are particularly at risk since surveys suggest that this group believes that there is not a problem playing sports with a concussion. Returning to sport before the concussion has been fully resolved can increase long-term injuries. Since adolescence is a time in which an individual's brain goes through a series of cortical reorganizations, brain insults at this time put the adolescent at greater risk for serious injury. For college and professional athletes, different pressures may cause players to ignore information concerning the effects of concussion. Overall, this can lead to a lack of candor when athletes at all levels describe their symptoms. Thus, it is critical to utilize measures that evaluate the effects of concussion beyond the traditional signs and symptoms seen with the disorder.

Acceleration/deceleration forces commonly lead to concussive injuries, which often produce diffuse microstructural injury. Due to the diffuse nature of these injuries, standard structural imaging, such as MRI and CT, may not be able to identify all abnormalities [3]. Instead of the gross structural damage or lesions found in penetrating head injury or severe traumatic brain injuries (TBIs), concussive episodes are characterized by their cognitive dysfunction, specifically in information processing and working memory [3].

Need for Physiologic Measurement in Clinical Concussion Diagnosis/Management

Athletic participation is unique in its requirement of the able bodied participant. Physicians and allied health professionals making recommendations for athletes returning to sport from concussion or mild traumatic brain injury (mTBI) must ultimately be comfortable with the concept of repeated injury. In other words, clinicians must ensure that an athlete recovering from concussion to full athletic participation be as resilient to head trauma as a non-head-injured healthy athlete. Ultimately, clinicians must be assured that the athletes' risk of short-term or long-term effects from their concussive episode has been minimized as best as possible.

With these important clinical considerations in mind, management of sports-related concussion or mTBI must evolve beyond the limitations in the currently accepted definition of concussion describing *functional* recovery from concussion being representative of clinical healing. Considering the number of mTBI-linked short-term and long-term physical and mental health issues [4–7], clinicians and researchers alike must take important steps to ensure proper management of the athlete recovering from mTBI. Intense scrutiny of residual physiological and functional deficits as well as measuring and monitoring the athlete's rate of pathophysiological recovery from concussive injuries must become our primary focus. By increasing our collective efforts we can look to reduce significant short- and long-term health issues. Yet despite this need, clinical management of the mild head-injured athlete has not changed in decades.

One of the reasons that clinical management of concussion has remained largely unchanged is due partly to a disproportionate focus on functional cognitive testing. Neuropsychological testing remains the mainstay in determining the clinical recovery for the concussed athlete. As neuropsychological testing is limited to cognitive functional performance, it has seemingly maximized its clinical utility at present. Therefore, clinical researchers need to push the constructs of other applicable and relevant diagnostic tools to provide athletes recovering from sports-related concussion with better assessment and management tools. These tools must be able to distinguish residual functional *and* structural (physiological) recovery from mTBI. As both diffuse functional and structural injuries are present in mTBI [8, 9] clinicians and researchers must develop and research both functional and structural diagnostic tools when treating the athlete recovering from concussion. Due to the diffuse nature of the injury and the consequential cognitive dysfunction, electroencephalographies (EEGs), which are able to systematically evaluate the underlying neural process that contributes to functional networks, are a sensitive and appropriate tool to evaluate the effects of concussive episodes.

Several organizations include the presence of pathophysiology in their definitions of concussion. Thus, it seems appropriate to utilize a physiological measure to denote the presence of concussion. One such measure capable of this is EEG. The EEG was first demonstrated in humans by Hans Berger in 1924 and published 5 years later [10]. Since the neurons of the brain and their connections are constantly active, EEG can be measured in an individual both during conscious and unconscious states as seen in sleep and brain trauma. As such, EEG was the first brain assessment tool that was able to establish an alteration in brain function in a TBI population [11–13] and has continued to be useful in the brain injury field.

Early EEG research with 300 patients clearly demonstrated the slowing of major frequency bands and focal abnormalities within 48 h post-injury [14]. A study by McClelland et al. has shown that EEG recordings performed during the immediate post-concussion period demonstrated a large amount of "diffusely distributed slow-wave potentials," which were markedly reduced when recordings were performed 6 weeks after injury [15]. Additionally, Tebano et al. showed a shift in the mean frequency in the alpha (8–10 Hz) band toward lower power and an overall decrease of beta (14–18 Hz) power in patients suffering from mTBI [16]. The reduction of theta power [17] accompanying a transient increase of alpha–theta ratios [18, 19] was identified as residual symptoms in mTBI patients.

At the beginning of the twenty-first century, Gaetz and Bernstein [3] cited electrophysiological techniques as the most commonly used method to evaluate brain functioning, noting the relatively low cost, noninvasive nature of the test, and the long, well-documented history dating back to the 1930s. Leon-Carrion et al. [20] echo the benefits defined by Gaetz and Bernstein and also speak to the uncomplicated procedure, high test–retest reliability, and characteristic stability of EEG as additional features that contribute to its appropriateness as a diagnostic testing tool.

The Nature of EEG

EEG reflects the electrical activity of the brain at the level of the synapse [21]. It is the product of changing excitatory and inhibitory currents. More specifically, graded postsynaptic potentials of the cell body and dendrites of vertically orientated pyramidal cells in cortical layers three to five give rise to the EEG recorded on the scalp. The ability to record the relatively small voltage at the scalp from these actions results from the fact that pyramidal cells tend to share a similar orientation and polarity and may be synchronously activated. Action potentials contribute very little to the EEG. However, since changes at the synapse do influence the production of action potentials, there is an association of EEG with spike trains [22]. The summation of these electrophysiological measures is precisely what makes EEGs better suited for the study of mTBI compared to several other types of brain imaging techniques.

Historically, the system of locating electrodes in EEG is referred to as the International 10–20 system [23]. The name 10–20 refers to the fact that electrodes in this system are placed at sites 10 and 20 % from four anatomical landmarks. One landmark is the front of the nasion (the bridge of the nose). In the rear of the head, the inion (the bump at the back of the head just above the neck) is used. The left and right landmarks are the preauricular points (depressions in front of the ears above the cheekbone). In this system, the letters refer to areas of the brain; O = occipital, P = parietal, C = central, F = frontal, and T = temporal. Numerical subscripts indicate laterality (odd numbers left, even right) and degree of displacement from the midline (subscripted z). Thus, C3 describes an electrode over the central region of the brain on the left side whereas Cz would refer to an electrode placed at the top of the scalp above the central area. With the development of dense array systems, the historical 10–20 system has been greatly expanded.

To record the EEG, electrical signals of only a few microvolts must be detected on the scalp. A signal can be found by amplifying the differential between two electrodes, at least one of which is placed on the scalp. Since the signal must be amplified almost one million times, care must be taken that the resulting signal is indeed actual EEG and not artifact. Where the electrodes are placed and how many are used depend on the purpose of the recording. Almost all EEG procedures currently use a variety of EEG caps with up to 256 electrodes built into the cap, although it is always possible to record EEG from only two electrodes.

Table 5.1 Frequency ranges for each given bandwidth

Bandwidth name	Frequency (Hz)
Delta	0–4
Theta	4–8
Alpha	8–13
Beta1	13–24
Beta2	24–32
Gamma	32–60

Those recording caps that use 128–256 electrodes are generally referred to as dense array EEG recordings and are used in most research settings. However, research in clinical situations, such as the hospital emergency room, has shown that as few as five electrodes can be used for the screening of mTBIs [24]. In this study, EEG showed a 94.7 % accuracy rate when compared with computed tomography for detecting mTBIs. This underlines the potential of using even simple EEG montages for detecting concussions in a sports setting.

EEG Frequency Bands

One important parameter of EEG is a determination of frequency. Although there are some minor discrepancies in the literature in terms of the beginning and ending of specific frequency band, a general template is presented in Table 5.1. Frequency bands are generally determined through signal processing technique such as Fourier analysis and wavelet analysis.

Alpha activity can be seen in about three-fourths of all individuals when they are awake and relaxed. Asking these individuals to further relax and close their eyes will result in recurring periods of several seconds in which the EEG consists of relatively large, rhythmic waves of about 8–12 Hz. This is the *alpha rhythm*, the presence of which has been related to relaxation and the lack of active cognitive processes. If someone who displays alpha activity is asked to perform cognitive activity such as solving an arithmetic problem in his or her head, alpha activity will no longer be present in the EEG. This is referred to as alpha blocking. Typically, cognitive activity causes the alpha rhythm to be replaced by high frequency, low amplitude EEG activity referred to as beta activity. Since the discovery of the alpha rhythm, a variety of studies have focused on its relationship to psychological processes and broad developments of the cognitive and affective neurosciences amplified this interest (see [25, 26] for reviews).

High frequency activity occurs when one is alert. Traditionally, lower-voltage variations ranging from about 18 to 30 Hz have been referred to as beta and higher frequency lower-voltage variations ranging from about 30 to 70 Hz or higher are referred to as gamma. Initial work suggests that gamma activity is related to the brain's ability to integrate a variety of stimuli into a coherent whole.

For example, Catherine Tallon-Baudry and her colleagues [27] showed individuals pictures of a hidden Dalmatian dog that was difficult to see because of the black and white background. After training individuals to see the dog, differences in the gamma band suggested meaningful and non-meaningful stimuli produced differential responses.

Additional patterns of spontaneous EEG activity include delta activity (0.5–4 Hz), theta activity (5–7 Hz), and lambda and K-complex waves and sleep spindles, which are not defined solely in terms of frequency. Theta activity refers to EEG activity in the 4–8 Hz range. Grey Walter [28], who introduced the term theta rhythm, suggested that theta was seen at the cessation of a pleasurable activity. More recent research associated theta with such processes as hypnagogic imagery, REM (rapid eye movement) sleep, problem solving, attention, and hypnosis. Source analysis of midline theta suggests that the anterior cingulate is involved in its generation [29]. In an early review of theta activity, Schacter [30] suggested that there are actually two different types of theta activity: First, there is theta activity associated with low levels of alertness as would be seen as one falls asleep. Secondly, there is theta activity associated with attention and active and efficient processing of cognitive and perceptual tasks. This is consistent with the suggestion of Vogel et al. [31] that there are two types of behavioral inhibition, one associated with a gross inactivation of an entire excitatory process resulting in less active behavioral states and one associated with selective inactivity as seen in overlearned processes.

Delta activity is low frequency (0.5–4 Hz) and has been traditionally associated with sleep in healthy humans as well as pathological conditions including cerebral infarct, contusion, local infection, tumor, epileptic foci, and subdural hematoma. The idea is that these types of disorders influence the neural tissue that in turn creates abnormal neural activity in the delta range by cutting off these tissues from major input sources. Although these observations were first seen with intracranial electrodes, more recent work has found similar result using MEG and EEG techniques. Additionally, EEG delta activity is the predominant frequency of human infants during the first 2 years of life.

EEG and Concussion

While conventional EEGs are not part of the current clinical "gold-standard" assessment battery, a number of studies show EEG differences in those individuals suffering from mTBI compared to healthy controls (see [32] for an overview). Of the differences observed on conventional EEGs, the most common abnormalities seen are generalized or focal slowing as well as weakened posterior alpha in mTBI patients [14, 33, 34]. These deficits were found in the immediate post-injury period (within a few hours of a concussive episode); however, similar findings have been reported even when there is a longer period between injury occurrence and injury evaluation.

These common abnormalities seen on conventional EEG recordings usually resolve within the first few months post-injury [35], similar to the resolution of functional and symptomatic deficits in typical concussive recovery. However, up to 10 % of individuals diagnosed with mTBI still show atypical electrophysiological readings in the late post-injury period [35, 36]. This small but significant portion of individuals who show electrophysiological abnormalities in the late post-injury period parallels those individuals who have atypical resolution of concussive symptoms and functioning.

Traditionally, in clinical settings, conventional EEGs were interpreted by the visual inspection of raw EEG signals. However, studies show that visual inspection of EEG lacks the sensitivity to detect changes following mTBI. With the advancement of computerized signal processing techniques, there is a growing body of literature that suggests more complex EEG paradigms may be used to assess changes in functional status after concussive injuries [3]. Compared to visually inspected EEGs, computerized EEG analyses are advantageous because they can detect subtle differences in signal patterns and shifts not visible to the naked eye [8]. Due to these benefits, Cannon et al. [37] indicated that the usefulness of EEG as an assessment tool for brain injury is due to its "direct signature of neural activity" and "ideal temporal resolution."

Several different types of variables can be isolated using quantitative EEG methods. Spectral analysis, relative amplitude and power in a particular frequency bandwidth, coherence, and phase are the most common types of analyses performed in EEGs. In terms of TBI, frequency and coherence analyses of particular cortical areas can offer important information [3, 8, 38]. By examining the pattern of activity between the cortical areas, it is also possible to delineate brain networks, see how they are involved in different types of tasks, and determine how they differ under certain conditions such as the presence of a concussion.

Coherence analysis describes how the EEG signal at each of two electrodes is related to one another. In simple terms, coherence reflects the manner in which two signals "covary" at a particular frequency. In specific, coherence measurements represent the correlation of signal phase stability between two different electrodes. Coherence measures within the same frequency band offer an estimate of the temporal relationships between adjacent neural systems. Like correlation, coherence is a measure between 0 and 1, where 1 represents a perfect phase correlation between two groups and 0 represents no correlation. Thus, in performing the coherence analysis, one can also obtain a measure of phase or synchrony.

The particular interest in EEG coherence is due to the biological nature of concussive injury. The brain structures involved in neural connectivity, such as the reticular system activation and thalamocortical tracts, are the structures most likely to be affected by mTBI. Considering the probability that these areas are altered following concussion, frequency and coherence analyses are likely to be the most sensitive electrophysiological measures to indicate deficits due to concussive injury.

According to Arciniegas [8], frequency measures can vary with the number of neurons (smaller number, smaller amplitude/power), the integrity of the thalamocortical circuits in which the neurons contribute (injury to the circuit causes slower frequencies), and the influence of activation from the reticular system (increases in reticular system activity cause higher frequencies, while decreases in reticular system activity cause lower frequencies).

Coherence, which by definition correlates the frequency measures between two different electrodes, may indicate the level of communication between different areas of the brain and signify neural network connectivity and dynamics [8]. Reduced coherence values can be attributed to damage in myelinated fibers and/or gray matter [38]. If lowered coherence values are seen in mTBI patients, it is still unknown which of these factors, or if a combination of all of them, produce these results.

Each concussive episode is individualized and may produce different changes in the brain. In turn, one might expect that the respective EEG measures would be different in each mTBI patient. While the electrophysiological deficits found for each concussive episode remain unique, several consistent EEG patterns have been identified. According to a review by Arciniegas [8], the most common EEG findings in mTBI include: (1) a decrease in mean alpha frequency [16, 19, 39–42], increase in theta activity [15, 17, 43, 44], or increased alpha–theta ratio [18, 19, 39, 42] and (2) lessened alpha and beta power between anterior and posterior regions, weakened alpha power (posterior region), and increased coherence between frontal and temporal regions [45–47].

Along with these findings, a literature review by Nuwer et al. [34] listed other common EEG findings after concussive episodes. These findings concluded that changes in EEG measures resolved along the same timeline as symptoms, with gradual changes mainly occurring over weeks to months. The researchers also found that left temporal slowing may correspond to lingering cognitive symptoms. In all the studies evaluated by Nuwer, coherence was not correlated to outcome or diffuse axonal injury. Due to how quickly EEG patterns can change in an mTBI population [8], it is critically important that research involving individuals being tested after a concussive injury are evaluated in as similar time points as possible.

Evidence provided by Thornton [48] and Thatcher et al. [49] indicates that the EEG patterns seen in a concussed athlete do not quickly change over time and, therefore, should be present at the initial time of injury. While this is useful in describing EEG as a possible tool in diagnosing and evaluating concussed individuals, it also indicates that concussive episodes, even "mild" or "typical" episodes, cause long lasting alterations in brain electrophysiology. Work by Barr et al. [50] showed that despite improvement or normal levels of cognitive functioning, brain patterns remain altered in mTBI patients. This further suggests that the brain may not completely heal from concussive episodes; instead the individual learns to compensate for the deficit in order to achieve normal performance. The idea of compensation instead of recovery has been examined in a study by Thornton [51] and discussed in a book chapter [38].

Two prominent studies have examined the reproducibility of EEG absolute measures. First, a study by Corsi-Cabrera et al. [52] tested nine subjects 11 times over a 1-month period. When looking at absolute amplitude, the median correlation coefficient over the 11 sessions was 0.94. Alpha and beta bands showed greater variability than any of the other bands. Pollock et al. [53] evaluated test–retest reliability in each bandwidth over a 20-week period on 46 normal controls.

Absolute amplitude in theta, alpha, and beta1 had correlation coefficients that exceeded 0.60. Beta2 and delta correlation coefficients were found to be lower, with delta showing the poorest correlation. The authors also found that absolute amplitude has higher correlation coefficients than relative power and is, therefore, recommended for use in future studies. The high levels of correlation found in these studies, combined with the varying intervals between testing sessions (a common feature in concussion testing), imply that absolute amplitude is an appropriate measure for research purposes.

Although related to amplitude, several studies have separately analyzed the reproducibility of power. Salinsky et al. [54] tested absolute and relative power and found correlation coefficients of 0.84. Tests were run between 12 and 16 weeks apart on 25 normal controls. Cannon et al. [37] examined test–retest EEG power reliability by examining 19 normative controls over a 30-day testing period. Each participant was recorded for a 4-min interval under an eyes open and eyes closed condition. Intraclass correlation coefficients (ICCs) for absolute power were 0.90 for eyes closed data and 0.77 for eyes open data. The results of these studies closely mimic those found when evaluating amplitude, with power having sufficiently high levels of reliability over both short (days) and long (months) testing periods.

Mathematically distinct from amplitude and power, researchers have spent time considering the reproducibility of coherence values. Studies by Harmony et al. [55] and Nikulin and Brismar [56] evaluated the reproducibility of coherence during rest and cognitive tasks in individuals. Both studies found good correlations within a given task or under resting state conditions but Harmony et al. reported much lower correlation values between sessions, even within the same subject during the same condition.

While these early tests show low levels of reproducibility, even within testing sessions, more recent research has provided vastly different results. The Cannon et al. [37] study mentioned earlier also examined coherence over a 30-day testing period. For eyes closed coherence measures, ICCs for delta, theta, alpha, and beta bandwidths were all greater than 0.90. For the eyes open condition, coherence in all bandwidths had ICCs above 0.85. This indicates "good" to "very good" reproducibility for all EEG variables examined and deems coherence as a reliable enough measure to use in both a research and clinical setting.

In all of the studies presented, roughly half of the variance seen in all EEG variables was reproducible within the given subject. These measures have all been determined to have a sufficient level of reproducibility to use in future research. However, it should be noted that these results do not necessarily indicate that EEG can currently be considered a reliable diagnostic tool and differentiate between concussed and healthy individuals.

Although there are many benefits to using EEGs in concussion research and a wealth of knowledge has been gained, the use of EEG in this type of research is not without its criticisms and limitations. Nuwer et al. [34] have questioned the use of EEG in concussion research, citing the lack of clear EEG features that are specifically unique to mTBI patients, especially late after injury. While there is merit to a lack of unique abnormalities, several studies [57, 58] have found deficits in concussed participants up to 3 years post-injury.

Most EEG and concussion research focus on lower frequency bands, but several studies by Thornton [38, 48, 51, 58] demonstrated that extending the frequency to include gamma bands provides important additional information, particularly between correlating EEG variables and the participant's cognitive deficits. Additionally, most research and, consequently, normative databases provide information solely about eyes closed conditions. This severely limits the type of cognitive testing that can be simultaneously completed; restricting neuropsychological testing to auditory-based tests. While auditory-based cognitive research has provided valuable EEG patterns, such as those outlined in Thorton and Carmody [38], several cognitive domains cannot be adequately assessed via auditory tasks. The link between EEG patterns and cognitive domains, such as visual memory and attention, remains poorly established and under-researched.

In summary, reviews by Arciniegas [8] and Nuwer et al. [34] have cited numerous studies that have proven EEG as a useful tool for identifying and managing concussive injuries. While EEGs are one of the least expensive and easiest to use neuroimaging tools, the expertise needed to administer and evaluate EEG results, as well as the lack of research between EEG and concussion, has kept EEG evaluations from becoming part of the current clinical gold standard. The most comprehensive EEG study using a database of 608 mTBI subjects that were followed up to 8 years post-injury revealed a number of findings. These include: (a) increased coherence in frontal–temporal regions; (b) decreased power differences between anterior and posterior cortical regions; and (c) reduced alpha power in the posterior cortical region, which was attributed to mechanical head injury [47]. A study by Thornton [58] has shown a similar data trend in addition to demonstrating the attenuation of EEG within the high frequency gamma cluster (32–64 Hz) in mTBI patients. Overall, resting EEG has demonstrated alterations in power dynamics across electrical spectra [8], increased short distance coherences [59], and decrease in connectivity across long-distance connections [59]. These consistent findings in resting EEG and mTBI research point to the sensitivity and validity of using EEG in the assessment and management of concussion. However, it should be noted that one controversial report concluded that no clear EEG features are unique to mTBI, especially late after injury [34].

Current Work from Our Lab

In our work, significant reduction of the cortical potentials amplitude and concomitant alteration of gamma activity (40 Hz) were observed in mTBI subjects performing force production tasks 3 years post-injury [57]. More recently, we showed a significant reduction of EEG power within theta and delta frequency bands during standing postures in subjects with single and multiple concussions up to 3 years post-injury [58] and reduced amplitude of cortical potentials (MRCP) up to 30 days post-injury [60]. Unfortunately, there is no systematic EEG research available in the literature on subjects suffering and recovering from multiple concussions.

We applied advanced *EEG-wavelet entropy* measures to detect brain functional deficits in mTBI subjects. These EEG measures were significantly reduced after the first and more significantly after the second mTBI far beyond 7 days post-injury. Most importantly, the rate of recovery of EEG entropy measures was significantly slower after second mTBI compared to the first concussion [61]. Recently, we reported the alteration of EEG signals in mTBI subjects detected by a novel measure of nonstationarity, named Shannon entropy of the peak frequency shifting [62]. These findings are complementary to our previously published concussion report indicating the presence of residual deficits in mTBI subjects detected by multichannel EEG signals classifier using support vector machine [63]. We also conducted an EEG resting state study and reported the alteration of cortical functional connectivity in mTBI subjects revealed by graph theory, ICA, and LORETA analyses. Overall, a clear departure from *small world-like network* was observed in mTBI subjects [59].

The presence of a residual disturbance of the neuronal network is involved in execution of postural movement in mTBI subjects incorporating EEG- and VR-induced measures [64]. There was a significant increase of *theta* power during the progression of a balance task. Specifically, this *theta* increment was obvious initially at central areas with further diffusion to frontal electrode sites bilaterally. Interestingly, no significant *theta* power was present in concussed subjects at either phase of postural task progression. Most recently we reported that 85 % of mTBI subjects who showed significant alteration of alpha power in acute phase of injury did not return to pre-injury status up to 12 months [65].

Compensatory Approach During Concussion Assessment Batteries

Several studies have found electrophysiological deficits in asymptomatic concussed participants [66–68]. In these studies, concussed participants displayed normal levels of cognitive functioning, yet continue to show physiological dysfunction on EEG measures. The authors cite an unknown compensatory mechanism as an explanation for the findings. As part of our research, we sought to investigate this compensatory mechanism in more detail. In order to assess this, we chose to record EEG signals while participants were completing clinical concussion assessment measures, specifically the Immediate Post-Concussion Assessment and Cognitive Testing (ImPACT) neuropsychological and VR balance and spatial navigation modules, as well as EEG resting state evaluations in order to highlight the differences between clinical cognitive and balance performance and neuroelectric measures.

In a sample of 13 normal volunteers and seven concussed participants, no differences were found between groups on ImPACT and VR composite outcome scores. When looking at sub-scores, the only significant difference was poorer stationary balance in the concussed group. However, several significant group differences were found when looking at the EEG variables. For EEG resting state and ImPACT conditions, the concussed group had significantly lower power in the theta and beta bandwidths. Additionally, the concussed group had significantly lower alpha power during the ImPACT conditions and significantly lower delta power in the VR conditions. Conversely, the concussed group displayed significantly higher levels of coherence during EEG resting state and ImPACT evaluations, but lower levels of coherence during VR balance and spatial navigation testing.

Overall, for EEG resting state and ImPACT, these results indicate that concussed participants could not establish enough local effort (seen via lower power), so they recruited additional long-distance network connections (seen via the increased coherence). By recruiting additional networks, the concussed participants were able to successfully compensate for their neuroelectric deficits and produce normal clinical results. For the VR modules, concussed participants were not able to compensate as successfully. This was seen via the inability to recruit additional long-distance networks and clinically in the overall poorer balance in the concussed group, specifically the significantly worse static balance. This research indicates a disconnect between cognitive and neuroelectric resolution. Future research projects aim at determining whether cognitive functions resolve before physiological function or if current clinical concussion assessments are not sensitive enough to detect the residual affects of concussion.

Return to Play and EEG Concussion Research

One specific area that is still lacking in research and is noted in second international consensus statement [69] and in the statement from the World Health Organization's (WHO) task force on mTBI [70] is the area of return to work or play. The WHO task force found no studies that demonstrate acceptable evidence to suggest when a person or athlete may safely return to work or the athletic field. As it has demonstrated its ability to identify physiological differences in the recovery from TBI, EEG should be considered as a feasible diagnostic tool for use within the "Return to Play" protocol and recommendations given to athletes returning to activity and sport.

As previously mentioned throughout this chapter, EEG has been used to study concussion or mTBI throughout all stages of recovery from acute, subacute to chronic or long term. One such clinical stage EEG has not been used is within the "Return to Play" stepwise progression back into athletic participation. The "Return to Play" protocol is the internationally accepted method for the safe return to activity of an athlete recovering from concussion [71]. This formalized "Return to Play" protocol has been in place since the original 2001 Concussion in Sport Group (CISG) Consensus Statement and remains unstudied and based on little to no scientific evidence, yet is still used as the "gold standard" for returning athletes to competition.

Under this procedure, "Return to Play" after a concussion follows a stepwise progression of increasing efforts and risk as outlined in Table 5.2. First the athlete must be completely asymptomatic at rest for a period of at least 24 h. Once asymptomatic and cleared by a supervising physician, the athlete may progress to a light

Table 5.2 Graduated "Return to Play" protocol

Rehabilitation stage	Functional exercise	Objective
No activity	Complete physical and cognitive rest	Recovery
Light aerobic exercise	Walking, swimming, or stationary cycling keeping intensity <70 % age-adjusted MHR. "No resistance training"	Increase heart rate
Sports-specific exercise	Skating drills in ice hockey, running drills in soccer. No head impact activities	Add movement
Non-contact training drills	Progression to more complex training drills (e.g., passing drills)	Exercise coordination
	"May start resistance training"	Cognitive load
Full contact practice	Following medical clearance participate in normal training activities	Restore confidence and assess functional skills by coaching staff
Return to play	Normal game play	

aerobic exercise such as walking or stationary cycling. This light aerobic challenge is limited by restricting athletes to <70 % of their calculated maximum heart rate.

With this activity progression, each stage of increasing efforts should be separated by 24 h with health professionals monitoring the athletes and their symptom status. If any of the athlete's post-concussion symptoms should manifest before, during, or after a stage within the protocol, the athlete is instructed to drop back to the previous asymptomatic stage and try to progress again after a further 24-h period of rest.

In our lab we investigated the use of EEG as a supplementary tool in the clinical assessment of concussion during the "Return to Play" phase of recovery. Specifically, we looked at the differential effect of exercise (modified YMCA bike protocol) on the quantitative EEG measures of spectral absolute power and coherence in normal volunteers vs. mTBI subjects. We hypothesized that the YMCA bike protocol would induce differential EEG measurement between each group. We also hypothesized that the YMCA bike protocol would induce similar physiologic measurements (heart rate, self-reported post-concussion symptoms) between groups performing the exercise protocol and that both groups would demonstrate clinically asymptomatic performances.

There were several major findings from this study. Of particular clinical significance was the clinical symptomatology surrounding the mTBI group. All mTBI subjects had all returned to clinical asymptomatic status at rest as determined by self-reported symptom scores (SRSS), clinical cognitive measures (SCAT-2), clinical balance measures (BESS), and computer-based neuropsychological test scores (CNS Vital Signs, ImPACT). These athletes had also been cleared by a sports medicine physician for the initiation of the "Return to Play" protocol as outlined above. All subjects met the clinical criteria for asymptomatic at rest [72] for a period of at least 24 h prior to exercise testing.

In addition, the modified YMCA bike protocol was capable of producing similar physiologic changes between groups in terms of heart rate dynamic changes during the bike with both exercise and post-exercise recovery; meaning there were no group differences in dynamic measures of heart rate throughout the bike protocol or post-bike recovery phase. In addition, both groups demonstrated no differences in the presentation of symptoms related to concussion and all subject participants were able to finish the exercise protocol without stopping due to excessive fatigue or the onset of exercise-induced post-concussion symptoms. These clinical findings are significant as they comply with a typical clinical progression back into activity without adverse clinical consequence. The absence of clinically significant symptoms allows the athlete to progress in stages of the "Return to Play" protocol as outlined by the CISG International Guidelines [69, 71]. As a result of the absence of clinical symptoms within each stage of the "Return to Play" protocol, the athletes within the mTBI group returned to normal sports participation within 4 days. They demonstrated no clinical abnormalities requiring a delay in their progression and were subsequently fully released based on current clinical standards. However, some differences were evident when reviewing the physiological data from the EEG evaluation.

Both groups (normal volunteers, mTBI) demonstrated no regional power differences at rest and at 24 h follow-up. In addition, both groups demonstrated no significant differences in mean or regional coherence values at rest or at 24 h follow-up. Historically within the literature, abnormal attenuation of alpha power and an increase in focal slow-wave distribution are short lasting and typically return to normal within the subacute phase of experimental concussion [73–75]. Further, in a recent quantitative EEG examination by McCrea et al., no resting state differences in athletes recovering from mTBI at days 8 and 45 post-injury were found when compared to age-matched controls [76]. Within the neural imaging research, resting-state fMRI findings of mTBI cohorts at rest do not vary significantly from normal volunteers [77]. This is an important finding as researchers look to develop the clinical significance of EEG as a diagnostic tool for mTBI. Resting state EEG measurement remains largely normal as reported throughout the literature.

With the introduction of exercise, physiologic differences were observed between groups. The modified YMCA bike protocol increased alpha, beta, theta, and delta absolute power amplitudes across all regions (frontal, central, and posterior) in the mTBI group vs. normal volunteers. Specifically, exercise significantly increased the power of theta and delta frequency ranges that are considered broadly to represent a pathological state that has been established in the literature. Theta power increases stem from injury and pathophysiologic changes in the cerebral cortex [17]. As is known, mTBI results in altered cerebral blood flow [78, 79], decreased energy metabolism [80], release of excitatory amino acids (EAA), and decreased postsynaptic function among other effects already mentioned. In work by Nagata, his group demonstrated that cortical blood flow (CBF) and oxygen (O_2) metabolism correlated negatively with delta and theta power [81]. Meaning, as CBF and O_2 metabolism decreased there was a subsequent increase in delta and theta power. In addition, increases in theta power have long been established in the mTBI literature [15, 44] and are indicative of pathology. Delta activity has been known to increase in many pathological states. This increase of delta power in resting EEG has been documented in different pathological conditions [82–84]. The lack of specificity of this effect linked with any range of pathological conditions suggests that increase of slow waves (delta/theta frequencies) represents a typical response to any brain injury, pathology, and disruption of neural homeostasis.

The specific findings of this investigation would suggest that the use of EEG within the "Return to Play" protocol for athletes recovering from concussion is feasible. Moreover, current clinical guidelines used to evaluate the athlete may not bring residual abnormalities to the forefront and lead to premature "Return to Play." The inclusion of EEG as a physiologic tool proves to have some worth in examining the recovering athlete and may provide clinicians with valuable data when making "Return to Activity" decisions. Furthermore as demonstrated by this investigation, exercise may be an effective mechanism for uncovering residual abnormalities in recovering athletes.

References

1. Roozenbeek B, Maas A, Menon D. Changing patterns in the epidemiology of traumatic brain injury. Nat Rev Neurol. 2013;9(4):231–6.
2. Jordan B. The clinical spectrum of sport-related traumatic brain injury. Nat Rev Neurol. 2013;9(4):222–30.
3. Gaetz M, Bernstein D. The current status of electrophysiologic procedures for the assessment of mild traumatic brain injury. J Head Trauma Rehabil. 2001;16(4):386–405.
4. Teasdale T, Engberg A. Suicide after traumatic brain injury: a population study. J Neurol Neurosurg Psychiatry. 2001;71(4):436–40.
5. Uryu K, Laurer H, McIntosh T, Praticò D, Martinez D, Leight S, Lee V, Trojanowski J. Repetitive mild brain trauma accelerates Abeta deposition, lipid peroxidation, and cognitive impairment in a transgenic mouse model of Alzheimer amyloidosis. J Neurosci. 2002; 22(2):446–54.
6. Blaylock R, Maroon J. Immunoexcitotoxicity as a central mechanism in chronic traumatic encephalopathy—a unifying hypothesis. Surg Neurol. 2011;2(1):107.
7. Barnes S, Walter K, Chard K. Does a history of mild traumatic brain injury increase suicide risk in veterans with PTSD? Rehabil Psychol. 2012;57(1):18–26.
8. Arciniegas D. Clinical electrophysiologic assessments and mild traumatic brain injury: state-of-the-science and implications for clinical practice. Int J Psychophysiol. 2011;82(1):41–52.
9. Bigler E, Maxwell W. Neuropathology of mild traumatic brain injury: relationship to neuroimaging findings. Brain Imaging Behav. 2012;6(2):108–36.
10. Berger H. Über das Elektronkephalogram des Menschen. Arch Psychiatry. 1929;87:527–70.
11. Glaser M, Sjaardem H. Value of the electroencephalogram in craniocerebral injuries. J Nerv Ment Dis. 1944;99(4):433.
12. Jasper H, Kershman J, Elvidge A. Electroencephalographic study in clinical cases of injury of the head. Arch Neurol Psychiatry. 1940;10:328–48.
13. Williams D. The significance of an abnormal electroencephalogram. J Neurol Psychiatry. 1941;4(3–4):257–68.
14. Geets W, Louette N. Early EEG in 300 cerebral concussions. Rev Electroencephalogr Neurophysiol Clin. 1985;14(4):333–8.
15. McClelland R, Fenton G, Rutherford W. The postconcussional syndrome revisited. J R Soc Med. 1994;87:508–10.

16. Tebano M, Cameroni M, Gallozzi G, Loizzo A, Palazzino G, Pezzini G, Ricci G. EEG spectral analysis after minor head injury in man. Electroencephalogr Clin Neurophysiol. 1988; 70(2):185–9.
17. Montgomery E, Fenton G, McClelland R, MacFlynn G, Rutherford W. The psychobiology of minor head injury. Psychol Med. 1991;21(2):375–84.
18. Pratar-Chand R, Sinniah M, Salem F. Cognitive evoked potential (P300): a metric for cerebral concussion. Acta Neurol Scand. 1988;78:185–9.
19. Watson M, Fenton G, McClelland R, Lumsden J, Headley M, Rutherford W. The post-concussional state: neurophysiological aspects. Br J Psychiatry. 1995;167:514–21.
20. Leon-Carrion J, Martin-Rodriguez J, Damas-Lopez J, Martin J, Dominguez-Morales M. A QEEG index of level of functional dependence for people sustaining acquired brain injury: the Seville Independence Index (SINDI). Brain Inj. 2008;22(1):61–74.
21. Nunez P, Srinivasan R. A theoretical basis for standing and traveling brain waves measured with human EEG with implications for an integrated consciousness. Clin Neurophysiol. 2006;117(11):2424–35.
22. Whittingstall K, Logothetis N. Frequency-band coupling in surface EEG reflects spiking activity in monkey visual cortex. Neuron. 2009;64(2):281–9.
23. Jasper H. The ten-twenty electrode system of the International Federation. Electroencephalogr Clin Neurophysiol. 1958;10:370–5.
24. O'Neil B, Prichep L, Naunheim R, Chabot R. Can quantitative brain electrical activity aid in the triage of mild traumatic brain-injured patients? Ann Emerg Med. 2011;58(4):208.
25. Shaw N. The neurophysiology of concussion. Prog Neurobiol. 2002;67(4):281–344.
26. Bazanova O, Vernon D. Interpreting EEG alpha activity. Neurosci Biobehav Rev. 2013; (epub ahead of print).
27. Tallon-Baudry C, Bertrand O, Delpuech C, Permier J. Oscillatory gamma-band (30–70 Hz) activity induced by a visual search task in humans. J Neurosci. 1997;17(2):722–34.
28. Walter W. The living brain. Oxford: W.W. Norton; 1953. p. 311.
29. Luu P, Tucker D. Regulating action: alternating activation of midline frontal and motor cortical networks. Clin Neurophysiol. 2001;112(7):1295–306.
30. Schacter D. EEG theta waves and psychological phenomena: a review and analysis. Biol Psychol. 1977;5(1):47–82.
31. Vogel W, Broverman D, Klaiber E. EEG and mental abilities. Electroencephalogr Clin Neurophysiol. 1968;24:166–75.
32. Slobounov S, Gay M, Johnson B, Zhang K. Concussion in athletics: ongoing clinical and brain imaging research controversies. Brain Imaging Behav. 2012;6(2):224–43.
33. Geets W, de Zegher F. EEG and brainstem abnormalities after cerebral concussion. Short term observations. Acta Neurol Belg. 1985;85(5):277–83.
34. Nuwer M, Hovda D, Schrader L, Vespa P. Routine and quantitative EEG in mild traumatic brain injury. Clin Neurophysiol. 2005;116(9):2001–25.
35. Koufen H, Dichgans J. Frequency and course of posttraumatic EEG-abnormalities and their correlations with clinical symptoms: a systematic follow up study in 344 adults (author's transl). Fortschr Neurol Psychiatr Grenzgeb. 1978;46(4):165–77.
36. Jacome D, Risko M. EEG features in post-traumatic syndrome. Clin Electroencephalogr. 1984;15(4):214–21.
37. Cannon R, Baldwin D, Shaw T, Diloreto D, Phillips S, Scruggs A, Riehl T. Reliability of quantitative EEG (qEEG) measures and LORETA current source density at 30 days. Neurosci Lett. 2012;518:27–31.
38. Thornton K, Carmody D. Traumatic brain injury rehabilitation: QEEG biofeedback treatment protocols. Appl Psychophysiol Biofeedback. 2009;34(1):59–68.
39. Chen X, Tao L, Chen A. Electroencephalogram and evoked potential parameters examined in Chinese mild head injury patients for forensic medicine. Neurosci Bull. 2006;22:165–70.

40. Coutin-Churchman P, Anez Y, Uzcategui M, Alvarez L, Vergara F, Mendez L, Fleitas R. Quantitative spectral analysis of EEG in psychiatry revisited: drawing signs out of numbers in a clinical setting. Clin Neurophysiol. 2003;114:2294–306.
41. Korn A, Golan H, Melamed I, Pascual-Marqui R, Friedman A. Focal cortical dysfunction and blood-brain barrier disruption in patients with postconcussion syndrome. J Clin Neurophysiol. 2005;22:1–9.
42. von Bierbrauer A, Weissenborn K, Hinrichs H, Scholz M, Kunkel H. Automatic (computer-assisted) EEG analysis in comparison with visual EEG analysis in patients following minor cranio-cerebral trauma (a follow-up study). EEG EMG Z Elektroenzephalogr Elektromyogr Verwandte Geb. 1992;23(3):151–7.
43. Fenton G, McClelland R, Montgomery A, MacFlynn G, Rutherford W. The postconcussional syndrome: social antecedents and psychological sequelae. Br J Psychiatry. 1993;162:493–7.
44. Fenton G. The postconcussional syndrome reappraised. Clin Electroencephalogr. 1996;22: 174–82.
45. Thatcher R. Maturation of the human frontal lobes: physiological evidence for staging. Dev Neuropsychol. 1991;7(3):397–419.
46. Thatcher R, North D, Curtin R, Walker R, Biver C, Gomez F, Salazar A. An EEG severity index of traumatic brain injury. J Neuropsychiatry Clin Neurosci. 2001;13(1):77–87.
47. Thatcher R, Walker R, Gerson I, Geisler F. EEG discriminant analyses of mild head trauma. Electroencephalogr Clin Neurophysiol. 1989;73(2):94–106.
48. Thornton K. Improvement/rehabilitation of memory functioning with neurotherapy/QEEG biofeedback. J Head Trauma Rehabil. 2000;15(6):1285–96.
49. Thatcher R, Biver C, McAlaster R, Salazar A. Biophysical linkage between MRI and EEG coherence in closed head injury. Neuroimage. 1998;8(4):307–26.
50. Barr W, Prichep L, Chabot R, Powell R, McCrea M. Measuring brain electrical activity to track recovery from sport-related concussion. Brain Inj. 2012;26(1):58–66.
51. Thornton K. The electrophysiological effects of a brain injury on auditory memory functioning. The QEEG correlates of impaired memory. Arch Clin Neuropsychol. 2003;18(4):363–78.
52. Corsi-Cabrera M, Solís-Ortiz S, Guevara M. Stability of EEG inter- and intrahemispheric correlation in women. Electroencephalogr Clin Neurophysiol. 1997;102(3):248–55.
53. Pollock V, Schneider L, Lyness S. Reliability of topographic quantitative EEG amplitude in healthy late-middle-aged and elderly subjects. Electroencephalogr Clin Neurophysiol. 1991;79(1):2026.
54. Salinsky M, Oken B, Morehead L. Test-retest reliability in EEG frequency analysis. Electroencephalogr Clin Neurophysiol. 1991;79(5):382–92.
55. Harmony T, Fernández T, Rodríguez M, Reyes A, Marosi E, Bernal J. Test-retest reliability of EEG spectral parameters during cognitive tasks: II. Coherence. Int J Neurosci. 1993; 68(3–4):263–71.
56. Nikulin V, Brismar T. Long-range temporal correlations in alpha and beta oscillations: effect of arousal level and test-retest reliability. Clin Neurophysiol. 2004;115(8):1896–908.
57. Slobounov S, Sebastianelli W, Simon R. Neurophysiological and behavioral concomitants of mild brain injury in collegiate athletes. Clin Neurophysiol. 2002;113(2):185–93.
58. Thompson J, Sebastianelli W, Slobounov S. EEG and postural correlates of mild traumatic brain injury in athletes. Neurosci Lett. 2005;377(3):158–63.
59. Cao C, Slobounov S. Alteration of cortical functional connectivity as a result of traumatic brain injury revealed by graph theory, ICA, and sLORETA analyses of EEG signals. IEEE Trans Neural Syst Rehabil Eng. 2010;18(1):11–9.
60. Slobounov S, Sebastianelli W, Moss R. Alteration of posture-related cortical potentials in mild traumatic brain injury. Neurosci Lett. 2005;383(3):251–5.
61. Slobounov S, Cao C, Sebastianelli W. Differential effect of first versus second concussive episodes on wavelet information quality of EEG. Clin Neurophysiol. 2009;120(5):862–7.

62. Cao C, Slobounov S. Application of a novel measure of EEG non-stationarity as 'Shannon-entropy of the peak frequency shifting' for detecting residual abnormalities in concussed individuals. Clin Neurophysiol. 2011;122(7):1314–21.
63. Cao C, Tutwiler R, Slobounov S. Automatic classification of athletes with residual functional deficits following concussion by means of EEG signal using support vector machine. IEEE Trans Neural Syst Rehabil Eng. 2008;16(4):327–35.
64. Slobounov S, Sebastianelli W, Newell K. Incorporating virtual reality graphics with brain imaging for assessment of sport-related concussions. Conf Proc IEEE Eng Med Biol Soc. 2011;2011:1383–6.
65. Slobounov S, Sebastianelli W, Hallett M. Residual brain dysfunction observed one year post-mild traumatic brain injury: combined EEG and balance study. Clin Neurophysiol. 2012;123(9):1755–61.
66. Broglio S, Pontifex M, O'Connor P, Hillman C. The persistent effects of concussion on neuro-electric indices of attention. J Neurotrauma. 2009;26(9):1463–70.
67. Gosselin N, Thériault M, Leclerc S, Montplaisir J, Lassonde M. Neurophysiological anomalies in symptomatic and asymptomatic concussed athletes. J Neurosurg. 2006;58(6):1151–61.
68. Thériault M, De Beaumont L, Gosselin N, Filipinni M, Lassonde M. Electrophysiological abnormalities in well functioning multiple concussed athletes. Brain Inj. 2009;23(11): 899–906.
69. McCrory P, Johnston K, Meeuwisse W, Aubry M, Cantu R, Dvorak J, Graf-Baumann T, Kelly J, Lovell M, Schamasch P. Summary and agreement statement of the 2nd International Conference on Concussion in Sport, Prague 2004. Br J Sports Med. 2005;39:196–204.
70. Cancelliere C, Cassidy D, Côté P, Hincapié C, Hartvigsen J, Carroll L, Marras C, Boyle E, Kristman V, Hung R, Stålnacke BM, Rumney P, Coronado V, Holm L, Borg J, Nygren-de Boussard C, Af Geijerstam JL, Keightley M. Protocol for a systematic review of prognosis after mild traumatic brain injury: an update of the WHO Collaborating Centre Task Force findings. Syst Rev. 2012;1(1):1–17.
71. McCrory P, Meeuwisse WH, Aubry M, Cantu RC, Dvořák J, Echemendia RJ, Engebretsen L, Johnston K, Kutcher JS, Raftery M, Sills A, Benson BW, Davis GA, Ellenbogen R, Guskiewicz KM, Herring SA, Iverson GL, Jordan BD, Kissick J, McCrea M, McIntosh AS, Maddocks D, Makdissi M, Purcell L, Putukian M, Schneider K, Tator CH, Turner M. Consensus statement on concussion in sport: the 4th International Conference on Concussion in Sport, Zurich, November 2012. J Athl Train. 2013;48(4):554–75.
72. Alla S, Sullivan J, McCrory P. Defining asymptomatic status following sports concussion: fact or fallacy? Br J Sports Med. 2012;46(8):562–9.
73. Ward A. The physiology of concussion. Clin Neurosurg. 1966;12:95–111.
74. Echlin F. Spreading depression of electrical activity in the cerebral cortex following local trauma and its possible role in concussion. Arch Neurol Psychiatry. 1950;63(5):830–2.
75. West M, Parkinson D, Havlicck V. Spectral analysis of the electroencephalographic response to experimental concussion in the rat. Electroencephalogr Clin Neurophysiol. 1982; 53:192–200.
76. McCrea M, Prichep L, Powell M, Chabot R, Barr W. Acute effects and recovery after sport-related concussion: a neurocognitive and quantitative brain electrical activity study. J Head Trauma Rehabil. 2010;25(4):283–92.
77. Zhang K, Johnson B, Gay M, Horovitz S, Hallett M, Sebastianelli W, Slobounov S. Default mode network in concussed individuals in response to YMCA physical stress test. J Neurotrauma. 2012;29(5):756–65.
78. Len T, Neary JP. Cerebrovascular pathophysiology following mild traumatic brain injury. Clin Physiol Funct Imaging. 2011;31:85–93.
79. Len T, Neary JP, Asmundson GJ, Goodman D, Bjornson B, Bhambhanis YN. Cerebrovascular reactivity impairment after sport-induced concussion. Med Sci Sports Exerc. 2011;43(12):2241–8.
80. Vagnozzi R, Signoretti S, Cristofori L, Alessandrini F, Floris R, Isgro E, Ria A, Marziale S, Zoccatelli G, Tavazzi B, Del Bolgia F, Sorge R, Broglio SP, McIntosh TK, Lazzarino G.

Assessment of metabolic brain damage and recovery following mild traumatic brain injury: a multicentre, proton magnetic resonance spectroscopic study in concussed patients. Brain. 2010;133:3232–42.

81. Nagata K. Metabolic and hemodynamic correlates of quantitative EEG mapping. Electroencephalogr Clin Neurophysiol. 1995;97(4):S49.

82. Bates A, Kiehl K, Laurens K, Liddle P. Low-frequency EEG oscillations associated with information processing in schizophrenia. Schizophr Res. 2009;115:222–30.

83. Babiloni C, Ferri R, Binetti G, Vecchio F, Frisoni G, Lanuzza B, Miniussi C, Nobili F, Rodriguez G, Rundo F, Cassarino A, Infarinato F, Cassetta E, Salinari S, Eusebi F, Rossini P. Directionality of EEG synchronization in Alzheimer's disease subjects. Neurobiol Aging. 2009;30:93–102.

84. Korb A, Cook I, Hunter A, Leuchter A. Brain electrical source differences between depressed subjects and healthy controls. Brain Topogr. 2008;21:138–46.

Chapter 6
The Relevance of Assessing Cerebral Metabolic Recovery for a Safe Return to Play Following Concussion

Stefano Signoretti, Barbara Tavazzi, Giuseppe Lazzarino, and Roberto Vagnozzi

Abstract Concussion, a peculiar type of mild traumatic brain injury (mTBI) frequently encountered in sports medicine, is characterized by complex molecular alterations of various important functions of neuronal cells, including mitochondrial-related energy supply, ionic homeostasis, neurotransmitters, N-acetylaspartate (NAA) homeostasis, and even gene expression. Most of these molecular and metabolic derangements are of limited duration (spontaneous recovery of metabolism and cell functions), representing the bases of the metabolic brain vulnerability occurring after mTBI. In this chapter, we describe results of experimental studies evidencing the connections among mTBI, energy metabolism, mitochondrial dysfunctions, and NAA, as well as we summarize results of clinical studies demonstrating that the monitoring of brain metabolism (NAA and creatine) by proton magnetic resonance spectroscopy (^{1}H-MRS) is a useful tool to increase the safety of return to play of athletes after a concussion. The application of ^{1}H-MRS in concussed athletes shows that clinical symptoms clear much faster than normalization of brain metabolism.

S. Signoretti, M.D., Ph.D.
Department of Neurosciences—Head and Neck Surgery, Division of Neurosurgery,
San Camillo Hospital, Circonvallazione Gianicolense 87, Rome 00152, Italy
e-mail: stefano.signoretti@tiscali.it

B. Tavazzi, Ph.D.
Institute of Biochemistry and Clinical Biochemistry, Catholic University of Rome,
Largo F. Vito 1, Rome 00168, Italy
e-mail: btavazzi@rm.unicatt.it

G. Lazzarino, Ph.D. (✉)
Department of Biology, Geology and Environmental Sciences, Division of Biochemistry
and Molecular Biology, University of Catania, Viale A. Doria 6, Catania 95125, Italy
e-mail: lazzarig@unict.it

R. Vagnozzi, M.D., Ph.D.
Department of Biomedicine and Prevention, Section of Neurosurgery, University of Rome
Tor Vergata, Via Montpellier 1, Rome 00133, Italy
e-mail: vagnozzi@uniroma2.it

S.M. Slobounov and W.J. Sebastianelli (eds.), *Concussions in Athletics: From Brain to Behavior*, DOI 10.1007/978-1-4939-0295-8_6,
© Springer Science+Business Media New York 2014

^{1}H-MRS allows to measure objective parameters of biochemical relevance and is suitable to determine the end of the period of brain vulnerability. This information cannot otherwise be obtained with clinical tests of current use and is important to minimize the risks related to an early return on the field of concussed athletes.

Keywords Brain concussion • Energy metabolism • Magnetic resonance spectroscopy • Mild traumatic brain injury • Mitochondrial dysfunctions • *N*-acetylaspartate

Introduction

Although traumatic brain injury (TBI) is one of the most important public health issues worldwide, despite countless scientific reports, the available epidemiological data are not easily comparable, varying greatly between countries [1, 2]. Some of the differences could be ascribed to the disparity in study years, inclusion criteria, and research methods along with admission policies, particularly in the case of mild traumatic brain injury (mTBI) [3]. As thoroughly reported elsewhere, the annual incidence of all TBI categories in European countries is estimated at between 100 and 1,967 per 100,000 persons [4, 5], with mild and moderate TBI accounting for 80–95 %, while the US result ranges even wider, with approximately 1.5–8 million people experiencing a TBI each year, 75–90 % of which are classified as "mildly" injured or "concussed." These broad margins of annual incidence are due to the fact that there is still confusion and inconsistency among researchers and organizations in defining and understanding this type of trauma and that an unknown proportion of mTBI victims do not seek any medical attention.

mTBI has indeed too many synonyms, including "brain concussion," "mild head injury," "minor head injury," and "minimal TBI" [6, 7]. Even the terms "head" and "brain" have been used interchangeably [1, 8]. The essential misleading aspect accompanying mTBI, however, is the label "mild." It originates from the most often used system for grading the severity of cranio-cerebral trauma, the Glasgow Coma Scale (GCS), a systematic score which grades a person's level of consciousness on a scale of 3–15 based on verbal, motor, and eye-opening reactions to stimuli. It is generally agreed that a TBI with a GCS of 13 or above is considered "mild," even if the scale per se only indicates a "mildly affected level of consciousness," giving no insight about the true brain disturbances. We all know in fact that different patients with the same GCS score may not function at the same level.

To confuse the picture, blended into the vast world of mTBI, lies the "concussion," a rather troubling, clinical entity recently considered by three International Consensus Conferences in which it had been defined and redefined by a panel of experts to reach a rather vague final definition (at least from a clinical point of view) such as "… a complex pathophysiological process affecting the brain, induced by traumatic biomechanical forces" [9–11].

Notwithstanding, some facts are certain about concussions: from many parts of the world, data consistently show that there is a peak incidence rate in children, young adults, and elderly people that males are injured 2–3 times as often as women, and that approximately 20 % of mTBI are sport-related. So, it has become more common to diagnose and follow concussion in athletes than in non-athletes, due to the intrinsic risks inherent in several types of contact and non-contact sports [12]. Athletes represent a group of people particularly at risk for concussive brain injury and in professional athletics, the economic interests are markedly related to the athlete's health and performance [13].

Basic science data, collected from many reported bench studies, have clarified some aspects of this particular clinical entity, suggesting that, after all, mTBIs are not always as "mild" as the name would suggest, and short-term as well as long-term consequences may very well be overcome simply by understanding the metabolic and molecular conditions of the injured brain cells. The importance of an in-depth look at molecules in the evaluation of the post-concussive period is evidenced by the application of a number of advanced neuroimaging techniques, such as proton magnetic resonance spectroscopy (^{1}H-MRS), functional magnetic resonance (fMR), diffuse tensor imaging (DTI), and positron emission tomography (PET), which all demonstrate structural and metabolic alterations after single and multiple concussions [14–18].

Energy Metabolism and Gene Modulation: Crucial Issues of Concussion-Induced Brain Vulnerability

Concussion can be caused by any direct bump, blow, or jolt to the head, but can also occur indirectly from a fall or a blow to the body. On the whole, every event that leads the head and brain to move quickly back and forth causes the brain to experience a mechanical "shake" by virtue of the action of the acceleration and deceleration forces transmitted to the head immediately after the impact. This apparently simple incident is capable of initiating a complex cascade of subsequent neurochemical and neurometabolic events.

The sudden stretching of the neuronal and axonal membranes sets off an indiscriminate flux of ions through previously regulated ion channels and transient physical membrane defects [19, 20]. This process is followed by a widespread release of a multitude of neurotransmitters, particularly excitatory amino acids (EAAs) [21–23] resulting in further changes of neuronal ionic homeostasis. Among the EAAs, glutamate plays the pivotal role by binding to the kainite, N-methyl-D-aspartate (NMDA), and D-amino-3-hydroxy-5-methyl-4-isoxazolepropionic acid ionic channels. NMDA receptor activation is responsible for a further depolarization, ultimately causing an influx of calcium ions into the cells. As clearly demonstrated in bench studies, this event occurs very rapidly, starting in the very early phases after trauma (1–5 min) and persisting for 24–48 h after injury [24, 25].

The subsequent mitochondrial calcium overloading represents one of the essential points of the aforementioned posttraumatic ionic cellular derangement.

Notwithstanding the impressive increase in the knowledge, the tremendously complex pathobiological mechanisms underlying the changes in cellular functions following mTBI lead to a still incomplete picture of the post-traumatized cerebral cells. However, some clearly evidenced alterations rely on mitochondrial calcium overfilling: this phenomenon is directly responsible for inducing changes of inner membrane permeability [26, 27], with consequent malfunctioning of the electron transport chain (ETC) and finally of the uncoupling of oxidative phosphorylation [28, 29]. To reestablish pre-trauma cellular ionic balance, the Na+/K+ adenosine triphosphate (ATP)-dependent pumps must work at their maximal capacities, and a high level of glucose oxidation is required to satisfy this sudden increased energy demand. Under normal aerobic conditions and correct mitochondrial functioning, most glucose consumption is coupled to oxygen consumption, thus optimizing ATP generation; that is, glucose consumption almost overlaps to glucose oxidation.

However, damaged by the calcium surplus, the electron flow from reduced coenzymes to molecular oxygen through the ETC is significantly altered and the mitochondria cannot maintain the correct phosphorylating capacity. Thus, it happens that during the time of maximum energy request, the concussion-induced transient mitochondrial malfunctioning causes an imbalance between ATP consumption and production. This scenario results in a rapid net decrease of all metabolites representative of the cell energy state (ATP and guanosine triphosphate—GTP) mirrored by a proportional increase of their dephosphorylated products (adenosine diphosphate—ADP, adenosine monophosphate—AMP, guanosine diphosphate—GDP, guanosine monophosphate—GMP, nucleosides, and oxypurines). The raise in some of these intracellular compounds (AMP, ADP, inorganic phosphorus) acts as an efficient positive signal on some of the key regulatory enzymes of glycolysis, such as phosphofructokinase, hexokinase, and pyruvatekinase, leading to an overall net increase in the glycolytic rate. Hence, neurons compensate, in part, the energy crisis triggered by mitochondrial malfunctioning by increasing glucose consumption via the more rapid, but less efficient, oxygen-independent glycolysis. The uncoupling between oxygen and glucose consumption and the yet unfulfilled energy requirement explain the paradoxical temporary increase in neuronal glucose consumption, notwithstanding a period of general metabolic depression. In fact, local cerebral metabolic rates for glucose are documented to increase by 46 % above control levels within the first 30 min after injury and may last from 30 min to 4 h [30–33]. The overall evidence from these studies demonstrates that the traumatic insult is directly responsible for sudden biochemical changes, beginning immediately after injury and leading to subsequent depression of the brain energy metabolism. It is important to emphasize that in these circumstances the metabolic switch in glucose metabolism leading to increased glycolysis is not related to hypoxic phenomena.

In line with the energy crisis caused by mitochondrial dysfunction and increased energy demand following mTBI, it has recently been demonstrated, in an in vitro study in organotypic hippocampal slice cultures, that a stretch injury capable of generating an mTBI-like insult [34] triggers a gene program of neuroprotection, similar to that found in hibernators [35]. In particular, a downregulation of genes encoding for several subunits of the ETC was observed, thus suggesting that neurons reduce mitochondrial activity in a period of mitochondrial malfunctioning, probably to avoid an overflow of reactive oxygen species (ROS) occurring during incorrect electron transfer through the ETC [36]. Authors also found that, to overcome this time interval of energy crisis, neurons activate a strategy of gene regulation aimed at minimizing ATP consuming reactions (downregulation of transcription and translation genes). Even the restoration of calcium homeostasis takes place via ATP-independent mechanisms by upregulating genes encoding for calmodulin-binding proteins [35].

As already said, such a pattern of gene regulation can be encountered in hibernators and also in ischemic preconditioning: the difference is that in ischemic preconditioning and hibernators, this occurs in response to the decreased oxygen and substrate availability to tissues, fast in ischemic preconditioning and slow in hibernators. This gene program of neuroprotection has been observed following a stretch injury equal to that caused by an mTBI in a pure "in vitro" system, with cells having full availability to substrates and oxygen at constant concentrations during the whole duration of the experiments. Therefore, it appears that following mTBI, mitochondria suffer transient malfunctioning specifically involving ETC and its capacity to correctly handle the tetravalent reduction of molecular oxygen, in spite of no change in oxygen and substrate availability to cells. This decreases the amount of ATP generation causing, if protracted, a dramatic increase in oxidative/nitrosative stress. Decrease in energy balance and, more importantly, signals derived from mitochondrially produced oxygen and nitrogen radicals are likely to be the factors triggering the gene program of neuroprotection, having in the decrease of electron flow through the ETC during transient mitochondrial malfunctioning, one of its main effects/target (downregulation of complexes I, III, and IV of the ETC) [37]. This finding contributes to further explain hyperglycolysis and demonstrate that the major molecular changes influencing the post-injury period are triggered by the trauma itself and do not require secondary ischemic damage.

Notwithstanding it is considered a "mild" form of TBI, concussion is able to cause profound biochemical and molecular changes, with the relevant peculiarity being that the described metabolic modifications are fully reversible [38]. As recently reported, the metabolic derangement and the post-mTBI "energy crisis" are considered chiefly responsible for the compromised synaptic plasticity and the subsequent cognitive deficits [39]. Furthermore, the aforementioned transient alterations of brain metabolism support the hypothesis that the ability to depress temporarily the basal metabolic rate and enter a hypometabolic or dormant state, through a targeted modulation of gene expression, is a necessary strategy for the traumatically injured brain. This adaptive physiological mechanism involving mitochondrial functions, energy metabolism and gene expression, represents the molecular bases of the period of time known as "window of brain vulnerability," originally suggested by Giza and Hovda [40].

A Surrogate Marker of the Post-concussive
Brain Damage: *N*-acetylaspartate

Two fundamental findings brought *N*-acetylaspartate (NAA) to the attention of neuroscientists during the past three decades; the first was that NAA, after having suppressed the proton signal of water, was found to be the most prominent compound detectable with ¹H-MRS in the human brain. The second was the connection to the rare but fatal hereditary genetic disorder known as Canavan disease. These findings captured the attention of the general neurosciences, dramatically accelerating the pace of research into the neurochemistry and neurobiology of a molecule indeed definable as "unique" [41].

Although the exact role of this compound within the cellular and subcellular milieus remains to be established, brain NAA was found in concentrations a 100-fold higher than in non-nervous tissues and therefore considered a brain-specific metabolite [42, 43] and as an in vivo marker of neuronal density. NAA metabolism involves different cell types: (1) neuronal mitochondria take care of its biosynthesis via the activity of the recently characterized *N*-acetyltransferase enzyme, named NAT8L, which is a protein encoded by a three-exon gene located on mouse chromosome 5 and human chromosome 4 (band 4p16.3) [44]; (2) oligodendrocytes mainly contribute to its degradation via the activity of the cytoplasmic hydrolase *N*-acetylaspartoacylase (ASPA). NAA homeostasis is finely regulated by at least four different velocities: (1) rate of neuronal biosynthesis by NAT8L activity; (2) rate of neuronal outflow in the extracellular space; (3) rate of oligodendrocyte uptake; (4) rate of oligodendrocyte degradation by activity of ASPA [45, 46]. Since NAA biosynthesis also requires a continuous import of aspartate into the mitochondrial compartment, an essential role in regulating NAA homeostasis is played by *aralar*, the mitochondrial transporter of aspartate–glutamate [47]. In general, due to the indirect high energetic cost needed, NAA production is also strictly dependent on the neuronal energy state and, therefore, on the correct mitochondrial functioning. In fact, NAA synthesis requires the availability and the energy of hydrolysis of acetyl-CoA ($\Delta G = -31.2$ kJ/mol), working as the acetyl group and energy donor in the acetylation reaction of aspartate catalyzed by NAT8L. It is of primary importance to understand that when acetyl-CoA is used for NAA synthesis, there is an indirect high-energy cost to the cell. In fact, since in this case acetyl-CoA will not enter the citric acid cycle (Krebs' cycle), there will be a decrease in the production of reducing equivalents (3 NADH and 1 FADH$_2$) as the fuel for the ETC. Since the oxidative phosphorylation is stoichiometrically coupled to the amount of electrons transferred to molecular oxygen by the ETC, the final result will be a net loss of 12 ATP molecules for each newly synthesized NAA molecule.

NAA concentration within neurons is comparable to that of glutamate (~10 mmol/L brain water) but, notwithstanding such a relevant amount and in spite of NAA is known since the late 1950s, there is no unanimity on the biochemical functions of this "enigmatic" molecule. According to different studies, NAA may act as storage form for aspartate, protein synthesis regulator, shuttle of acetate, and "amino-nitrogen" from the mitochondria to the cytoplasm, breakdown product or precursor of the neurotransmitter N-acetylaspartylglutamate (NAAG), metabolically inert pool regulating the anion deficit balance, and metabolically active pool involved in the production of glutamate. Most likely NAA might play a marginal role in any of the aforementioned processes, but recent studies have suggested that the main roles of NAA are to operate as an acetyl group donor in lipid myelin biosynthesis [41], and to be involved in neuronal osmoregulation against cytotoxic swelling by acting as a "molecular water pump" [45].

Physiologically, NAA concentration is kept within a strict oscillation range even though it is regenerated 1.44 times/24 h (with a calculated turnover rate of approximately 0.75 mmol/L water/hour). Therefore, it appears evident that either the continuous energy requirement to ensure NAA turnover or the perfect balance of the different velocities is involved in its homeostasis. Pathologically, NAA has been observed to increase only in the fatal brain neurodegeneration known as Canavan disease in which, due to mutations in the gene encoding for ASPA [48, 49], a defective enzyme with no (or minimal) catalytic activity is synthesized [50]. This causes a relatively modest increase in cerebral NAA since this compound, instead of being accumulated within the cerebral tissue, is released into the blood stream (where it is modestly increased over the physiologic value) and finally excreted in the urine in concentrations 100 to 1000 times higher than the normal value [51, 52]. Vice versa, the pathologic NAA decrease has been observed in a single case known to date of hereditary NAT8L deficiency [44] as well as in association with many neurological diseases causing neuronal and axonal degeneration such as tumors, epilepsy, dementia, stroke, hypoxia, multiple sclerosis, and many leukoencephalopathies [53].

In the field of TBI, however, a very innovative hypothesis, according to which NAA reduction was believed to be proportional to the severity of trauma, seemed to attribute to this compound the putative role of biomarker with profound biochemical and clinical implications [54]. By measuring via high-performance liquid chromatography [55, 56] the time-course changes in whole brain levels of NAA and several high-energy compounds including ATP in three different levels of experimental, closed, and diffuse TBI (mild, severe, and severe + hypoxia-hypotension), it was clearly demonstrated that the reduction in NAA and ATP correlated to the severity of the insult (see Fig. 6.1), revealing spontaneous recovery with lower levels of trauma and irreversible decrease in the others [54].

In this study, an impressive similarity in the time-course modifications in these two compounds after graded injury was observed and it was shown that 48 h postinjury was the minimal time point at which one can clearly distinguish the severity of TBI, from a metabolic point of view [54]. These bench data strongly supported the indication for a potential role of NAA in quantifying neuronal damage and predicting neuropsychological outcome after TBI and being of high clinical relevance since the use of ^{1}H-MRS allows for the measurement of NAA noninvasively in vivo [57–60]. In addition, the metabolic recovery observed in the mTBI animals implied that the process leading to the reversible NAA and ATP reductions was attributable to transient biochemical changes and not simply to cell death. Beyond showing the profound TBI-induced modification in NAA homeostasis, this finding clearly

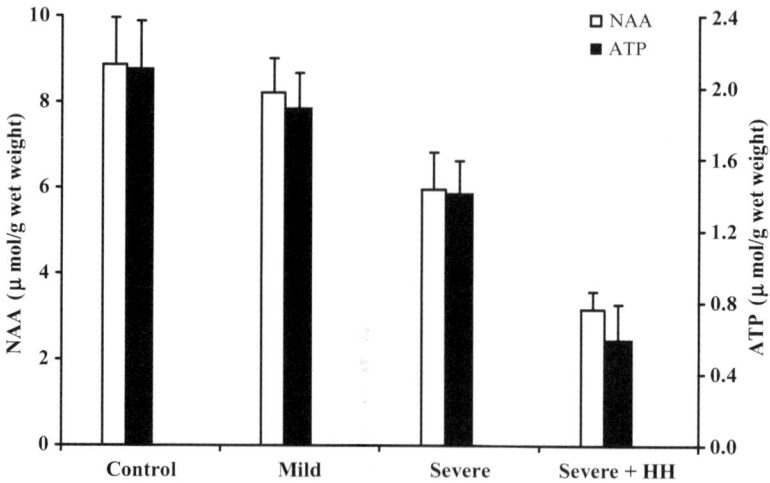

Fig. 6.1 Bar graph showing the association between the changes in NAA and ATP cerebral concentrations as a function of the severity of TBI. Rats underwent different traumatic insults (mild, severe, severe + hypoxia-hypotension) using the weight drop model with diffuse axonal injury. Animals were sacrificed 48 h after TBI and metabolites of interest were assayed by HPLC on deproteinized whole brain homogenates. Each histogram is the mean of six animals. Standard deviations are represented by *vertical bars*. NAA and ATP in severe and severe + hypoxia-hypotension rats were different from either values recorded in controls ($p < 0.01$) or from those recorded in mild-injured animals ($p < 0.01$)

demonstrated that different levels of "physical" injury correlated with different levels and kinetics of "biochemical" damage, which are reversible in mTBI and irreversible in severe TBI (sTBI) [37, 54].

Substantial evidence indicates that NAA synthesis takes place exclusively in neurons, that it is strictly tied to neuronal energy metabolism and mitochondrial functions, and that the distribution pattern of NAA closely parallels the distribution of "respiratory activity" [41–46]. It has been clearly evidenced that in the general posttraumatic metabolic derangement, acetyl-CoA homeostasis is affected by graded head injury, following a pattern very similar to those observed for both ATP and NAA [61]. Therefore, in metabolic conditions of low ATP availability, when all of the pathways and cycles devoted to energy supply are operating at their maximal activity with the aim of replenishing ATP levels, acetyl-CoA will not be accessible for NAA synthesis. Only when the ATP deficiency is fully restored will acetyl-CoA become available again to be shifted into the NAA "production" pathway.

With this in mind, a decrease in NAA concentration can be seen as an indirect marker of posttraumatic metabolic energy impairment. According to these concepts, it is evident that if NAA is still below the physiological values after an mTBI, the concussive biochemical derangement involving more complex pathways than simple NAA homeostasis [34–37] cannot be considered to be resolved. Thus, NAA embodies a biochemical surrogate marker to monitor the overall cerebral metabolic status, and it appears that under conditions of decreased NAA, the cells are functional yet are still experiencing energetic imbalance. It is important to emphasize that these results on brain energy metabolism following an mTBI are consequences of the recently discovered gene program of neuroprotection discussed above [35].

Post-concussion Brain Vulnerability

The basic pathophysiological paths explored thus far have clarified some aspects of this particular clinical entity, suggesting that albeit concussion is considered a form of mTBI, should not to be considered so "mild." With the exception of the almost always punctual reversibility of all the metabolic and molecular modifications induced, it is probably not prudent to use the adjective "mild" when referring to a traumatic event that can have so many consequences involving fundamental functions of neuronal cell metabolism. However, while all of these biochemical modifications are scientifically interesting, they might appear, at a first glance, of negligible clinical utility because they are all spontaneously and fully reversible; moreover, patients with mTBI show no or minimal focal neurological problems and generally show a "radiologically" normal brain.

Despite the apparently "calm" clinical scenario and the reversible biochemical/metabolic damage, a reasonable body of evidence clearly demonstrated that "concussed" brain cells, although still perfectly functioning, during this period of molecular and biochemical alterations are truly under a peculiar state of "vulnerability," originally proposed by Hovda and colleagues [62]. If during this limited period of time neuronal cells sustain a second, typically nonlethal, insult in a close temporal proximity from the first, they would suffer irreversible damage and die [62]. Subsequent studies have strongly corroborated these original findings showing that during this transient period of altered brain metabolism, a second concussive episode may cause significant additional neuronal damage [63, 64]. In other words, concussion induces a pathophysiologic condition, mainly manifested by mitochondrial malfunctioning and energetic metabolic perturbations, that makes the brain more susceptible to a second trauma, even if of modest entity. This occurrence is capable of causing severe and sometimes irreversible cellular injury, thereby creating a disproportion between the trauma severity and the subsequent cerebral damage. It is worth recalling that, in the clinical setting, the possibility of having a second concussive injury within a not yet defined period of time from the first (i.e., days or weeks) has been reported to be even fatal in some instances [65–69], a phenomenon also known as the second impact syndrome (SIS), occasionally encountered in sports medicine [70].

Several studies in animals in which investigators focused on mTBI-induced dysfunction have been published, and current data support the concept of transient biochemical and physiologic alterations that may be exacerbated by repeated mild injuries within specific time windows of vulnerability [61, 63, 64]. In a rat weight drop experiment performed by applying a new and easily reproducible protocol to

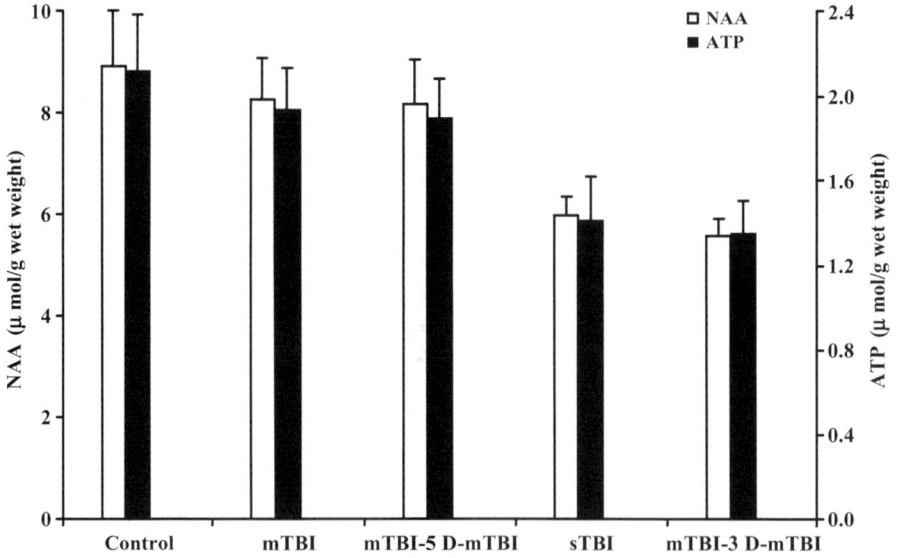

Fig. 6.2 Bar graph showing the changes in NAA and ATP cerebral concentrations in rats subjected to single mild or sTBI, or to repeat mTBI spaced by different time intervals (3 or 5 days). The traumatic insults were induced using the weight drop model with diffuse axonal injury. Animals were sacrificed 48 h after the last TBI and metabolites of interest were assayed by HPLC on deproteinized whole brain homogenates. Each histogram is the mean of six animals. Standard deviations are represented by *vertical bars*. No differences in both NAA and ATP were observed between a single mTBI and a repeat mTBI with 5-day interval (also no different from controls), as well as between a single sTBI and a repeat mTBI with 3-day interval (metabolites in these two groups of animals were significantly different from those recorded in controls, $p < 0.01$). This indicates that a second mTBI has no cumulative effects with the first one when falling outside the window of brain vulnerability; otherwise, the effects on brain metabolism are those observed after a single sTBI (cumulative effects in the case of two repeat mTBIs spaced by 3 days or more specifically the second injury occurs inside the window of brain vulnerability)

simulate a "second impact" condition, it was clearly demonstrated that levels of NAA, ATP, and the ATP/ADP ratio decreased significantly as a function of the time interval between two repeat concussions [61]. Maximal metabolic abnormalities were seen when the occurrence of two mild injuries was separated by a 3-day interval; in fact, the metabolic abnormalities in these animals were similar to those occurring after a single sTBI. However, when the two concussions were spaced by 5 days, results of the biochemical parameters were identical to those recorded in rats experiencing a single episode of mTBI (see also Fig. 6.2).

The other astonishing observation about this study was that of an identical 10 % mortality rate in animals subjected to a single sTBI and animals doubly injured by mTBI with a 3-day trauma interval; on the contrary, no animals died when subjected to a single mTBI or double-impact mTBI with a 5-day interval [61]. In a follow-up study, similar perturbations were found to persist as late as 7 days after double impact in animals receiving two mTBIs spaced by 3 days, indicating cumulative effects from repeat mTBI caused irreversible modifications of brain metabolism equal to those provoked by a single sTBI. Similar data were reported by Laurer et al. [71] in a histopathology study in which they described the important cumulative effects of two episodes of mTBI (24 h apart) in mice, which led to pronounced cellular damage when compared with animals that sustained a single trauma only. The authors concluded that although the brain was not morphologically damaged after a single concussive insult, its vulnerability to a second concussive impact was dangerously increased [71]. These results were reproduced in additional studies, either in the juvenile [72] or in the adult rat [73] thus corroborating the initial findings suggesting that the metabolic alterations can persist for days after concussion, creating no morphological damage but representing the pathological basis of the brain's vulnerability [62, 74].

According to the results of these studies, it may be affirmed that if the second concussion finds the cells fully committed to recover from the first insult, but still in a perfectly reversible energetic failure, it will cause further mitochondrial malfunctioning, leading to the same irreversible metabolic damage (characterized by permanent energetic failure) observed after a single severe injury [61, 73]. Thus, two mTBIs that occur too close in temporal proximity can replicate the effects of a single sTBI. The key biochemical issue of the vulnerable brain lies in the incomplete resolution of the initially reversible energetic crisis triggered by the first insult and, very probably, by the profound changes in the pattern of gene expression aimed at neuroprotection [35]. The foremost clinical implication of these experimental data is that within days after injury, the metabolic effects of two concussions can be dangerously additive. This information might not be surprising; however, similar human data regarding brain metabolites currently are not available. The second clinical implication of this notion is again remarkable because it is very difficult to establish how long the aforementioned period of brain vulnerability will last and when the occurrence of a second trauma would be uneventful.

In summary, all these preclinical data provide the experimental demonstration of the exquisitely metabolic nature of "brain vulnerability" kicked off by an mTBI, and offer a unique contribution to the complex biochemical damage underlying the clinical scenario of repeated concussive trauma, sometimes leading to catastrophic brain injury. Moreover, these data highlight that concussion triggers changes in cerebral cell homeostasis that can be evaluated at the molecular level, therefore representing key parameters with which to monitor the recovery of cell functions in post-concussed subjects.

"Imaging" the Brain's Biochemistry: The Role of Proton Magnetic Resonance Spectroscopy (¹H-MRS)

The above-described alterations of central energy metabolism might well represent a reasonable explanation of the striking and unpredictable discordance often observed between the minimal findings on conventional imaging [75] and the extent of neurocognitive deficits exhibited by patients with mTBI [76, 77]. As a fact, none of the currently available diagnostic tests [77–80] is capable of measuring this unique, transient, and potentially dangerous state of metabolic vulnerability of the "concussed" brain tissue, since changes during such a period are "visible" at the molecular level only.

The relevance of NAA as a biochemical marker of the metabolic neuronal "wealth" brings in a valid possibility to investigate changes in brain metabolism, stating that NAA and other groups of metabolites can be noninvasively measured "in vivo" by ^{1}H-MRS. This technique is based on the ability to localize the MRS signal into a specific volume of tissue, therefore providing a real-time "image" of the neurochemistry of certain brain regions, which in pathological states, differs from healthy tissue. The hardware for MRS is similar to standard MRI, requiring only additional software to suppress the signal of water, to capture the signal of various compounds at variable wavelength, and to provide analysis and imaging. Data can be obtained from either a single volume of brain, known as the single voxel spectroscopy, or a 2- or 3D analysis simultaneously acquired over a wider region, known as the multi-voxel spectroscopy or chemical shift imaging (CSI). Briefly, when subtracting the spectral signal of the ^{1}H of water (the most abundant molecule containing an atom with an unpaired proton, which is a prerequisite to allow to detect a molecule by MRS), the ^{1}H-NAA resonance returns one of the best defined peaks at approximately 2 ppm. By using the clinically safe magnetic fields of the MR apparatuses (1.5 or 3.0 T) in the range from 1.8 to 3.4 ppm two additional, well-resolved, resonance peaks are obtained, one at approximately 3.2 ppm referring to "choline" (Cho) and the other at approximately 2.9 ppm referring to "creatine" (Cr). It is worth recalling that the relatively low magnetic fields of 1.53.T currently used (with no clinical side effects) do not allow to discriminate the NAAG signal in the NAA peak or the creatine phosphate (CrP) signal in the Cr peak or to resolve about the ten different compounds containing the choline moiety in their molecule in the Cho peak [53].

However, when referring to NAA and Cr, this is of limited relevance since, in the brain tissue, NAA and Cr are about ten times more concentrated than the respective related compounds NAAG [51, 56] and CrP [81, 82] and the areas of these two peaks can generally be considered as legitimate measurements of NAA and Cr. Since the Cho peak is mainly composed by phosphocholine, glycerophosphocholine, and phosphatidylcholine, quantification of this peak area is not in direct correlation with one compound only. In summary, in a typical ^{1}H-MRS spectrum, the NAA peak represents the NAA-containing compounds (with NAA contributing for 90 % to the peak signal) and it is used as a marker of energy state and neuronal integrity, and the Cr peak represents creatine-containing compounds (with creatine accounting for 90 % of the intensity signal) and thought to be a further marker of cellular energy, while the Cho peak represents the choline-containing compounds (with phosphocholine, glycerophosphocholine, and phosphatidylcholine accounting for about 90 % of the intensity peak signal) the biological meaning of which is that of being related to the cell membrane turnover/density.

Unless determining the water content within the voxel(s) for a calculation of the absolute concentrations of the different metabolites [53, 83], it is always necessary to quantify at the same time all the three peak areas and carry out a semiquantitative evaluation of these metabolites expressed by the NAA/Cr and NAA/Cho and Cho/Cr ratios [84–89].

In a pilot study carried out in a cohort of ten concussed athletes, examined by ^{1}H-MRS for their NAA cerebral content at different time points after the concussive event, it was demonstrated that there was a significant decrease in NAA (either in terms of the NAA/Cr or NAA/Cho ratios) during the first 15 days post-injury with a subsequent normalization occurring 30 days after concussion [90]. An important finding of this study was that all athletes declared to be symptom-free within the first 15 days following the traumatic insult when brain metabolism was far to get normalized, i.e., disappearance of symptoms and metabolism rescue did not correlate. Furthermore, notwithstanding it was mandatory to restrain from physical activity before normalization of brain metabolism, three additional athletes enrolled in this study, prompted by the clearance from post-concussive symptoms, returned to play and experienced a second concussion between the tenth and the thirteenth day after the first insult. Although they were not affected by SIS nor showed signs of sTBI, they showed a significant delay in NAA normalization.

The results of this pilot study were confirmed by a recent multicenter clinical trial involving 40 concussed athletes and 30 healthy volunteers [91]. Thanks to the involvement of three neuroradiologic centers, we were initially able to demonstrate that, despite different combinations of field strengths (1.5 or 3.0 T) and modes of spectrum acquisition (single- or multi-voxel), results on relative NAA quantification did not depend on the scanners currently in use in most neuroradiology centers, confirming that NAA determination represents a quick (15-min), easy-to-perform, noninvasive tool to accurately measure changes in cerebral biochemical damage occurring after a concussion. The cohort of 40 concussed athletes was evaluated at 3, 15, 22, and 30 days post-impact by ^{1}H-MRS for the evaluation of brain metabolism. Patients exhibited the most significant decrease in NAA (evaluated in terms of metabolite ratios) at day 3 post-injury, showing a gradual nonlinear recovering, initially slow and, following day 15, faster.

At 30 days post-injury, all subjects showed complete recovery, having metabolite ratios not different from values detected in controls (see also Fig. 6.3). It is very important to underline that all these 40 patients self-declared symptom clearance between 3 and 15 days after concussion, confirming results of the pilot study [90] and strongly demonstrating differential times of disappearance of clinical gross signs and of normalization of NAA levels.

As clearly indicated in Fig. 6.4, it is also worth mentioning that the individual rate of NAA recovery varied from athlete to athlete, thus suggesting that this variation might have been due to possible differences in the severity of each concussion.

Bearing in mind results obtained in brain-injured rats, demonstrating the close similarity between NAA and ATP recovery following TBI, it is possible to affirm that the overall meaning of the aforementioned studies is that concussion in humans causes an evident energy failure detectable by ^{1}H-MRS in terms of NAA and opening a window of metabolic brain vulnerability the closure of which (normalization of brain NAA) occurs much later than clinical healing.

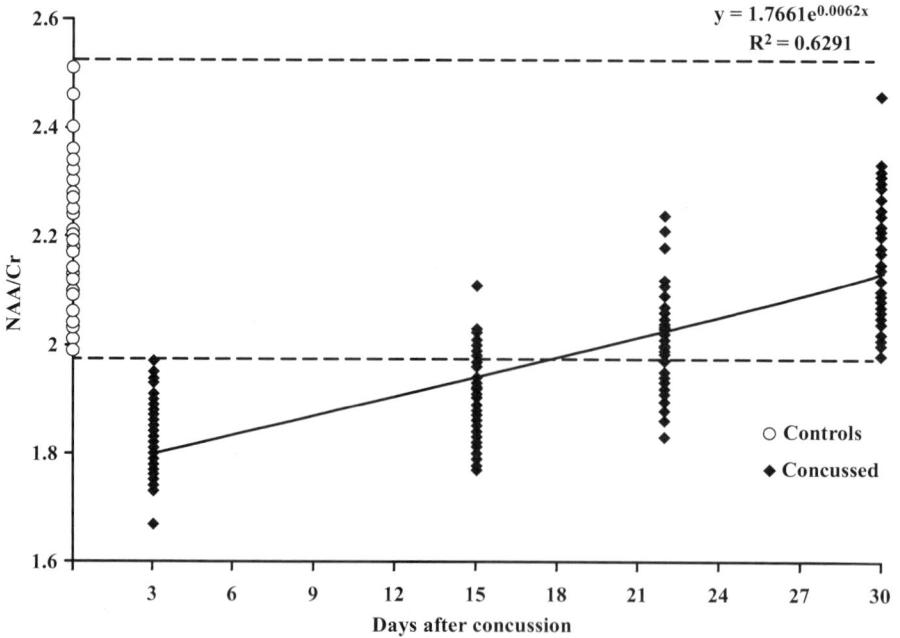

Fig. 6.3 Time-course changes in the NAA/Cr ratio recorded in 40 concussed athletes using proton magnetic resonance spectroscopy (^{1}H-MRS). Control values of the NAA/Cr ratio were obtained in a group of 30 age- and sex-matched healthy subjects, having no prior history of concussions. Recovery of brain metabolism followed a nonlinear trend, according to the exponential equation reported in the figure and suggested a slow recovery in the first 15 days and a much faster recovery in the second 15 days. In this group of athletes, 30 days was the time necessary to have the NAA/Cr ratio in all subjects fall within the range of variability of controls. It is very important to note that ALL athletes declared to be symptom-free at the time of the second ^{1}H-MRS when only 5/40 had values of the NAA/Cr ratio similar to those of controls, concluding that there was no correlation between clinical healing and normalization of brain metabolism

Recently, we had the opportunity to collect ^{1}H-MRS data from a group of six athletes who returned to play on symptom disappearance and received a second concussive episode when brain metabolism was still depressed [92]. The first impressive finding of this study was that while athletes were symptom-free in 5.8 ± 2.1 days after the first injury, 41.2 ± 13.0 days were necessary for symptom disappearance after the second concussion. The second very relevant observation (see Fig. 6.5) was that the time required to measure values of the NAA/Cr ratio similar to those recorded in controls was of 81.2 ± 24.4 days after the second concussion, i.e., again twice a longer time than that needed for clinical healing [92]. Last but not least, the NAA/Cr ratio recorded in these athletes in the next days after the second concussion was almost as low as that measured in severely injured patients [89].

It is well known that restraint from physical activity following concussion should be mandatory until the symptoms persist, to avoid the risk of insurgence of SIS, with SIS being interpreted as an acute, fatal disease caused by uncontrolled brain swelling.

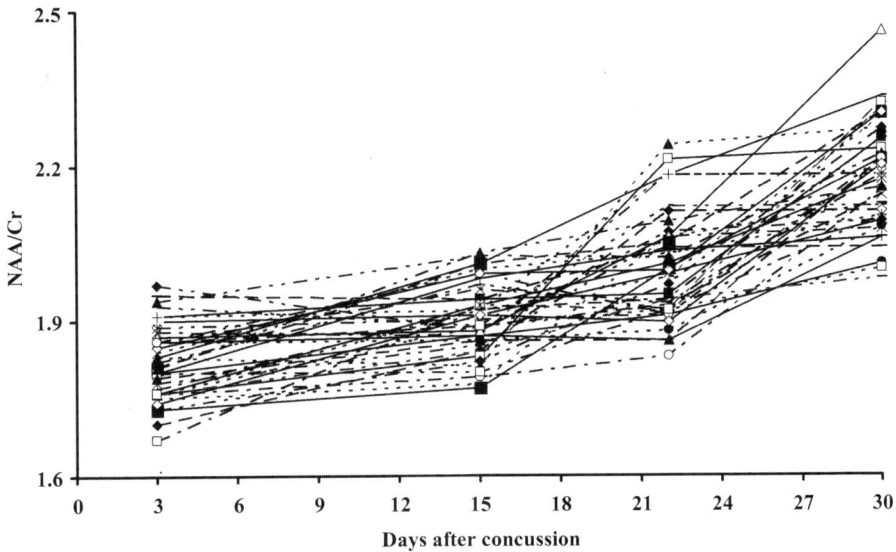

Fig. 6.4 Individual recovery of brain metabolism, evaluated in terms of NAA/Cr ratio by ^{1}H-MRS, occurring in the 40 concussed athletes shown in Fig. 6.3. As it is evident from this re-plotting, the rate of recovery, the time needed to restore normal concentration of metabolites related to brain energy metabolism, varies from subject to subject thus meaning that full normalization may occasionally be obtained earlier than 30 days after injury

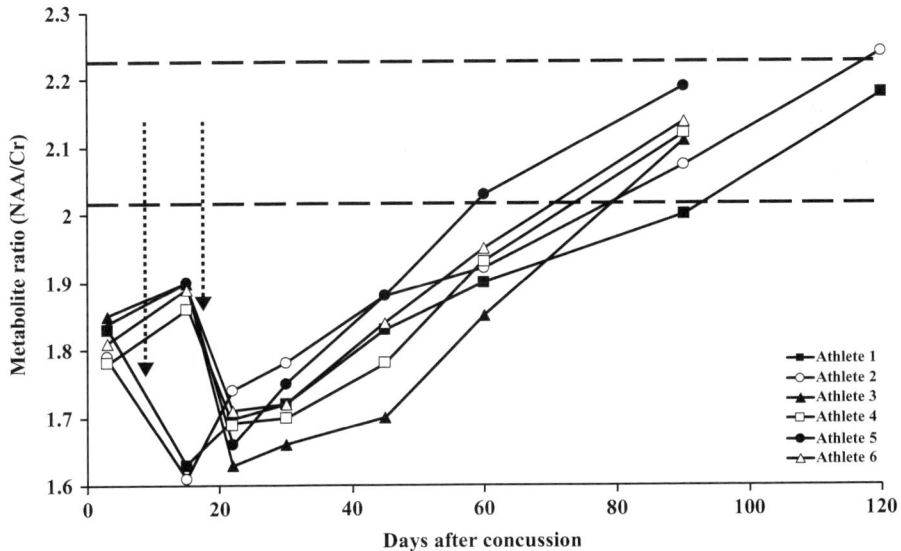

Fig. 6.5 Effect of two repeat concussions on the recovery of brain metabolism, evaluated in terms of NAA/Cr ratio by ^{1}H-MRS, in six athletes who received the second injury inside the window of metabolic brain vulnerability. The second concussive event, indicated by the arrows, occurred when athletes were symptom-free but had NAA/Cr ratio below the normal ranges (indicated in the figure by *horizontal dotted lines*). It is worth recalling that while duration of symptoms lasted 5.8 ± 2.1 days after the first injury, 41.2 ± 13.0 days were necessary for symptom disappearance after the second concussion. Analogously, it was observed a much longer time (81.2 ± 24.4 days) to obtain normalization of cerebral energy metabolism after the second concussion

A handful of previously published cases have been reported on patients (mostly involved in sports-related activities) who experienced a second injury that unexpectedly and unpredictably led to sustained intracranial hypertension and catastrophic outcomes [93].

Nowadays, by virtue of all the aforementioned studies, we can state with reasonable confidence that, during symptoms permanence after an mTBI, the brain, in that very time, is certainly still vulnerable to a hypothetic second concussion. The topic, however, is much more complicated by the fact that the resolution of clinical symptoms does not coincide with the "closure" of the temporal window of brain metabolic imbalance "opened" by the first trauma. Thus, it appears dramatically clear that the question of whether the brain had fully recovered from the metabolic disturbances caused from the first concussive injury must not remain unanswered and it is also difficult to imagine that a symptom-free, post-concussed athlete is allowed to go back on the field with the quasi certainty that his brain is still suffering from metabolic abnormalities.

The restricted cohort of doubly concussed athletes described above certainly opens a further discussion. In fact, although all athletes received two repeat concussions approximately of the same severity (for each athlete, both events were characterized by the same acute symptoms with no change in GCS and a negative MRI), clinical symptoms after the second impact lasted much longer than the first one. In other words, the effects of the second concussion were not fatal, but they were somehow not proportionate to the entity of the second concussive insult. Most likely, the second concussion occurred when the brain cells were completing the recovery of impaired metabolic functions, and thus it only produced a limited cumulative effect with moderate worsening of the clinical pictures.

Hence, it is conceivable to infer that, in the case of repeat concussions, it is the time interval between the two concussions that drives the clinical and metabolic evolution. The reason why SIS is, fortunately, an extremely rare condition is probably because it represents a sort of "perfect storm" [94], an extremely random and hardly predictable situation generated by the odd combination of the severity of the initial concussion, the time interval between the two traumas, and the metabolic state of the brain at the time of the second concussion. However, from the results obtained in our doubly concussed athletes, it is conceivable to sustain that SIS may be a concept to revise and not to limit the rare cases with fatal prognosis. Possibly, SIS of lower grades is encountered any time a disproportion between the entity of the second concussion and normalization of brain metabolism (but also of clinical healing) is observed.

Once again the question of whether the brain has completed its metabolic healing from the initial insult cannot be left unanswered. Furthermore, it is also hard to imagine that a concussed athlete measured by ^{1}H-MRS and found metabolically depressed (low NAA/Cr or NAA/Cho ratios) is allowed to return to play instead of waiting for brain energy metabolism normalization.

In a very recent paper describing 11 cases of concussed athletes, it was also pointed out that in some instances, alteration of brain metabolism goes deeper, involving not only NAA but Cr too [95]. This group of athletes suffered from a more severe concussive event, causing longer time in both clinical and metabolic recovery and a more pronounced imbalance of metabolism (change in both NAA and Cr concentrations). These clinical results were corroborated by previous data from a bench study. In fact, in rats following mTBI, in addition to NAA and ATP, Cr underwent a reversible 44.5 % decline, which was accompanied by a less than 15 % CrP diminution at the same time point (24 h post-mTBI). Altogether, the sum of Cr + CrP in brain of these mTBI rats accounted for a 42 % decrease at 24 h post-injury [96]. This transient depletion of the cerebral Cr compound pool was restored following 120 h from mTBI. In the same animal study, it was also showed that mTBI did not affect the concentration of phosphatidylcholine, i.e., one of the main compounds responsible for the intensity signal of the Cho peak in the ^{1}H-MRS spectrum. Recent data seem to indicate that the Cr–CrP system plays an important role in performing the translocation of newly synthesized ATP from the mitochondrial to the cytoplasmic compartment [97, 98] and that Cr may act as a neurotransmitter [99].

The decrease in total Cr levels observed in those athletes may well be explained by the experimentally documented general depression of brain metabolism after mTBI and the correspondence to the window of metabolic brain vulnerability that may have occurred in coincidence of concussive episodes of severity higher than that causing NAA decrease only. If this were true, the ^{1}H-MRS evaluation of brain metabolism may open the possibility to biochemically grade concussion that may be associated either to the time necessary for the metabolic recovery or to the simultaneity in the decrease of NAA and Cr. One example of grading concussion on the basis of the time needed for the metabolic recovery occurred in four athletes, for whom the return to play was based not only on symptom disappearance but mainly on NAA normalization, is given in Fig. 6.6.

All data presented question the validity of clinical criteria, neuropsychological tests, and balance tests to determine the safe return of athletes to play since demonstrating that the recovery of brain metabolism certainly occurs much later than disappearance of post-concussive symptoms and normalization of other currently used tests. Apart from signs and symptoms, which of course play a fundamental role to diagnose and to initially manage the concussion, there is a desperate need to "biologically" grade the "severity" of a concussion and this can only be done by using objective, quantifiable parameters of biological relevance in the understanding of the recovery following the traumatic event and the closure of the window of brain vulnerability.

^{1}H-MRS allows the monitoring of a real time-course of NAA, Cr, and Cho following mTBI, demonstrating the transient cerebral hypometabolism (decrease in NAA and Cr) and the metabolic brain vulnerability period. ^{1}H-MRS is a potent, unique tool with which one can monitor the "closure" of the window of metabolic brain vulnerability. Furthermore, the very recent report carried out in a cohort of 24 symptom-free concussed athletes (as assessed by clinical self-reported symptom resolution, cognitive and clinical balance testing (SCAT-2 and BESS), and clearance from a medical professional for the first stage of aerobic activity) showed significant alterations in brain metabolism (decrease in NAA in the genu but not in the splenium of the corpus callosum) strongly support the concept that clinical healing is not coincidental with normalization of brain metabolism [100].

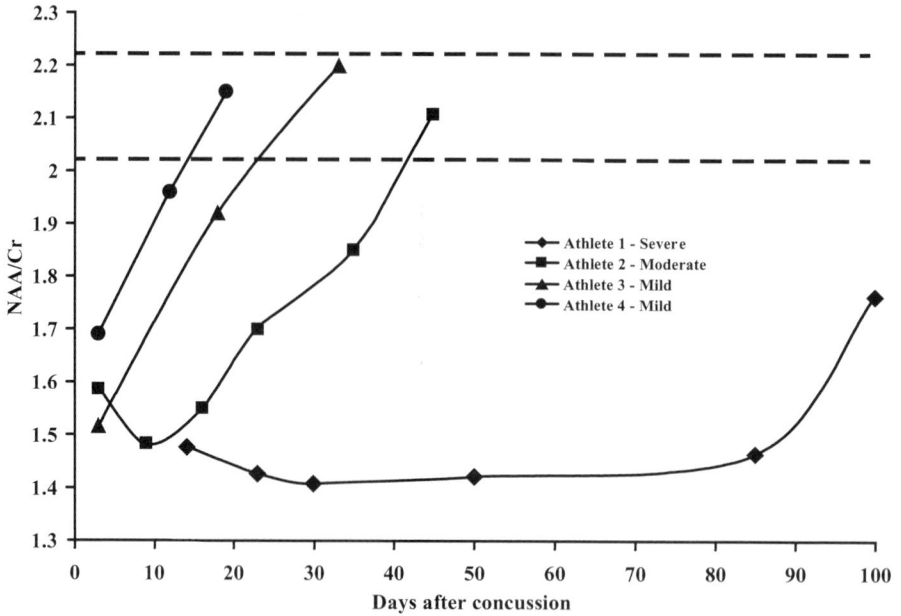

Fig. 6.6 Glaring example of the potentiality in the use of ¹H-MRS to grade concussion by means of the semiquantitative determination of an objective, biochemical parameter. According to the time of recovery of NAA, it was possible to discriminate severe (athlete 1), moderate (athlete 2), and mild concussion (athletes 3 and 4) in these four concussed soccer players (three "Serie A" top players and one semiprofessional player)

Furthermore, recent studies also questioned the validity of determining the return to play upon the simple normalization of neuropsychological tests [101, 102], thus reinforcing the concept that different objective diagnostic approaches in the evaluation of post-concussed athletes are necessary. In athletes affected by sports-related concussions, the use of ¹H-MRS should be highly recommended to evaluate recovery of their cerebral metabolism for a more secure return to the field.

Conclusions

Experimental studies demonstrated that concussion, which is a peculiar type of mTBI frequently encountered in sports medicine, is characterized by complex alterations of various important functions of neuronal cells, including mitochondrial-related energy supply, ionic homeostasis, neurotransmitters, NAA homeostasis, and even gene expression, leading to questions about the appropriateness of the term *mild*. Particular emphasis was given to the fact that most of the molecular and metabolic derangements are of limited duration (spontaneous recovery of metabolism and cell functions), representing the bases of the metabolic brain vulnerability occurring after mTBI. From a metabolic point of view, it was shown that changes in ATP induced by mTBI mirror those occurring to NAA, rendering this molecule a surrogate marker to monitor brain energy metabolism following concussion.

The application of the so-called advanced neuroimaging techniques (^{1}H-MRS, fMR, DTI, PET) in clinical studies allows improvement of our understanding of the pathophysiology of concussions by producing objective data of relevance in assessing normalization of brain functions. The open question on when to allow the return of a concussed athlete to play certainly received important answers by the use of ^{1}H-MRS to monitor disturbances and recovery of brain metabolism in concussed athletes. Thanks to the solidity of the preclinical data and to the parameters measured which are of exquisite biochemical importance, ^{1}H-MRS currently represents the sole technique with which to study the recovery of brain metabolism in the subacute phases following concussion, capable to intercept compounds related to energy metabolism and mitochondrial functions (NAA and Cr). The application of ^{1}H-MRS allows for the determination of the closure of the dangerous temporal window of metabolic brain vulnerability therefore increasing the safeness of athletes' return to play.

References

1. de Kruijk JR, Twijnstra A, Leffers P. Diagnostic criteria and differential diagnosis of mild traumatic brain injury. Brain Inj. 2001;15:99–106.
2. Bruns J, Hauser WA. The epidemiology of traumatic brain injury: a review. Epilepsia. 2003;44 Suppl 10:2–10.
3. Roozenbeek B, Maas A, Menon DK. Changing patterns in the epidemiology of traumatic brain injury. Nat Rev Neurol. 2013;9:231–6.
4. van der Naalt J. Prediction of outcome in mild to moderate head injury: a review. J Clin Exp Neuropsychol. 2001;23:837–51.
5. Vos PE, Battistin L, Birbamer G, Gerstenbrand F, Potapov A, Prevec T, et al. EFNS guideline on mild traumatic brain injury report of an EFNS task force. Eur J Neurol. 2002;9:207–19.
6. Kushner D. Mild traumatic brain injury toward understanding manifestations and treatment. Arch Intern Med. 1998;158:1617–24.
7. McCrea M, Kelly JP, Randolph C, Cisler R, Berger L. Immediate neurocognitive effects of concussion. Neurosurgery. 2002;50:1032–42.
8. Esselman PC, Uomoto JM. Classification of the spectrum of mild traumatic brain injury. Brain Inj. 1995;9:417–24.
9. Aubry M, Cantu R, Dvorak J, Graf-Baumann T, Johnston K, Kelly J, et al. Summary and agreement statement of the first international conference on concussion in sport, Vienna 2001. Recommendations for the improvement of safety and health of athletes who may suffer concussive injuries. Br J Sports Med. 2002;36:6–10.
10. McCrory P, Johnston K, Meeuwisse W, Aubry M, Cantu R, Dvorak J, et al. Summary and agreement statement of the 2nd international conference on concussion in sport, Prague 2004. Br J Sports Med. 2005;39:196–204.
11. McCrory P, Meeuwisse W, Johnston K, Dvorak J, Aubry M, Molloy M, et al. Consensus statement on concussion in sport 3rd international conference on concussion in sport held in Zurich, November 2008. Clin J Sport Med. 2009;19:185–200.
12. Meehan WP, Bachur RG. Sport-related concussion. Pediatrics. 2009;123:114–23.

13. Maroon JC, Lovell MR, Norwig J, Podelek K, Powell JW, Hartl R. Cerebral concussion in athletes: evaluation and neuropsychological testing. Neurosurgery. 2000;47:659–69.

14. Sinson G, Bagley LJ, Cecil KM, Torchia M, McGowan JC, Lenkinski RE, McIntosh TK, Grossman RI. Magnetization transfer imaging and proton MR spectroscopy in the evaluation of axonal injury: correlation with clinical outcome after traumatic brain injury. AJNR Am J Neuroradiol. 2001;22:143–51.

15. Johnson B, Zhang K, Gay M, Horovitz S, Hallett M, Sebastianelli W, et al. Alteration of brain default network in subacute phase of injury in concussed individuals resting-state fMRI study. Neuroimage. 2012;59:511–8.

16. Zhang K, Johnson B, Pennell D, Ray W, Sebastianelli W, Slobounov S. Are functional deficits in concussed individuals consistent with white matter structural alterations combined FMRI and DTI study. Exp Brain Res. 2010;204:57–70.

17. Lipton ML, Gellella E, Lo C, Gold T, Ardekani BA, Shifteh K, et al. Multifocal white matter ultrastructural abnormalities in mild traumatic brain injury with cognitive disability, a voxel-wise analysis of diffusion tensor imaging. J Neurotrauma. 2008;25:1335–42.

18. Kou Z, Wu Z, Tong KA, Holshouser B, Benson RR, Hu J, et al. The role of advanced MR imaging findings as biomarkers of traumatic brain injury. J Head Trauma Rehabil. 2010; 25:267–82.

19. Farkas O, Lifshitz J, Povlishock JT. Mechanoporation induced by diffuse traumatic brain injury: an irreversible or reversible response to injury? J Neurosci. 2006;26:3130–40.

20. Barkhoudarian G, Hovda DA, Giza CC. The molecular pathophysiology of concussive brain injury. Clin Sports Med. 2011;30:33–48.

21. Faden AI, Demediuk P, Panter SS, Vink R. The role of excitatory amino acids and NMDA receptors in traumatic brain injury. Science. 1989;244:798–800.

22. Katayama Y, Becker DP, Tamura T, Hovda DA. Massive increases in extracellular potassium and the indiscriminate release of glutamate following concussive brain injury. J Neurosurg. 1990;73:889–900.

23. Reger ML, Poulos AM, Buen F, Giza CC, Hovda DA, Fanselow MS. Concussive brain injury enhances fear learning and excitatory processes in the amygdala. Biol Psychiatry. 2012;71: 335–43.

24. Smith SL, Andrus PK, Zhang JR, Hall ED. Direct measurement of hydroxyl radicals, lipid peroxidation, and blood-brain barrier disruption following unilateral cortical impact head injury in the rat. J Neurotrauma. 1994;11:393–404.

25. Vagnozzi R, Marmarou A, Tavazzi B, Signoretti S, Di Pierro D, Del Bolgia F, et al. Changes of cerebral energy metabolism and lipid peroxidation in rats leading to mitochondrial dysfunction after diffuse brain injury. J Neurotrauma. 1999;16:903–13.

26. Zoratti M, Szab I. The mitochondrial permeability transition. Biochim Biophys Acta. 1995;1241:139–76.

27. Paradies G, Paradies V, Ruggiero FM, Petrosillo G. Changes in the mitochondrial permeability transition pore in aging and age-associated diseases. Mech Ageing Dev. 2013;134:1–9.

28. Schinder AF, Olson EC, Spitzer NC, Montal M. Mitochondrial dysfunction is a primary event in glutamate neurotoxicity. J Neurosci. 1996;16:6125–33.

29. Lifshitz J, Friberg H, Neumar RW, Raghupathi R, Welsh FA, Janmey P, et al. Structural and functional damage sustained by mitochondria after traumatic brain injury in the rat: evidence for differentially sensitive populations in the cortex and hippocampus. J Cereb Blood Flow Metab. 2003;23(2):219–31.

30. Yoshino A, Hovda DA, Kawamata T, Becker DP. Dynamic changes in local cerebral glucose utilization following cerebral conclusion in rats: evidence of a hyper and subsequent hypo-metabolic state. Brain Res. 1991;561:106–19.

31. Kawamata T, Katayama Y, Hovda DA, Yoshino A, Becker DP. Administration of excitatory amino acid antagonists via microdialysis attenuates the increase in glucose utilization seen following concussive brain injury. J Cereb Blood Flow Metab. 1992;12:12–24.

32. Andersen BJ, Marmarou A. Post-traumatic selective stimulation of glycolysis. Brain Res. 1992;585:184–9.

33. Marklund N, Sihver S, Hovda DA, Långström B, Watanabe Y, Ronquist G, et al. Increased cerebral uptake of [18F] fluoro-deoxyglucose but not [1-14C] glucose early following traumatic brain injury in rats. J Neurotrauma. 2009;26:1281–93.
34. Di Pietro V, Amin D, Pernagallo S, Lazzarino G, Tavazzi B, Vagnozzi R, et al. Transcriptomics of traumatic brain injury gene expression and molecular pathways of different grades of insult in a rat organotypic hippocampal culture model. J Neurotrauma. 2010;27:349–59.
35. Di Pietro V, Amorini AM, Tavazzi B, Hovda DA, Signoretti S, Giza CC, et al. Potentially neuroprotective gene modulation in an in vitro model of mild traumatic brain injury. Mol Cell Biochem. 2013;375:185–98.
36. Tavazzi B, Vagnozzi R, Signoretti S, Amorini AM, Belli A, Cimatti M, et al. Temporal window of metabolic brain vulnerability to concussions oxidative and nitrosative stresses—part II. Neurosurgery. 2007;61:390–6.
37. Harris LK, Black RT, Golden KM, Reeves TM, Povlishock JT, Phillips LL. Traumatic brain injury-induced changes in gene expression and functional activity of mitochondrial cytochrome C oxidase. J Neurotrauma. 2001;18:993–1009.
38. Tavazzi B, Signoretti S, Lazzarino G, Amorini AM, Delfini R, Cimatti M, et al. Cerebral oxidative stress and depression of energy metabolism correlate with severity of diffuse brain injury in rats. Neurosurgery. 2005;56:582–9.
39. Wu A, Ying Z, Gomez-Pinilla F. The salutary effects of DHA dietary supplementation on cognition, neuroplasticity, and membrane homeostasis after brain trauma. J Neurotrauma. 2011;28:2113–22.
40. Giza CC, Hovda DA. The neurometabolic cascade of concussion. J Athl Train. 2001; 36:228–35.
41. Moffett JR, Ross B, Arun P, Madhavarao CN, Namboodiri AM. N-acetylaspartate in the CNS: from neurodiagnostics to neurobiology. Prog Neurobiol. 2007;81:89–131.
42. Rigotti DJ, Kirov II, Djavadi B, Perry N, Babb JS, Gonen O. Longitudinal whole-brain N-acetylaspartate concentration in healthy adults. AJNR Am J Neuroradiol. 2011;32: 1011–5.
43. Moffett JR, Arun P, Ariyannur PS, Garbern JY, Jacobowitz DM, Namboodiri AM. Extensive aspartoacylase expression in the rat central nervous system. Glia. 2011;59:1414–34.
44. Wiame E, Tyteca D, Pierrot N, Collard F, Amyere M, Noel G, et al. Molecular identification of aspartate N-acetyltransferase and its mutation in hypoacetylaspartia. Biochem J. 2010;425: 127–36.
45. Baslow MH. Brain N-acetylaspartate as a molecular water pump and its role in the etiology of Canavan disease: a mechanistic explanation. J Mol Neurosci. 2003;21:185–90.
46. Baslow MH. N-acetylaspartate in the vertebrate brain: metabolism and function. Neurochem Res. 2003;28:941–53.
47. Satrústegui J, Contreras L, Ramos M, Marmol P, del Arco A, Saheki T, et al. Role of aralar, the mitochondrial transporter of aspartate-glutamate, in brain N-acetylaspartate formation and Ca(2+) signaling in neuronal mitochondria. J Neurosci Res. 2007;85:3359–66.
48. Kaul R, Gao GP, Aloya M, Balamurugan K, Petrosky A, Michals K, et al. Canavan disease mutations among Jewish and non-Jewish patients. Am J Hum Genet. 1994;55:34–41.
49. Elpeleg ON, Shaag A. The spectrum of mutations of the aspartoacylase gene in Canavan disease in non-Jewish patients. J Inherit Metab Dis. 1999;225:315–34.
50. Di Pietro V, Gambacurta A, Amorini AM, Finocchiaro A, D'Urso S, Ceccarelli L, et al. A new T677C mutation of the aspartoacylase gene encodes for a protein with no enzymatic activity. Clin Biochem. 2008;41:611–5.
51. Tavazzi B, Lazzarino G, Leone P, Amorini AM, Bellia F, Janson CG, et al. Simultaneous high performance liquid chromatographic separation of purines, pyrimidines, N-acetylated amino acids, and dicarboxylic acids for the chemical diagnosis of inborn errors of metabolism. Clin Biochem. 2005;38:997–1008.
52. Cozzolino M, Augello B, Carella M, Palumbo O, Tavazzi B, Amorini AM, et al. Chromosomal 17p13.3 microdeletion unmasking recessive Canavan disease mutation. Mol Genet Metab. 2011;104:706–7.

53. Rigotti DJ, Inglese M, Gonen O. Whole-brain N-acetylaspartate as a surrogate marker of neuronal damage in diffuse neurologic disorders. AJNR Am J Neuroradiol. 2007; 2818:43–9.
54. Signoretti S, Marmarou A, Tavazzi B, Lazzarino G, Beaumont A, Vagnozzi R. N-acetylaspartate reduction as a measure of injury severity and mitochondrial dysfunction following diffuse traumatic brain injury. J Neurotrauma. 2001;18:977–91.
55. Lazzarino G, Di Pierro D, Tavazzi B, Cerroni L, Giardina B. Simultaneous separation of malondialdehyde, ascorbic acid, and adenine nucleotide derivatives from biological samples by ion-pairing high-performance liquid chromatography. Anal Biochem. 1991;197:191–6.
56. Tavazzi B, Vagnozzi R, Di Pierro D, Amorini AM, Fazzina G, Signoretti S, et al. Ion-pairing high-performance liquid chromatographic method for the detection of N-acetylaspartate and N-acetylglutamate in cerebral tissue extracts. Anal Biochem. 2000;277:104–8.
57. Benedetti B, Rigotti DJ, Liu S, Filippi M, Grossman RI, Gonen O. Reproducibility of the whole-brain N-acetylaspartate level across institutions, MR scanners, and field strengths. AJNR Am J Neuroradiol. 2007;287:2–5.
58. Cohen BA, Inglese M, Rusinek H, Babb JS, Grossman RI, Gonen O. Proton MR spectroscopy and MRI-volumetry in mild traumatic brain injury. AJNR Am J Neuroradiol. 2007;28: 907–13.
59. Govindaraju V, Gauger G, Manley G, Ebel A, Meeker M, Maudsley AA. Volumetric proton spectroscopic imaging of mild traumatic brain injury. AJNR Am J Neuroradiol. 2004;25: 730–7.
60. Govind V, Gold S, Kaliannan K, Saigal G, Falcone S, Arheart KL, et al. Whole-brain proton MR spectroscopic imaging of mild-to moderate traumatic brain injury and correlation with neuropsychological deficits. J Neurotrauma. 2010;27:483–96.
61. Vagnozzi R, Tavazzi B, Signoretti S, Amorini AM, Belli A, Cimatti M, et al. Temporal window of metabolic brain vulnerability to concussions: mitochondrial-related impairment—part I. Neurosurgery. 2007;61:379–89.
62. Hovda DA, Badie H, Karimi S, Thomas S, Yoshino A, Kawamata T. Concussive brain injury produces a state of vulnerability for intracranial pressure perturbation in the absence of morphological damage. In: Avezaat CJJ, van Eijndhoven JHM, Maas AIR, Tans JT, editors. Intracranial pressure VIII. New York: Springer; 1983. p. 469–72.
63. Longhi L, Saatman KE, Fujimoto S, Raghupathi R, Meaney DF, Davis J, et al. Temporal window of vulnerability to repetitive experimental concussive brain injury. Neurosurgery. 2005;56:364–74.
64. Vagnozzi R, Signoretti S, Tavazzi B, Cimatti M, Amorini AM, Donzelli S, et al. Hypothesis of the postconcussive vulnerable brain experimental evidence of its metabolic occurrence. Neurosurgery. 2005;57:164–71.
65. Bowen AP. Second impact syndrome: a rare, catastrophic, preventable complication of concussion in young athletes. J Emerg Nurs. 2003;29(3):287–9.
66. Cantu RC. Second-impact syndrome. Clin Sports Med. 1998;17:37–44.
67. Cobb S, Battin B. Second-impact syndrome. J Sch Nurs. 2004;20:262–7.
68. Logan SM, Bell GW, Leonard JC. Acute subdural hematoma in a high school football player after 2 unreported episodes of head trauma: a case report. J Athl Train. 2001;36:433–6.
69. Mori T, Katayama Y, Kawamata T. Acute hemispheric swelling associated with thin subdural hematomas: pathophysiology of repetitive head injury in sports. Acta Neurochir Suppl. 2006;96:40–3.
70. Saunders RL, Harbaugh RE. The second impact in catastrophic contact-sports head trauma. JAMA. 1984;252:538–9.
71. Laurer HL, Bareyre FM, Lee VM, Trojanowski JQ, Longhi L, Hoover R, et al. Mild head injury increasing the brain's vulnerability to a second concussive impact. J Neurosurg. 2001;95:859–70.
72. Prins ML, Hales A, Reger M, Giza CC, Hovda DA. Repeat traumatic brain injury in the juvenile rat is associated with increased axonal injury and cognitive impairments. Dev Neurosci. 2010;32:510–8.

73. Prins ML, Alexander D, Giza CC, Hovda DA. Repeated mild traumatic brain injury: mechanisms of cerebral vulnerability. J Neurotrauma. 2013;30:30–8.
74. Doberstein CE, Hovda DA, Becker DP. Clinical considerations in the reduction of secondary brain injury. Ann Emerg Med. 1993;22:993–7.
75. Kurca E, Sivk S, Kucera P. Impaired cognitive functions in mild traumatic brain injury patients with normal and pathologic magnetic resonance imaging. Neuroradiology. 2006; 486:61–9.
76. Hunt T, Asplund C. Concussion assessment and management. Clin Sports Med. 2010;29: 5–17.
77. McCrea M, Guskiewicz KM, Marshall SW, Barr W, Randolph C, Cantu RC, et al. Acute effects and recovery time following concussion in collegiate football players: the NCAA Concussion Study. JAMA. 2003;290:2556–63.
78. Schatz P, Pardini JE, Lovell MR, Collins MW, Podell K. Sensitivity and specificity of the ImPACT Test Battery for concussion in athletes. Arch Clin Neuropsychol. 2006;21:9–19.
79. Broglio SP, Macciocchi SN, Ferrara MS. Sensitivity of the concussion assessment battery. Neurosurgery. 2007;60:105–8.
80. Register-Mihalik JK, Mihalik JP, Guskiewicz KM. Balance deficits after sports-related concussion in individuals reporting posttraumatic headache. Neurosurgery. 2008;63:76–80.
81. Galbraith RA, Furukawa M, Li M. Possible role of creatine concentrations in the brain in regulating appetite and weight. Brain Res. 2006;1101:85–91.
82. Seidl R, Stöckler-Ipsiroglu S, Rolinski B, Kohlhauser C, Herkner KR, Lubec B, Lubec G. Energy metabolism in graded perinatal asphyxia of the rat. Life Sci. 2000;67:421–35.
83. Barker PB, Soher BJ, Blackband SJ, Chatham JC, Mathews VP, Bryan RN. Quantitation of proton NMR spectra of the human brain using tissue water as an internal concentration reference. NMR Biomed. 1993;6:89–94.
84. Friedman SD, Brooks WM, Jung RE, Chiulli SJ, Sloan JH, Montoya BT, Hart BL, Yeo RA. Quantitative proton MRS predicts outcome after traumatic brain injury. Neurology. 1999;52: 1384–91.
85. Brooks WM, Stidley CA, Petropoulos H, Jung RE, Weers DC, Friedman SD, Barlow MA, Sibbitt Jr WL, Yeo RA. Metabolic and cognitive response to human traumatic brain injury: a quantitative proton magnetic resonance study. J Neurotrauma. 2000;17:629–40.
86. Garnett MR, Blamire AM, Corkill RG, Cadoux-Hudson TA, Rajagopalan B, Styles P. Early proton magnetic resonance spectroscopy in normal-appearing brain correlates with outcome in patients following traumatic brain injury. Brain. 2000;123:2046–54.
87. Brooks WM, Friedman SD, Gasparovic C. Magnetic resonance spectroscopy in traumatic brain injury. J Head Trauma Rehabil. 2001;16:149–64.
88. Mitsumoto H, Ulug AM, Pullman SL, Gooch CL, Chan S, Tang MX, et al. Quantitative objective markers for upper and lower motor neuron dysfunction in ALS. Neurology. 2007; 68:1402–10.
89. Signoretti S, Marmarou A, Aygok GA, Fatouros PP, Portella G, Bullock RM. Assessment of mitochondrial impairment in traumatic brain injury using high-resolution proton magnetic resonance spectroscopy. J Neurosurg. 2008;108:42–52.
90. Vagnozzi R, Signoretti S, Tavazzi B, Floris R, Ludovici A, Marziali S, et al. Temporal window of metabolic brain vulnerability to concussion: a pilot 1H-magnetic resonance spectroscopic study in concussed athletes—part III. Neurosurgery. 2008;62:1286–96.
91. Vagnozzi R, Signoretti S, Cristofori L, Alessandrini F, Floris R, Isgr E, et al. Assessment of metabolic brain damage and recovery following mild traumatic brain injury: a multicentre, proton magnetic resonance spectroscopic study in concussed patients. Brain. 2011;33: 3232–42.
92. Vagnozzi R, Signoretti S, Manara M, Tavazzi B, Floris R, Amorini AM, et al. The importance of restriction from physical activity in the metabolic recovery of concussed brain. In: Agrawal A, editor. Brain injury: pathogenesis, monitoring, recovery and management. Rijeka, Croatia: InTech; 2012. p. 501–22. ISBN 978-953-51-0265-6.

93. Cantu RC, Gean AD. Second-impact syndrome and a small subdural hematoma uncommon catastrophic result of repetitive head injury with a characteristic imaging appearance. J Neurotrauma. 2010;27:1557–64.
94. Signoretti S, Lazzarino G, Tavazzi B, Vagnozzi R. The pathophysiology of concussion. PM R. 2011;3 Suppl 2:S359–68.
95. Vagnozzi R, Signoretti S, Floris R, Marziali S, Manara M, Amorini AM, et al. Decrease in N-acetylaspartate following concussion may be coupled to decrease in creatine. J Head Trauma Rehabil. 2013;28(4):284–92. doi:10.1097/HTR.0b013e3182795045.
96. Signoretti S, Di Pietro V, Vagnozzi R, Lazzarino G, Amorini AM, Belli A, D'Urso S, Tavazzi B. Transient alterations of creatine, creatine phosphate, N-acetylaspartate and high-energy phosphates after mild traumatic brain injury in the rat. Mol Cell Biochem. 2010;333: 269–77.
97. Tachikawa M, Fujinawa J, Takahashi M, Kasai Y, Fukaya M, Sakai K, et al. Expression and possible role of creatine transporter in the brain and at the blood cerebrospinal fluid barrier as a transporting protein of guanidinoacetate, an endogenous convulsant. J Neurochem. 2008; 107:768–78.
98. Beard E, Braissant O. Synthesis and transport of creatine in the CNS: importance for cerebral functions. J Neurochem. 2010;115:297–313.
99. Royes LF, Fighera MR, Furian AF, Oliveira MS, Fiorenza NG, Ferreira J, et al. Neuromodulatory effect of creatine on extracellular action potentials in rat hippocampus: role of NMDA receptors. Neurochem Int. 2008;53:33–7.
100. Johnson B, Gay M, Zhang K, Neuberger T, Horovitz SG, Hallett M, et al. The use of magnetic resonance spectroscopy in the subacute evaluation of athletes recovering from single and multiple mild traumatic brain injury. J Neurotrauma. 2012;29:2297–304.
101. Randolph C. Baseline neuropsychological testing in managing sport-related concussion. Does it modify risk? Curr Sports Med Rep. 2011;10:21–6.
102. Mayers LB, Redick TS. Clinical utility of ImPACT assessment for postconcussion return-to-play counseling psychometric issues. J Clin Exp Neuropsychol. 2012;34:235–42.

Part II
Biomechanical Mechanisms of Concussion and Helmets

Chapter 7
The Biomechanics of Concussion: 60 Years of Experimental Research

Stefan M. Duma and Steven Rowson

Abstract Over the past 60 years, researchers across the planet have worked to understand the biomechanics of concussion and associated brain injuries. This chapter presents a summary of these efforts that begin with the human cadaver research performed in the 1950s and served as the foundation for the severity index and head injury criterion injury metrics. Following this research, experiments were performed on primates in order to quantify the injury physiology associated with concussion. More recently, the National Football League reconstructed concussive impacts and presented the first injury risk functions for concussion. The fourth dataset includes over two million head impacts measured with helmet instrumentation on volunteers playing football. By analyzing all of these data together, researchers have presented an array of injury risk functions for concussion that use both linear and rotational head acceleration parameters. Laboratory experiments utilize these risk functions to evaluate the performance of helmets and their ability to reduce the risk of concussion. Clinical studies have been performed that support and confirm the laboratory findings. The future of helmet testing will utilize a new impact system that more accurately reflects the head and neck kinematics the players experience during head impacts in sports.

Keywords Concussion • Biomechanics • mTBI • Sports • Acceleration • Brain • Helmet • Criteria • Linear acceleration • Rotational acceleration • Injury risk function

S.M. Duma, Ph.D. (✉) • S. Rowson, Ph.D.
School of Biomedical Engineering and Sciences, Virginia Tech—Wake Forest University,
313 Kelly Hall, 325 Stanger Street, MC 0298, Blacksburg, VA 24061, USA
e-mail: headbiomed@vt.edu

S.M. Slobounov and W.J. Sebastianelli (eds.), *Concussions in Athletics:*
From Brain to Behavior, DOI 10.1007/978-1-4939-0295-8_7,
© Springer Science+Business Media New York 2014

Introduction

Concussions are an injury of increasing public health concern. An estimated 1.7 million people sustain a traumatic brain injury (TBI) in the United States each year [1]. Of these injuries, 52,000 result in death, 275,000 result in hospitalization, and 1.365 million are treated and released from the emergency department. The direct medical costs and indirect costs, such as loss of productivity, are estimated to be on the order of $60 billion annually in the United States [2]. However, this esti- mate only takes into account the incidence of TBI that is reported by hospitals. Of the 1.7 million TBIs that are recorded each year, 75 % are classified as mild trau- matic brain injuries (mTBIs), or concussions [3]. The incidence of concussion is thought to be vastly underestimated as many of these injuries receive no medical attention [1, 4–6]. Recent estimates that account for this have suggested that there are as many as 3.8 million concussions associated with sports participation alone in the United States annually [4]. While sports-related concussion was once consid- ered to only result in immediate neurocognitive impairment and symptoms that are transient in nature, recent research is correlating long-term neurodegenerative effects with a history of sports-related concussion [7–9]. Furthermore, there is con- cern that repetitive sub-concussive head impacts in sports may lead to neurocogni- tive deficits [10–12]. Increased awareness and current media attention to these issues have contributed to concussion injuries becoming a primary health concern.

This review focuses on the experimental work related to the understanding of biomechanics associated with concussion. With the improved understanding of con- cussive biomechanics, the possibility of preventing these injuries exists through improved safety devices and techniques. Traditionally, the majority of brain injury biomechanics research has defined concussion as a severe and life-threatening injury. Concussive brain injury is unique in that the injury has a graded response that can vary from minor confusion to death [13]. Annually in the United States, there are only an estimated 300,000 concussions that result in loss of consciousness, with the remaining injuries resulting in less severe symptoms [4, 14]. However, the vary- ing grades of concussion are likely a scaled result of the varying mechanical stimuli input to the head [13]. Previous experiments involved investigating brain injury mechanisms, and how these mechanisms relate to the kinematics of the head. Kinematic parameters of the head are related to brain injury because they are thought to be indicative of the inertial response of the brain. Ideally, the head kine- matics of a human surrogate could be measured in a safety testing scenario and used to predict the tissue level response of the brain in an effort to evaluate injury poten- tial. With this goal in mind, many researchers have studied the relationship between head kinematics and brain injury.

Historically, investigating concussion in the laboratory has been challenging, given that the injury is identified by a physiologic response that most experimental models cannot reproduce. However, a vast amount of valuable research has been performed over the last 60 years that has helped us better understand the biomechan- ics associated with brain injury (Fig. 7.1). The data resulting from these works fall

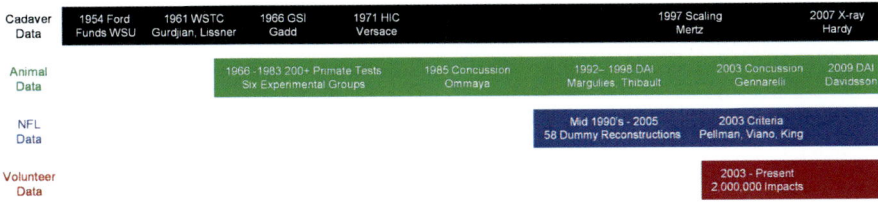

Fig. 7.1 Timeline of cadaver, animal, dummy, and volunteer head injury research performed over the past 60 years

under four research paths: cadaver research, animal research, dummy research, and volunteer research. Each of these research modalities is addressed individually in the subsequent sections of this review. The majority of these experiments have investigated linear and rotational kinematics independently, as these inputs have long been thought to result in different injury mechanisms [15]. Brain injury associated with the linear kinematics of the head is thought to result from a transient intracranial pressure gradient. Brain injury associated with the rotational kinematics of the head is thought to result from a strain response within the neural tissue. Explanations of these theories have been previously documented in great detail [16].

Whether brain injury is the result of linear or rotational kinematics of the head has been debated among scientists for the last 60 years, and is still debated to this day. In actuality, there are both linear and rotational head kinematics resulting from every head impact, and both likely contribute to injury risk [13]. This topic will be discussed with greater detail in the subsequent sections of the review. Furthermore, it should be stated that this review focuses on concussion resulting from direct head impacts. While it has been suggested that an impact to the chest or abdomen may result in concussion-like symptoms, there are no published data to support this as a primary injury mechanism. With the exception of a few primate tests, all of the research presented in this review investigates brain injury resulting from direct head impact. The following review sections will provide an overview of the past 60 years of biomechanics research focusing on brain injury, characterize the current state of helmets and their ability to reduce concussion risk, and discuss the direction of future experimental work related to reducing concussion incidence.

Cadaver Data

Traditionally, the automobile industry has led the majority of injury biomechanics research. Research specific to investigating the biomechanical mechanisms of head injury has been ongoing since the 1950s. This work began with cadaver experiments focusing on skull fracture and TBI, but the resulting injury prediction tools have also been used for the development of injury risk curves for mTBI.

The basic premise of this research has been to relate biomechanical measures with injury outcome to develop tools that can be used to evaluate the safety of products. The kinematic response of the head due to impact is commonly used to assess the likelihood of head injury due to the strong correlation with the injury mechanisms and ease of measurement.

In 1954, Ford funded Wayne State University to investigate head injury through a series of cadaver experiments. The Wayne State tolerance curve (WSTC) assesses the potential of catastrophic head injuries, such as skull fracture and severe brain injury. Drop tests of embalmed cadaver heads were used to correlate peak acceleration to skull fracture for impacts of durations between 1 and 6 ms [17]. Shortly after, the WSTC was extended from 6 to 10 ms based on comparative animal and cadaver tests investigating the relationships between head acceleration and transient intracranial pressure gradients [18]. To finalize the WSTC, a longer duration asymptote based on data from non-injurious volunteer accelerative sled tests [19]. Later work supported these findings through additional testing of human cadaver skulls and primates [20]. Enabled by additional funding from General Motors and Ford, several injury metrics were developed from retrospective analyses of the WSTC. Severity index (SI) is a weighted impulse criterion based on a linear approximation of the WSTC plotted on a log–log scale [21]. From a mathematical review of the relationship between the WSTC and SI, head injury criterion (HIC) was developed in an effort to account for the high tolerance of humans to long duration, low magnitude head accelerations [22]. Over the next several decades, these original data were scaled to generate risk functions for multiple populations and injury severities, such as mTBI [23, 24]. The WSTC, SI, and HIC relate peak linear head acceleration to probability of catastrophic head injury and serve as the basis of every head injury standard that is currently in regulation in the United States. Furthermore, these injury prediction tools have been thought to correlate with severe brain injury. The head injury standards result in safer product designs by allowing manufacturers to optimize product design to lower peak linear head acceleration, which in turn reduces the risk of head injury.

More recently, brain injury was specifically investigated using a cadaver model [25, 26]. In these experiments, neutral density targets were inserted into cadaver brains and a high-speed biplane X-ray was used to examine brain displacement and deformation during head impacts thought to be associated with concussion. Intracranial pressure was also measured for each test. This seminal work demonstrated that as linear and rotational head kinematics increase, the intracranial pressure gradients and brain motion relative to the skull increase. Furthermore, this work showed that the brain moves very little during concussive impacts and doesn't "slosh around" in the skull, with total brain excursions in the direction of impact on the order of 7 mm.

In summary, cadaver experiments were some of the first works to relate head kinematic measures to head injury risk. This work demonstrated that as the linear and rotational head kinematics increase, brain loading and the associated risk of injury also increase.

Animal Data

Acknowledging the obvious physiologic limitations of the cadaver model, a series of experiments were conducted with in vivo animal brain injury models. Throughout a two-decade period, over 200 experimental tests on subhuman primates investigated brain injury. These works specifically examined the roles of linear and rotational head acceleration in relation to brain injury [13, 15, 27–37].

In the 1960s, Ommaya et al. [37] investigated the role of whiplash in cerebral concussion (sudden traumatic unconsciousness with retrograde and posttraumatic amnesia following a blow to the head) and suggested that multiple mechanisms are involved in injury, including rotational acceleration, intracranial pressure gradients, and flexion–extension–tension of the neck. Ommaya and Hirsch [34] followed this work up in 1971 by quantifying tolerances for cerebral concussion from head impacts and whiplash and reported that only half potential for brain injury is related to head rotation. It was suggested that the remaining potential for cerebral concussion was related to the contact phenomena associated with impact. Around this same time, Gennarelli et al. [27] compared linear and rotational head motions associated with cerebral concussion. The scientists reported that concussion was only produced when the monkeys experienced a combination of linear and rotational motion, and not when only linear motion was experienced. However, both scenarios produced visible brain lesions. This same group followed this work up investigating the pathophysiologic responses to linear and rotational head accelerations. They reported that visible brain lesions were present in both the linear only group and the combined linear and rotational group, but that combined group had lesions that were more severe and diffuse [32].

In a separate set of experiments occurring parallel to the aforementioned work, Unterharnscheidt [15] also investigated linear and rotational acceleration's role in brain injury. Similar results to Gennarelli were reported, where the linear and combined groups both produced brain lesions, but of different characteristics. In 1980, Ono et al. [20] reported on a series of monkey experiments that largely agreed with the previous work of Ommaya, Hirsch, Gennarelli, and Thibault—in that linear and rotational acceleration, and contact phenomena play role in producing brain lesions. However, Ono et al.'s results suggested that rotational acceleration of the head did not correlate with concussion in monkeys, but linear acceleration was highly correlated to concussion.

Throughout the early 1980s, Gennarelli's group further investigated brain injury by developing a new system capable of inducing brain injuries from mild concussions to instantaneous death in primates [29]. This system induced a combination of linear and rotational acceleration on the head and was used to study the directional dependence of brain injury, diffuse axonal injury (DAI), coma, and subdural hematomas [28–31, 38]. Around this same time, Hodgson et al. [33] also investigated the role of impact location on cerebral concussion and reported that higher linear and rotational accelerations were associated with longer periods of unconsciousness of impacts to the side of the head than any other location.

These works have provided great insight to brain injury and its relation to head kinematics. Unfortunately, it is challenging to apply these data to humans. Due to anatomical, physiologic, and size differences between humans and primates, the data cannot be directly applied. Researchers have proposed various ways to scale the primate data to make them applicable to man [23, 39], but these attempts have been characterized as "completely speculative" [13].

The primate research is often referenced in the biomechanics community as showing that concussion is a result of rotational acceleration. It is often overlooked that all these tests also consisted of a large linear acceleration that accompanied the rotational acceleration. As long as the head is attached to a neck, it is impossible to put a head under pure rotational loading. This research demonstrates that both linear and rotational accelerations of the head contribute to injury.

NFL Data

In the mid-1990s, researchers began investigating concussive impacts experienced by professional football players in the National Football League (NFL) [40–47]. Film of concussive impacts was reviewed and impacts in which the boundary conditions of the impact could be determined were identified. Researchers then conducted full-scale reconstructions of these impacts using instrumented crash test dummies. A total of 58 cases were reconstructed from 31 events, including 25 concussive cases [47]. The full 3D kinematics of the head were measured for each case. The researchers found that linear and rotational accelerations were both significantly correlated to concussion risk (Fig. 7.2).

This dataset has proved to be very valuable in advancing our current understanding of concussive biomechanics. These data have been reanalyzed multiple times using finite element models to investigate the tissue level response of these

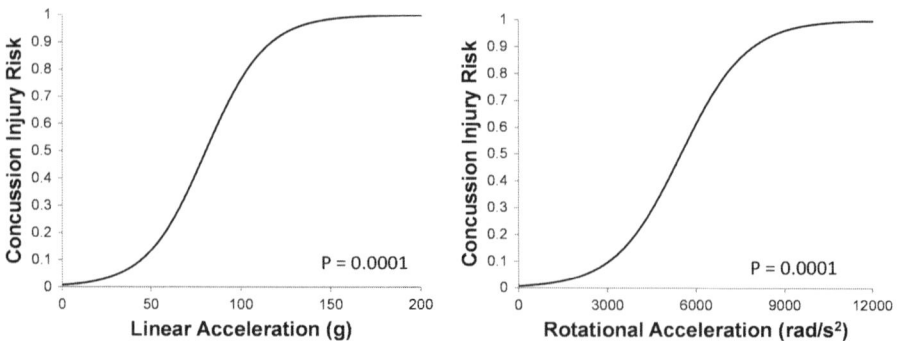

Fig. 7.2 Concussion risk curves for linear and rotational acceleration derived from the NFL dataset [47]

concussive events [48–50]. While valuable, the limitations of this study were that data were collected from dummies rather than humans, and that the generated dataset is biased towards concussive impacts, which will be discussed later.

Volunteer Data

The high occurrence of concussions in football provides a unique opportunity to collect biomechanical data to characterize mTBI. Competitive football has been used as an experimental environment for collecting head acceleration data directly from humans since the 1970s. Several early studies have had football players wear headbands instrumented with accelerometers to measure head acceleration during football games [51–53]. Another study instrumented football helmets directly to measure helmet acceleration [54]. While laying the groundwork for future research and providing a proof of concept, these older studies were limited in their ability to measure head acceleration and measured only a single player. Later, Naunheim et al. [55] instrumented the helmets of one high school hockey player and two high school football players (both linemen) with accelerometers to measure linear head acceleration. However, there were no documented incidents of concussion in these limited datasets.

In the early 2000s, the head impact telemetry (HIT) system was developed. The HIT system is a commercially available accelerometer array that is designed to integrate into existing football helmets. The device consists of six accelerometers that are oriented normal to the surface of the head. The accelerometers are elastically decoupled from the helmet so that they remain in contact with the head throughout impact. This ensures that the acceleration of the head, rather than the helmet, is measured [56]. The device is intended to be installed in helmets during play in games and practices, and continuously samples acceleration at 1,000 Hz using a circular buffer. Any time a single accelerometer exceeds 14.4 g, data acquisition is triggered and the data are wirelessly transmitted to a computer on the sideline. Resultant linear acceleration, resultant rotational acceleration, and impact location are computed using algorithms [57–59]. Axis-specific peak linear accelerations and the temporal response of resultant linear acceleration are also computed using the HIT system. Given the limitation of the commercially available HIT system not being able to measure the complete 3D kinematics of the head throughout an impact, a custom 6 degree of freedom (6DOF) head acceleration measurement device was developed using the same technology. The 6DOF measurement device is unique in that it consists of 12 accelerometers with their sensing axes oriented tangential to the skull. Acceleration data collected with the 6DOF measurement device can be used to compute the temporal response of linear and rotational acceleration to impact using a novel algorithm [60]. Both the HIT system and 6DOF measurement device have undergone extensive laboratory validation [61–63]. These systems have been used to collect head acceleration data from human

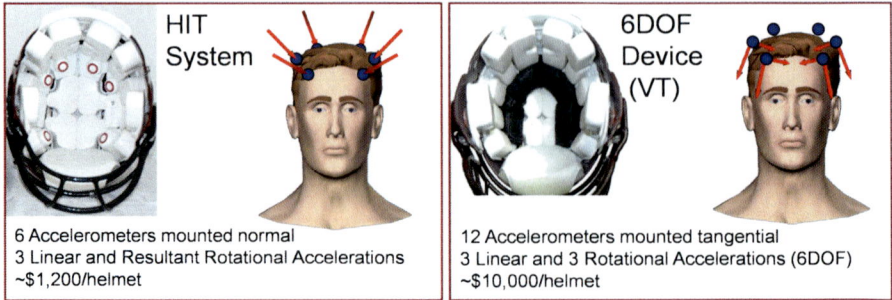

HIT System	6DOF Device (VT)
6 Accelerometers mounted normal 3 Linear and Resultant Rotational Accelerations ~$1,200/helmet	12 Accelerometers mounted tangential 3 Linear and 3 Rotational Accelerations (6DOF) ~$10,000/helmet

Fig. 7.3 Two different systems have been used in parallel to collect head acceleration directly from football players: the commercially available HIT system (*left*) and the custom 6DOF measurement device (*right*). Both systems have been well validated [61–63]

volunteers throughout the past decade. The majority of data collected to date have been collected with the commercially available HIT system due to the high cost of the custom 6DOF measurement device (Fig. 7.3). These technologies have since been adapted to other sports to collect head acceleration data from human volunteers in boxing, hockey, soccer, and skiing [64–70].

Duma et al. [71] presented the first study to quantify head acceleration in collegiate football players by collecting over 3,000 impacts from 38 players using eight HITS measurement devices, in which one concussive event was measured. A subsequent study expanded this dataset to include over 27,000 impacts (four concussions) and analyzed risk using a unique statistical analysis [72]. The nominal injury values reported representing 10 % risk of concussion were a peak linear acceleration of 165 g and HIC of 400. In separate studies, Schnebel et al. [73] presented data for over 62,000 (six concussions) head impacts experienced by 56 collegiate and high school football players recorded using HITS. Guskiewicz et al. [74] collected over 104,000 impacts (13 concussions) from 88 collegiate football players. Mihalik et al. [75] analyzed more than 57,000 impacts from 72 players to look at positional differences in impacts. Broglio et al. [76] recorded over 54,000 head impacts (including 13 concussions) experienced by 78 high school athletes. These initial studies provided great insight to the head kinematics associated with head impacts in football, but have largely been descriptive studies with small concussive sample sizes that made it difficult to draw conclusions about injury.

A larger NIH-funded collaborative study between Virginia Tech, Brown, and Dartmouth began in 2007 to specifically investigate the biomechanics associated with concussion through instrumenting a large cohort of collegiate athletes with the HIT system. Over 500,000 head impacts were collected in this study and a series of papers completely describing the exposure to head impact of the collegiate football player were produced [77–79]. Furthermore, concussion risk curves for linear and rotational acceleration were generated from these data [58, 80, 81]. By 2011, researchers from all institutions instrumenting football players had collectively

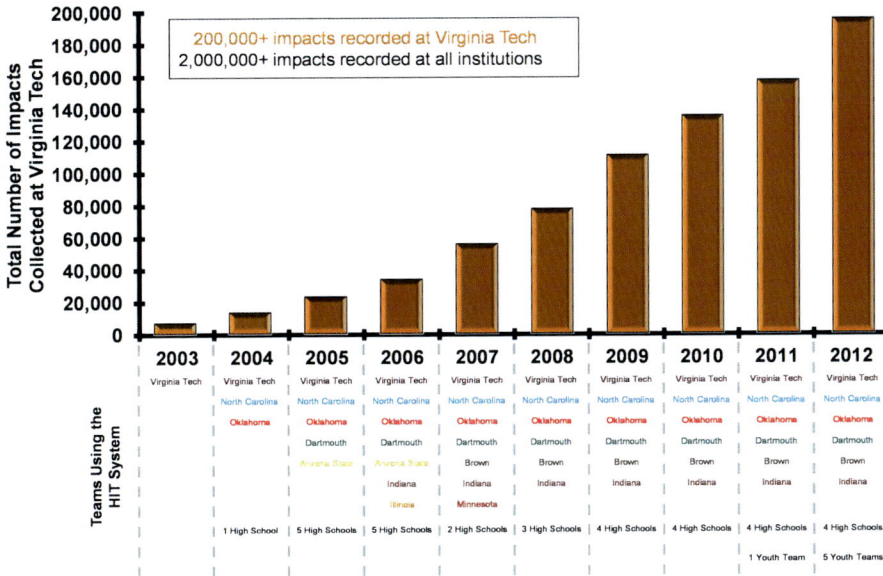

Fig. 7.4 Since 2003, over 2,000,000 head impacts have been collected between all institutions using the HIT system. Subjects have ranged in age from 6 to 23 years

recorded over 100 concussions. Through collaborative papers, the effect of head impact exposure on concussion and timing of concussion diagnosis relative to impact have been investigated [82, 83]. Researchers at Virginia Tech and Wake Forest have expanded this research by instrumenting youth football players to investigate concussive biomechanics in a pediatric population [84]. To date, acceleration data resulting from over 2,000,000 head impacts collected directly from humans ranging in age from 6 to 23 years have been analyzed (Fig. 7.4).

By collecting data directly from human volunteers, the limitations of the cadaver, animal, and dummy experiments are eliminated. These data represent the best available dataset on concussion in humans. The following section in this review will discuss how these data have been used to model brain injury. Interestingly, the concussive data collected in the cadaver, animal, dummy, and human volunteer datasets are remarkably similar. The average linear acceleration associated with concussion collected with the HIT system has been reported to be 105 ± 27 g [80]. This is statistically no different from the linear acceleration magnitudes associated with concussion (98 ± 28 g) reported in the NFL reconstructions [47]. Furthermore, the rotational kinematic concussive data described in the volunteer and NFL reconstructions overlap perfectly, and are agreeable with data collected in the animal experiments (Fig. 7.5). The powerful nature of overlapping data from completely different experimental methodologies suggests great confidence in the acceleration ranges used to characterize concussion in humans.

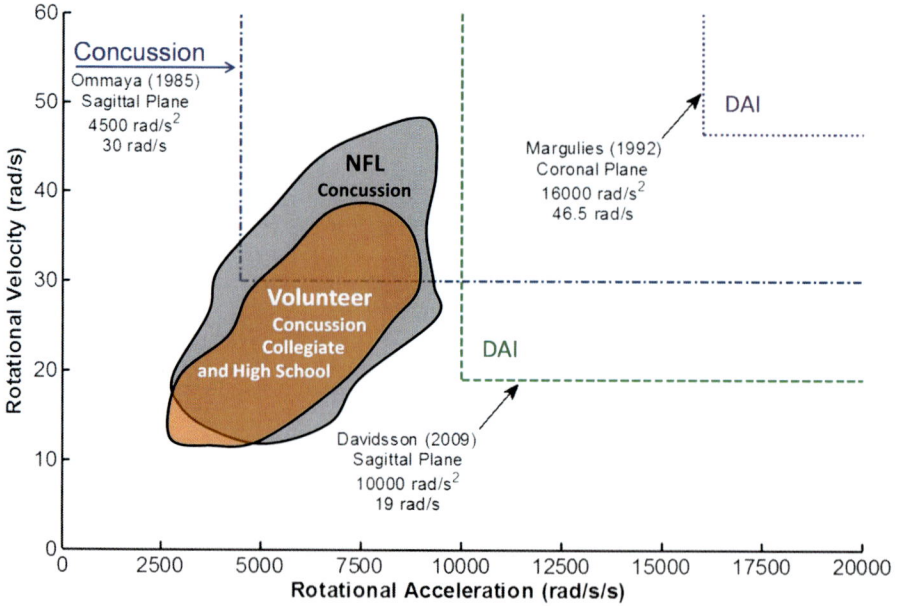

Fig. 7.5 Acceleration data describing concussion collected from animal models, NFL reconstructions, and human volunteers are consistent. This agreement provides great confidence in the acceleration ranges that have been used to describe concussion

Concussion Injury Criteria

In order to review the published concussion injury criteria, one must first discuss the differences between injury risk functions and injury thresholds. This is a basic concept that applies to the broad field of injury biomechanics for any specific body region, organ, or tissue level injury criteria. Due to the underlying variation in human tolerance from one person to the next, it is most accurate to discuss injury criteria relative to risk functions rather than specific thresholds. All set thresholds are tied to a defined risk of injury. For example, a vehicle that gets 5-star rating from the federal New Car Assessment Program (NCAP) testing is defined as a 10 % or less risk of serious injury for the given car crash test conditions. In other words, if ten people get in the same crash in that vehicle, it is probable that one of them will sustain a serious injury. The same risk analysis applies to concussion research as a specific head impact will result in risk of injury to some segment of the population. Any set threshold for concussion will be linked to a risk of concussion. This concept is critical to understand when evaluating published injury criteria.

As discussed in the previous sections, this risk of concussion injury is significantly correlated to head acceleration. All published research with primates, NFL dummy reconstructions, and volunteer data has demonstrated the same fact: the risk of concussion increases as head acceleration increases. This relationship applies to both linear and rotational head acceleration components.

While the primate research focused on rotational acceleration, it is important to note that all of those experiments also included linear acceleration components. In 1992, Margulies and Thibault [85] published a study based on the primate data that presented 16,000 rad/s^2 as the threshold for DAI using rotational acceleration as the injury metric. A more recent study by Davidsson et al. [86] used a rat model and suggested 10,000 rad/s^2 as the DAI threshold. Although DAI is much more severe than concussion injury, these studies are useful for setting a higher bound. A concussion-specific threshold of 4,500 rad/s^2 was presented by Ommaya based on his analysis of the primate data [13]. Gennarelli et al. [87] confirmed and expanded on Ommaya's concussion threshold in a study that presented three values associated with different concussion severity levels: 3,000 rad/s^2 for mild concussion, 4,500 rad/s^2 for classical concussion, and 8,000 rad/s^2 for severe concussion. The research clearly show the range of rotational acceleration associated with concussion (Fig. 7.5).

The NFL reconstructions presented 58 cases (25 concussion injury and 33 non-injury) that were used to develop injury risk functions for concussion [46, 48]. These studies found that linear and rotational accelerations are significantly correlated with risk of concussion (Fig. 7.2). The risk functions presented by Pellman et al. show a 50 % risk of concussion at 81 g for linear acceleration and 5,500 rad/s^2 for rotational acceleration. While the values for the 25 concussion cases match well to the primate data (Fig. 7.5), it is important to note that the relative sample size of the injury to non-injury cases is not representative of the actual exposure. Considering the complete head impact exposure of a football player, there are vastly more concussive cases relative to non-injury cases. This results in a dataset biased towards concussion. Not taking a random sample of the exposure has the effect of overestimating risk, since the actual field exposure is not represented in the case distribution [88]. The reason for this small sample size is that the reconstructions were very difficult and time-consuming, so that it was not practical to reconstruct all the impacts of every game. Without accounting for the actual head impact exposure, these risk functions should be considered to overestimate risk.

The 10 years of volunteer data collection has eliminated the limitations of the NFL reconstructions in that the complete head exposure was recorded for the instrumented players. The concussion cases for the volunteer data are nearly identical to the NFL concussion cases and fit as expected relative to the primate data (Fig. 7.5). Beyond the advantages of recorded data from human subjects, the complete exposure profile allows for the development of concussion risk functions that accurately reflect a player's risk for a given impact. From this dataset, separate risk functions for linear acceleration and rotational acceleration were developed [58, 80]. Most recently, Rowson and Duma presented a study in 2013 that presents a combined probability risk function that incorporates both linear and rotational acceleration components for the prediction of concussion risk [81]. Their analysis utilized both the NFL and the volunteer datasets in order to develop the combined risk equation (Fig. 7.6). The study also accounted for the underreporting of concussions. Given that all head impacts include both linear and rotational acceleration components, this new risk function will be very useful for evaluating concussion risk. Data from the Hybrid III or a modified National Operating Committee on Standards for

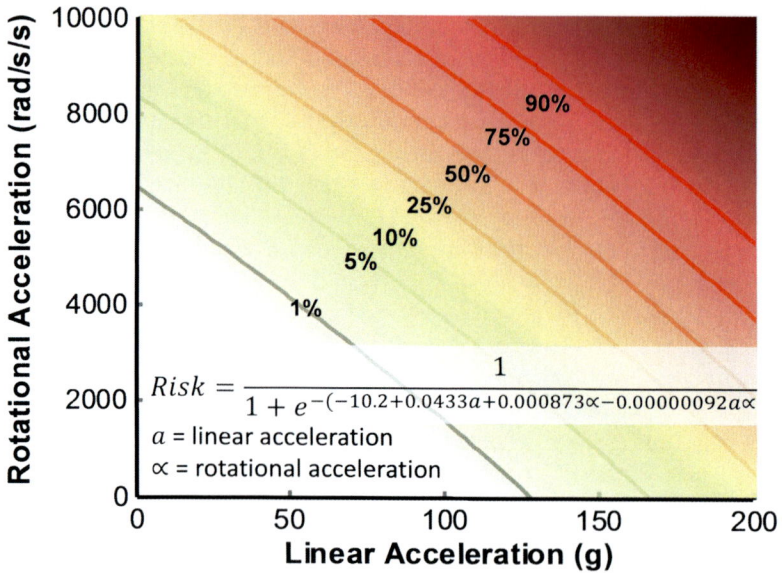

Fig. 7.6 Concussion injury risk function based on the combination of linear and rotational acceleration developed using the NFL and volunteer datasets [81]

Athletic Equipment (NOCSAE) head form can be analyzed with this equation. It is anticipated that this will be used not only in the area of sports-related concussions but also in automobile safety and military restraint applications.

Helmet Performance

During the 1960s, head injuries during sporting events were increasing as participation in sports overall increased. At that time there were no governing bodies to oversee the safety of sporting equipment. In 1968 alone, there were 32 fatalities in sporting events—a startlingly high number that is difficult to comprehend in today's safety conscious society. Because of this, the NOCSAE was created as a mechanism to fund research and develop standards for improved helmet design in 1969. As the NOCSAE helmet test standards were developed and implemented, helmet designs were improved and subsequently there was a dramatic reduction in sports-related fatalities over the next several years [89–91]. The basic NOCSAE test for football helmets involves testing the helmet on the NOCSAE head form in controlled linear drop tests at a range of energy levels (drop heights) and a range of impact locations (Fig. 7.7). Accelerometers placed at the center of gravity of the NOCSAE head form measure linear acceleration along three orthogonal directions. These data are processed to calculate the severity index (SI). As long as the peak SI value is below

Fig. 7.7 Standard NOCSAE
drop test configuration for
evaluating the performance of
football helmets.
Accelerometers inside the
head form evaluate the
helmet's ability to manage
the impact energy

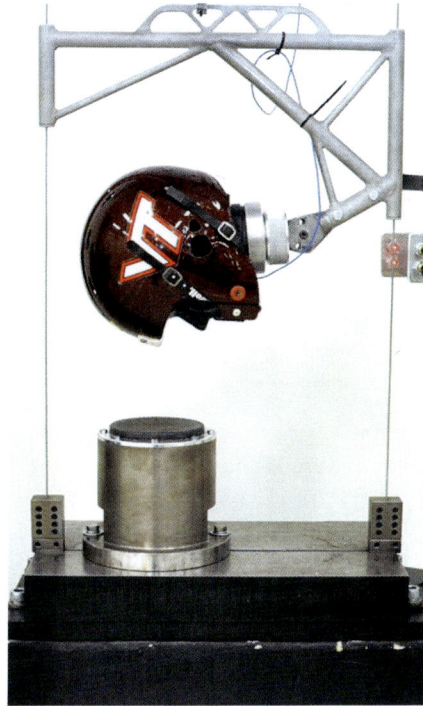

1,200 for all impact tests, then the helmet passes the NOCSAE standard. Without
question, NOCSAE should be praised and credited for leading the efforts that have
nearly eliminated skull fractures and fatal injuries in modern sports. For those that
suggest the helmet should be removed from the game, the fatality data from 1968
suggest otherwise.

More recently, focus has shifted to sports-related concussion and a helmet's ability to reduce the risk of concussion. Given that concussion risk is correlated to head
acceleration, new research is examining the ability of a helmet to manage the impact
energy and lower head acceleration. This is the critical limitation of the NOCSAE
standard which treats all helmets the same as long as they pass the 1,200 SI threshold. To illustrate this limitation, one can examine acceleration data from two helmets that both pass the NOCSAE standard (Fig. 7.8). For a 60 in. drop test on the
top location, the Adams A2000 helmet just barely passes the NOCSAE standard
with a peak SI value of 1,134. In contrast, the Riddell 360 results in a strikingly
lower SI value of 416. The differences are even more substantial when considering
the peak resultant linear acceleration values. The Adams A2000 shows a peak value
of 190 g compared to the Riddell 360 peak value of only 84 g. These two helmets
are clearly not the same, as the Riddell 360 design is far superior at managing the
impact energy and therefore resulting in substantially lower head acceleration values. In terms of concussion risk, the risk functions in the previous section calculate
that the Adams A2000 would show nearly 100 % risk of concussion, compared to

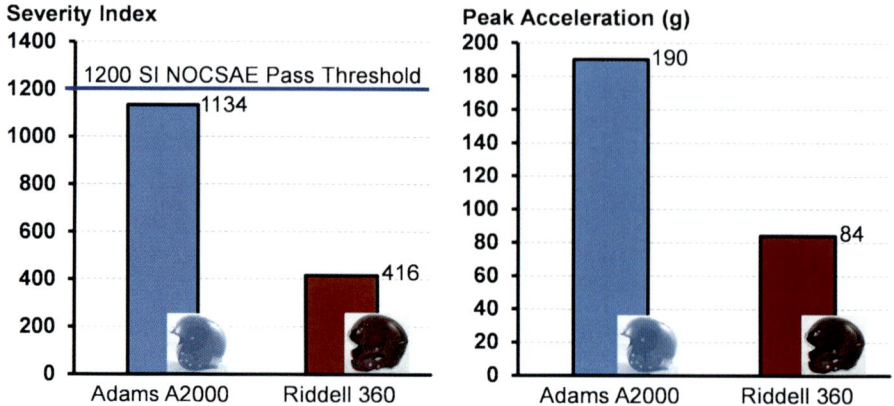

Fig. 7.8 Acceleration results from NOCSAE style tests on the top location from 60 in. drops. Both helmets pass the NOCSAE threshold, but Riddell 360 results in substantially lower head accelera-tion values

the Riddell 360 which would predict less than 10 % risk for this high energy impact. This dramatic risk reduction illustrates the vast differences in the performance of the two helmets.

A new formula for evaluating helmet performance was published in 2011 by Rowson and Duma, entitled the Summation of Tests for the Analysis of Risk (STAR) equation [80]. This formula (7.1) combined years of on-field head impact exposure data with helmet-specific acceleration data from laboratory tests. Four different impact locations (front, top, back, side) are evaluated at six energy (height) levels using the NOCSAE test configuration. The peak acceleration from each test is used to calculate the concussion risk for that impact and then multiplied by the exposure value for the impact direction and energy level. All the test values are summated to simulate one season of player head impact exposure. All testing details are public (www.sbes.vt.edu/nid).

$$STAR = \sum_{l=1}^{4}\left(\sum_{h=1}^{6}E\left(l,h\right)\cdot R\left(a\right)\right) \tag{7.1}$$

In the spring of 2011, 2012, and 2013, Virginia Tech has released the STAR val-ues for adult football helmets using the STAR equation. Given that Virginia Tech has no financial ties to any helmet manufacturer or NOCSAE, these ratings are the only independent dataset that is publically available for consumers to utilize when purchasing football helmets. As illustrated in Fig. 7.8, football helmets can be very different in their ability to reduce head acceleration. In 2011 only one helmet was given a 5-star rating. By 2013 a total of four helmets by three manufacturers were given a 5-star rating (Fig. 7.9). Using a more complex test methodology, the NFL found similar results [92, 93]. In the future, the STAR system will be expanded to utilize both linear and rotational acceleration parameters [81].

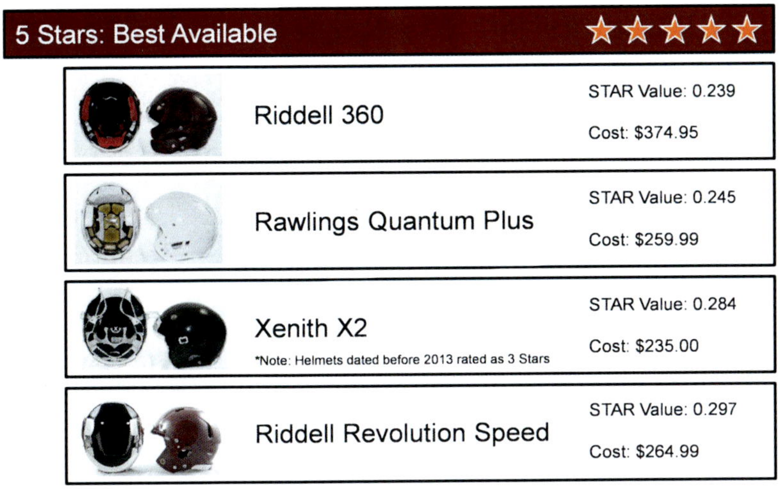

5 Stars: Best Available	★ ★ ★ ★ ★
Riddell 360	STAR Value: 0.239 Cost: $374.95
Rawlings Quantum Plus	STAR Value: 0.245 Cost: $259.99
Xenith X2 *Note: Helmets dated before 2013 rated as 3 Stars	STAR Value: 0.284 Cost: $235.00
Riddell Revolution Speed	STAR Value: 0.297 Cost: $264.99

Fig. 7.9 By reducing head acceleration, four helmet models developed by three manufacturers achieved a 5-star rating in model year 2013 with STAR values below 0.300 (www.SBES.vt.edu/nid)

Clinical Validation of Helmet Performance

While laboratory tests have documented the differences in helmet performance, it is important to support these laboratory tests with clinical studies. To date, three clinical studies have been performed that each found statistically significant reduction in concussion risk between helmet models. This concussion risk on the field is corresponding to the acceleration reduction as measured in the laboratory tests. The studies compare the newer design of the Riddell Revolution to the older design of the Riddell VSR4 (Fig. 7.10). The Revolution design has an augmented shell and increased padding compared to the VSR4. The laboratory tests give the Revolution a 4-star rating compared to the 1-star rating of the VSR4 based on the Revolution's ability to lower head acceleration. Both helmets are very popular models and that is the primary reason they were utilized in these studies.

The first study evaluated 2,141 high school athletes over a 3-year period. The data showed a statistically significant 31 % reduction in concussion risk for players wearing the Revolution helmet compared to those in the standard helmets [94]. The study was peer reviewed and published in the journal Neurosurgery along with six opinion letters. Five of the six letters were generally positive and supported the research; however, one letter by Dr. Cantu was sharply critical of the study in several aspects. Primarily, Dr. Cantu stated that the study was flawed because the standard helmets were older than the Revolution helmets, and that older helmets perform worse than newer helmets. It is important to note that there are no published data to support this statement by Dr. Cantu, and he later withdrew this primary criticism. Additional criticisms involved potential conflict of interests with the authors, and the limitation that the concussions were not diagnosed by physicians. In 2012, the

Fig. 7.10 Three separate
clinical studies have found
that the Riddell Revolution
(*top*) significantly reduces the
risk of concussion compared
to standard helmets such as
the Riddell VSR4 (*bottom*)

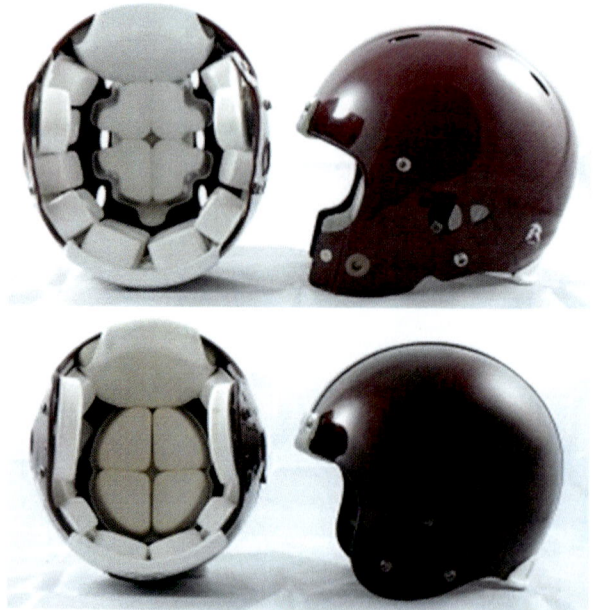

Federal Trade Commission (FTC) investigated Riddell based on their claims of the Revolution helmet's ability to reduce concussion risk through citing this study. In 2013, the FTC closed the investigation and took no action.

The second clinical study published in 2012 evaluated the risk of concussion in over 300 Virginia Tech football players over a 9-year period (2003–2011) [63]. The unique aspect of this study was that all of the players were instrumented with the HIT system, which allowed for the complete head impact exposure to be accounted for in the analysis. For each helmet type, the number of impacts not resulting in diagnosed concussion was compared to the number of impacts that resulted in diagnosed concussion. This study found a statistically significant 85 % reduction in concussion risk for players wearing the Revolution helmets compared to those in the VSR4 helmets. This study addresses the limitations that Dr. Cantu raised in that helmet age was controlled, as each player was provided with his own new helmet of either type. In addition, there are no conflicts of interests with the authors, and the same physician made each concussion diagnosis throughout the 9 years.

The third and largest clinical study will be published in spring 2014. It also compares the performance of the Revolution helmet to the VSR4 across eight collegiate football teams including the University of North Carolina, University of Oklahoma, Brown University, Dartmouth College, University of Minnesota, Indiana University, University of Illinois, and Virginia Tech. All subjects in this study also wore helmets instrumented with the HIT system so that the full head impact exposure could be analyzed. Again, a statistically significant reduction in concussion risk for the Revolution compared to the VSR4 was observed.

Overall, three separate clinical studies have found a significant reduction in concussion risk between players wearing the Riddell Revolution compared to players wearing the Riddell VSR4. Interestingly, the STAR system predicts a 54 % reduction in concussion risk between these two helmet models, and the clinical studies show significant risk reductions between 31 and 85 %.

Future Testing and Dummy Head Forms

The future of helmet testing will involve systems that can simulate the complete kinematics of on-field head impacts for any given sport. While the original NOCSAE style drop test proved very successful at minimizing the risk of skull fractures, it is limited with a rigid neck to measuring only linear acceleration. Over the past 10 years, the NFL and NOCSAE worked together to develop the next generation of impact test device, known as the linear impactor [95, 96]. In this system, the energy source is a pneumatic piston that accelerates a ram to impact a head form attached to a Hybrid III neck mounted to a slider table (Fig. 7.11). This configuration allows the head to translate and rotate upon impact and therefore more accurately simulate the kinematics observed in sporting impacts. A variety of instrumentation techniques, such as a nine accelerometer array or a combination of accelerometer and angular rate sensors, can be utilized inside the head form in order to capture both linear and rotational acceleration components. The NFL has utilized this system extensively to evaluate football helmet performance [92, 93, 96, 97]. This system can be purchased from Biokinetics (Ottawa, Canada) and is currently being utilized by many testing labs across the world.

The head and neck assembly in the linear impact system can be modified to use the Hybrid III head form or the NOCSAE head form with both attaching to the

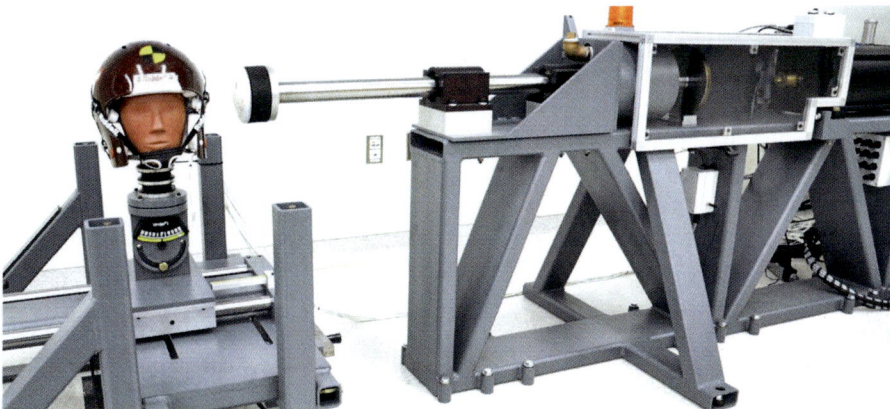

Fig. 7.11 Linear pneumatic impactor provides high velocity impacts that result in similar linear and rotational kinematics as on-field impacts

Fig. 7.12 The HIII and
NOCSAE head forms with
sectioned football helmet,
illustrating the poor fit of the
HIII head in the posterior
head/neck region as
compared to the NOCSAE
head

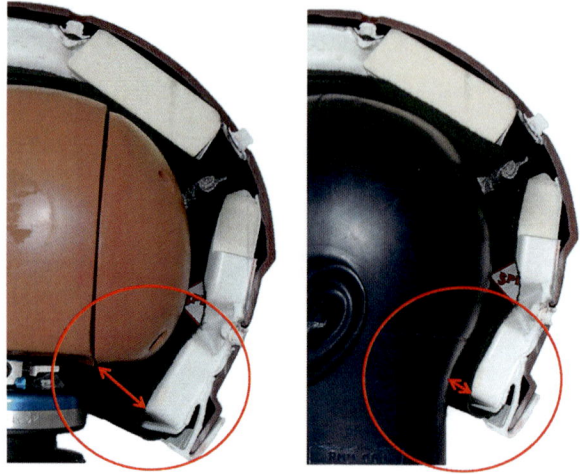

Hybrid III neck. There is much debate as to which head form is best given the differences in the construction design and materials. In the simplest terms, the Hybrid III is a hollow head form while the NOCSAE head form is fluid filled. Perhaps the most important difference relative to helmet design is the fact that the external geometries of the two head forms are very different and this can have a dramatic effect on helmet fit parameters. The Hybrid III head form was never designed for helmet testing so the biofidelity of its specific geometry was not a critical aspect of its development. There are two specific areas in which the Hybrid III head form differs from the NOCSAE head form and those of humans. First, the Hybrid III does not have fully formed facial bones in the maxilla region while the NOCSAE head form does. This results in large gaps near the check pads when putting a helmet on the Hybrid III, and this difference is not seen with the NOCSAE head form or when players wear the helmets. Second, the largest difference is observed in the posterior section as the Hybrid III cuts off dramatically near the neck attachment (Fig. 7.12). In contrast, the NOCSAE system has continuous geometry into the neck attachment and this results in more realistic helmet fit. Because of these differences, helmet testing on the Hybrid III can be prone to confounding fit issues. For these reasons, future testing will include the NOCSAE head form on the Hybrid III neck [95, 96]. Ongoing research is examining the neck attachment location relative to the center of gravity of the NOCSAE head form.

In closing, it is important to note that while extensive research allows for the characterization of concussion risk, the helmet design alone cannot be considered the only solution. A player in even the very best helmet may sustain a concussion given that player's history and genetic makeup. The best approach to reducing the risk of concussion in all sports is to adopt a three-part approach. First, proper rules and regulations are needed to discourage head impacts when at all possible. Second, proper coaching techniques are needed to help players learn the proper impact methods. Third, players should utilize the best helmet and protection devices as proven with biomechanical test data.

Acknowledgments We acknowledge the tremendous efforts and contributions of all researchers who contributed to advancing the understanding of brain injury over the past 60 years. Over the past 10 years we are very grateful to the agencies that sponsored our research projects that contributed to this chapter. Externally, we acknowledge funding from the National Institutes of Health (National Institute for Child Health and Human Development) (Contract No. R01HD048638), National Highway Traffic Safety Administration, Toyota Motor Corporation, Toyota Central Research and Development Laboratory, and the Department of Defense. Internally, we acknowledge support from the Institute for Critical Technologies and Applied Sciences, Via College of Osteopathic Medicine, and the Virginia Tech—Wake Forest University School of Biomedical Engineering and Sciences.

References

1. Faul M, Xu L, Wald MM, Coronado VG. Traumatic brain injury in the United States: emergency department visits, hospitalizations, and deaths. Atlanta, GA: Centers for Disease Control and Prevention, National Center for Injury Prevention and Control; 2010.
2. Finkelstein E, Corso P, Miller T, associates. The incidence and economic burden of injuries in the United States. New York, NY: Oxford University Press; 2006.
3. Centers for Disease Control and Prevention (CDC) National Center for Injury Prevention and Control. Report to congress on mild traumatic brain injury in the United States: steps to prevent a serious public health problem. Atlanta, GA: Centers for Disease Control and Prevention; 2003.
4. Langlois JA, Rutland-Brown W, Wald MM. The epidemiology and impact of traumatic brain injury: a brief overview. J Head Trauma Rehabil. 2006;21(5):375–8.
5. Langburt W, Cohen B, Akhthar N, O'Neill K, Lee JC. Incidence of concussion in high school football players of Ohio and Pennsylvania. J Child Neurol. 2001;16(2):83–5.
6. McCrea M, Hammeke T, Olsen G, Leo P, Guskiewicz K. Unreported concussion in high school football players: implications for prevention. Clin J Sport Med. 2004;14(1):13–7.
7. Gavett BE, Stern RA, McKee AC. Chronic traumatic encephalopathy: a potential late effect of sport-related concussive and subconcussive head trauma. Clin Sports Med. 2011;30(1): 179–88.
8. Omalu BI, DeKosky ST, Hamilton RL, Minster RL, Kamboh MI, Shakir AM, et al. Chronic traumatic encephalopathy in a national football league player: part II. Neurosurgery. 2006;59(5):1086–92.
9. Omalu BI, DeKosky ST, Minster RL, Kamboh MI, Hamilton RL, Wecht CH. Chronic traumatic encephalopathy in a National Football League player. Neurosurgery. 2005;57(1):128–34.
10. Guskiewicz KM, Marshall SW, Bailes J, McCrea M, Cantu RC, Randolph C, et al. Association between recurrent concussion and late-life cognitive impairment in retired professional football players. Neurosurgery. 2005;57(4):719–26.
11. Guskiewicz KM, Marshall SW, Bailes J, McCrea M, Harding Jr HP, Matthews A, et al. Recurrent concussion and risk of depression in retired professional football players. Med Sci Sports Exerc. 2007;39(6):903–9.
12. Janda DH, Bir CA, Cheney AL. An evaluation of the cumulative concussive effect of soccer heading in the youth population. Inj Control Saf Promot. 2002;9(1):25–31.
13. Ommaya AK. Biomechanics of head injuries: experimental aspects. In: Nahum AM, Melvin J, editors. Biomechanics of trauma. Eat Norwalk, CT: Appleton-Century-Crofts; 1985.
14. Thurman DJ, Branche CM, Sniezek JE. The epidemiology of sports-related traumatic brain injuries in the United States: recent developments. J Head Trauma Rehabil. 1998;13(2):1–8.
15. Unterharnscheidt FJ. Translational versus rotational acceleration: animal experiments with measured inputs. In: Proceedings of the 15th Stapp Car Crash Conference, SAE 710880; 1971.

16. Hardy WN, Khalil TB, King AI. Literature review of head injury biomechanics. Int J Impact Eng. 1994;15(4):561–86.
17. Lissner HR, Lebow M, Evans FG. Experimental studies on the relation between acceleration and intracranial pressure changes in man. Surg Gynecol Obstet. 1960;111:329–38.
18. Gurdjian E, Lissner H, Evans F, Patrick L, Hardy W. Intracranial pressure and acceleration accompanying head impacts in human cadavers. Surg Gynecol Obstet. 1961;113:185.
19. Patrick LM, Lissner HR, Gurdijan ES. Survival by design-head protection. In: Proceedings of the 7th Stapp Car Crash Conference; 1963. p. 483–99.
20. Ono K, Kikuchi A, Nakamura M, Kobayashi H, Nadamura H. Human head tolerance to sagittal impact reliable estimation deduced from experimental head injury using sub-human primates and human cadaver skulls. In: Proceedings of the 24th Stapp Car Crash Conference; 1980. p. 101–60.
21. Gadd CW. Use of a weighted-impulse criterion for estimating injury hazard. In: Proceedings of the 10th Stapp Car Crash Conference, SAE 660793; 1966.
22. Versace J. A review of the severity index. In: SAE technical paper series, SAE 710881; 1971.
23. Mertz HJ, Irwin AL, Prasad P. Biomechanical and scaling bases for frontal and side impact injury assessment reference values. Stapp Car Crash J. 2003;47:155–88.
24. Mertz HJ, Prasad P, Irwin AL, editors. Injury risk curves for children and adults in frontal and rear collisions. In: SAE technical paper series; 1997.
25. Hardy WN, Foster CD, Mason MJ, Yang KH, King AI, Tashman S. Investigation of head injury mechanisms using neutral density technology and high-speed biplanar x-ray. Stapp Car Crash J. 2001;45:337–68.
26. Hardy WN, Mason MJ, Foster CD, Shah CS, Kopacz JM, Yang KH, et al. A study of the response of the human cadaver head to impact. Stapp Car Crash J. 2007;51:17–80.
27. Gennarelli T, Ommaya A, Thibault L, editors. Comparison of translational and rotational head motions in experimental cerebral concussion. In: Proceedings of the 15th Stapp Car Crash Conference; 1971.
28. Gennarelli TA. Head injury in man and experimental animals: clinical aspects. Acta Neurochir Suppl (Wien). 1983;32:1–13.
29. Gennarelli TA, Adams JH, Graham DI. Acceleration induced head injury in the monkey. The model, its mechanical and physiological correlates. Acta Neuropathol Suppl. 1981;7:23–5.
30. Gennarelli TA, Thibault LE. Biomechanics of acute subdural hematoma. J Trauma. 1982;22(8):680.
31. Gennarelli TA, Thibault LE, Adams JH, Graham DI, Thompson CJ, Marcincin RP. Diffuse axonal injury and traumatic coma in the primate. Ann Neurol. 1982;12(6):564–74.
32. Gennarelli TA, Thibault LE, Ommaya AK. Pathophysiologic responses to rotational and translational accelerations of the head. In: SAE technical paper series 720970; 1972. p. 296–308.
33. Hodgson V, Thomas L, Khalil T, editors. The role of impact location in reversible cerebral concussion. In: Twenty-seventh Stapp Car Crash Conference proceedings (P-134) with International Research Committee on Biokinetics of Impacts (IRCOBI); 1983.
34. Ommaya A, Hirsch A. Tolerances for cerebral concussion from head impact and whiplash in primates. J Biomech. 1971;4(1):13–21.
35. Ommaya AK, Gennarelli TA. Cerebral concussion and traumatic unconsciousness. Correlation of experimental and clinical observations of blunt head injuries. Brain. 1974;97(4):633–54.
36. Ommaya AK, Hirsch AE, Flamm ES, Mahone RH. Cerebral concussion in the monkey: an experimental model. Science. 1966;153(732):211–2.
37. Ommaya AK, Hirsch AE, Martinez JL, editors. The role of whiplash in cerebral concussion. In: Proceedings of the 10th Stapp Car Crash Conference; 1966.
38. Gennarelli T, Thibault L, Tomei G, Wiser R, Graham D, Adams J, editors. Directional dependence of axonal brain injury due to centroidal and non-centroidal acceleration. In: 31st Stapp Car Crash Conference; 1987.
39. Ommaya AK, Yarnell P, Hirsch AE, Harris EH. Scaling of experimental data on cerebral concussion in sub-human primates to concussion threshold for man. In: Proceedings of the 11th Stapp Car Crash Conference, SAE 670906; 1967.

40. Newman JA, Barr C, Beusenberg MC, Fournier E, Shewchenko N, Welbourne E, et al., editors. A new biomechanical assessment of mild traumatic brain injury. Part 2: results and conclusions. In: Proceedings of the International Research Conference on the Biomechanics of Impacts (IRCOBI). Montpellier, France: IRCOBI; 2000.
41. Newman JA, Beusenberg MC, Fournier E, Shewchenko N, Withnall C, King AI, et al., editors. A new biomechanical assessment of mild traumatic brain injury. Part 1: methodology. In: Proceedings of the International Research Conference on the Biomechanics of Impacts (IRCOBI). Barcelona, Spain: IRCOBI; 1999.
42. Newman JA, Beusenberg MC, Shewchenko N, Withnall C, Fournier E. Verification of biomechanical methods employed in a comprehensive study of mild traumatic brain injury and the effectiveness of American football helmets. J Biomech. 2005;38(7):1469–81.
43. Newman JA, Shewchenko N, Welbourne E. A proposed new biomechanical head injury assessment function—the maximum power index. Stapp Car Crash J. 2000;44:215–47.
44. Pellman EJ, Powell JW, Viano DC, Casson IR, Tucker AM, Feuer H, et al. Concussion in professional football: epidemiological features of game injuries and review of the literature— Part 3. Neurosurgery. 2004;54(1):81–94.
45. Pellman EJ, Viano DC, Casson IR, Tucker AM, Waeckerle JF, Powell JW, et al. Concussion in professional football: repeat injuries—Part 4. Neurosurgery. 2004;55(4):860–73.
46. Pellman EJ, Viano DC, Tucker AM, Casson IR. Concussion in professional football: location and direction of helmet impacts—Part 2. Neurosurgery. 2003;53(6):1328–40.
47. Pellman EJ, Viano DC, Tucker AM, Casson IR, Waeckerle JF. Concussion in professional football: reconstruction of game impacts and injuries. Neurosurgery. 2003;53(4):799–812.
48. King AI, Yang KH, Zhang L, Hardy W, Viano DC, editors. Is head injury caused by linear or angular acceleration? In: Proceedings of the International Research Conference on the Biomechanics of Impact (IRCOBI), Lisbon, Portugal; 2003.
49. Kleiven S. Predictors for traumatic brain injuries evaluated through accident reconstructions. Stapp Car Crash J. 2007;51:81–114.
50. Zhang L, Yang KH, King AI. A proposed injury threshold for mild traumatic brain injury. J Biomech Eng. 2004;126(2):226–36.
51. Moon DW, Beedle CW, Kovacic CR. Peak head acceleration of athletes during competition— football. Med Sci Sports. 1971;3(1):44–50.
52. Reid SE, Epstein HM, O'Dea TJ, Louis MW, Reid Jr SE. Head protection in football. J Sports Med. 1974;2(2):86–92.
53. Reid SE, Tarkington JA, Epstein HM, O'Dea TJ. Brain tolerance to impact in football. Surg Gynecol Obstet. 1971;133(6):929–36.
54. Morrison WE. Calibration and utilization of an instrumented football helmet for the monitoring of impact accelerations [microform]. University Park, PA: Penn State University; 1983.
55. Naunheim RS, Standeven J, Richter C, Lewis LM. Comparison of impact data in hockey, football, and soccer. J Trauma. 2000;48(5):938–41.
56. Manoogian S, McNeely D, Duma S, Brolinson G, Greenwald R. Head acceleration is less than 10 percent of helmet acceleration in football impacts. Biomed Sci Instrum. 2006;42:383–8.
57. Crisco JJ, Chu JJ, Greenwald RM. An algorithm for estimating acceleration magnitude and impact location using multiple nonorthogonal single-axis accelerometers. J Biomech Eng. 2004;126(6):849–54.
58. Rowson S, Duma SM, Beckwith JG, Chu JJ, Greenwald RM, Crisco JJ, et al. Rotational head kinematics in football impacts: an injury risk function for concussion. Ann Biomed Eng. 2012;40(1):1–13.
59. Greenwald RM, Gwin JT, Chu JJ, Crisco JJ. Head impact severity measures for evaluating mild traumatic brain injury risk exposure. Neurosurgery. 2008;62(4):789–98.
60. Chu JJ, Beckwith JG, Crisco JJ, Greenwald R. A novel algorithm to measure linear and rotational head acceleration using single-axis accelerometers. J Biomech. 2006;39 Suppl 1:S534.
61. Beckwith JG, Greenwald RM, Chu JJ. Measuring head kinematics in football: correlation between the head impact telemetry system and hybrid III headform. Ann Biomed Eng. 2012;40(1):237–48.

62. Rowson S, Beckwith JG, Chu JJ, Leonard DS, Greenwald RM, Duma SM. A six degree of freedom head acceleration measurement device for use in football. J Appl Biomech. 2011;27(1):8–14.
63. Rowson S, Duma SM. The virginia tech response. Ann Biomed Eng. 2012;40(12):2512–8.
64. Beckwith JG, Chu JJ, Greenwald RM. Validation of a noninvasive system for measuring head acceleration for use during boxing competition. J Appl Biomech. 2007;23(3):238–44.
65. Brainard LL, Beckwith JG, Chu JJ, Crisco JJ, McAllister TW, Duhaime AC, et al. Gender differences in head impacts sustained by collegiate ice hockey players. Med Sci Sports Exerc. 2012;44(2):297–304.
66. Greenwald RM, Durham SR, Beckwith JB, Stephens T. Biomechanics of head impacts in pediatric snowboarders. In: 18th international symposium on ski trauma and skiing safety conference, Garmisch-Partenkirchen, Germany; 2009. p. 24.
67. Hanlon E, Bir C. Validation of a wireless head acceleration measurement system for use in soccer play. J Appl Biomech. 2010;26(4):424–31.
68. Hanlon EM, Bir CA. Real-time head acceleration measurement in girls' youth soccer. Med Sci Sports Exerc. 2012;44(6):1102–8.
69. Mihalik JP, Guskiewicz KM, Marshall SW, Blackburn JT, Cantu RC, Greenwald RM. Head impact biomechanics in youth hockey: comparisons across playing position, event types, and impact locations. Ann Biomed Eng. 2012;40(1):141–9.
70. Stojsih S, Boitano M, Wilhelm M, Bir C. A prospective study of punch biomechanics and cognitive function for amateur boxers. Br J Sports Med. 2010;44(10):725–30.
71. Duma SM, Manoogian SJ, Bussone WR, Brolinson PG, Goforth MW, Donnenwerth JJ, et al. Analysis of real-time head accelerations in collegiate football players. Clin J Sport Med. 2005;15(1):3–8.
72. Funk JR, Duma SM, Manoogian SJ, Rowson S. Biomechanical risk estimates for mild traumatic brain injury. In: Annual proceedings of the Association for the Advancement of Automotive Medicine, vol. 51; 2007. p. 343–61.
73. Schnebel B, Gwin JT, Anderson S, Gatlin R. In vivo study of head impacts in football: a comparison of National Collegiate Athletic Association Division I versus high school impacts. Neurosurgery. 2007;60(3):490–5.
74. Guskiewicz KM, Mihalik JP, Shankar V, Marshall SW, Crowell DH, Oliaro SM, et al. Measurement of head impacts in collegiate football players: relationship between head impact biomechanics and acute clinical outcome after concussion. Neurosurgery. 2007;61(6):1244–53.
75. Mihalik JP, Bell DR, Marshall SW, Guskiewicz KM. Measurement of head impacts in collegiate football players: an investigation of positional and event-type differences. Neurosurgery. 2007;61(6):1229–35.
76. Broglio SP, Schnebel B, Sosnoff JJ, Shin S, Fend X, He X, et al. Biomechanical properties of concussions in high school football. Med Sci Sports Exerc. 2010;42(11):2064–71.
77. Crisco JJ, Fiore R, Beckwith JG, Chu JJ, Brolinson PG, Duma S, et al. Frequency and location of head impact exposures in individual collegiate football players. J Athl Train. 2010;45(6):549–59.
78. Crisco JJ, Wilcox BJ, Beckwith JG, Chu JJ, Duhaime AC, Rowson S, et al. Head impact exposure in collegiate football players. J Biomech. 2011;44(15):2673–8.
79. Crisco JJ, Wilcox BJ, Machan JT, McAllister TW, Duhaime AC, Duma SM, et al. Magnitude of head impact exposures in individual collegiate football players. J Appl Biomech. 2012;28(2):174–83.
80. Rowson S, Duma SM. Development of the STAR Evaluation System for football helmets: integrating player head impact exposure and risk of concussion. Ann Biomed Eng. 2011;39(8):2130–40.
81. Rowson S, Duma SM. Brain injury prediction: assessing the combined probability of concussion using linear and rotational head acceleration. Ann Biomed Eng. 2013;41(5):873–82.
82. Beckwith JG, Greenwald RM, Chu JJ, Crisco JJ, Rowson S, Duma SM, et al. Timing of concussion diagnosis is related to head impact exposure prior to injury. Med Sci Sports Exerc. 2013;45(4):747–54.

83. Beckwith JG, Greenwald RM, Chu JJ, Crisco JJ, Rowson S, Duma SM, et al. Head impact exposure sustained by football players on days of diagnosed concussion. Med Sci Sports Exerc. 2013;45(4):737–46.

84. Duma SM, Rowson S, Cobb B, MacAllister A, Young T, Daniel R. Effectiveness of helmets in the reduction of sports-related concussions in youth. Institute of Medicine, Commissioned paper by the Committee on Sports-Related Concussion in Youth; May 2013.

85. Margulies SS, Thibault LE. A proposed tolerance criterion for diffuse axonal injury in man. J Biomech. 1992;25(8):917–23.

86. Davidsson J, Angeria M, Risling MG, editors. Injury threshold for sagittal plane rotational induced diffuse axonal injuries. In: Proceedings of the International Research Conference on the Biomechanics of Impact (IRCOBI), York, UK; 2009.

87. Gennarelli TA, Pintar FA, Yoganandan N, editors. Biomechanical tolerances for diffuse brain injury and a hypothesis for genotypic variability in response to trauma. In: Annual proceedings/Association for the Advancement of Automotive Medicine. Association for the Advancement of Automotive Medicine; 2003.

88. Funk JR, Rowson S, Daniel RW, Duma SM. Validation of concussion risk curves for collegiate football players derived from HITS data. Ann Biomed Eng. 2012;40(1):79–89.

89. NOCSAE. Standard performance specification for newly manufactured baseball/softball catcher's helmets with faceguard. Overland Park, KS: National Operating Committee on Standards for Athletic Equipment; 2010.

90. NOCSAE. Standard performance specification for newly manufactured football helmets. Overland Park, KS: National Operating Committee on Standards for Athletic Equipment; 2011.

91. NOCSAE. Standard test method and equipment used in evaluating the performance characteristics of protective headgear/equipment. Overland Park, KS: National Operating Committee on Standards for Athletic Equipment; 2011.

92. Viano DC, Halstead D. Change in size and impact performance of football helmets from the 1970s to 2010. Ann Biomed Eng. 2012;40(1):175–84.

93. Viano DC, Withnall C, Halstead D. Impact performance of modern football helmets. Ann Biomed Eng. 2012;40(1):160–74.

94. Collins M, Lovell MR, Iverson GL, Ide T, Maroon J. Examining concussion rates and return to play in high school football players wearing newer helmet technology: a three-year prospective cohort study. Neurosurgery. 2006;58(2):275–86.

95. NOCSAE. Standard linear impactor test method and equipment used in evaluating the performance characteristics of protective headgear and face guards. Overland Park, KS: National Operating Committee on Standards for Athletic Equipment; 2006.

96. Pellman EJ, Viano DC, Withnall C, Shewchenko N, Bir CA, Halstead PD. Concussion in professional football: helmet testing to assess impact performance—Part 11. Neurosurgery. 2006;58(1):78–96.

97. Viano DC, Withnall C, Wonnacott M. Effect of mouthguards on head responses and mandible forces in football helmet impacts. Ann Biomed Eng. 2012;40(1):47–69.

Chapter 8
Acute and Lingering Impairments in Post-concussion Postural Control

Thomas A. Buckley

Abstract The fourth International Consensus Statement on Concussion in Sport reports that 80–90 % of concussions recover in 7–10 days. Impairments in postural control are a cardinal symptom following a sports-related concussion; however, many studies suggest that these impairments resolve within 3–5 days post-injury. Multiple recent studies, utilizing diverse and sophisticated research paradigms, are suggesting that this may be premature and that prolonged recovery could be normal. Therefore, the overarching purpose of the studies reported herein is to investigate impairments in postural control following a concussion and to identify recovery. We investigated the efficacy of "non-novel" tasks including gait initiation, gait variability, gait termination, and static stance and track the individual's performance across time to identify residual impairments compared to performance on the standard clinical assessment battery. In the acute aftermath of a concussion, the subjects demonstrated substantial impairments in postural control across all tasks which are consistent with a multiple previous investigations. However, the novel findings were the identification of persistent and lingering impairments in postural control which were present despite apparent full recovery on all clinical measures. Specifically, the impairments were more apparent when evaluating central control mechanisms (e.g., movement strategies and anticipatory postural adjustments) as standard kinematic variables returned to premorbid values in a timelier manner. These results suggest that individuals may be returning to sports participation prior to complete concussion recovery and could be a mechanism for the high recurrent concussion rate as well as recent speculation associating concussions and other sports-related injuries.

Keywords Postural control • Concussion • Gait • Recovery

T.A. Buckley, Ed.D. (✉)
Department of Health and Kinesiology, Georgia Southern University,
62 Georgia Avenue, Box 8076, Statesboro, GA 30460, USA
e-mail: Tbuckley@Georgiasouthern.edu

S.M. Slobounov and W.J. Sebastianelli (eds.), *Concussions in Athletics:*
From Brain to Behavior, DOI 10.1007/978-1-4939-0295-8_8,
© Springer Science+Business Media New York 2014

Introduction

As discussed throughout this text, sports-related concussion has reached epidemic levels with estimates of up to 3.8 million concussions occurring annually in the United States [1]. However, some estimate that this may only reflect the tip of the iceberg as over half to three-quarters of all concussions may go unreported [2–4]. In order to appropriately manage sports-related concussions accurate, sensitive, and specific diagnostic tools are required. Ideally, athletes would be forthcoming about symptoms following a potential injury, but many athletes are clearly unaware of common concussion symptoms [2, 3, 5]. Further, numerous high-profile cases exist of athletes opening lying about concussion symptoms (e.g., New York Jets quarterback Greg McElroy), admitting they would lie about symptoms (e.g., Brian Urlacher), not report symptoms (e.g., Troy Polamalu), downplaying the seriousness of the injury (e.g., Maurice Jones Drew), indicating a necessity to play through a concussion (e.g., Calvin Johnson), or intentionally trying to sandbag the baseline testing protocol to hasten return to participation (e.g., Peyton Manning) [6]. While standard imaging technology (e.g., MRI, CT) is effective in identifying structural pathology, these same procedures are not sensitive to the largely physiological pathology of concussion [7, 8]. Recent imaging advances including functional MRI (fMRI), diffusion tensor imaging, MR spectroscopy, and others hold promise for future utilization; however, they remain as research tools and are not recommended for routine clinical care [7–11]. Similarly, there have been multiple attempts at identifying a blood biomarker (e.g., 100-B, UCH-L1) of concussion which, although promising, is likely not ready to move beyond research utilization [12–15]. Neuropsychological testing, while a valuable contribution to concussion management, has limitations including low to moderate test–retest reliability, low sensitivity, a small practice/learning effect, potential "sandbagging" of the test, and test administration differences [16–25].

Accurate and timely recognition of a sports-related concussion is critical in preventing associated sequelae. Specifically, the failure to acutely identify the presence of a concussion potentially exposes the individual to the rare, but often fatal, second impact syndrome (SIS) [26–28]. While the specific neurophysiology of SIS remains elusive, it is generally believed to result from altered cerebral autoregulation following a head injury whereby the brain is unable to regulate cerebral and intracranial pressure [26]. This loss of autoregulation results in rapid cerebral vascular congestion, increased intracranial pressure, brain herniation, and often death within minutes [26, 27]. SIS occurs when an athlete who has suffered an initial concussion suffers a second concussion before the symptoms associated with the first concussion have fully cleared [29]. A recent review of catastrophic head injuries highlighted the need to restrict participation until symptom-free as almost 60 % of football players suffering catastrophic head injuries had a previous head injury and almost 40 % admitted to playing despite residual symptoms of the prior head injury [28].

Fortunately, SIS is an extraordinarily rare condition; however, appropriate concussion management is vital to reduce the risk of repeat concussion. Once the individuals suffer a single concussion, they are at a three- to sixfold increased risk of suffering a second same-season concussion and over 90 % of the repeat injuries occur within the first 10 days post-injury, potentially suggestive of a window of increased vulnerability [30–33]. Further, this repeat concussion is likely to present worse and has a prolonged recovery time [34, 35]. Finally, recent evidence identified over the last decade has suggested an association between concussions and later-life neuropathologies including mild cognitive impairment [36], clinically diagnosed depression [37], potentially earlier onset of Alzheimer disease [36], chronic traumatic encephalopathy [38, 39], and amyotrophic lateral sclerosis [40]. Thus, it is clearly imperative for health care providers to accurately identify concussions acutely as well as properly manage the condition post-injury. Therefore, this chapter will explore the utilization of postural control as a biomarker of both concussion diagnosis and recovery.

Postural Control and Concussion

The phrases postural control, postural stability or instability, balance, and equilibrium are unfortunately frequently used interchangeably in both the lay vernacular and, occasionally, the professional literature [41, 42]. Postural control involves regulating the body's position in space for the dual purposes of stability and orientation whereas postural stability is the ability to control the center of mass (COM) in relationship to the base of support [43]. The COM refers to the weighted average, in 3D space, of each of the body segments and is generally considered to be the key variable in the postural control system [42–44]. The control of the COM during either static or dynamic tasks is generally categorized into three neurological components: (1) motor processes, (2) sensory processes, and (3) supraspinal or cognitive processes [43]. The motor processes include the organization of muscles throughout the body into neuromuscular synergies [43]. The sensory processes comprise three systems: (1) visual system, (2) vestibular system, and (3) somatosensory system [42]. The visual system is primarily involved in planning locomotion and avoiding obstacles; the vestibular system, sometimes referred to as the body's gyro, senses linear and angular acceleration [42, 45]. Finally, the somatosensory system has multiple responsibilities including sensing the position and velocity of bodily segments, their contact with external objects, and the orientation of the body relative to gravity [42, 45]. The role of the cognitive processes in postural control is an emerging area of research with focus on "attentional resources" [43]. There are two primary theories underlying cognitive control of posture: (1) "Capacity theory" which is based on the sharing of a limited set of neurological resources and (2) "Bottleneck theory" which suggests there is a competition between tasks for limited neurological resources and a prioritization occurs [43]. Overall, postural control is the resultant of complex interactions between multiple bodily systems which have to work cooperatively to control the orientation and stability of the body [43].

Nearly all neuromuscular disorders result in some degeneration in the postural control systems and concussions are not an exception [42]. Indeed, the adverse effects of a concussion on postural control have been well elucidated in the literature [46]. Briefly, a deficit in the interaction between the visual, vestibular, and somatosensory systems is generally considered to be the underlying post-concussion neuropathology [47, 48]. Specifically, post-concussion it is believed that the individual is unable to appropriately integrate sensory input, ignore altered environmental conditions, and apply the appropriate motor control strategies to maintain precise postural control [47–49]. Recently, an increased focus on vestibular considerations for post-concussion balance impairments had evolved and led to recommend for vestibular therapy in cases of delayed or prolonged recovery [50, 51]. Finally, others have speculated that either diffuse axonal injury or the post-concussion neurometabolic cascade plays either a primary or secondary role in post-concussion impairments in postural control [30, 52]. Current clinical assessment batteries of postural control, utilizing either the balance error scoring system (BESS) or sensory organization test (SOT), have suggested that postural control recovers within 1–5 days post-injury, frequently prior to symptom resolution or achieving baseline values on computerized neuropsychological tests [47, 53].

Post-concussion Postural Control Assessment Battery

The original assessment of postural control following a concussion incorporated the Romberg test [54, 55]. The Romberg test, originally developed in 1853, was designed to subjectively assess somatosensory impairment in individuals with neurological conditions [56, 57]. However, the Romberg test was criticized for failing to objectively identifying subtle post-concussion balance deficits [49]. More recently, force plate measures have been developed to assess postural control and are valid and reliable and numerous metrics have been investigated [41, 58–63]. One commonly used research system, occasionally referred to as the "gold-standard," is the SOT which is thoroughly reviewed in separate chapter in this textbook. Generally, the SOT is both valid and reliable with impairments in postural control noted for 3–5 days post-injury and suggested that the vestibular system of the sensory processes is most commonly impaired [41, 46, 64–68]. However, force plate (>$10,000) and sophisticated balance systems (SOT: >$75,000) are expensive, likely cost-prohibitive for the overwhelming majority of sports medicine clinical sites, and may require extensive additional training or the addition of a biomechanist to the sports medicine staff. Indeed, even amongst NCAA Division I athletic trainers, less than 1 % reported utilizing the SOT [69]. Thus, a cost-effective and practical postural control assessment paradigm was required to appropriately assess post-concussion impairments.

Current consensus of appropriate concussion management, both during the sideline or acute concussion assessment or when tracking recovery, calls for a multifaceted assessment battery as no single test is highly sensitive [7, 20, 70]. The fourth International Consensus Statement on Concussion in Sport (4th CIS) recommends a two-component balance assessment: (1) a modified BESS (mBESS) and/or

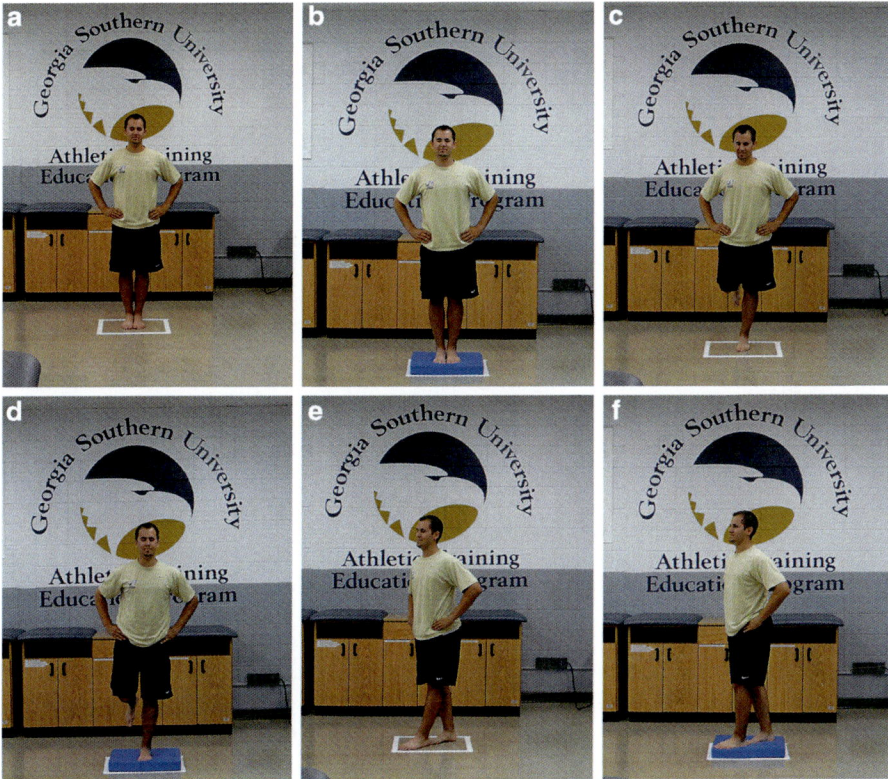

Fig. 8.1 The six stances of the balance error scoring system (BESS) test. Conditions (**a**)–(**c**) are on a firm surface while conditions (**d**)–(**f**) are on a foam surface. Conditions (**a**) and (**d**) have both feet on the surface and in contact, conditions (**b**) and (**e**) are single leg, and conditions (**c**) and (**f**) are tandem stance. Each stance is performed for 20 s and the total numbers of errors per stance (maximum of 10 per stance) are summed for a total score

(2) tandem gait [7]. The mBESS consists of three stances (double, single, tandem) on a single surface which is solid [7]. The mBESS has received limited attention in the literature; however, normative data suggests the scores increase (worsen) with aging and obesity [71]. The tandem gait assessment consists of a heel-to-gait for 3 m along a 38 mm wide piece of tape, a 180° turn, and returning along the same walkway [7]. The test is repeated four times and the best trial time is recorded as the individuals score [7]. While this test has not been evaluated post-concussion, some evidence suggests a dynamic gait assessment may be more reliable and less influenced by fatigue than a static test such as BESS [72].

While the mBESS and tandem gait are the current recommendations of the 4th CIS, the more commonly used postural control assessment post-concussion remains the original BESS test [69, 73–75]. The original BESS consists of three stances (double, single, and tandem) on two surfaces (firm and foam) with errors being counted for deviations from the test position [56, 65]; see also Fig. 8.1.

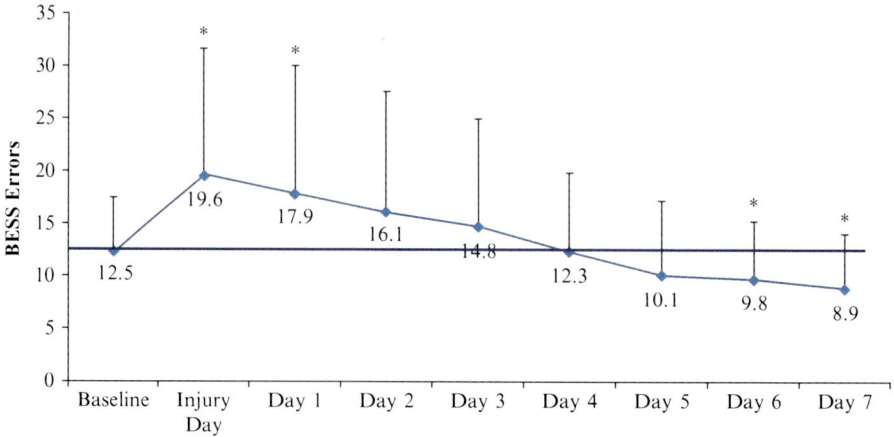

Fig. 8.2 BESS scores across time. There was a significant increase (worsening) in BESS score at immediate post-injury ($p=0.001$) and day 1 post-injury ($p=0.010$). There was a significant decrease (improvement) in BESS score at day 6 ($p=0.045$) and day 7 ($p=0.012$) despite over 20 % of participants still endorsing symptoms for at least 6 days

The BESS appears sensitive to acute concussion with an increase of 6–8 errors post-injury being commonly reported [53, 76]. The specificity of the BESS remains >0.91 through the first week post-injury; however, the sensitivity is low immediately post-injury, 0.34, and continues to decrease to 0.16 over the first 3 days post-injury [76, 77]. Unfortunately, the minimal detectable change values for the BESS test range from 7.3 (intrarater) to 9.4 (interrater) [78]. An additional considerable limitation to the BESS is a noted practice effect, potentially due to the test's utilization of foam to perturb the somatosensory system [79]. Repeat administration, as quickly as the second administration of the test, has repeatedly demonstrated a significant reduction in the number of errors committed [80–82]. Further, this improvement has been noted to persist for the duration of a fall athletic season, 90 days [83]. Our post-concussion assessment protocol involves daily BESS testing, as is common amongst athletic trainers [69], and, similar to previous studies [53], shows an increase (worsening) of BESS score in the immediate 24 h post-injury; however, with repeat administration there was a significant decrease (improvement) of BESS score, as compared to baseline, within a week post-injury, often prior to symptom resolution (Fig. 8.2).

This would inappropriately suggest that balance actually improves post-concussion. These limitations have resulted in the suggestion to conduct multiple baseline testing sessions [80, 84]; however, this is not being incorporated by most athletic trainers likely due to time constraints [69]. Additional limitations of the BESS include fatigue, dehydration, functional ankle instability, neuromuscular training, and testing environment [85–92]. Finally, the influences of previous common sports injuries (e.g., ankle or knee sprains) which occur after the baseline testing but prior to a post-concussion assessment have not currently been elucidated.

Overall, the current utilization of the BESS test, despite being the most commonly used postural control assessment tool, is fundamentally flawed as there is scant evidence that multiple baseline tests are occurring nor that the post-injury limitations are being considered [69].

These assessment batteries are typically performed in a single-task manner (i.e., only a motor task without concurrent cognitive tasks); however, an emerging line of research suggests that dual-task testing may be advantageous in the post-concussion population [93–96]. This is the next logical step in concussion assessment as Winter has suggested that the central nervous system is capable of adapting for a loss of function following a pathology until the patient is deprived of the compensating system [42]. This is consistent with recent findings related to compensatory strategies seen in diverse testing paradigms post-concussion [97–105]. Currently, most post-concussion dual-task testing protocols utilize sophisticated computerized equipment to perform the assessment with balance assessments performed with the SOT and either an auditory or visual switch task as the cognitive challenge [94, 106]. Unfortunately, as previously discussed, these tests are likely impractical for most clinicians as they lack both equipment and training to perform the assessments [69]. A second line of dual-task motor and cognitive challenges involves gait and working memory tasks which will be discussed in the next section.

Postural Control During Motor Tasks Post-concussion

Early evidence of gait impairments following concussion were reported by McCrory based on video analysis of concussions sustained in the mid-1990s by competitors in Australian rules football [107]. Gait impairments, operationally defined as ataxic, stumbling, or unsteady gait, were noted post-injury in 41 % of concussed athletes with the majority manifesting symptoms immediately post-injury; however, a small percentage, 14 %, had a minimal delay of 10–20 s prior to the onset of gait unsteadiness [107]. While not specifically studied, it was speculated that gait unsteadiness involved a brainstem pathology and was multifactorial including postural tone, cerebellar, and labyrinthine function [107]. This study, while limited to gross video observations without true biomechanical assessment, provided foundational evidence of post-concussion gait impairments.

Compared to other commonly investigated neurological pathologies (e.g., Parkinson disease, elderly fallers, stroke, amputee), investigations of gait to identify impairments in postural control post-concussion have been fairly limited. Indeed, there are more review articles (e.g., systematic reviews, meta-analyses) on gait in the elderly than original research articles related to concussion and gait. The majority of gait studies were performed at one laboratory and were largely delimited to grade II concussions, as defined by the American Academy of Neurology (no LOC and symptoms persisting longer than 15 min) [108], had fairly homogeneous and small ($n = 10$–17/group) participant populations for most studies, lacked within-subject pre-injury data, and have involved a variety of gait tasks including single-task gait, dual-task gait with working memory challenges, and obstacle avoidance tasks [98–104, 109–111]. Finally, not all raw data is provided for all dependent variables of interest limiting the ability to perform a meta-analysis of the findings.

Utilizing traditional clinical measures of balance (e.g., BESS), large cohort investigators have suggested that postural control returns to its baseline value within 3–5 days post-injury [53]. The post-concussion gait studies which have been currently published are limited by lack of within-subjects baseline data; however, they are generally tightly matched to otherwise healthy control subjects. Within this context, gait velocity generally appears to return to a normal value by day 5 or 6 post-injury despite still experiencing concussion-related symptoms [99–101, 111], although in one study it had not recovered by day 28 [110]. This finding and other similar findings need to be taken in context as an apparent practice effect was potentially a confounding variable as the gait velocity steadily increased with each testing session in the healthy control group. However, by day 28 the concussion subjects had still not reached the initial and lowest gait velocity of the control subjects [110]. Similar findings were noted in the stepping characteristics (stride time, width, and length) [111] and sagittal plane COM measurements (anterior displacement and velocity of the COM and the anterior center of pressure [COP]–COM separation) [99, 111]. Frontal plane kinematics may be a more challenging task post-concussion as there is a limited base of support during the single-support phase of gait [112]. During single-task gait, post-concussion participants demonstrated limited increases in the medial to lateral COM range of motion and velocity [98, 102, 104, 111]. These impairments appear to persist for up to 28 days post-injury despite apparent recovery on the traditional clinical assessment battery [104, 111]. Interestingly, in many of these studies there was an apparent recovery on many dependent variables by day 5 post-injury, but significant differences reemerged 2–4 weeks later. These findings suggest either potential differences on day 5 are not statistically significant due to small groups and the possibility of the study being underpowered or some residual consequence of delayed impairment following a concussion. Overall, these gait studies suggest that a conservative gait strategy has been adopted post-concussion, although the rationale for these strategies remains unknown.

Adopting from methodologies utilized with elderly and diseased state patients, the addition of a cognitive challenge to the motor task of gait is beginning to be explored post-concussion. Both impairments in postural control and cognitive processing are known acute consequences of a concussion and thus not surprisingly both are abnormal when tested within 24 h of the injury. Post-concussion gait studies utilizing a dual-task paradigm have largely focused on utilizing working memory challenges (e.g., reciting the months of the year backwards) from the mini mental examination to assess cognitive performance while performing either level over ground gait or obstacle avoidance [113]. A recent systematic review and meta-analysis by Lee et al. [96] suggested that gait velocity and frontal plane range of motion are sensitive markers of dual-task interference in post-concussion individuals (Fig. 8.3).

Specifically, a pooled mean decrease in gait velocity of 0.13 m/s was noted across the meta-analysis which is similar to a noted decrease of 0.17 m/s across a

a Concussed

Study or Subgroup	Dual task Mean [m/s]	SD [m/s]	Total	Single task Mean [m/s]	SD [m/s]	Total	Weight	Mean Difference IV, Random, 95% CI [m/s]	Mean Difference IV, Random, 95% CI [m/s]
Catena et al.[15]	1.097	0.166	14	1.219	0.137	14	32.1%	-0.12 [-0.23, -0.01]	
Parker et al.[16]	1.097	0.113	10	1.25	0.122	10	38.5%	-0.15 [-0.26, -0.05]	
Parker et al.[26] (AT)	1.101	0.174	14	1.227	0.15	14	28.2%	-0.13 [-0.25, -0.01]	
Parker et al.[26] (NAT)	1.321	0.114	14	1.27	1.127	14	1.2%	0.05 [-0.54, 0.64]	
Total (95% CI)			**52**			**52**	**100.0%**	**-0.13 [-0.20, -0.07]**	

Heterogeneity: Tau^2 = 0.00; Chi^2 = 0.56, df= 3 (P = 0.90); I^2 = 0%
Test for overall effect: Z = 4.08 (P < 0.0001)

-0.5 -0.25 0 0.25 0.5

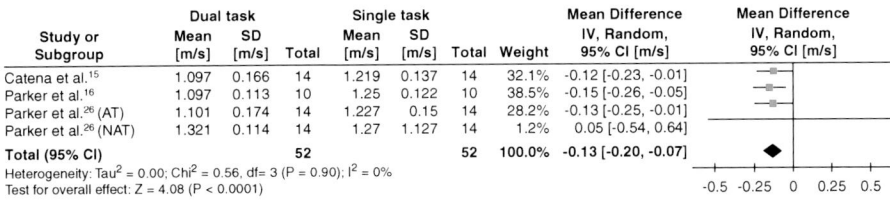

b Non-Concussed

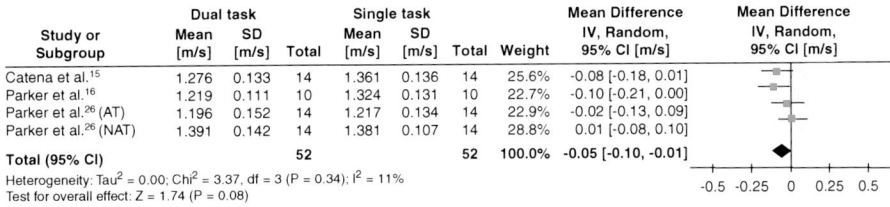

Study or Subgroup	Dual task Mean [m/s]	SD [m/s]	Total	Single task Mean [m/s]	SD [m/s]	Total	Weight	Mean Difference IV, Random, 95% CI [m/s]	Mean Difference IV, Random, 95% CI [m/s]
Catena et al.[15]	1.276	0.133	14	1.361	0.136	14	25.6%	-0.08 [-0.18, 0.01]	
Parker et al.[16]	1.219	0.111	10	1.324	0.131	10	22.7%	-0.10 [-0.21, 0.00]	
Parker et al.[26] (AT)	1.196	0.152	14	1.217	0.134	14	22.9%	-0.02 [-0.13, 0.09]	
Parker et al.[26] (NAT)	1.391	0.142	14	1.381	0.107	14	28.8%	0.01 [-0.08, 0.10]	
Total (95% CI)			**52**			**52**	**100.0%**	**-0.05 [-0.10, -0.01]**	

Heterogeneity: Tau^2 = 0.00; Chi^2 = 3.37, df = 3 (P = 0.34); I^2 = 11%
Test for overall effect: Z = 1.74 (P = 0.08)

-0.5 -0.25 0 0.25 0.5

Fig. 8.3 Meta-analysis of dual task. Forest plots for concussed (**a**) and non-concussed (**b**) groups for gait velocity at day 2. (◇): pooled mean estimate of the differences between ST and DT conditions; (□): difference between ST and DT conditions for individual studies; *AT* athletes, *NAT* non-athletes; *horizontal bars* represent 95 % confidence intervals. Lee H, Sullivan SJ, Schneiders AG. The use of the dual-task paradigm in detecting gait performance deficits following a sports-related concussion: A systematic review and meta-analysis. J Sci Med Sport. 2013:16(1): 2–7 (Permission received from publisher)

diverse population of neurologically impaired participants [96, 114]. In the acute recovery phase following a concussion, similar to single-task gait, multiple impairments are noted during dual-task gait. Specifically, when compared to tightly matched control subjects, reductions in stride length, anterior velocity of the COM, and COM displacement in the frontal plane have been reported [98–103, 110]. Consistent with many dual-task paradigms, most kinematic characteristics of gait were reduced with the addition of a cognitive task in both the recently concussed and healthy control groups [98–103, 110]. The recovery patterns of dual-task gait were similar to, but expand upon, the single-task gait with apparent lingering deficits still present up to 28 days post-injury [99–101, 110]. Once again, the frontal plane kinematics appeared most sensitive to the identification of delayed recovery following a concussion [112]. These findings support the necessity of a multifaceted concussion assessment as most cognitive and postural control assessments are recovered far before 28 days post-injury [53]. Further, when compared to a commonly utilized computerized neuropsychological test, there was little relationship with the dual-task gait performance [99]. The authors speculated that dynamic motor tasks, such as dual-task gait, are potentially more complex and challenging than traditional computerized neuropsychological tests and may better approximate the demands experienced during sports participation [99].

The results of these combined studies suggest that impairments in postural control persist for up to 1 month post-injury despite resolution on the traditional clinical assessment battery. Further, an interesting, but unexplained, finding was the apparent recovery within a week post-injury, but residual impairment in performance which persisted up to a month. Future research needs to elucidate the reasons for this altered performance.

Experimental Post-concussion Postural Control

The remaining postural control data presented in this chapter is derived from the Georgia Southern University Concussion Management research protocol. This data represents 84 participants (Ht: $1.74 + 0.13$ m; weight: $79.7 + 23.5$ kg; age: $19.6 + 1.4$ years; 50.7 % with a previous history of concussion [$0.8 + 1.1$ overall]) who suffered a sports-related concussion. The concussion initial presentations (9.5 % LOC; 34.5 % posttraumatic amnesia) and recovery timelines (symptom-free: $4.8 + 3.1$ days; BESS recovery: $2.9 + 2.8$ days; standard assessment of concussion recovery [SAC]: $2.2 + 1.8$ days) are consistent with previous large epidemiological studies [32, 33, 53]. All participants completed a graduated and progressive return to participation exercise protocol, generally consistent with the third International Consensus Statement on Concussion in Sport (3rd CIS) [7], and the average time to unrestricted return to participation was $12.6 + 5.1$ days.

The post-injury assessment protocol has been modified over the years as new information and recommendations have been incorporated. Specifically, the protocol was established in the late 2008 and did not incorporate computerized neuropsychological testing until 2010. The postural control testing occurred in the biomechanics laboratory which contains four force plates (AMTI, Watertown, MA) and an instrumented walkway (GAITRite; CIR Systems, Sparta, NJ); see also Fig. 8.4. Following a concussion, injured student-athletes performed the BESS,

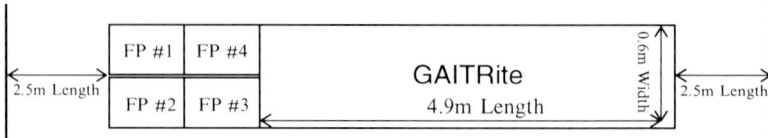

Fig. 8.4 Biomechanics laboratory set-up. The gait initiation trials began with the participant standing on force plates (FP) #1 and #2, having the first football impact on either force plates #3 or #4, and continuing down the instrumented walkway to a target end line 2.5 m beyond the walkway. Gait termination trials transversed the instrumented walkway and terminated with the penultimate step impacting force plates #3 or #4 and the termination step occurring on force plates #1 and #2. Stepping kinematics were recorded from the instrumented walkway during both initiation and termination trials. Buckley TA, Munkasy BA, Tapia-Lovler TG, Wikstrom EA. Altered Gait Termination Strategies Following a Concussion. Gait and Posture. (epub March 11, 2013) (Permission received from publisher)

SAC, and a graded symptom checklist (22-items, 0–6 Likert scale) daily until they achieved their baseline values on each specific test. Participants were tested daily with over 90 % compliance.

Acute Concussion Response

The control of posture and locomotion are interdependent at several levels of the central nervous system [115]. Therefore, impaired posture and gait components may contribute to deficits in locomotion due to adaptive changes in neural control [115]. Many post-concussion balance assessments (e.g., BESS, SOT) are novel challenges and, as described, are subject to a substantial practice effect with repeat administration [79–83]. Thus, we have opted to utilize what we refer to as "non-novel" tasks—these are tasks which are performed as regular activities of daily living and therefore not subject to a practice or learning effect. One task commonly utilized to investigate the interactions between posture and locomotion components is gait initiation (GI). Indeed, GI, the phase between motionless standing and steady state locomotion requiring the generation of propulsive forces, has been shown to be a sensitive indicator of balance dysfunction [116]. GI challenges the postural control systems as it is a volitional transition from a large stable base of support to a smaller continuously unstable posture during gait [117]. From a motor control perspective, GI requires the central nervous system to regulate the spatial and temporal relationship between the position and motion of the COM [118]. Therefore, GI has been used to quantify impairments in postural instability amongst elderly, Parkinson disease, stroke, and amputee patient groups [119–125].

During static stance, the COP and COM are tightly coupled and located just anterior to the malleolus [124]. To initiate gait, they must decouple to generate forward momentum while maintaining upright balance [124, 126]. Initially, the COP moves posteriorly and laterally towards the initial swing limb (Fig. 8.5). This anticipatory postural adjustment (APA), controlled by the supplementary motor area and/or premotor area, involves bilateral tibialis anterior activation and soleus inhibition [127–129]. The initial posterior COP movement generates the forward momentum needed to separate the COP and COM while the lateral COP displacement, controlled by the gluteus medias, propels the COM towards the initial stance limb [130]. This momentum generation is necessary to achieve successful forward locomotion while maintaining upright balance. Thus, the initial posterior and lateral COP displacements are sensitive indicators of balance dysfunction [119, 120, 125, 131].

Following a sports-related concussion, impairments in GI have been noted. A typical healthy adult will displace his or her COP approximately 5–7 cm both posteriorly and laterally during the APA phase of GI. One day post-concussion, the otherwise healthy adults' APA posterior displacement was 2.59 + 1.62 cm; a 131 % decrease compared to a normal healthy adult. Similarly, the lateral displacement of the COP post-concussion is reduced to 3.43 + 1.92 cm; a decrease of ~75 % from a healthy adult. As the posterior and lateral displacement during the APA is believed

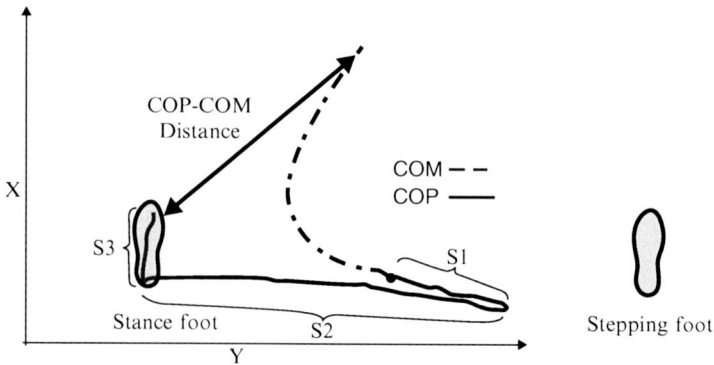

Fig. 8.5 The center of pressure (COP) and center of mass (COM) displacement during GI. When standing quietly, the COP is roughly equally distributed between the 2 ft. Upon movement initiation, the COP is displaced posterior and lateral towards the initial swing limb (S1). The S1 phase is the anticipatory postural adjustment (APA) phase of GI. As the initial swing limb leaves the ground, the COP is then displaced laterally towards the initial stance limb (S2). Finally, as the initial stance limb leaves the ground, the COP moves anteriorly under the foot (S3). Hass CJ, Waddell DE, Fleming RP, Juncos JL, Gregor RJ. Gait initiation and dynamic balance control in Parkinson's disease. Archives of Physical Medicine and Rehabilitation. 2005 Nov;86(11):2172–6 (Permission received from publisher)

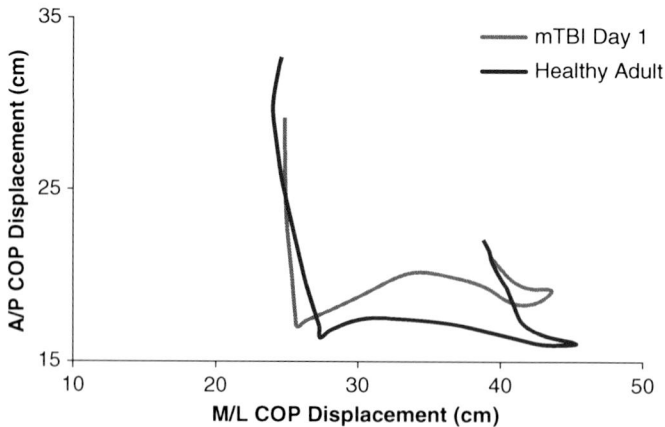

Fig. 8.6 COP exemplar trace for day 1 post-injury and a healthy control subject. The APA phase represents the posterior and lateral shift, towards the initial swing limb, which occurs prior to movement. The normal healthy adult typically has 5–7 cm of displacement in both the posterior and lateral directions; however, the post-concussion reduced both the posterior (2.59 + 1.62 cm) and lateral (3.43 + 1.92 cm) displacements by 131 % and 75 %, respectively

to generate the momentum needed to accelerate the COM forward, it is not surprising that the initial step length (0.60 m) and velocity (0.58 m/s) are substantially reduced compared to population norms [125]. An exemplar COP displacement trace is provided in Fig. 8.6 and particular attention should be paid to the APA phase noting that the COP at movement initiation is nearly identical between traces.

This postural conservative strategy, unlikely to be associated with a fear of falling as is commonly suggested in neurologically impaired older adults, is consistent with gait-based studies comparing post-concussion postural control to healthy adults.

While comparison to healthy individuals is valid, comparing the individuals to their own premorbid performance is ideal. While the observed differences may appear small (i.e., only a few centimeters), the effect size of these differences needs to be considered. Effect size is a measure of the magnitude of the difference between groups and a value of 0.2 is considered a small effect, 0.5 a medium effect size, and 0.8 a large effect size. There is some debate on using effect size on within-subjects measures, but this is largely focused on varying treatment effects which are not present within this data set [132]. Following a sports-related concussion, individuals reduce their APA posterior displacement from a premorbid value of 5.46–2.34 cm, statistically significant ($p < 0.001$) with a large effect size (d) of 1.99. Similarly, the lateral displacement during the APA phase is reduced from 5.55 to 3.25 cm, statistically significant ($p < 0.001$) with a moderate effect size of 0.51. The reductions in APA COP displacement are likely associated with the reduction in initial step length (PRE: $0.68 + 0.11$ m and day 1: $0.60 + 0.09$, $p = 0.001$, $d = 0.37$) and step velocity (PRE: $0.67 + 0.17$ m/s and day 1: $0.58 + 0.15$ m/s, $p = 0.021$, $d = 0.27$). These results suggest that the largest impairments are noted in the APA component of GI as opposed to the resulting stepping characteristics. This likely occurs as the APA component is a supraspinal or central control process whereas the stepping characteristics are likely controlled at multiple levels including supraspinal (motor cortex), spinal (central pattern generators), and peripheral (local neuromuscular adaptations) [127–129, 133–135].

The post-concussion response to gait has been well established through a series of studies conducted in Li-Shan Chou's lab at the University of Oregon and has been discussed previously [98–105, 109–111]. Our data is similar with noted deficits on the day following the concussion. Specifically, substantial decrements in performance were noted in gait velocity (PRE: $1.49 + 0.13$ m/s and day 1: $1.17 + 0.13$ m/s, $p < 0.001$, $d = 0.77$), mean step length (PRE: $0.76 + 0.04$ m and day 1: $0.64 + 0.05$ m, $p = 0.002$, $d = 0.76$), percentage of the gait cycle in double support (PRE: $22.48 + 2.38$ % and day 1: $24.59 + 2.23$, $p = 0.035$, $d = 0.42$), and percentage of the gait cycle in the swing phase (PRE: $38.75 + 1.12$ % and day 1: $37.7 + 1.21$ %, $p = 0.05$, $d = 0.41$). In a small subgroup, increases in gait variability, expressed as a coefficient of variation, have been identified post-concussion. Gait variability is an indicator of the rhythmicity and gait stability and is known to be impaired in elderly individuals or those with neurological impairments [136–139]. A variability of greater than 7 % has been associated with impairments in postural control in older individuals with neurological impairments; however, in healthy adults normal variability is below 3 % [140–144]. While the post-concussion individuals in this study did not exceed the 7 % threshold, there were increases from baseline (<3 %) to day 1 post-injury (>3 %). Consistent with the Oregon findings, these results suggest a conservative gait strategy is adopted following a concussion. However, the neurophysiological explanation has not been fully elucidated.

These previous findings suggest that, acutely post-concussion, impairments in postural control are identified with single (motor)-task challenges; however, emerging evidence suggests that reallocation of attentional resources and/or neural plasticity may allow the individual to overcome simple single-task challenges [62, 97, 145]. Dual-task challenges examine the effect of executing a secondary cognitive task (e.g., mental processing) on the concurrent performance of a primary motor task (e.g., walking) [145]. Even routine motor activities, such as sitting, standing quietly, or walking, require cognitive processing [146]. Previous investigations noted impaired postural control during both quiet stance and gait in healthy young adults under dual-task conditions [147, 148]. Simultaneous performance of a motor task and a cognitive task may interfere with the performance of one or both, probably due to competing demands for inherently limited attentional resources [149–151]. Utilizing working memory challenges (e.g., serial 7's), post-concussion participants had further reductions in the displacement of the COP during the APA phase of GI and took shorter and slower steps than during single-task GI. Consistent with the findings from the Oregon studies, those differences were also present during gait with significant reductions in gait velocity, stride length, single-support phase, and swing phase when compared to healthy young adults. Interestingly, there were no differences noted within subjects when comparing single- and dual-task gait; potentially due to an inverted "ceiling" effect whereby individual's performance during single task was already dramatically impaired. Indeed, both single- (1.17 m/s) and dual-task (1.15 m/s) gait velocities fell below the 1.2 m/s threshold often cited for a healthy gait in elderly and neurologically impaired individuals [152, 153].

Gait termination (GT) is not a mirror image of GI [154]. Rather, GT is a process by which the central nervous system anticipates, controls, and arrests the forward momentum of the COM without exceeding the borders of the base of support [155, 156]. Further, GT has a known and invariant set of parameters that constrains the multiple degrees of freedom within the lower extremity [157–159]. However, GT poses a unique challenge to the postural control systems because the COM is often located outside the base of support at the onset of GT [126]. As a result, GT is an excellent model for investigating alterations in motor programming and neurologic dysfunction. The central neurophysiologic control of GT is more elusive than GI; however, an fMRI study has suggested that the prefrontal area, specifically the inferior frontal gyrus and the pre-supplementary motor area, likely controls GT [154]. Indeed, GT has quantified impairments in postural control amongst the aging, people with Parkinson disease, amputee groups, chronic ankle instability, and those with general balance disorders [158–168].

The termination of gait requires the coordinated activity of both legs. Indeed, force production is modulated bilaterally such that the lead limb (limb behind the COM) reduces foot push-off propulsive forces as the swing limb (limb in front of the COM) concurrently increases vertical and anteroposterior braking forces [157, 158, 169]. Reduced propulsive forces are caused by soleus inhibition and increased activation of the tibialis anterior while concurrent increases in braking forces are due to an increased soleus activity and inhibition of the tibialis anterior [166, 170].

Table 8.1 Means, standard deviations, 95 % confidence intervals, and effect sizes for gait termination performance

	Control (n = 26)	Day 1 post-concussion (n = 15)	Control to day-1 post hoc p-values (effect size)	Day 10 post-concussion (n = 12)	Control to day-10 post hoc p-values (effect size)
Gait velocity (m/s)	1.32 ± 0.14 (1.26–1.38)	1.16 ± 0.14[a,b] (1.08–1.23)	0.01 (1.14)	1.33 ± 0.19 (1.21–1.46)	0.97 (0.06)
Propulsive (%)	−0.25 ± 0.53 (−0.41 to −0.10)	0.44 ± 0.17[a] (0.24–0.64)	<0.01 (0.85)	0.46 ± 0.13[a] (0.23–0.69)	<0.01 (0.85)
Braking (%)	−0.30 ± 0.20 (−0.39 to −0.21)	−0.05 ± 0.27[a,b] (−0.17 to 0.07)	<0.01 (0.54)	0.16 ± 0.23[a] (0.03–0.29)	<0.01 (0.95)

From Buckley TA, Munkasy BA, Tapia-Lovler TG, Wikstrom EA. Altered Gait Termination Strategies Following a Concussion. Gait and Posture. (epub March 11, 2013); used with permission
[a]Significant difference from the control group
[b]Significant difference from the day-10 time point

Failure to reduce lead limb propulsive forces results in an increased reliance on a single-limb stopping strategy and subsequently longer termination times and a greater number of steps required to control the COM [160]. Therefore, increases in propulsive and braking forces have been identified as sensitive indicators of balance dysfunction and alterations in the cortical control of GT [158, 160, 165]; see also Table 8.1.

In the aftermath of a concussion, GT performance is clearly impaired [171]. Initially, the reduced gait velocity, as previously described, may mask the task performance and, therefore, normalization to gait velocity is required. Further, to more clearly understand the postural strategies utilized, GT variables are compared to performance during standard gait trials. One would naturally expect the penultimate step during GT to have a reduced propulsive force and the terminal step to have an increased braking force relative to normal gait. Conversely, post-concussion the individuals actually increased their propulsive force during the penultimate step and reduced their braking force during the termination step [171]. This highly inefficient pattern of performing GT is suggestive of a central deficit and the selection of an inappropriate motor program to perform the GT task.

While measures of dynamic postural control are insightful in understanding impairments in postural control following a concussion, static stance assessments can also provide additional clarity. Several attempts have been made to quantify static post-concussion postural control utilizing approximate entropy measures but have generally failed to identify differences or noted decreased randomness [63, 172, 173]. The authors speculated that the reduced randomness was secondary to either distorted interactions in the brain or increased co-contraction of the lower extremity musculature; however, these conclusions were drawn from relatively

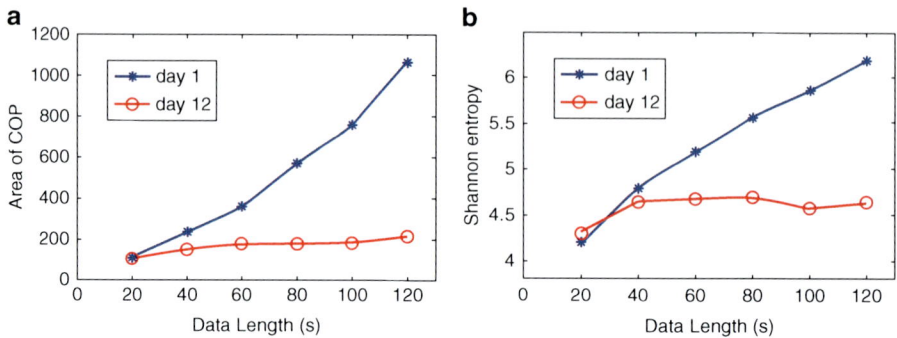

Fig. 8.7 COP area measures and Shannon entropy measures across time. There were no differences between day 1 and day 12 post-injury when the data was sampled for less than 60 s. Gao J, Hu J, Buckley TA, White K, Hass CJ. Shannon and Renyi entropies to classify effects of Mild Traumatic Brain Injury on postural sway. PLoS One. 2011;6(9):e24446 (PLoS One does not require a permission release to republish materials and the article citation is provided above)

short (20–30 s) data sets [173]. When a longer data set (120 s) was investigated, a greater than linear increase in COP area was noted across time suggesting that longer time frames are required for analysis [59]. Specifically, visual analysis clearly shows that at 20–40 s, there would be no differences between groups, but at 120 s clear differences are apparent [59]. Additionally, applying more sophisticated entropy measures, such as Shannon and Renyi measures, successfully identified impairments in postural control [59]. Unfortunately, this study lacks premorbid data, but some early analysis suggests that these trends continue when compared to baseline tests (Fig. 8.7).

Postural Control and Recovery

As discussed, the traditional post-concussion clinical assessment battery suggests that postural control recovers within 3–5 days post-injury [46, 53]. However, this apparent recovery often occurs prior to symptom resolution or achieving baseline values on computerized neuropsychological test batteries [53]. This suggests that while the current clinical battery may be sufficient to identify the presence of a concussion [70], it may lack the sensitivity to identify residual impairments which persist over time. Each of the non-novel tasks which show impairments in the immediate aftermath of a concussion has also demonstrated residual impairments which persist long after recovery based on standard clinical balance tests as well as self-reported symptoms, cognitive testing, and computerized neuropsychological testing.

A healthy young adult has approximately a 5–7 cm displacement of the COP in both the posterior and lateral directions during the APA phase of GI. However, on the day the individuals pass their BESS test (2.9 + 2.8 days post-injury), which clinically suggests their balance has returned to premorbid levels, substantial significant

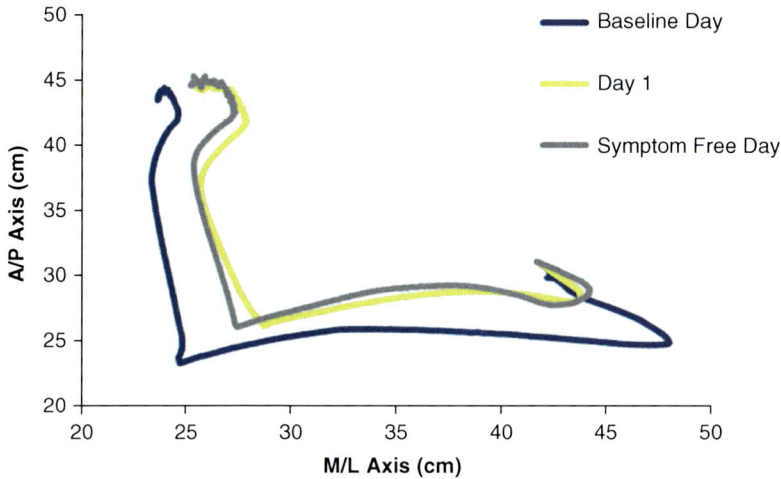

Fig. 8.8 Exemplar changes in COP displacement. The normal healthy adult typically has 5–7 cm of displacement in both the posterior and lateral directions. The posterior APA phase is reduced following a concussion (2.59 + 1.62 cm) and remains reduced at the time (4.8 + 3.1 days) the individual self-reports symptom-free (3.58 + 1.88 cm). Similarly, the lateral displacement is reduced immediately following a concussion (3.43 + 1.92 cm) and remains reduced at the time the individual self-reports symptom-free (4.51 + 2.31 cm)

deficits are noted in both the posterior (PRE: 5.46 + 1.82 cm and BESS: 2.54 + 1.28 cm, $p < 0.001$, $d = 0.68$) and lateral (PRE: 5.55 + 2.13 cm and BESS: 2.93 + 1.63 cm, $p < 0.001$, $d = 0.57$) directions. Similarly, on the day the individual self-reports being symptom-free (4.8 + 3.1 days) there were still impairments in the posterior APA COP displacement (3.58 + 1.88 cm, $p = 0.008$, $d = 0.45$); see Fig. 8.8. Even by 12 days post-injury, the most common time frame for return to participation, the posterior COP displacement was still reduced (4.23 cm) compared to baseline values, although this is within one standard deviation of the baseline. In each case, the standard kinematic stepping characteristics had achieved baseline values thus suggesting the APA phase is a better discriminator of impaired postural control. At no point during the testing protocol, on average, did the posterior COP displacement during the APA phase achieve a value equal to or greater than the baseline value.

The Oregon gait studies interestingly found that most gait kinematic variables returned to baseline values by day 5/6 post-injury and then demonstrated limited impairments at the 2- and 4-week follow-up testing. Conversely, standard gait kinematic stepping characteristics largely returned to baseline values for our subjects prior to return to participation status; however, gait variability assessment remained impaired throughout the recovery process. Specifically, at both self-selected normal pace and at face-paced gait, the variability increased post-injury and either remained flat-lined across time or continued to increase throughout the recovery process. Considering the normal healthy variability is typically below 3 %, the normal self-selected paced step length and step time variability as well as the fast-paced step length, step time, and step width variability all exceeded 3 % at

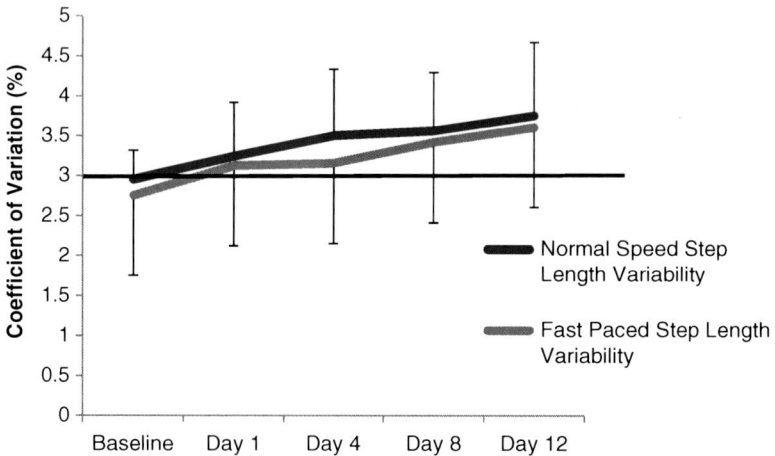

Fig. 8.9 Step length variability. There was a significant increase in step length variability at day 12 post-concussion compared to baseline. Normal healthy adults typically have step length variability at or below 3 %

return to participation (see Fig. 8.9). Similar to previous findings, these results suggest that despite apparent recovery on all clinical assessments, central neurological impairments may still persist.

Consistent with the lingering and persistent deficits noted during gait initiation and gait variability, gait termination remained impaired despite recovery on clinical assessment batteries [171]. By 10 days post-injury, all participants, in this subset, were fully recovered based on BESS, SAC, self-report symptoms, and ImPACT testing; however, clear impairments persisted during GT. Specifically, while gait velocity returned to normal values (actually exceeding the velocity of the control subjects), the post-concussion individuals continued to present with an altered motor strategy for terminating gait. Relative to normal gait trials, the post-concussion individuals continued to have abnormally increased propulsive forces during the penultimate step and decreased braking forces on the termination step—in both cases the motor strategy was actually less efficient than their performance on day 1 post-concussion [171]. While current studies have not elucidated the reasons for this altered movement strategy, it is likely a postural conservative strategy potentially secondary to lingering post-concussion impairments in the prefrontal area [154].

Finally, and consistent with the other reported measures, the impairments in postural control are also noted during static stance trials using sophisticated entropy measures [59]. Once again, despite all participants having achieved baseline values on all clinical measures, impairments in static postural control were still present at least 10 days post-injury; see Fig. 8.10. While this study focused more on the scientific applications of varying entropy metrics, as opposed to clinical application, the underlying mechanisms for the impairments in postural control were not investigated. However, *the results do support the emerging evidence that based on more sophisticated assessment protocols, most concussions do not recover within 7–10 days post-injury.*

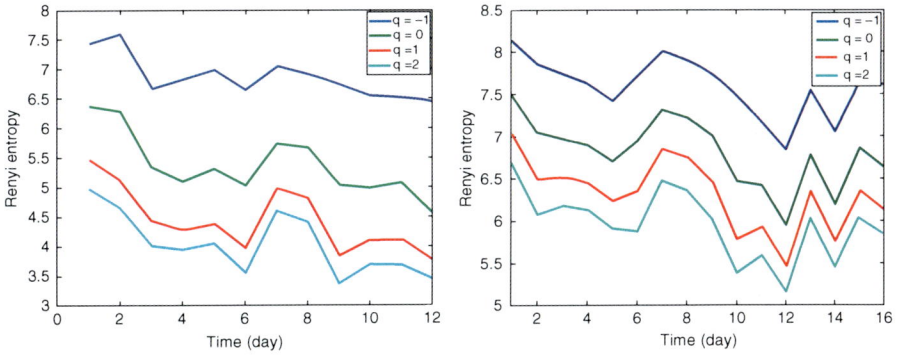

Fig. 8.10 Temporal variations of Renyi entropies for two subjects. Gao J, Hu J, Buckley TA, White K, Hass CJ. Shannon and Renyi entropies to classify effects of Mild Traumatic Brain Injury on postural sway. PLoS One. 2011;6(9):e24446 (PLoS One does not require a permission release to republish materials and the article citation is provided above)

Conclusion

The 4th CIS reports that 80–90 % of concussions in adults resolve within 7–10 days of the injury; however, this is presumably based on earlier epidemiological studies which operationally defined recovery based on self-reported symptoms, SAC, and the BESS [7, 53]. However, a growing body of evidence, utilizing diverse research paradigms including the postural control studies presented herein, has suggested that recovery is prolonged well beyond a couple of weeks [99–101, 104, 111, 174–177]. While the evidence may not fully support the recommendation yet, McKee has proposed a 4- to 6-week recovery period post-concussion to facilitate optimal healing [38]. While it is medically appropriate and ethical to treat concussions conservatively given the emerging association between repeated head injuries and later-life neuropathologies, this is complicated by an already unacceptably low (~50 %) concussion reporting rate [2–4]. Whereas fractures, dislocations, and sprains/strains are often obvious and easy to identify, concussions frequently rely on the individual to self-report the symptoms as severe confusion or disorientation and loss of consciousness are infrequent [32]. Anecdotal evidence suggests that a longer period of time before the student-athlete received medical clearance to return to participation would likely lower the current reporting rate and result in many student-athletes continuing to participate despite having a concussion. Conversely, allowing the injured student-athlete to return prematurely may expose the individual to increased risk of re-injury with potential later-life complications. This paradox will likely continue to challenge sports medicine clinicians for the foreseeable future; however, it is becoming clear that lingering post-concussion impairments persist longer than just 7–10 days.

References

1. Langlois JA, Rutland-Brown W, Wald MM. The epidemiology and impact of traumatic brain injury: a brief overview. J Head Trauma Rehabil. 2006;21(5):375–8.
2. McCrea M, Hammeke T, Olsen G, Leo P, Guskiewicz K. Unreported concussion in high school football players: implications for prevention. Clin J Sport Med. 2004;14(1):13–7.
3. Llewellyn TA, Burdette GT, Joyner AB, Buckley TA. Concussion reporting rates at the conclusion of an intercollegiate athletic career. Clin J Sport Med. 2013;24(1):76–9.
4. Meehan WP, 3rd, Mannix RC, O'Brien MJ, Collins MW. The prevalence of undiagnosed concussions in athletes. Clin J Sport Med. 2013;23(5):339–342.
5. Kaut KP, DePompei R, Kerr J, Congeni J. Reports of head injury and symptom knowledge among college athletes: implications for assessment and educational intervention. Clin J Sport Med. 2003;13(4):213–21.
6. Players still willing to hide head injuries. Associated Press; 2011 [cited 5 June 2013]. Available from http://espn.go.com/nfl/story/_/id/7388074/nfl-players-say-hiding-concussions-option.
7. McCrory P, Meeuwisse WH, Aubry M, Cantu B, Dvorak J, Echemendia RJ, et al. Consensus statement on concussion in sport: the 4th International Conference on Concussion in Sport held in Zurich, November 2012. Br J Sports Med. 2013;47(5):250–8.
8. Davis GA, Iverson GL, Guskiewicz KM, Ptito A, Johnston KM. Contributions of neuroimaging, balance testing, electrophysiology and blood markers to the assessment of sport-related concussion. Br J Sports Med. 2009;43(1):36–45.
9. Kutcher JS, McCrory P, Davis G, Ptito A, Meeuwisse WH, Broglio SP. What evidence exists for new strategies or technologies in the diagnosis of sports concussion and assessment of recovery [Review]? Br J Sports Med. 2013;47(5):299–303.
10. Dashnaw ML, Petraglia AL, Bailes JE. An overview of the basic science of concussion and subconcussion: where we are and where we are going. Neurosurg Focus. 2012;33(6):E5.
11. Henry LC, Tremblay S, Leclerc S, Khiat A, Boulanger Y, Ellemberg D, et al. Metabolic changes in concussed American football players during the acute and chronic post-injury phases. BMC Neurol. 2011;11:105.
12. Unden J, Romner B. Can low serum levels of S100B predict normal CT findings after minor head injury in adults?: an evidence-based review and meta-analysis. J Head Trauma Rehabil. 2010;25(4):228–40.
13. Liu MC, Akinyi L, Scharf D, Mo JX, Larner SF, Muller U, et al. Ubiquitin C-terminal hydrolase-L1 as a biomarker for ischemic and traumatic brain injury in rats. Eur J Neurosci. 2010;31(4):722–32.
14. Papa L, Akinyi L, Liu MC, Pineda JA, Tepas III JJ, Oli MW, et al. Ubiquitin C-terminal hydrolase is a novel biomarker in humans for severe traumatic brain injury. Crit Care Med. 2010;38(1):138–44.
15. Jeter CB, Hergenroeder GW, Hylin MJ, Redell JB, Moore AN, Dash PK. Biomarkers for the diagnosis and prognosis of mild traumatic brain injury/concussion. J Neurotrauma. 2013; 30(8):657–70.
16. Barr WB. Neuropsychological testing of high school athletes—preliminary norms and test-retest indices. Arch Clin Neuropsychol. 2003;18(1):91–101.
17. Broglio SP, Ferrara MS, Macciocchi SN, Baumgartner TA, Elliott R. Test-retest reliability of computerized concussion assessment programs. J Athl Train. 2007;42(4):509–14.
18. Randolph C. Baseline neuropsychological testing in managing sport-related concussion: does it modify risk? Curr Sports Med Rep. 2011;10(1):21–6.
19. Schatz P. Long-term test-retest reliability of baseline cognitive assessments using ImPACT. Am J Sports Med. 2010;38(1):47–53.
20. Register-Mihalik JK, Guskiewicz KM, Mihalik JP, Schmidt JD, Kerr ZY, McCrea MA. Reliable change, sensitivity, and specificity of a multidimensional concussion assessment battery: implications for caution in clinical practice. J Head Trauma Rehabil. 2013;28(4): 274–83.

21. Iverson GL, Lovell MR, Collins MW. Interpreting change on ImPACT following sport concussion. Clin Neuropsychol. 2003;17(4):460–7.
22. Erdal K. Neuropsychological testing for sports-related concussion: how athletes can sandbag their baseline testing without detection. Arch Clin Neuropsychol. 2012;27(5):473–9.
23. Glatts C, Schatz P. "Sandbagging" baseline concussion testing on ImPACT is more difficult than it appears. Arch Clin Neuropsychol. 2012;27(6):621–9.
24. Moser RS, Schatz P, Neidzwski K, Ott SD. Group versus individual administration affects baseline neurocognitive test performance. Am J Sports Med. 2011;39(11):2325–30.
25. Resch J, Driscoll A, McCaffrey N, et al. impact test-retest reliability: reliably unreliable? J Athl Train. 2013;48(4):506–11.
26. Bey T, Ostick B. Second impact syndrome. West J Emerg Med. 2009;10(1):6–10.
27. Cantu RC. Second-impact syndrome. Clin Sports Med. 1998;17(1):37–44.
28. Boden BP, Tacchetti RL, Cantu RC, Knowles SB, Mueller FO. Catastrophic head injuries in high school and college football players. Am J Sports Med. 2007;35(7):1075–81.
29. Cantu RC. Recurrent athletic head injury: risks and when to retire. Clin Sports Med. 2003;22(3):593–603.
30. Giza CC, Hovda DA. The neurometabolic cascade of concussion. J Athl Train. 2001; 36(3):228–35.
31. Zemper ED. Two-year prospective study of relative risk of a second cerebral concussion. Am J Phys Med Rehabil. 2003;82(9):653–9.
32. Guskiewicz KM, Weaver NL, Padua DA, Garrett Jr WE. Epidemiology of concussion in collegiate and high school football players. Am J Sports Med. 2000;28(5):643–50.
33. Guskiewicz KM, McCrea M, Marshall SW, Cantu RC, Randolph C, Barr W, et al. Cumulative effects associated with recurrent concussion in collegiate football players: the NCAA Concussion Study. JAMA. 2003;290(19):2549–55.
34. Collins MW, Lovell MR, Iverson GL, Cantu RC, Maroon JC, Field M. Cumulative effects of concussion in high school athletes. Neurosurgery. 2002;51(5):1175–9.
35. Eisenberg MA, Andrea J, Meehan W, Mannix R. Time interval between concussions and symptom duration. Pediatrics. 2013;132:8–17.
36. Guskiewicz KM, Marshall SW, Bailes J, McCrea M, Cantu RC, Randolph C, et al. Association between recurrent concussion and late-life cognitive impairment in retired professional football players. Neurosurgery. 2005;57(4):719–26; discussion 719–26.
37. Guskiewicz KM, Marshall SW, Bailes J, McCrea M, Harding Jr HP, Matthews A, et al. Recurrent concussion and risk of depression in retired professional football players. Med Sci Sports Exerc. 2007;39(6):903–9.
38. McKee AC, Cantu RC, Nowinski CJ, Hedley-Whyte ET, Gavett BE, Budson AE, et al. Chronic traumatic encephalopathy in athletes: progressive tauopathy after repetitive head injury. J Neuropathol Exp Neurol. 2009;68(7):709–35.
39. Schwartz A. Suicide reveals signs of a disease seen in N.F.L. New York Times, 14 Sept 2010.
40. McKee AC, Gavett BE, Stern RA, Nowinski CJ, Cantu RC, Kowall NW, et al. TDP-43 proteinopathy and motor neuron disease in chronic traumatic encephalopathy. J Neuropathol Exp Neurol. 2010;69(9):918–29.
41. Cavanaugh JT, Guskiewicz KM, Stergiou N. A nonlinear dynamic approach for evaluating postural control: new directions for the management of sport-related cerebral concussion. Sports Med. 2005;35(11):935–50.
42. Winter DA. Human balance and posture control during standing and walking. Gait Posture. 1995;3(4):193–214.
43. Shumway-Cook A, Woollacott MH. Motor control: translating research into clinical practice. 4th ed. Philadelphia: Lippincott Williams & Wilkins; 2012.
44. Scholz JP, Schoener G, Hsu WL, Jeka JJ, Horak F, Martin V. Motor equivalent control of the center of mass in response to support surface perturbations. Exp Brain Res. 2007;180(1): 163–79.
45. Highstein SM, Holstein GR. The anatomical and physiological framework for vestibular prostheses. Anat Rec. 2012;295(11):2000–9.

46. Guskiewicz KM. Balance assessment in the management of sport-related concussion. Clin Sports Med. 2011;30(1):89–102.

47. Guskiewicz KM, Ross SE, Marshall SW. Postural stability and neuropsychological deficits after concussion in collegiate athletes. J Athl Train. 2001;36(3):263–73.

48. Guskiewicz KM. Postural stability assessment following concussion: one piece of the puzzle. Clin J Sport Med. 2001;11(3):182–9.

49. Ellemberg D, Henry LC, Macciocchi SN, Guskiewicz KM, Broglio SP. Advances in sport concussion assessment: from behavioral to brain imaging measures [Review]. J Neurotrauma. 2009;26(12):2365–82.

50. Chandrasekhar SS. The assessment of balance and dizziness in the TBI patient. Neurorehabilitation. 2013;32(3):445–54.

51. Lei-Rivera L, Sutera J, Galatioto JA, Hujsak BD, Gurley JM. Special tools for the assessment of balance and dizziness in individuals with mild traumatic brain injury. Neurorehabilitation. 2013;32(3):463–72.

52. Mouzon B, Chaytow H, Crynen G, Bachmeier C, Stewart J, Mullan M, et al. Repetitive mild traumatic brain injury in a mouse model produces learning and memory deficits accompanied by histological changes. J Neurotrauma. 2012;29(18):2761–73.

53. McCrea M, Guskiewicz KM, Marshall SW, Barr W, Randolph C, Cantu RC, et al. Acute effects and recovery time following concussion in collegiate football players: the NCAA Concussion Study. JAMA. 2003;290(19):2556–63.

54. Jansen EC, Larsen RE, Olesen MB. Quantitative romberg test—measurement and computer calculation of postural stability. Acta Neurol Scand. 1982;66(1):93–9.

55. Thyssen HH, Brynskov J, Jansen EC, Munsterswendsen J. Normal ranges and reproducibility for the quantitative romberg test. Acta Neurol Scand. 1982;66(1):100–4.

56. Riemann BL, Guskiewicz KM, Shields EW. Relationship between clinical and forceplate measures of postural stability. J Sport Rehabil. 1999;8(2):71–82.

57. Khasnis A, Gokula RM. Romberg's test. J Postgrad Med. 2003;49(2):169–72.

58. Riemann BL, Guskiewicz KM. Assessment of mild head injury using measures of balance and cognition: a case study. J Sport Rehabil. 1997;6(3):283–9.

59. Gao J, Hu J, Buckley T, White K, Hass C. Shannon and Renyi entropies to classify effects of mild traumatic brain injury on postural sway. PLoS One. 2011;6(9):e24446.

60. Slobounov S, Cao C, Sebastianelli W, Slobounov E, Newell K. Residual deficits from concussion as revealed by virtual time-to-contact measures of postural stability. Clin Neurophysiol. 2008;119(2):281–9.

61. Slobounov S, Sebastianelli W, Hallett M. Residual brain dysfunction observed one year post-mild traumatic brain injury: combined EEG and balance study. Clin Neurophysiol. 2012;123(9):1755–61.

62. Slobounov S, Tutwiler R, Sebastianelli W, Slobounov E. Alteration of postural responses to visual field motion in mild traumatic brain injury. Neurosurgery. 2006;59(1):134–9.

63. Cavanaugh JT, Guskiewicz KM, Giuliani C, Marshall S, Mercer V, Stergiou N. Detecting altered postural control after cerebral concussion in athletes with normal postural stability. Br J Sports Med. 2005;39(11):805–11.

64. Mrazik M, Ferrara MS, Peterson CL, Elliott RE, Courson RW, Clanton MD, et al. Injury severity and neuropsychological and balance outcomes of four college athletes. Brain Inj. 2000;14(10):921–31.

65. Riemann BL, Guskiewicz KM. Effects of mild head injury on postural stability as measured through clinical balance testing. J Athl Train. 2000;35(1):19–25.

66. Peterson CL, Ferrara MS, Mrazik M, Piland T, Elliott T. Evaluation of neuropsychological stability following cerebral domain scores and postural concussion in sports. Clin J Sport Med. 2003;13(4):230–7.

67. Cavanaugh JT, Guskiewicz KM, Stergiou N, editors. Detecting altered postural control after cerebral concussion in athletes without postural instability. Philadelphia, PA: Lippincott Williams & Wilkins; 2004.

68. Register-Mihalik JK, Mihalik JP, Guskiewicz KM. Balance deficits after sports-related concussion in individuals reporting posttraumatic headache. Neurosurgery. 2008;63(1):76–80; discussion 80–2.

69. Kelly KA, Jordan EM, Burdette GT, Buckley TA. NCAA Division I athletic trainers concussion management practice patterns. J Athl Train. 2013 [epub ahead of print].

70. Broglio SP, Macciocchi SN, Ferrara MS. Sensitivity of the concussion assessment battery. Neurosurgery. 2007;60(6):1050–7.

71. Iverson GL, Koehle MS. Normative data for the modified balance error scoring system in adults. Brain Inj. 2013;27(5):596–9.

72. Schneiders AG, Sullivan SJ, Handcock P, Gray A, McCrory PR. Sports concussion assessment: the effect of exercise on dynamic and static balance. Scand J Med Sci Sports. 2012;22(1):85–90.

73. Ferrara MS, McCrea M, Peterson CL, Guskiewicz KM. A survey of practice patterns in concussion assessment and management. J Athl Train. 2001;36(2):145–9.

74. Notebaert AJ, Guskiewicz KM. Current trends in athletic training practice for concussion assessment and management. J Athl Train. 2005;40(4):320–5.

75. Covassin T, Elbin R, Stiller-Ostrowski JL. Current sport-related concussion teaching and clinical practices of sports medicine professionals. J Athl Train. 2009;44(4):400–4.

76. McCrea M, Barr WB, Guskiewicz K, Randolph C, Marshall SW, Cantu R, et al. Standard regression-based methods for measuring recovery after sport-related concussion. J Int Neuropsychol Soc. 2005;11(1):58–69.

77. Mulligan IJ, Boland MA, McIlhenny CV. The balance error scoring system learned response among young adults. Sports Health. 2013;5(1):22–6.

78. Finnoff JT, Peterson VJ, Hollman JH, Smith J. Intrarater and interrater reliability of the balance error scoring system (BESS). PM R. 2009;1(1):50–4.

79. Pagnacco G, Carrick FR, Pascolo PB, Rossi R, Oggero E. Learning effect of standing on foam during posturographic testing preliminary findings. Biomed Sci Instrum. 2012;48:332–9.

80. Hunt TN, Ferrara MS, Bornstein RA, Baumgartner TA. The reliability of the modified balance error scoring system. Clin J Sport Med. 2009;19(6):471–5.

81. McLeod TCV, Perrin DH, Guskiewicz KM, Shultz SJ, Diamond R, Gansneder BM. Serial administration of clinical concussion assessments and learning effects in healthy young athletes. Clin J Sport Med. 2004;14(5):287–95.

82. Valovich TC, Perrin DH, Gansneder BM. Repeat administration elicits a practice effect with the balance error scoring system but not with the standardized assessment of concussion in high school athletes. J Athl Train. 2003;38(1):51–6.

83. Burk JM, Munkasy BA, Joyner AB, Buckley TA. Balance error scoring system performance changes after a competitive athletic season. Clin J Sport Med. 2013;23(4):312–7.

84. Broglio SP, Zhu W, Sopiarz K, Park Y. Generalizability theory analysis of balance error scoring system reliability in healthy young adults. J Athl Train. 2009;44(5):497–502.

85. Susco TM, McLeod TCV, Gansneder BM, Shultz SJ. Balance recovers within 20 minutes after exertion as measured by the balance error scoring system. J Athl Train. 2004;39(3):241–6.

86. Wilkins JC, McLeod TCV, Perrin DH, Gansneder BM. Performance on the balance error scoring system decreases after fatigue. J Athl Train. 2004;39(2):156–61.

87. Fox ZG, Mihalik JP, Blackburn JT, Battaglini CL, Guskiewicz KM. Return of postural control to baseline after anaerobic and aerobic exercise protocols. J Athl Train. 2008;43(5):456–63.

88. Onate JA, Beck BC, Van Lunen BL. On-field testing environment and balance error scoring system performance during preseason screening of healthy collegiate baseball players. J Athl Train. 2007;42(4):446–51.

89. Weber AF, Mihalik JP, Register-Mihalik JK, Mays S, Prentice WE, Guskiewicz K. Dehydration and performance on clinical concussion measures in collegiate wrestlers. J Athl Train. 2013;48(2):153–60.

90. Docherty CL, McLeod TCV, Shultz SJ. Postural control deficits in participants with functional ankle instability as measured by the balance error scoring system. Clin J Sport Med. 2006;16(3):203–8.

91. McLeod TCV, Armstrong T, Miller M, Sauers JL. Balance improvements in female high school basketball players after a 6-week neuromuscular-training program. J Sport Rehabil. 2009;18(4):465–81.

92. Erkmen N, Taskin H, Kaplan T, Sanioglu A. The effect of fatiguing exercise on balance performance as measured by the balance error scoring system. Isokinet Exerc Sci. 2009;17(2):121–7.

93. Broglio SP, Tomporowski PD, Ferrara MS. Balance performance with a cognitive task: a dual-task testing paradigm. Med Sci Sports Exerc. 2005;37(4):689–95.

94. Resch JE, May B, Tomporowski PD, Ferrara MS. Balance performance with a cognitive task: a continuation of the dual-task testing paradigm. J Athl Train. 2011;46(2):170–5.

95. Teel EF, Register-Mihalik JK, Troy Blackburn J, Guskiewicz KM. Balance and cognitive performance during a dual-task: preliminary implications for use in concussion assessment. J Sci Med Sport. 2013;16(3):190–4.

96. Lee H, Sullivan SJ, Schneiders AG. The use of the dual-task paradigm in detecting gait performance deficits following a sports-related concussion: a systematic review and meta-analysis. J Sci Med Sport. 2013;16(1):2–7.

97. Chen JK, Johnston KM, Frey S, Petrides M, Worsley K, Ptito A. Functional abnormalities in symptomatic concussed athletes: an MRI study. Neuroimage. 2004;22(1):68–82.

98. Parker TM, Osternig LR, Lee HJ, van Donkelaar P, Chou LS. The effect of divided attention on gait stability following concussion. Clin Biomech. 2005;20(4):389–95.

99. Parker TM, Osternig LR, van Donkelaar P, Chou L-S. Recovery of cognitive and dynamic motor function following concussion. Br J Sports Med. 2007;41(12):868–73.

100. Catena RD, van Donkelaar P, Chou L-S. The effects of attention capacity on dynamic balance control following concussion. J Neuroeng Rehabil. 2011;8:8.

101. Catena RD, van Donkelaar P, Chou L-S. Different gait tasks distinguish immediate vs. long-term effects of concussion on balance control. J Neuroeng Rehabil. 2009;6:25.

102. Catena RD, van Donkelaar P, Chou L-S. Altered balance control following concussion is better detected with an attention test during gait. Gait Posture. 2007;25(3):406–11.

103. Catena RD, van Donkelaar P, Chou L-S. Cognitive task effects on gait stability following concussion. Exp Brain Res. 2007;176(1):23–31.

104. Catena RD, van Donkelaar P, Halterman CI, Chou L-S. Spatial orientation of attention and obstacle avoidance following concussion. Exp Brain Res. 2009;194(1):67–77.

105. Howell D, Osternig L, Van Donkelaar P, Mayr U, Chou L-S. Effects of concussion on attention and executive function in adolescents. Med Sci Sports Exerc. 2013;45(6):1030–7.

106. Okumura MS, Cooper SL, Ferrara MS, Tomporowski PD. Global switch cost as an index for concussion assessment: reliability and stability. Med Sci Sports Exerc. 2013;45(6):1038–42.

107. McCrory PR, Berkovic SF. Video analysis of acute motor and convulsive manifestations in sport-related concussion. Neurology. 2000;54(7):1488–91.

108. Kelly JP, Rosenberg JH. Diagnosis and management of concussion in sports. Neurology. 1997;48(3):575–80.

109. Parker TM, Osternig LR, Van Donkelaar P, Chou LS. Gait stability following concussion. Med Sci Sports Exerc. 2006;38(6):1032–40.

110. Parker TM, Osternig LR, Van Donkelaar P, Chou LS. Balance control during gait in athletes and non-athletes following concussion. Med Eng Phys. 2008;30(8):959–67.

111. Parker TM, Osternig LR, Van Donkelaar P, Chou LS. Gait stability following concussion. Med Sci Sports Exerc. 2006;38(6):1032–40.

112. Van Donkelaar P, Osternig L, Chou LS. Attentional and biomechanical deficits interact after mild traumatic brain injury. Exerc Sport Sci Rev. 2006;34(2):77–82.

113. Bell R, Hall RCW. Mental status examination. Am Fam Physician. 1977;16(5):145–52.

114. Al-Yahya E, Dawes H, Smith L, Dennis A, Howells K, Cockburn J. Cognitive motor interference while walking: a systematic review and meta-analysis. Neurosci Biobehav Rev. 2011;35(3):715–28.

115. Mille ML, Hilliard MJ, Martinez KM, Simuni T, Rogers MW. Acute effects of a lateral postural assist on voluntary step initiation in patients with Parkinson's disease. Mov Disord. 2007;22(1):20–7.
116. Chang HA, Krebs DE. Dynamic balance control in elders: gait initiation assessment as a screening tool. Arch Phys Med Rehabil. 1999;80(5):490–4.
117. Hass CJ, Gregor RJ, Waddell DE, Oliver A, Smith DW, Fleming RP, et al. The influence of Tai Chi training on the center of pressure trajectory during gait initiation in older adults. Arch Phys Med Rehabil. 2004;85(10):1593–8.
118. Mille ML, Johnson ME, Martinez KM, Rogers MW. Age-dependent differences in lateral balance recovery through protective stepping. Clin Biomech. 2005;20(6):607–16.
119. Hass CJ, Waddell DE, Wolf SL, Juncos JL, Gregor RJ. Gait initiation in older adults with postural instability. Clin Biomech. 2008;23(6):743–53.
120. Hass CJ, Waddell DE, Fleming RP, Juncos JL, Gregor RJ. Gait initiation and dynamic balance control in Parkinson's disease. Arch Phys Med Rehabil. 2005;86(11):2172–6.
121. Brunt D, Vanderlinden DW, Behrman AL. The relation between limb loading and control parameters of gait initiation in persons with stroke. Arch Phys Med Rehabil. 1995;76(7):627–34.
122. Halliday SE, Winter DA, Frank JS, Patla AE, Prince F. The initiation of gait in young, elderly, and Parkinson's disease subjects. Gait Posture. 1998;8(1):8–14.
123. Tokuno CD, Sanderson DJ, Inglis JT, Chua R. Postural and movement adaptations by individuals with a unilateral below-knee amputation during gait initiation. Gait Posture. 2003;18(3):158–69.
124. Polcyn AF, Lipsitz LA, Kerrigan DC, Collins JJ. Age-related changes in the initiation of gait: degradation of central mechanisms for momentum generation. Arch Phys Med Rehabil. 1998;79(12):1582–9.
125. Vallabhajosula S, Buckley TA, Tillman MD, Hass CJ. Age and Parkinson's disease related kinematic alterations during multi-directional gait initiation. Gait Posture. 2013;37(2):280–6.
126. Jian Y, Winter DA, Ishac MG, Gilchrist L. Trajectory of the body COG and COP during initiation and termination of gait. Gait Posture. 1993;1(1):9–22.
127. Brunt D, Short M, Trimble M, Liu SM. Control strategies for initiation of human gait are influenced by accuracy constraints. Neurosci Lett. 2000;285(3):228–30.
128. Massion J. Movement, posture and equilibrium—interaction and coordination. Prog Neurobiol. 1992;38(1):35–56.
129. Chang W-H, Tang P-F, Wang Y-H, Lin K-H, Chiu M-J, Chen S-HA. Role of the premotor cortex in leg selection and anticipatory postural adjustments associated with a rapid stepping task in patients with stroke. Gait Posture. 2010;32(4):487–93.
130. Winter DA, Prince F, Frank JS, Powell C, Zabjek KF. Unified theory regarding A/P and M/L balance in quiet stance. J Neurophysiol. 1996;75(6):2334–43.
131. Hass CJ, Buckley TA, Pitsikoulis C, Barthelemy EJ. Progressive resistance training improves gait initiation in individuals with Parkinson's disease. Gait Posture. 2012;35(4):669–73.
132. Vincent WJ. Statistics in kinesiology. 3rd ed. Champaign, IL: Human Kinetics; 2005.
133. Tate JJ, Milner CE. Real-time kinematic, temporospatial, and kinetic biofeedback during gait retraining in patients: a systematic review. Phys Ther. 2010;90(8):1123–34.
134. Prochazka A, Ellaway P. Sensory systems in the control of movement. Compr Physiol. 2012;2(4):2615–27.
135. Cheron G, Duvinage M, De Saedeleer C, Castermans T, Bengoetxea A, Petieau M, et al. From spinal central pattern generators to cortical network: integrated BCI for walking rehabilitation. Neural Plast. 2012;2012:375148.
136. Roemmich RT, Nocera JR, Vallabhajosula S, Amano S, Naugle KM, Stegemoller EL, et al. Spatiotemporal variability during gait initiation in Parkinson's disease. Gait Posture. 2012;36(3):340–3.
137. Hausdorff JM. Gait dynamics in Parkinson's disease: common and distinct behavior among stride length, gait variability, and fractal-like scaling. Chaos. 2009;19(2):026113.

138. Wittwer JE, Andrews PT, Webster KE, Menz HB. Timing variability during gait initiation is increased in people with Alzheimer's disease compared to controls. Dement Geriatr Cog Disord. 2008;26(3):277–83.

139. Lindemann U, Klenk J, Becker C, Moe-Nilssen R. Assessment of adaptive walking performance. Med Eng Phys. 2013;35(2):217–20.

140. Nakamura T, Meguro K, Sasaki H. Relationship between falls and stride length variability in senile dementia of the Alzheimer type. Gerontology. 1996;42(2):108–13.

141. Hausdorff JM, Zemany L, Peng CK, Goldberger AL. Maturation of gait dynamics: stride-to-stride variability and its temporal organization in children. J Appl Physiol. 1999;86(3): 1040–7.

142. Hausdorff JM, Edelberg HK, Mitchell SL, Goldberg AL, Wei JY. Increased gait unsteadiness in community-dwelling elderly fallers. Arch Phys Med Rehabil. 1997;78(3):278–83.

143. Beauchet O, Annweiler C, Lecordroch Y, Allali G, Dubost V, Herrmann FR, et al. Walking speed-related changes in stride time variability: effects of decreased speed. J Neuroeng Rehabil. 2009;6:32.

144. Frenkel-Toledo S, Giladi N, Peretz C, Herman T, Gruendlinger L, Hausdorff JM. Effect of gait speed on gait rhythmicity in Parkinson's disease: variability of stride time and swing time respond differently. J Neuroeng Rehabil. 2005;2:23.

145. Armieri A, Holmes JD, Spaulding SJ, Jenkins ME, Johnson AM. Dual task performance in a healthy young adult population: results from a symmetric manipulation of task complexity and articulation. Gait Posture. 2009;29(2):346–8.

146. Silsupadol P, Lugade V, Shumway-Cook A, van Donkelaar P, Chou LS, Mayr U, et al. Training-related changes in dual-task walking performance of elderly persons with balance impairment: a double-blind, randomized controlled trial. Gait Posture. 2009;29(4):634–9.

147. Kerr B, Condon SM, McDonald LA. Cognitive spatial processing and the regulation of posture. J Exp Psychol Hum Percept Perform. 1985;11(5):617–22.

148. Ebersbach G, Dimitrijevic MR, Poewe W. Influence of concurrent tasks on gait—a dual-task approach. Percept Mot Skills. 1995;81(1):107–13.

149. Shumway-Cook A, Woollacott M. Attentional demands and postural control: the effect of sensory context. J Gerontol A Biol Sci Med Sci. 2000;55(1):10–6.

150. Plummer-D'Amato P, Altmann LJP, Saracino D, Fox E, Behrman AL, Marsiske M. Interactions between cognitive tasks and gait after stroke: a dual task study. Gait Posture. 2008;27(4):683–8.

151. Woollacott M, Shumway-Cook A. Attention and the control of posture and gait: a review of an emerging area of research. Gait Posture. 2002;16(1):1–14.

152. Langlois JA, Keyl PM, Guralnik JM, Foley DJ, Marottoli RA, Wallace RB. Characteristics of older pedestrians who have difficulty crossing the street. Am J Public Health. 1997;87(3): 393–7.

153. Hoxie RE, Rubenstein LZ, Hoenig H, Gallagher BR. The older pedestrian. J Am Geriatr Soc. 1994;42(4):444–50.

154. Wang JJ, Wai YY, Weng YH, Ng KK, Huang YZ, Ying LL, et al. Functional MRI in the assessment of cortical activation during gait-related imaginary tasks. J Neural Transm. 2009;116(9):1087–92.

155. Perry SD, Santos LC, Patla AE. Contribution of vision and cutaneous sensation to the control of centre of mass (COM) during gait termination. Brain Res. 2001;913(1):27–34.

156. Sparrow WA, Tirosh O. Gait termination: a review of experimental methods and the effects of ageing and gait pathologies. Gait Posture. 2005;22(4):362–71.

157. Bishop MD, Brunt D, Pathare N, Patel B. The interaction between leading and trailing limbs during stopping in humans. Neurosci Lett. 2002;323(1):1–4.

158. Bishop MD, Brunt D, Kukulka C, Tillman MD, Pathare N. Braking impulse and muscle activation during unplanned gait termination in human subjects with parkinsonism. Neurosci Lett. 2003;348(2):89–92.

159. O'Kane FW, McGibbon CA, Krebs DE. Kinetic analysis of planned gait termination in healthy subjects and patients with balance disorders. Gait Posture. 2003;17(2):170–9.

160. Bishop M, Brunt D, Marjama-Lyons J. Do people with Parkinson's disease change strategy during unplanned gait termination? Neurosci Lett. 2006;397(3):240–4.
161. Menant JC, Steele JR, Menz HB, Munro BJ, Lord SR. Rapid gait termination: effects of age, walking surfaces and footwear characteristics. Gait Posture. 2009;30(1):65–70.
162. Vrieling AH, van Keeken HG, Schoppen T, Otten E, Halbertsma JPK, Hof AL, et al. Gait termination in lower limb amputees. Gait Posture. 2008;27(1):82–90.
163. Vrieling AH, van Keeken HG, Schoppen T, Hof AL, Otten B, Halbertsma JPK, et al. Gait adjustments in obstacle crossing, gait initiation and gait termination after a recent lower limb amputation. Clin Rehabil. 2009;23(7):659–71.
164. Miff SC, Childress DS, Gard SA, Meier MR, Hansen AH. Temporal symmetries during gait initiation and termination in nondisabled ambulators and in people with unilateral transtibial limb loss. J Rehabil Res Dev. 2005;42(2):175–82.
165. Wikstrom EA, Bishop MD, Inamdar AD, Hass CJ. Gait termination control strategies are altered in chronic ankle instability subjects. Med Sci Sports Exerc. 2010;42(1):197–205.
166. Tirosh O, Sparrow WA. Age and walking speed effects on muscle recruitment in gait termination. Gait Posture. 2005;21(3):279–88.
167. Oates AR, Frank JS, Patla AE, VanOoteghem K, Horak FB. Control of dynamic stability during gait termination on a slippery surface in Parkinson's disease. Mov Disord. 2008;23(14):1977–83.
168. Cameron D, Murphy A, Morris ME, Raghav S, Iansek R. Planned stopping in people with Parkinson. Parkinsonism Relat Disord. 2010;16(3):191–6.
169. Crenna P, Cuong DM, Breniere Y. Motor programmes for the termination of gait in humans: organisation and velocity-dependent adaptation. J Physiol. 2001;537(3):1059–72.
170. Hase K, Stein RB. Analysis of rapid stopping during human walking. J Neurophysiol. 1998;80(1):255–61.
171. Buckley TA, Munkasy BA, Tapia-Lovler TG, Wikstrom EA. Altered gait termination strategies following a concussion. Gait Posture. 2013;38(3):549–51.
172. Sosnoff JJ, Broglio SP, Shin S, Ferrara MS. Previous mild traumatic brain injury and postural-control dynamics. J Athl Train. 2011;46(1):85–91.
173. Cavanaugh JT, Guskiewicz KM, Giuliani C, Marshall S, Mercer VS, Stergiou N. Recovery of postural control after cerebral concussion: new insights using approximate entropy. J Athl Train. 2006;41(3):305–13.
174. Mayers L. Return-to-play criteria after athletic concussion—a need for revision. Arch Neurol. 2008;65(9):1158–61.
175. Dupuis F, Johnston KM, Lavoie M, Lepore F, Lassonde M. Concussions in athletes produce brain dysfunction as revealed by event-related potentials. Neuroreport. 2000;11(18):4087–92.
176. Gosselin N, Theriault M, Leclerc S, Montplaisir J, Lassonde M. Neurophysiological anomalies in symptomatic and asymptomatic concussed athletes. Neurosurgery. 2006;58(6):1151–60.
177. De Beaumont L, Brisson B, Lassonde M, Jolicoeur P. Long-term electrophysiological changes in athletes with a history of multiple concussions. Brain Inj. 2007;21(6):631–44.

Chapter 9
Biomechanical Studies of Impact and Helmet Protection

Andrew S. McIntosh

Abstract There has been an increasing focus on the role of helmets in reducing the risk of concussion in sport. Helmets in some sports have a well-established effect on reducing the risk of moderate to severe head injury, but the additional potential for helmets that have satisfied that objective to prevent concussion is unclear. Furthermore, the risk of moderate to severe head injury in some sports is low, e.g., rugby union and Australian rules football; however, there is clear risk of concussion in these sports, which presents an opportunity for helmets to mitigate that risk only. This chapter addresses the biomechanical studies of impact and helmet protection in sport.

Keywords Concussion • Helmets • Biomechanics of concussion

Introduction

Definitions of concussion have evolved over time and these definitions should inform our interpretation of past research. Studies on concussion in the not too distant past may have examined a constellation of brain injuries that are more severe than those currently considered as concussion in sport. The current definition, signs, and symptoms of concussion in sport have been informed substantially by the four consensus statements on concussion in sport, the most recent of which was published in 2013 [1].

Developing effective helmets for sport is challenging. Intrinsic and extrinsic factors and the exposure profile of the inciting event all require consideration and realization in an affordable, light-weight, and comfortable device that does not impede

A.S. McIntosh, Ph.D., M.Biomed.E., B.App.Sci. (P.T.) (✉)
Centre for Healthy and Safe Sports, The University of Ballarat,
SMB Campus, Lydiard Street South, Ballarat, VIC 3353, Australia
e-mail: as.mcintosh@bigpond.com

S.M. Slobounov and W.J. Sebastianelli (eds.), *Concussions in Athletics:*
From Brain to Behavior, DOI 10.1007/978-1-4939-0295-8_9,
© Springer Science+Business Media New York 2014

athletic performance or enjoyment. Intrinsic risk factors include age, gender, injury history, anatomy, and behavior. Extrinsic risk factors include the laws of the game (especially around head contact), the environment (e.g., the playing surface from soft ground to ice), and the use of personal protective equipment. The inciting event might be summarized into a small predictable pattern (e.g., in soccer head-to-head or arm-to-head impacts during aerial contest for the ball), be broad or even unknown. In the context of concussion in sport this chapter will describe current knowledge regarding helmet performance, and consider helmet design characteristics and standards, human factors, research and development needs, and opportunities.

Epidemiological Approaches: Effectiveness and Efficacy

There have been two systematic reviews of the effectiveness of helmets in preventing concussion in sport as well as other expert reviews on helmets in sport [2–4]. Table 9.1 summarizes the results of those reviews.

The epidemiological studies show that at present helmets cannot be relied upon as the primary method to prevent concussion. In a sporting team or organization it is not possible to satisfy a duty of care by only mandating helmet use. In some sports, e.g., Australian rules football, rugby union, rugby league, and soccer, there is no evidence that helmets, referring to padded headgear, prevent concussion. In American football and ice hockey, the epidemiological evidence regarding the benefits of helmets in preventing concussion is inconclusive. In both these sports there is evidence that helmets are effective in preventing head injuries overall.

One of the major impediments to the use of epidemiological methods to assess the role of helmets in sports that have mandatory helmet use, e.g., American

Table 9.1 Summary of effectiveness of helmets in preventing concussion

Sport	Concussion rate (games)	Proportion of injuries (%)	Helmet mandatory	Effective in reducing concussion
Rugby union	4.1–6.9 per 1,000 player hours (all levels)	5–15	No	No
American football	0.5–5.3 per 1,000 athletic exposures (high school and collegiate)	5	Yes	Inconclusive
Football (soccer)	0.06–1.08 per 1,000 player hours	3	No	No
Ice hockey	0.2–6.5 per 1,000 player hours (collegiate and professional)	2–19	Yes, including face shields in some competitions	Inconclusive
Bicycle riding	Not quantified	Depends on sample inclusion criteria	City, state, country dependent	Yes

There are variations in injury rate measures based on injury definitions, exposure measurements, chosen denominator, level of play, and age groups assessed football, is that comparisons can only be made between types of helmets, not between athletes assigned randomly to a helmet group and a no helmet group. In 2013, McGuine's study reported no difference in concussion risk by helmet brand or year of manufacture amongst high school football players [5]. In an earlier study, Collins observed that a smaller proportion of high school football players wearing the then new Riddell Revolution® helmet were concussed (5.3 %) than players wearing standard helmets (7.6 %) [6]. A comparison between players wearing and not wearing a helmet is not possible. Thus, the overall benefit remains unclear. To this end one American football helmet manufacturer advises the public that: "No helmet system can prevent concussions while playing football" [7].

Other issues, e.g., non-compliance, confound the conduct, results, and analysis of epidemiological studies. Non-compliance may arise in sports where helmet use is not mandatory and athletes are randomized to a helmet wearing group but do not normally wear a helmet. In the largest randomized control trial of helmets in sport, the author and colleagues found actual helmet wearing compliance to be poor in each of the three study arms, which may have weakened the positive trend observed with the "modified" helmet for those players who stuck with wearing the helmet during the study [8]. In a compliance analysis, wearers of the "modified" headgear compared to non-wearers had a non-significant reduction of greater than 50 % in the likelihood of concussion causing one missed game. Players reported that the "modified" helmet, which was thicker and heavier than the "standard" design, felt stiff and uncomfortable. Although helmets in rugby union are substantially lighter than in American football, the perception relative to experience of an even lighter headgear or no headgear influenced compliance.

Bicycle helmets have been shown to reduce the likelihood of concussion when the injury patterns of helmet wearing bicycle riders are compared to non-wearers. In a recent analysis of admissions to a major metropolitan trauma center bicycle riders wearing helmets were observed to have a 54 % reduction in the likelihood of concussion and a 66 % reduction in the likelihood of intracranial injury (including concussion) compared to bicycle riders not wearing a helmet [9]. In bicycle crashes with motor vehicles, a training hazard for professional and recreational sports cyclists, the majority of brain injuries (79 %) were concussive or involved loss-of-consciousness [10]. Moderate concussive injuries were associated with a 46 % reduction if a helmet was worn. Concussion cases in trauma admission data may be based on different diagnostic criteria, e.g., the International Classification of Disease (ICD) or the Abbreviated Injury Scale (AIS), than those in many helmet studies in football where the sports concussion consensus guidelines have been applied.

Helmet Characteristics

The most important functional characteristic of a helmet in the context of concussion is impact energy attenuation; a characteristic that has also been referred to as acceleration management. Ideally, the impact will cause the helmet to deform a substantial proportion of its thickness, without fully deforming or "bottoming out." The liner of the helmet or, in the case of padded headgear worn in rugby union the entire helmet, largely determines the impact energy attenuation performance. In short, the greater the deformation of the helmet the greater the reduction in impact force as well as in head acceleration. The helmet can also distribute the impact force over an area larger than the contact area. In helmets with a well-established role in transport and sport, e.g., bicycle and motorcycle helmets, the helmet is designed for a single crash event. In contrast, American football, rugby union, and ice hockey helmets are designed to provide protection throughout a season or more of multiple head impact exposures. The general properties of helmets and their function have been addressed well by many authors, e.g., Newman (1993) and Hoshizaki and Brien (2004), and will not be repeated in this chapter [11, 12].

The next most important functional characteristics are the mass, mass distribution, fit, restraint system, and vision. Sports helmets need to be wearable during extreme physical activities; therefore, helmet mass must be minimized. The mass distribution of the helmet and attachments is important in reducing the flexion moment that the helmet may apply to the head and neck. A flexion moment will be counteracted by neck extensor activation leading to muscle fatigue and increased joint reaction forces. It is imperative to ensure that the helmet and all components are correctly selected and adjusted for the individual athlete. Providing a kit bag with a few helmets to fit all the team is not best practice. Vision and the restraint system characteristics are usually addressed in sports helmet standards. Where faceguards (visors) are mounted to helmets to prevent projectile to face or head impacts, the adjustment of the faceguard is important as apertures may permit a projectile travelling at speed to strike the face directly. Some helmet styles permit adjustment of the faceguard, e.g., cricket helmets, where others do not, e.g., baseball helmets. The former introduces the potential for injury due to misuse.

Performance Requirements and Standards

Helmet performance is assessed in the laboratory by examining the capacity of the helmet to minimize headform acceleration in impact tests. These tests are conducted against set criteria, e.g., a linear acceleration pass criterion, or to derive an injury risk estimate. During a test a selected amount of impact energy is delivered to the helmet–headform system via a drop rig, pendulum, or mechanical device. The headform's linear and, in some cases, angular acceleration is measured during the impact. The input characteristics of the tests, e.g., energy, dimensions of impact interface, and headform, have gradually evolved to reflect knowledge on impact exposures in specific sports. The output characteristics, e.g., headform dynamic responses, have also evolved to reflect knowledge on injury mechanisms and human tolerance. However, requirements in many helmet standards are not currently aligned to maximize the potential for standard compliant helmets to prevent concussion. This would require the lowering of pass levels, e.g., to well below 100 g, and consideration for angular acceleration criteria and related test methods. As will be presented in this section, more valid assessments of helmet performance are observed when the laboratory tests reflect the impact exposures in the specific sport (impact location, impact severity, interface characteristics, and frequency) and the biofidelity of the head–neck system is considered. A range of headforms is used in research and standards testing: Hybrid III headforms, rigid ISO headforms, and NOCSAE headforms. Each has a distinct influence on the test outcomes. In an otherwise equivalent impact, head acceleration will be greater with a rigid ISO headform in comparison to a Hybrid III headform.

The author and others have conducted baseline tests on bare headforms. These reveal a clear risk of concussion related to linear head acceleration even in impacts equivalent to the head falling 0.5 m [3]:

- Hybrid II dropped onto a flat rigid anvil at 3.13 m/s has a peak linear acceleration of 282 g and Head Injury Criterion (HIC) of 906 [13].
- Projectile impacts (ice hockey puck, baseball, and cricket ball) into a Hybrid III headform mean peak linear accelerations were in the range of 233–316 g for 19 m/s impacts and 342–426 g for 27 m/s impacts [14].
- Hybrid III headform mean peak linear headform accelerations in flat rigid anvil were in the range 241–261 g (HIC 493–741) at 3.1.3 m/s and 368–512 g (HIC 1,620–2,789) at 4.43 m/s [9].
- Hybrid III headform peak linear accelerations in padded linear impactor tests were in the range 42–67 g at 3.6 m/s and 100–110 g at 7.4 m/s [15].

In the context of laboratory impact tests, helmets need to reduce both linear and angular headform acceleration. As a guide the 15 % likelihood of concussion for adult males is 45 g and the 50 % likelihood is 75 g for resultant linear acceleration at the head's center of gravity [16]. For the bare headform impacts described above helmets need to reduce the linear acceleration in the range two- to tenfold to prevent concussion. Angular acceleration tolerance thresholds vary; Rowson et al. reported in 2012 that the 75 % likelihood of concussion for resultant angular acceleration is 6.9 krad/s^2 [17].

How Well Do Helmets Perform?

Rugby—Helmets (padded headgear) in rugby must comply with the International Rugby Board's (IRB) performance regulations [18]. The helmet properties are restricted to an undeformed thickness of 10 mm and a foam density of 45 kg/m^3. The IRB's impact performance requirements state that in a 13.8 J rigid (EN 960) headform impact onto a rigid flat anvil the peak headform acceleration shall not be less than 200 g. The mandated performance requirements exclude headgear from preventing concussion due to the biomechanical criteria and are inconsistent with the philosophy of many helmet standards.

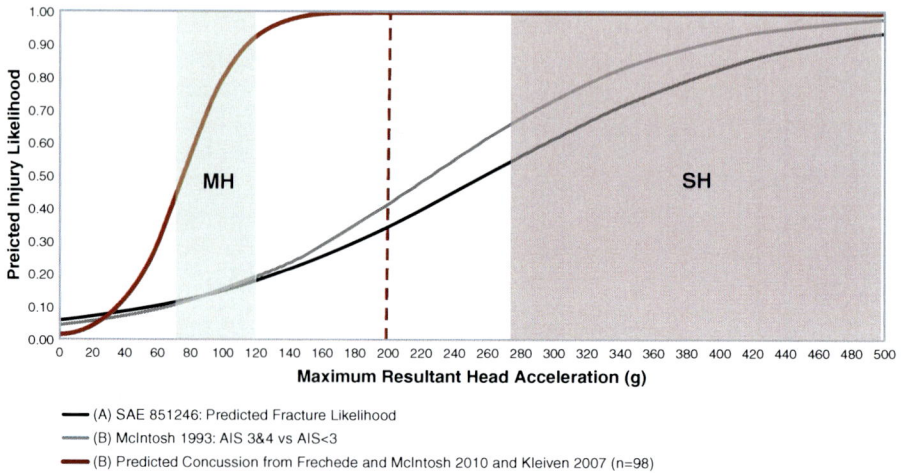

- (A) SAE 851246: Predicted Fracture Likelihood
- (B) McIntosh 1993: AIS 3&4 vs AIS<3
- (B) Predicted Concussion from Frechede and McIntosh 2010 and Kleiven 2007 (n=98)

Fig. 9.1 The range of laboratory test results for standard rugby headgear (SH) and modified headgear (MH) in 0.3 m drop tests is presented with reference to injury tolerance data. In the randomized control trial, no effect on concussion was observed for standard headgear. In contrast there was a greater than 50 % non-significant reduction in concussion leading to a missed game based on a compliance analysis. The *vertical red dashed line* is the IRB's acceleration criterion. Line (A) is the SAE 851246 skull fracture likelihood curve, line (B) is the likelihood of AIS 3 and 4 versus AIS < 3 severity head injury, and line (C) is the concussion likelihood formed by pooling NFL and Australian (unhelmeted) football reconstructed injury and non-injury concussion cases

Impact tests on helmets meeting the IRB's requirements ("standard") and a "modified" version were conducted by the author [19]. The modified headgear was 16 mm thick and made from 60 kg/m^3 polyethylene foam. The standard headgear was 10 mm thick and made from 45 kg/m^3 polyethylene foam. Tests using a rigid headform from a 0.3 m drop height produced peak accelerations in the range 276–689 g for standard headgear and 69–123 for modified headgear. At 0.4 m peak accelerations for the modified headgear were 110–273 g. Figure 9.1 shows a level of consistency between the laboratory tests and the results of the randomized controlled trial superimposed onto injury likelihood curves [16]. The performance of the modified headgear in laboratory tests identified a potential in low severity impacts for the headgear to reduce the linear acceleration to a tolerable range. In the epidemiological study there was a greater than 50 % non-significant reduction in missed game concussions based on a compliance analysis. With greater compliance, this may have been a significant association. The epidemiological study was of players aged under 13 years to under 20 years; therefore, the tolerance data presented in Fig. 9.1 may not be suitable, but the impact exposure may be less severe than observed in adult rugby union and Australian football and more reflective of the laboratory tests, noting also that a rigid headform was used. These highlight the intrinsic and extrinsic factors described in the introduction.

Projectile sports (cricket/baseball)—Helmets in cricket and baseball are intended to prevent head injury and provide a structure for mounting a faceguard or visor.

Table 9.2 Cricket and baseball helmet projectile impact results

Ball speed (m/s)	Bare Hybrid III headform		Helmet		Percent reduction relative to bare headform (%)	
	Cricket (average MAcc (g))	Baseball (average MAcc (g))	Cricket (average MAcc (g))	Baseball (average MAcc (g))	Cricket	Baseball
19	278	316	67	72	76	77
27	347	426	160	139	54	67

Average of the maximum headform acceleration (MAcc) is presented for all impact sites combined for bare headform and helmeted impacts with the appropriate ball

The faceguard prevents facial and ocular injury, as well as other head injuries. Despite the similar hazards in the two sports, cricket helmets tend to have a thin relatively stiff liner in contrast to thick and compliant baseball liner. The success of helmets in managing the head impact acceleration in projectile impacts was assessed in a selection of helmets over a decade ago [14]. Standards for cricket helmets have changed little in the intervening period, but proposals are being considered to introduce a projectile test as opposed to the current drop tests. Our work indicated little correlation between the magnitude of headform accelerations in equivalent impact energy tests conducted using drop tests onto a rigid anvil (as per the standard) and projectile tests for cricket helmets. In contrast, there was better correlation between projectile test results and drop tests onto a modular elastomeric programmer anvil for baseball and ice hockey helmets. This demonstrates that impact tests can be developed that do not necessarily resemble sports-specific impact characteristics, but are indicative of helmet performance in sports-specific impacts. At that time, baseball helmets demonstrated a greater capacity to reduce headform acceleration than cricket helmets, although the results did not indicate that a baseball or cricket helmet would prevent concussion if the projectile struck the head in an impact directed radially (or centric) to the head's center of gravity (Table 9.2). However, it is more common in match situations to observe a glancing ball-to-helmet impact.

Ice hockey—Recent ice hockey head impact tests have highlighted the relationship between sports-specific impacts and helmet performance in terms of head dynamics [20]. Realistic shoulder-to-head and head-to-ice impacts were simulated using an instrumented Hybrid III head and neck. The peak resultant linear and angular head accelerations were 264 g and 11 krad/s^2 for "ice" impacts and 113 g and 0.97 krad/s^2 for "shoulder" impacts. The head accelerations exceeded concussion thresholds. Predicted brain loading patterns demonstrated relationships with the impact severity and the direction of loading. The results demonstrate:

- The importance of helmet test methods reflecting impact exposure patterns and injury risks in the sport. If hypothetically, 90 % of concussions occurred because of a shoulder impact, but the most serious head injuries occurred due to impacts with the ice, then test methods need to address both injury risks without creating mutually exclusive requirements.

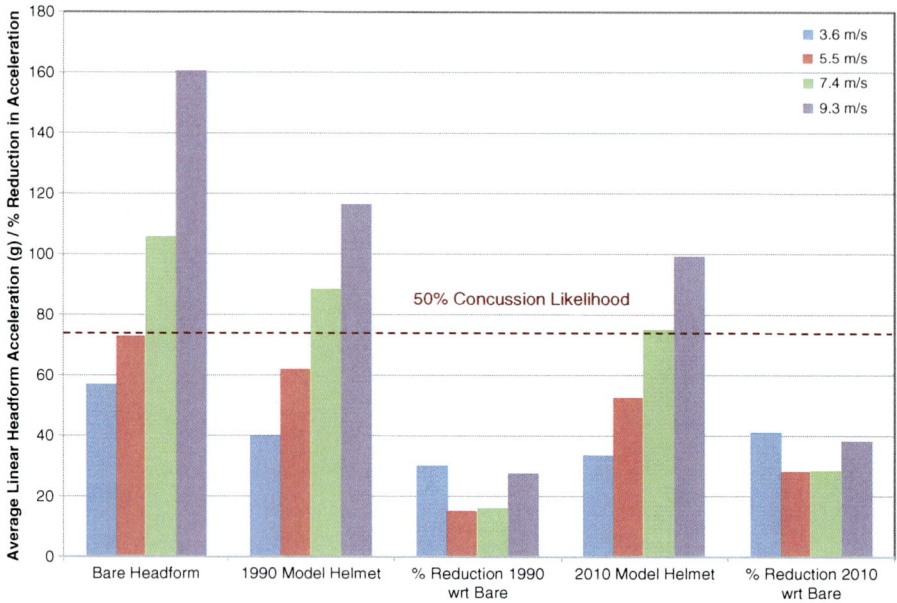

Fig. 9.2 Comparison of averaged results for bare headform and 1990 and 2010 model American football helmets [15]

- Brain loading patterns need to be considered more thoroughly in order to derive injury tolerance data and to understand the spectrum of concussion presentations.
- Consideration of the ability of helmets to modify brain loading patterns in sports-specific impacts can provide valuable information for the development of helmets and helmet test methods.

American football—Viano and Halstead compared representative American football helmets from the years 2010, 1990, 1980, and 1970 and performed bare Hybrid III headform impacts [15]. The average mass for the 2010 model helmets (including the faceguard) was 1.95 kg. In relative terms the 2010 helmets reduced the linear headform acceleration compared to bare headform tests on average by 42 %, 28 %, 29 %, and 38 % at 3.6, 5.5, 7.4, and 9.3 m/s, respectively. In absolute terms, the 50 % likelihood threshold for concussion of 75 g is exceeded on average in the 7.4 m/s impacts. Therefore, 2010 American football helmets may reduce the risk of concussion noticeable in impacts up to 7.4 m/s, if those impacts are equivalent to the test method. In relative terms the 2010 helmets are slightly better than the 1990 helmets, but in absolute terms a similar concussion risk exists with the average linear head acceleration of 89 g at 7.4 m/s (Fig. 9.2). When the average reduction in acceleration (helmet to bare headform) is averaged across all test speeds, the 1990 helmet reduced acceleration by 22 % compared to 34 % for the 2010 helmets; there is a relative risk reduction of 54 % for the newer helmets. This contrasts to a relative risk reduction of 31 % for all players and 41 % for those without a concussion history in the study by Collins et al. [6]. Therefore, some clear parallels can be seen in laboratory test performance and on-field performance. In contrast, an American football helmet manufacturer advises, "Scientists have not reached agreement on how the results of impact absorption tests relate to concussions. No conclusions about a reduction of risk or severity of concussive injury should be drawn from impact absorption tests" [7].

The STAR evaluation system presents a conceptual difference to many standard approaches and fills an important need for consumer-related helmet data. The latter may assist players, families, and teams in purchasing decisions and may stimulate helmet developments. The STAR system summarizes the exposure-weighted impact performance of helmets [21]. The validity of the STAR system could be enhanced by epidemiological studies.

Cycling—Bicycle riding is a major sport, recreational activity, and means of transport. The hazards and injury risks in bicycle riding are broad. A cyclist may fall off while cycling and hit the road surface and in a more severe crash may collide with a moving car. As per American football, the initial rationale for bicycle helmets was to prevent a more severe spectrum of injury, including skull fracture and intracranial hemorrhage, rather than sports concussion. Recent comparative crash simulation tests have demonstrated that the laboratory performance of bicycle helmets is a reasonable predictor of the real world performance [22]. In comparison to helmeted impacts across all impact configurations mean maximum headform acceleration was 2.8–6.7 times greater without a helmet and angular accelerations were between 2.0 and 7.3 times greater without a helmet, depending on the exact impact characteristics (Fig. 9.3). An analysis of the oblique test results using biomechanical injury likelihood relationships again paralleled well the results of epidemiological studies. The analyses showed a significant effect of helmets on reducing the likelihood of severe head injury, but a potential for concussion to occur across a range of impacts. In contrast, the bare headform tests predicted a high risk of severe skull and brain injuries even in the more benign crash scenarios (Fig. 9.3).

Heading in football/soccer: why current helmets are not needed—Helmets are available and marketed for soccer. Their performance is not governed by a standard and there are no convincing epidemiological or laboratory studies that demonstrate their effectiveness or efficacy. Although there is a risk of concussion in soccer, it is relatively low. Despite concerns that heading itself may cause brain injury through a cumulative dose effect, the evidence suggests that during the aerial contest for the ball, head impacts causing immediate injury occur because of head-to-head impacts or arm-to-head impacts [23]. These intentional or accidental impacts can be controlled through the laws of the game. Arguably, helmets would reduce the ability of a player to head a ball and may lead to players compensating for the loss of ball rebound by changing their head–neck dynamics. This in turn might result in higher speed head-to-head impacts; although this is speculative. Unlike contact football codes where accidental head contact does occur frequently, soccer has other opportunities to prevent concussion through its laws, law enforcement, training, and supervision.

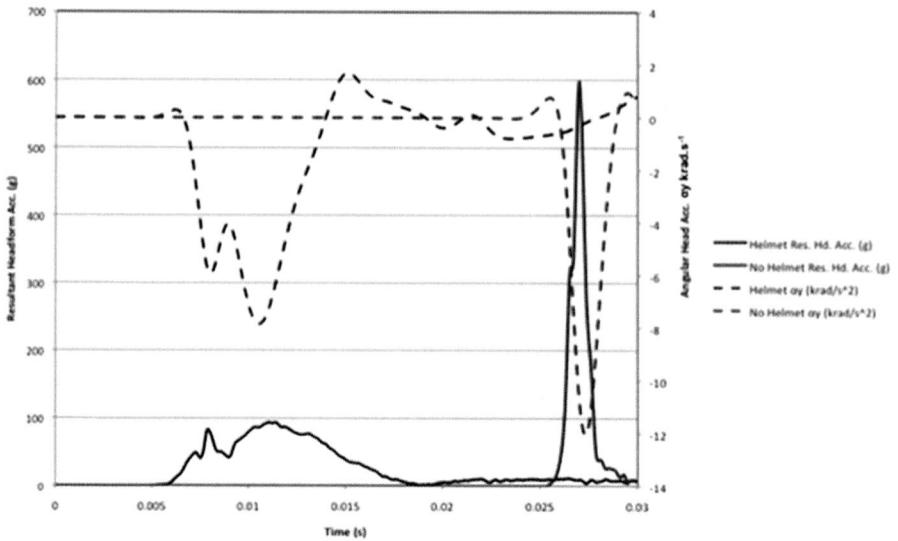

Fig. 9.3 Comparison of head linear and angular acceleration time histories in oblique impacts using a Hybrid III head and neck. Occipital impacts were conducted with a drop height of 1 m and striker (*horizontal*) speed of 15 km/h. The resultant headform acceleration was around 100 g for the bicycle helmet impact compared to 600 g for the bare headform impact. Peak angular acceleration in the helmet impact was almost half the bare headform impact

Future Development

There is a need for general and sports-specific research and development to improve the protection offered by current helmets. Our understanding of the mechanisms of concussion generally and in specific sports, as well as human tolerance levels, has improved enormously over the last 15 years. Knowledge in these areas is consistent with established injury criteria for more severe head injuries. When this knowledge is applied to helmet test methods, standards and helmet design improvements in the ability of helmets to prevent concussion can be expected.

Correlations between biomechanical test data for helmets and epidemiological studies are generally good: the trends in improved impact energy attenuation are paralleled between the lab and the field; and absolute measures of head acceleration can predict on-field helmet performance, albeit imperfectly. The strengths of the correlations are affected by the intrinsic and extrinsic factors and the nature of the inciting event that influence injury likelihood and injury severity on field. These are not necessarily considered fully in laboratory test methods.

Current tolerance data treat concussion as one single pathology although the clinical symptoms and variation in cognitive impairments suggest differences within the umbrella term of concussion. Age-specific tolerance data are not available. It is also becoming clearer that impact direction and location influence concussion tolerance.

In this context, the use of resultant head linear or angular acceleration criteria may not be optimal. Therefore, test methods will need to develop further.

The role of angular acceleration in concussion is gradually being resolved. It is rare for high angular acceleration to occur without high linear acceleration or impact force. Therefore, these characteristics are typically coupled. Despite the focus of helmet testing on linear acceleration management, helmets do reduce angular acceleration. Further improvements in this area are possible but require suitable test methods and standards, without compromising linear acceleration performance.

If a causal relationship between cumulative head impact exposure and brain injury is conclusively proven, i.e., the so-called sub-concussive impacts, then helmets in those sports that permit intentional head impact or have a high incidence of accidental head impact will need to offer even greater protection in comparison to protection against a single overload event. At present the objective should be to prevent concussion, because it is a known risk and there are known consequences of repeat concussions.

It is imperative that biomechanical laboratory studies and well-designed epidemiological studies are conducted together. Both forms of investigation are invaluable. In comparison to epidemiological studies, laboratory studies are inexpensive and variations can be made and assessed rapidly. Confidence in laboratory studies that can be gained through validation through epidemiological studies assists in a cycle of improvement. Video analysis of games coupled with on-field monitoring of head impact biomechanics, behavioral surveys and usability studies, can further enhance knowledge gained from epidemiological studies, as these assist in the interpretation of the main epidemiological results.

As the final note, there has been an enormous expansion of biomechanical knowledge in the field of concussion and helmets in sport over the last 15 years. As research findings are translated into helmet design and as new helmet technologies develop, improvements in the ability of helmets to prevent concussion can be expected. This requires the support of the major sports, equipment manufacturers, research groups, public funding bodies, and athletes.

References

1. McCrory P, Meeuwisse W, Aubry M, Cantu B, Dvorak J, et al. Consensus statement on concussion in sport—The 4th international conference on concussion in sport held in Zurich, November 201. Br J Sports Med. 2013;47:250–8.
2. Benson B, Hamilton G, Meeuwisse W, McCrory P, Dvorak J. Is protective equipment useful in preventing concussion? A systematic review of the literature. Br J Sports Med. 2009;43(1): i56–67.
3. Benson BW, McIntosh AS, Maddocks D, Herring SA, Raftery M, et al. What are the most effective risk reduction strategies in sport concussion? From protective equipment to policy. Br J Sports Med. 2013;47:321–6.
4. McIntosh AS, Andersen TE, Bahr R, Greenwald R, Kleiven S, et al. Sports helmets now and in the future. Br J Sports Med. 2011;45:1258–65.

5. McGuine, Brooks A, Hetzel S, Rasmussen J, McCrea M. The association of the type of football helmet and mouth guard with the incidence of sport related concussion in high school football players. Proceedings of the American Orthopedic Society for Sports Medicine Annual General Meeting, Chicago, USA; 2013.
6. Collins M, Lovell MR, Iverson GL, Ide T, Maroon J. Examining concussion rates and return to play in high school football players wearing newer helmet technology: a three-year prospective cohort study. Neurosurgery. 2006;58:275–86.
7. Shutt Helmets Website. http://www.schuttsports.com/Default.aspx. 2013.
8. McIntosh AS, McCrory P, Finch CF, Best JP, Chalmers DJ, et al. Does padded headgear prevent head injury in rugby union football? Med Sci Sports Exerc. 2009;41:306–13.
9. McIntosh AS, Curtis K, Rankin T, Cox M, Pang TY, et al. Associations between helmet use and brain injuries amongst injured pedal- and motor-cyclists: a case series analysis of trauma centre presentations. Australas Coll Road Saf. 2013;24:11–20.
10. Bambach MR, Mitchell RJ, Grzebieta RH, Olivier J. The effectiveness of helmets in bicycle collisions with motor vehicles: a case-control study. Accid Anal Prev. 2013;53:78–88.
11. Newman J. The biomechanics of head trauma: head protection. In: Nahum AM, Melvin JW, editors. Accidental injury biomechanics and prevention. New York: Springer; 1993. p. 292–310.
12. Hoshizaki TB, Brien SE. The science and design of head protection in sport. Neurosurgery. 2004;55:956–67.
13. Benz G, McIntosh AS, Kallieris D, Daum R. A biomechanical study of bicycle helmet effectiveness in childhood. Eur J Pediatr Surg. 1993;3:259–63.
14. McIntosh AS, Janda D. Cricket helmet performance evaluation and comparison with baseball and ice hockey helmets. Br J Sports Med. 2003;37:325–30.
15. Viano DC, Halstead D. Change in size and impact performance of football helmets from the 1970s to 2010. Ann Biomed Eng. 2012;40:175–84.
16. McIntosh AS. Biomechanical considerations in the design of equipment to prevent sports injury. J Sports Eng Technol. 2012;226:193–9.
17. Rowson S, Duma S, Beckwith J, Chu JJ, Greenwald RM, et al. Rotational head kinematics in football impacts: an injury risk function for concussion. Ann Biomed Eng. 2012;40:1–13.
18. International Rugby Board Handbook 2013. Dublin: International Rugby Board.
19. McIntosh AS, McCrory P, Finch C. Performance enhanced headgear—a scientific approach to the development of protective headgear. Br J Sports Med. 2004;38:46–9.
20. Kendall M, Post A, Rousseau P, Oeur A, Gilchrist MD, et al. A comparison of dynamic impact response and brain deformation metrics within the cerebrum of head impact reconstructions representing three mechanisms of head injury in ice hockey. Proc IRCOBI Conf. 2012;2012: 430–40.
21. Rowson S, Duma SM. Development of the STAR evaluation system for football helmets: integrating player head impact exposure and risk of concussion. Ann Biomed Eng. 2011; 39:2130–40.
22. McIntosh AS, Lai A, Schilter E. Bicycle helmets: head impact dynamics in helmeted and unhelmeted oblique impact tests. Traffic Inj Prev. 2013;14(5):501–8.
23. Andersen TE, Arnason A, Engebretsen L, Bahr R. Mechanisms of head injuries in elite football. Br J Sports Med. 2004;38:690–6.

Part III
Neural Substrates, Biomarkers, and Brain Imaging of Concussion Research

Chapter 10
Neuropathology of Mild Traumatic Brain Injury: Relationship to Structural Neuroimaging Findings

Erin D. Bigler

Abstract The basics of structural neuroimaging identified neuropathological changes that may be identified on computed tomography and magnetic resonance imaging associated with mild traumatic brain injury (mTBI) are reviewed. Emphasis is placed on understanding the subtle nature of neuropathology that may accompany mTBI and its detection with neuroimaging. The role of diffusion tensor imaging is overviewed with numerous examples provided that illustrates neuroimaging techniques that detect mTBI abnormalities.

Keywords Mild traumatic brain injury (mTBI) concussion • Neuropsychology neuroimaging • Biomarkers • Neuropathology brain damage cognitive and neurobehavioral sequelae

Introduction

The limits of neuroimaging specify what types of neuropathology can be detected in traumatic brain injury (TBI), especially if the injury is mild. Fortunately, tremendous advances in neuroimaging technologies especially with magnetic resonance imaging (MRI) have been made over the last decade, even in detection of subtle pathology following mild traumatic brain injury (mTBI). Most conventional MRI studies configure anatomical images with millimeter resolution, meaning MRI detects pathology at a similar level of resolution, although submillimeter resolution

E.D. Bigler, Ph.D. (✉)
Department of Psychology and Neuroscience Center, Brigham Young University,
1190D Kimball Tower, Provo, UT 84602, USA

Department of Psychiatry, University of Utah, Salt Lake City, UT, USA
e-mail: erin_bigler@byu.edu

S.M. Slobounov and W.J. Sebastianelli (eds.), *Concussions in Athletics:*
From Brain to Behavior, DOI 10.1007/978-1-4939-0295-8_10,
© Springer Science+Business Media New York 2014

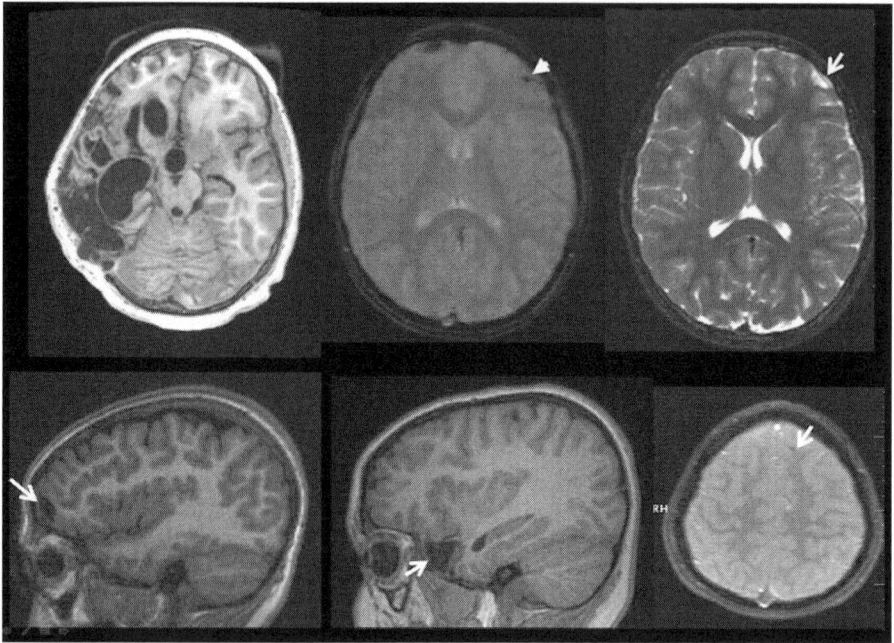

Fig. 10.1 The subtleness and diversity of MRI identified chronic (>6 months post-injury) brain lesions in four mTBI patients, all with a GCS of 15, compared to the massive structural pathologies associated with severe TBI are presented in this figure. The mTBI case shown in the *top middle* and *right* shows characteristic area of small focal encephalomalacia with increased region of CSF (*arrow*) in the T2-weighted image (*top right*) associated with residual hemosiderin (*arrowhead*) in the gradient-recalled echo (GRE) sequence (*top middle*). These pathological changes were originally the result of a focal frontal contusion. In the sagittal image in the *bottom left*, focal frontal encephalomalacia is evident (*arrow*) and encephalomalacia in the temporal lobe (*arrow*) in the *middle* image with the *bottom right* image showing an axial scan with subtle hemosiderin right at the gray-white junction (*arrow*). In contrast, the child with severe injury (axial view, *upper left*) has massive structural pathology. From Bigler ED, Abildskov TJ, Petrie J, Dennis M, Simic N, Taylor HG, et al. Heterogeneity of brain lesions in pediatric traumatic brain injury. *Neuropsychology*. 27(4), 438-451, 2013; used with permission

is now possible [1, 2]. However, the fundamental pathological changes that occur from TBI happen at the micron and nanometer cellular level [3, 4]. This means for brain injuries in the mild range, with the subtlest of neural injury that the macroscopic lesions characteristic of more severe injury are simply not visible in most cases. Straightforwardly, the contrast in gross visible detection of pathology from mild to severe TBI is demonstrated in Fig. 10.1.

In Fig. 10.1 all of the individuals with mTBI had a post-resuscitation Glasgow Coma Scale [5] score of 15 and were part of the Social Outcomes of Brain Injury in Kids (SOBIK [6]) investigation. Although all children in the SOBIK investigation who sustained mTBI had positive day-of-injury (DOI) computed tomography (CT), only about two-thirds of the 41 mTBI children had identifiable abnormalities when followed up approximately a year or more post-injury. As demonstrated in the Bigler et al. [6] investigation a number of the children with subtle hemorrhage and/ or localized edema on the DOI CT did not evidence visibly detectable abnormalities on follow-up MRI performed at least a year post-injury. While not possible in human mTBI studies, animal investigations that model mTBI where acute neuroimaging abnormalities become non-detectable over time nonetheless may show histological pathology [7, 8]. As such, it is safe to assume that DOI pathology like petechial hemorrhages that are not detected on follow-up imaging nonetheless indicate significant shear forces were present in the brain at the time of injury and likely do reflect where residual pathology may be present at the cellular level, just not detectable with contemporary neuroimaging methods.

Because of these limitations with neuroimaging resolution in detecting abnormalities, a simple dichotomy in structural imaging may be developed between lesions or abnormalities visibly identified at the macroscopic level and those more empirically or quantitatively derived from scan metrics. This distinction between visible versus empirically derived quantitative metrics will be further explored in this chapter but first some mention of the role of CT in TBI will be discussed because it is the most common initial or emergently performed imaging modality performed in TBI, including mTBI [9, 10]. As such, typically the first neuroimaging findings in TBI are CT based, providing important baseline information even when entirely negative. This chapter will not cover functional neuroimaging or magnetic resonance (MR) spectroscopy (MRS) as these techniques will be covered elsewhere and have previously been reviewed by Slobounov et al. [11]. Also, fundamentals of imaging will not be covered in this chapter as a variety of publications provide such information [12–14].

Heterogeneity of MTBI

As already alluded to in Fig. 10.1, no two head injuries are identical [15]. Even with the careful precision of animal models no two injuries can ever be identically replicated [16]. If one now adds to the complexity individual differences in human development and experience (the brain is an experience/age-dependent organ), combined with genetic endowment and whatever unique circumstances that occur with each injury, an incredible mix of events and circumstance accompanies every injury. So the pathology that is detectable via neuroimaging techniques will never be identical across individuals but there are common pathologies. As will be explained in greater detail throughout this chapter, particular vulnerability of white matter (WM) underlies much of the pathology associated with mTBI. Many axons are myelinated; with the vulnerability of WM damage from trauma the WM designation infers that the axon element of the neuron is particularly vulnerable in TBI. Interneuronal connection occurs via axons; thus, WM pathology in TBI may be considered a problem of neural connectivity. With a neuron's cell body densely compacted within the neuropil

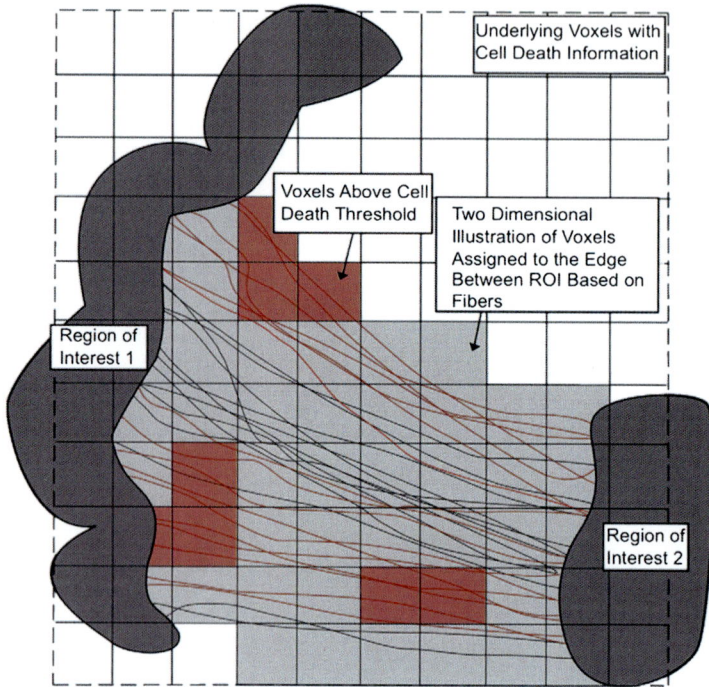

Fig. 10.2 This schematic shows how different axon trajectories may or may not be vulnerable to injury. As can be seen, there are only certain sectors where the biomechanical deformation sufficiently alters brain parenchyma to damage axons. *Lines* represent hypothetical axon projections from one gray matter structure to another. Note that even though all connect region of interest (ROI) 1 with ROI 2, and that out of all sectors where these hypothetical axons project, only eight of the sectors experienced sufficient deformation to damage axons, because of the differences in crossing routes and trajectories numerous axons were affected. From Kraft RH, McKee PJ, Dagro AM, Grafton ST. Combining the finite element method with structural connectome-based analysis for modeling neurotrauma: connectome neurotrauma mechanics. (*PLoS Comput Biol.* 2012; 8(8): e1002619; used with permission

of the gray matter and held tightly within this matrix of cell bodies, the axon extension becomes vulnerable because WM pathways course in multiple directions of various lengths creating a bend and interwoven lattice work of projecting axons making WM especially vulnerable to stretch, strain, and tensile effects following the mechanical deformation that occurs with impact injury [17, 18]. This is depicted in Fig. 10.2 which shows that only certain WM tracts are actually damaged within a particular biomechanical strain field (see [19]). Watanabe et al. [20] have shown how with each individual impact injury, unique influences occur from the biomechanical movement of the brain within the cranium. These unique individual differences, when coupled with the fact that neural tissue has different elastic properties that are region and structure dependent [21, 22], demonstrate that no two injuries from mTBI will ever produce identical pathology detectable by neuroimaging.

Time Sequence of Neuropathology Associated with MTBI

There can be no dispute that an acute brain injury has occurred in a witnessed traumatic event associated with positive loss of consciousness (LOC) and obvious biomechanical forces. Therefore, such cases represent the best model for understanding the time sequence of symptom resolution and return to baseline function. The case shown in Fig. 10.3, which displays a negative DOI CT scan, provides such an example. This young adult female sustained an mTBI in an auto-pedestrian accident.

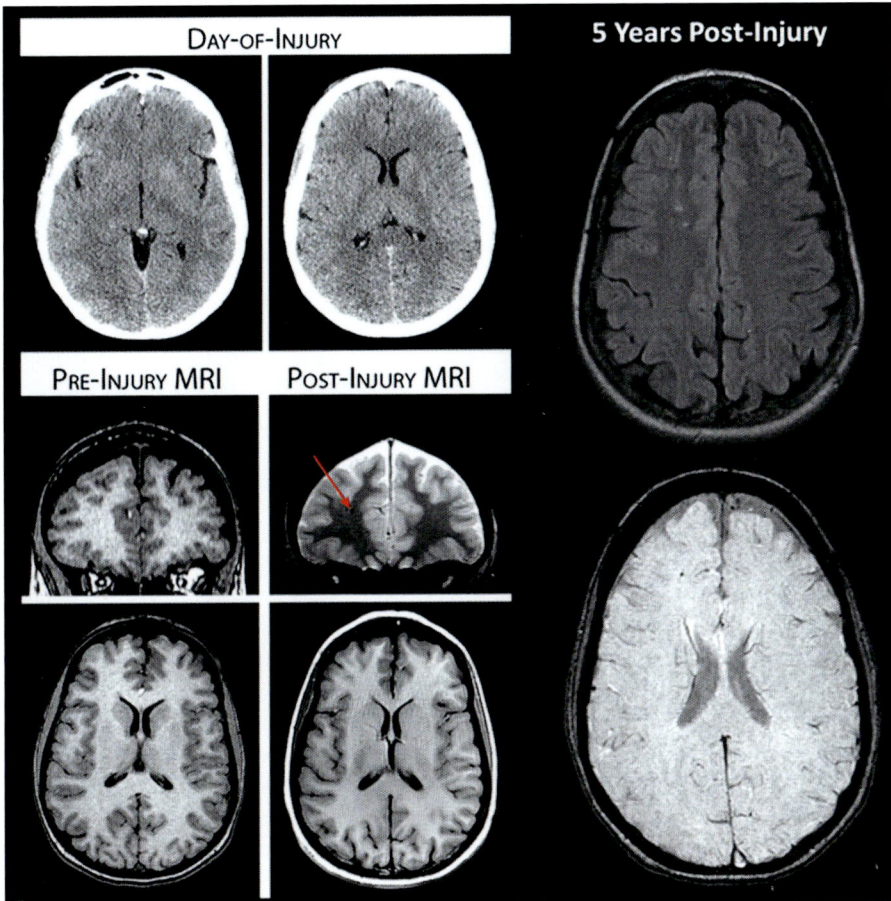

Fig. 10.3 This young adult sustained a significant mTBI in an auto-pedestrian injury where she had positive LOC, but the DOI CT revealed no abnormality. However, as symptoms persisted this patient was assessed with MRI which revealed hemosiderin and focal white matter hyperintensities. Interestingly, this patient had participated as a research subject prior to the injury, confirming no prior brain abnormalities, as shown in the pre-injury MRI, although only a T1-weighted MRI had been performed (courtesy of Geri Hanten, Ph.D.)

She was struck by a passing car while standing next to her vehicle with family members nearby, but no other family member was struck or injured. She was thrown into the air striking her head on the curb, resulting in immediate LOC (no skull fracture), which lasted 2–3 min according to eyewitness family members present at the time of the accident. Emergency medical services were on the scene within 10 min, where they found her conscious but confused. She had orthopedic injuries to her legs (ligament knee injuries), was stabilized and transported to the emergency department (ED) with a GCS of 15 noted on intake. During ED observation over the next couple of hours, GCS fluctuated between 13 and 15. With the head CT being negative (see Fig. 10.3), but given the severity of the impact, positive LOC and fluctuating level of GCS she was monitored overnight and discharged the next day, with outpatient follow-up provided through the hospital concussion care program. Interestingly, her post-concussive symptoms (PCS) of headache, mental confusion, lethargy, and sleepiness increased in the days that followed. Some have speculated that PCS reaches its apex on the DOI and then dissipates. While true for some, peak symptoms following mTBI may occur hours to days post-injury [23, 24], which was the case with this patient. She was a student and attempted to go back to her studies approximately 3 weeks post-injury but experienced major cognitive challenges, especially in terms of problems with focused and sustained attention. Because of the persistence in symptoms and that MRI studies had not been done, an MRI was obtained which demonstrated residual hemosiderin deposition scattered in the right frontal region as shown in Fig. 10.3, that also corresponded with scattered WM hyperintensities. These abnormalities remained stable over the next 5 years and represent common neuroimaging sequelae associated with mTBI. The follow-up scans objectively document the damage from the mTBI and also demonstrate the insensitivity of CT in detecting some micro-hemorrhages associated with mild injury as well as other pathologies that undoubtedly, given the MRI findings, were present on the DOI but below the threshold for CT detection. With regard to the timeline of symptom onset, what is of particular interest as demonstrated in this case is that it took several days for the full effects of the mTBI to be manifested and weeks to diminish but chronic deficits remained as would be expected given the MRI findings, consistent with shear damage within the frontal lobes.

Although the positive LOC in mTBI is abrupt and an obvious indicator of TBI, by definition for mTBI it has to be brief and transient or otherwise, the injury would no longer be considered "mild." The evolution of symptoms/problems associated with the initial injury likely has much to do with complex cellular responses to the mechanical deformation of brain parenchyma following injury which is overviewed in Fig. 10.4. [25]. Review of Fig. 10.4 clearly indicates that while mTBI is initiated by an event involving traumatic deformation of neural tissue, the event does not induce a singular pathological event, but initiates the most complex array of structural and physiological changes in brain parenchyma. If the biomechanical deformation is minimal, only transient disruption in neuron integrity occurs [26]. This is depicted in Fig. 10.5 [27], based on cultured neurons, that have been mechanically stretched to mimic injury, from minimal and transient to maximal with permanent damage. This illustration provides a nice heuristic, albeit simplistic, to visualize

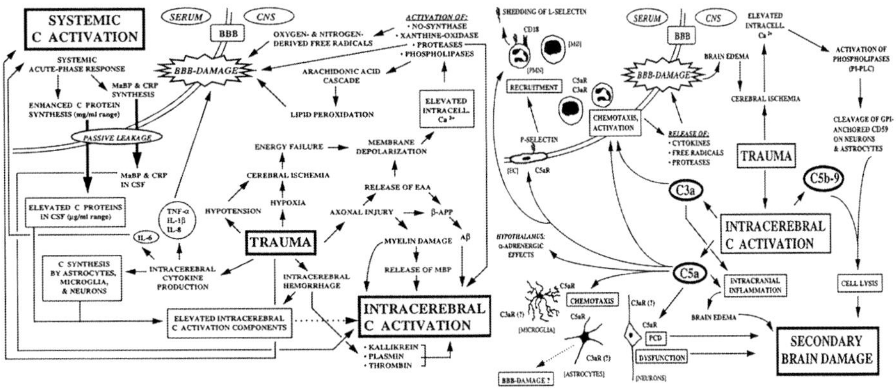

Fig. 10.4 These illustrations depict the primary (A-*left*) and secondary (B-*right*) mechanisms of pathology that occur from TBI. (A-*left schematic*) Cascade of pathophysiological events following traumatic brain injury: mechanisms of elevated complement levels and complement activation within the injured brain (the "C" abbreviation stands for the complement system, an important effector arm of the immune system in the defense against invading pathogens; see Stahel et al. [25] for details and additional explanations of the abbreviations and explanations about their interactions). (B-*right schematic*) Potential mechanisms of complement-mediated secondary brain damage following intrathecal complement activation in head trauma. *EC* endothelial cells, *MØ* monocytes/macrophages, *PMN* polymorphonuclear leukocytes; *?*, cell type-specific function unknown at present; again see Stahel et al. [25] for other abbreviations and explanations. From Stahel PF, Morganti-Kossmann MC, Kossmann T. The role of the complement system in traumatic brain injury—review. *Brain Res Brain Res Rev.* 1998; 27(3): 243–256; used with permission

what may occur following mTBI. Note in this heuristic, transient injury may not lead to structural damage. In such a scenario, the injury did not reach a severity threshold where reparative influences could not overcome the initial cascade of potentially permanent damaging effects from the traumatic pathophysiological events. However, with more significant perturbation, the deformation may begin a process that results in irregular axon morphology and synaptic discontinuities to complete axonal degradation.

Even the briefest viewing of Figs. 10.4 and 10.5 demonstrates the complexity of what attends even a mild injury but the timing of when pathology is expressed further complicates what may be detected with neuroimaging techniques. For example, Morrison et al. [28] show the complexity of the pathobiology of TBI based on severity and time post-injury in an in vitro model of stretch injury as depicted in Fig. 10.6. In this model immature hippocampi are removed, cultured, and then subjected to stretch injury. Dependent on the severity of stretch and time post-injury reflects differences in damage, some damage may be immediately sufficient to cause cell death whereas other cells may just be rendered physiologically instable but with the potential to return to baseline whereas others die.

However, if an injury is to be but a transient perturbation of physiological integrity, a large array of cellular functions, as depicted in Fig. 10.4, must overtime return

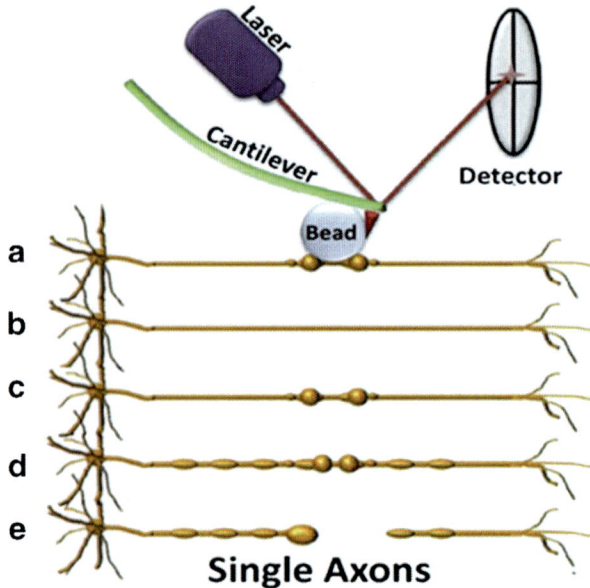

Fig. 10.5 This illustration depicts various potential axonal outcomes following stretch injury in an in vitro TBI model. (**a**) Shows stretch sufficient to create axon beading, which may have transient effect if minimal enough and as shown in (**b**) where axon morphology returns to baseline with no identifiable structural abnormality. However, initial beading may progress, as shown in (**c**) and (**d**), resulting in axon discontinuity and degeneration as shown in (**e**). From Magdesian MH, Sanchez FS, Lopez M, Thostrup P, Durisic N, Belkaid W, et al. Atomic force microscopy reveals important differences in axonal resistance to injury. *Biophys J*. 2012; 103(3): 405–414; used with permission

to homeostatic baseline. Translating this into what may occur in human mTBI, Fig. 10.7 shows how cognitive and neuroimaging findings change over time in mTBI during the first 8 days [29]. All of these mTBI patients had experienced an "uncomplicated" mTBI meaning that no abnormalities were identified in the DOI CT scan, almost all with a GCS of 15 and all the result of some type of motor vehicle accident. All subjects were assessed within 2 days of injury, and serially at days 3–4, 5–6, and 7–8 post-injury. Alternate forms of the Hopkins Verbal Learning Test-Recall (HVLT-R) were administered at each time point and as can be seen in Fig. 10.7, memory performance typically dipped between days 3–6, suggesting the confluence of primary and secondary effects from mTBI reaching their apex at this point. Interestingly, these subjects were also assessed at each time point with MRI and diffusion tensor imaging (DTI), where the fractional anisotropy (FA) measurement was obtained on each occasion. As plotted in Fig. 10.7, FA exhibited variable fluctuations within each individual as did memory function over the first 8 days post-injury. In mTBI acute increases in FA may reflect neuroinflammation [30] and as seen in Fig. 10.7, several mTBI patients showed FA peaks between days 3–4 and 7–8. Decrease in FA may reflect axon damage and without pre-injury neuroimaging

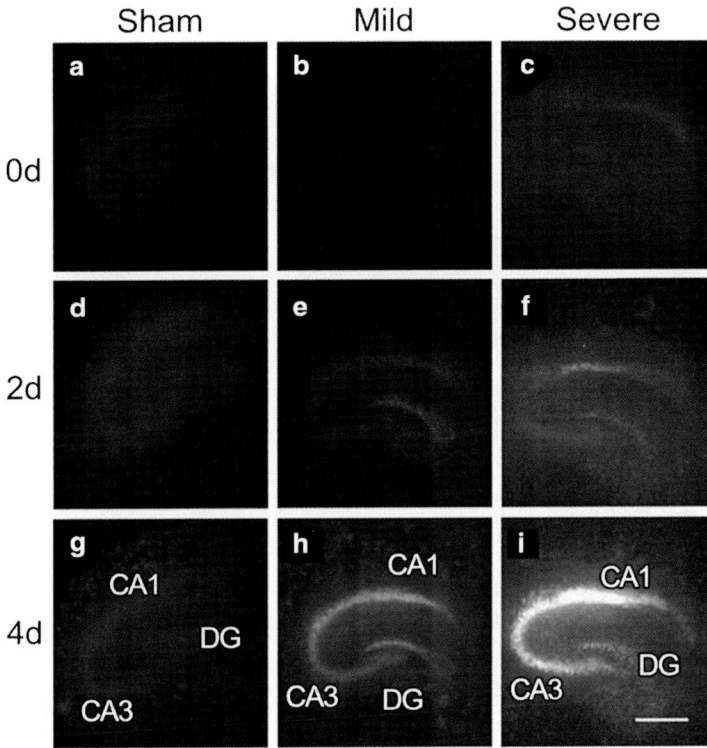

Fig. 10.6 The severity and timing of pathological changes is critical in understanding the effects of TBI. This in vitro cultured hippocampal study shows that neuronal pathology from injury takes days to be expressed and is proportional to severity of injury (mild, moderate, and severe stretch injury). *0d* represents the time point immediately after injury, *2d* represents the second-day post-injury and *4d* indicates the fourth-day post-injury. The images on day 0 show no distinct fluorescence and but a fuzzy appearance by the second day. However, by the fourth day extensive changes had occurred, distinctly more prominent in the severe injury sample. These investigators used propidium iodide fluorescence to microscopically detect cell damage where only damaged cells fluoresce with the degree of fluorescence reflective of the amount of damage. Clearly evident is that it took 4 days for cell damage to be prominently expressed, but even in the mild stretch condition cellular pathology occurred. Such findings support the development of symptoms associated with mTBI to take hours to days to reach an apex (scale bar = 1 mm). From Morrison B, Cater HL, Benham CD, Sundstrom LE. An in vitro model of traumatic brain injury utilising two-dimensional stretch of organotypic hippocampal slice cultures. *J Neurosci Methods.* 2006;150(2): 192–201; used with permission

to know precisely where each individual's FA baseline made it difficult to fully interpret these findings. However, from a memory performance perspective, almost all showed a decrease after day 1–2, with PCS symptoms reaching their peak around day 3. This does suggest that the variability in FA during this acute/subacute time frame may reflect instability of WM microstructure associated with the injury.

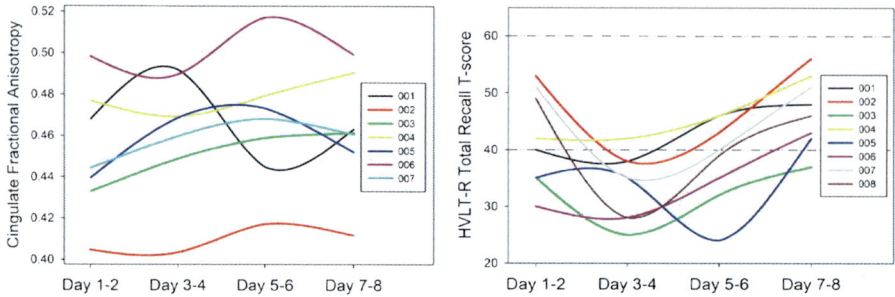

Fig. 10.7 Fractional anisotropy (FA) serial plots over the first 8 days post-injury for seven mTBI patients plotted with corresponding memory performance on the Hopkins Verbal Learning Test-Recall (HVLT-R) performed on the same day as the neuroimaging (note one patient did not have the serial neuroimaging performed). Note the fluctuation in FA, but also the general reduction in memory performance between days 3–4 and 7–8. From Wilde EA, McCauley SR, Barnes A, Wu TC, Chu Z, Hunter JV, et al. Serial measurement of memory and diffusion tensor imaging changes within the first week following uncomplicated mild traumatic brain injury. *Brain Imaging Behav.* 2012; 6(2): 319–328; used with permission

Computed Tomography in MTBI

CT imaging is especially rapid and with contemporary technology can be completed within seconds to minutes in the acutely injured individual. Since it uses X-ray beam technology, it is not influenced by paramagnetic objects like MRI and therefore life-support and other medical assist devices do not interfere with image acquisition or preclude the use of MRI. Likewise, metallic fragments from injury that may be paramagnetic can be imaged without concern about displacement by the strong magnetic fields generated by MRI. Excellent contrast between bone and brain parenchyma can be achieved with CT, where CT clearly has the advantage over MRI in demonstrating the presence and location of skull fractures, common sequelae with head injury. CT also provides methods for examining cerebrovasculature and inflammation in TBI.

In mTBI the commonly identified abnormalities are surface contusions typically at the brain–skull interface, petechial hemorrhages, and/or localized edema. The presence of petechial hemorrhage in TBI is considered a marker of DAI [31, 32], two examples of which are shown in Fig. 10.8. Skull fracture is also readily identifiable with CT and must be considered as an indicator of potential brain injury because the distinct forces necessary to fracture bone are certainly sufficient to injury brain parenchyma. Often because of the limited resolution of CT, even in the presence of some type of skull fracture in an individual with mTBI, parenchyma may appear normal on CT. Of course, just because neural tissue may appear "normal" does not mean normal microstructure and function because that is beyond the scope of what CT may detect.

When an abnormality is present on the DOI CT, as stated earlier, often the classification of "complicated mild TBI" is made. However, given contemporary advances

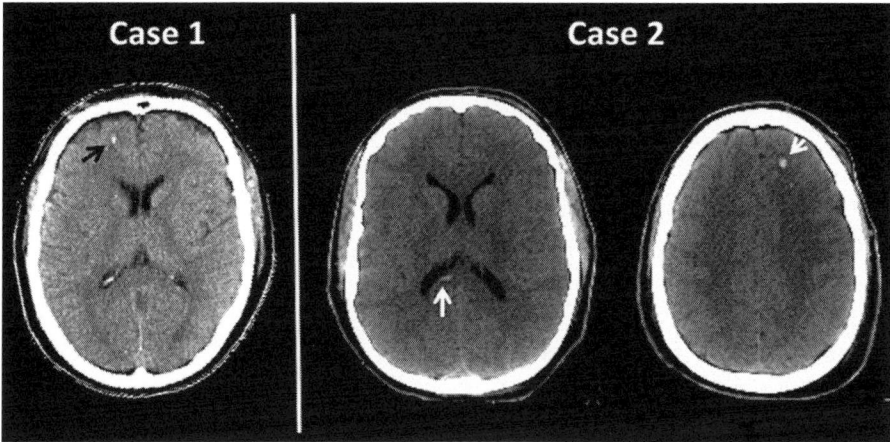

Fig. 10.8 CT appearance of petechial hemorrhage in two separate cases. Note the proximity of the lesion within the white matter but at the border of where the gray boundary is located. Both cases were adults and involved high-speed motor vehicle accidents. Note the *black arrow* in *Case 1* and the *top white arrow* in *Case 2* point to the hemorrhage which occurs right at the gray-white junction. In *Case 2* there is a contrecoup hemorrhagic lesion in the posterior corpus callosum, *bottom arrow*

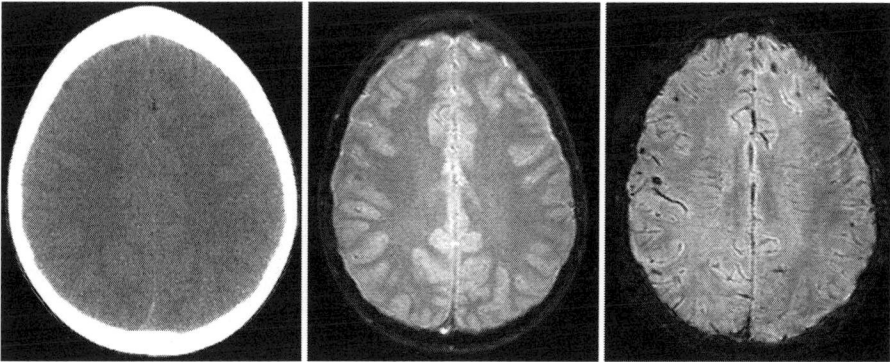

Fig. 10.9 The insensitivity of CT (A) and conventional gradient recalled echo (GRE, B) sequences to detect petechial hemorrhage is shown. The CT scan was interpreted to be within normal limits with no hemorrhage identified yet this individual agreed to participate in a research study and therefore was scanned with MRI procedures including susceptibility weighted imaging (SWI) as shown in (C) and magnetization transfer imaging (MTI, not shown) both show frontal abnormality and residual hemorrhage. From Bigler ED. Neuropsychology and clinical neuroscience of persistent post-concussive syndrome. *J Int Neuropsychol Soc.* 2008; 14(1): 1–22; used with permission

that identify mTBI abnormalities that simply are not detected by CT imaging, this classification is mostly meaningless. Figure 10.3 demonstrated this point and another case is shown in Fig. 10.9. The presence of hemosiderin deposition is presumed to be the best marker for the existence of traumatic shear injury [31, 32].

Currently, the superior MRI method for detecting hemorrhagic shear lesions in mTBI is susceptibility weighted imaging (SWI).

CT imaging readily identifies more serious acute injuries or evolving TBI pathologies that require neurosurgical intervention and is of critical importance in the initial triage and medical management of TBI, including mTBI. With that being said, however, it is of limited utility in mTBI although some perfusion techniques as markers of initial neuroinflammation have shown an ability to detect mTBI abnormalities not identified on conventional DOI CT imaging [33, 34].

Visible Macroscopic Abnormalities

To best understand what information may be gathered from MRI in TBI, it is important to understand that the abnormalities are, in part, time dependent and differ by primary as well as secondary injury effects. Bigler and Maxwell [3, 4] have outlined a time frame depicting the potential pathological changes that occur as presented in the schematic shown in Fig. 10.10. Figure 10.11 shows how visibly detectable lesions change over time. Characteristic primary and secondary pathologies can be readily defined when sequential imaging is performed, typically a combination of CT and MRI, as shown in Fig. 10.11.

In Fig. 10.11 the acute CT findings depict the faint appearance of blood, mostly likely indicative of a traumatic subarachnoid hemorrhage. The presence of hemorrhage in TBI, whether detected by CT or MRI, is commonly considered the best indicator of intracranial traumatic shear forces sufficient to produce traumatic axonal injury (TAI) [3, 4]. However, even with the best of resolution that CT imaging provides precise detection and localization of the significance of this type of pathology is limited as demonstrated Fig. 10.11. By 8 days post-injury, edema is identified, but the hemorrhage has basically resolved where phagocytosis has removed degraded blood by-products. By 2 months post-injury, CT imaging demonstrates what appears to be resolution. However, when scanned 4 years later with MRI, hemosiderin deposition is distinctly apparent not in the subarachnoid space, but within brain parenchyma. Imaging of the gyri where the hemorrhage was identified also distinctly demonstrates signal abnormality beyond the hemosiderin foci. When viewed with MRI and knowing the sequence of events, the initial impact forces in this region likely sheared both blood vessels and neural tissue, resulting in DAI and focal WM changes. However, the DOI CT mostly depicts subarachnoid hemorrhage, with little indication of underlying WM damage. Only through sequential imaging does the true clinical significance of this injury become apparent.

From Fig. 10.11 the primary and secondary effects of TBI can be inferred. At the point of impact, the primary injury occurs and given the follow-up MRI findings there likely was traumatic shear injury resulting in primary axotomy. However, considerable secondary injury also likely occurred because of the edema as well as vascular injury and whatever local pathologic, metabolic, and neurotransmitter derangements and aberrations that occurred. Sheared blood vessels can no longer

Programmed cell death (Apoptosis)

Reduction in caliber of axon. compaction of neurofilaments over 30 – 50 μm of axon length.

Watery or dark degeneration. Proteolysis of neurofilaments of axonal cytoskeleton but myelin figures remain for a period. Invasion by immune-responsive cells.

(24 hours – 12 weeks)
PROXIMAL PORTION OF AXON

WALLERIAN DEGENERATION OF DISTAL PORTION OF AXON

SECONDARY AXOTOMY
(minimum of 2 hours in animals, 12 hours in human beings
(4 hours – 12 weeks)
Axonal disconnection

Enlarged periaxonal space, focal compaction of neurofilaments, disruption of the axolemma, focal proteolysis of neurofilaments, foci of separation of myelin lamellae within internode

10-15% strain (1.5 – 6 hours)
Axonal swelling, influx of Ca^{2+},
Loss of fast axonal transport

Depolymerization of microtubules, μM calpain/phosphatase/kinase activation compaction of neurofilaments collapse/loss of neurofilament sidearms, foci of separation of myelin lamellae

Reverse pumping by Na/Ca exchanger, Ca^{2+} influx, injury to mitochondria, reduced ATP production, failure of ATP dependent membrane pumps, increased calcium influx, release of cyto-c, widespread activation of calpains related to the subaxolemma cytoskeleton

PRIMARY AXOTOMY
More than 20% strain

Membrane renting/fragmentation Proteolysis of axonal cytoskeleton in zone of axotomy

Sodium channel leakiness, Na^+ and Ca^{2+} influx, direct mechanical failure of microtubules

Membrane recovery

5% or less strain (seconds)
Transient depolarisation

Recovery

5 – 10% strain (15 min – 24 hours)
Functional and structural damage to the axolemma
depolarization and loss of ionic homeostasis

INJURY   Transient mechanical strain or Hypoxic-Ischemic-Injury

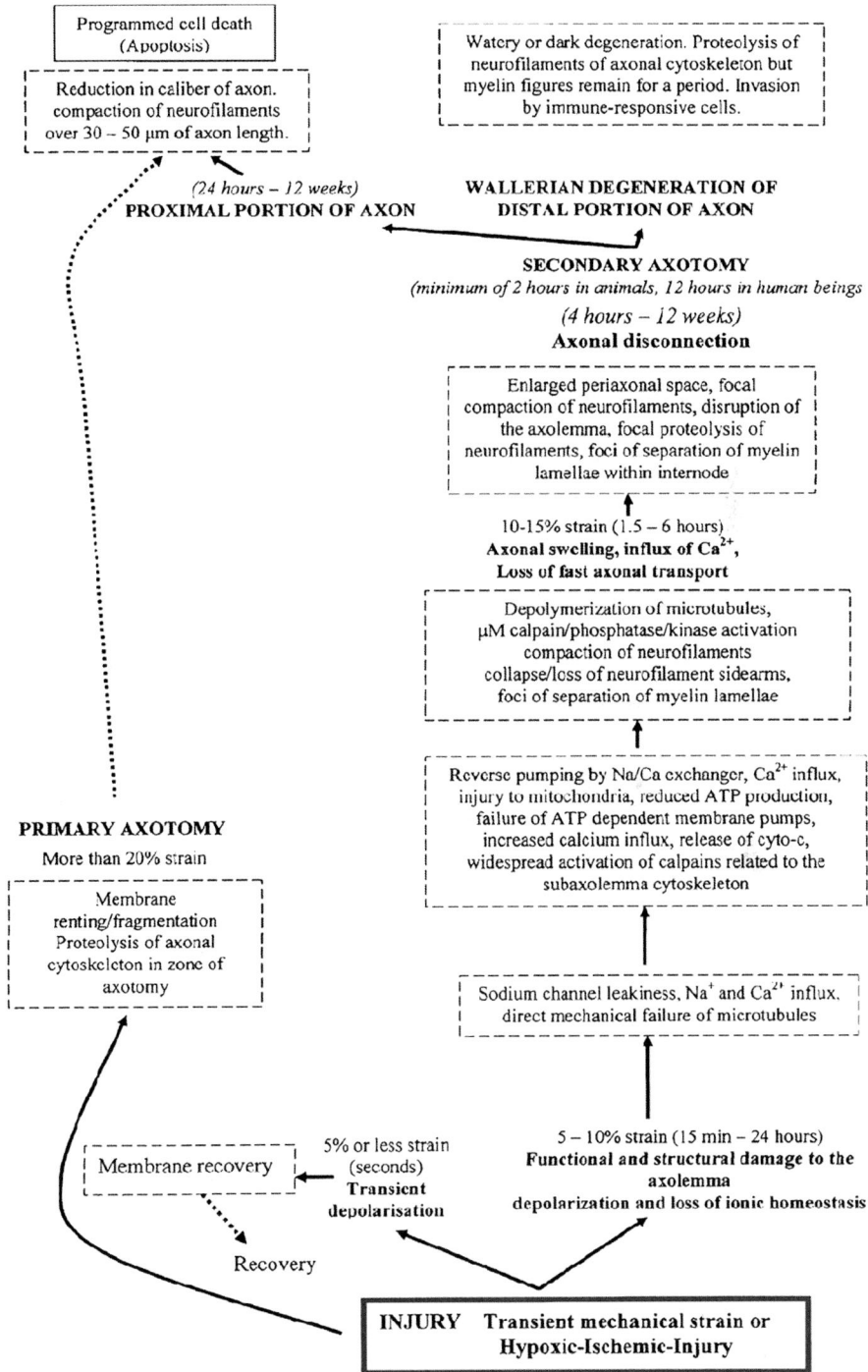

Fig. 10.10 Schematic overview of current thinking with regard to axonal injury in human DAI and animal diffuse traumatic brain injury. Modified from Biasca N, Maxwell WL. Minor traumatic brain injury in sports: a review in order to prevent neurological sequelae. Prog Brain Res 2007; 16: 263–291. From Bigler ED, Maxwell WL. Neuropathology of mild traumatic brain injury: relationship to neuroimaging findings—review. *Brain Imaging Behav.* 2012; 6(2): 108–136; used with permission

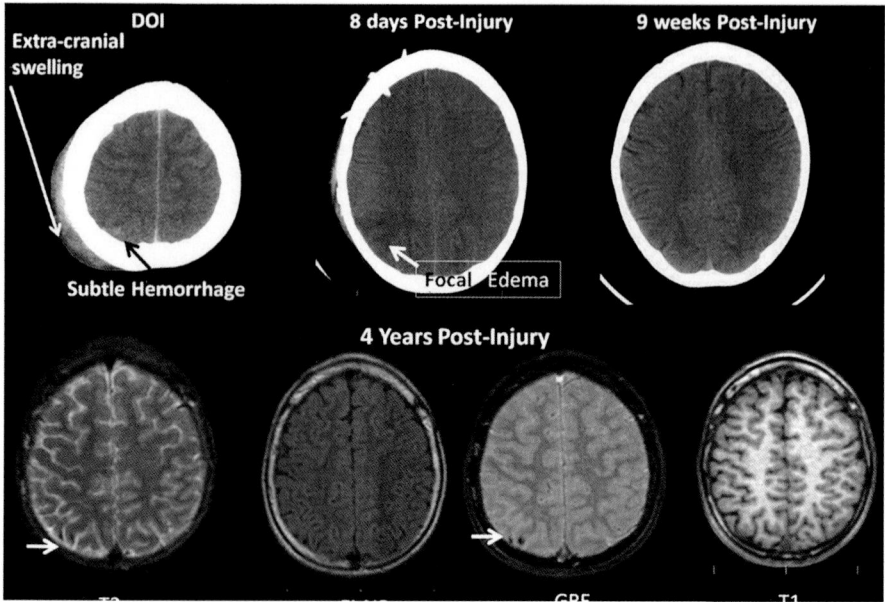

Fig. 10.11 Starting with the DOI CT scans, various lesion types are identified and using the DOI scan as baseline, changes from DOI to chronic state may be shown. The "lesion" starts off as a subtle subarachnoid hemorrhage but by 8 days post-injury is seen as edema which appears to resolve by 9 weeks post-injury. However, with follow-up MRI, subtle hemosiderin deposition is identified

provide oxygenated blood to the neuropil resulting in additional neural tissue (both neurons and glial cells) compromise, degradation, and potential death. Neuronal degeneration ensues which cannot be detected by CT imaging but is revealed by MRI. This potential sequence of events and its adverse influence on the axon is depicted in Fig. 10.12 [35].

Fig. 10.12 (continued) and local mitochondrial damage can follow, which, if unabated, collectively alters/impairs axonal transport illustrated in panel E. Alternatively, if these abnormalities do not progress, recovery is possible (F). When progressive, these events not only impair axonal transport but also lead to rapid intra-axonal change in the paranodal and perhaps internodal domains that elicit the collapse of the axolemma and its overlying myelin sheath to result in lobulated and disconnected axonal segments (G) that, over the next 15 min–2 h, fully detach (H). The proximal axonal segment in continuity with the cell body of origin now continues to swell from the delivery of vesicles and organelles via anterograde transport while the downstream fiber undergoes Wallerian change (I). Lastly, with the most severe forms of injury, the above identified calcium-mediated destructive cascades are further augmented by the poration of the axolemma, again primarily at the nodal region (J). The resulting calcium surge, together with potential local microtubular damage and disassembly, pose catastrophic intra-axonal change that converts anterograde to retrograde axonal transport, precluding continued axonal swelling, while the distal axonal segment fragments and disconnects (K), with Wallerian degeneration ensuing downstream (L). From Smith DH, Hicks R, Povlishock JT. Therapy development for diffuse axonal injury. *J Neurotrauma*. 2013; 30(5): 307–323; used with permission

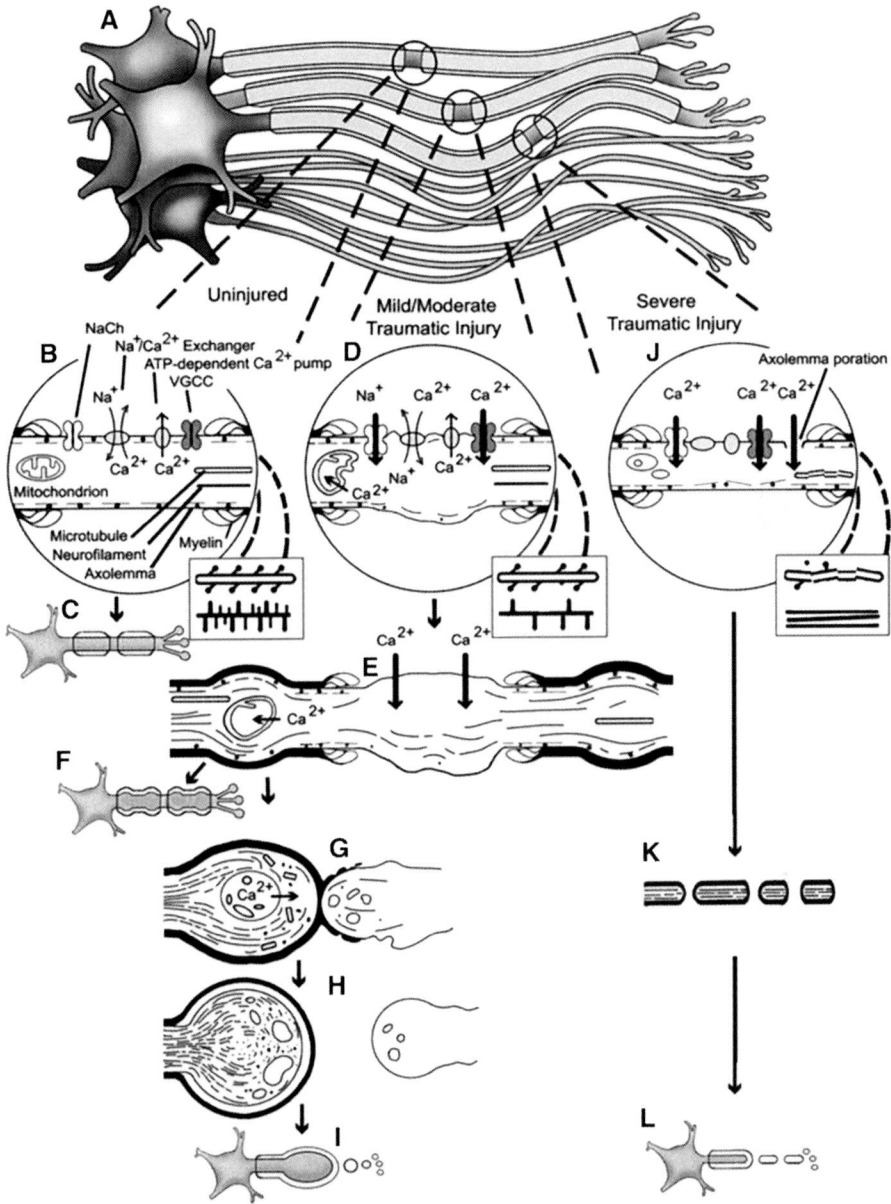

Fig. 10.12 Evolving pathophysiology of traumatic injury in myelinated axons. In this figure, the author's attempt, in an abbreviated fashion, to illustrate some of the key events believed to be involved in the pathobiology of traumatic axonal injury and, thereby, identify potential therapeutic targets. Although framed in the view of primary nodal involvement (A), this focus does not preclude comparable change ongoing in other regions of the axon. Panels B and C show normal axonal detail including the paranodal loops and the presence of intra-axonal mitochondria, microtubules, and neurofilaments, together with the presence of multiple axolemmal channels localized primarily to the nodal domain. Mild to moderate traumatic brain injury in panel D is observed to involve a mechanical dysregulation of the voltage-sensitive sodium channels, which contribute to increased calcium influx via reversal of the sodium calcium exchanger and the opening of voltage-gated calcium channels. This also impacts on the proteolysis of sodium channel inactivation that contributes further to local calcium dysregulation. Microtubular loss, neurofilament impaction,

Empirically Derived Quantitative MR Abnormalities

The common images generated from MR technology, like those shown in the various figures up to this point have all been generated by MR metrics that form the basis for the image display. However, these quantitative MR metrics permit analyses separate from just the anatomical image display. For example, Fig. 10.13 shows the appearance of a DTI MR sequence with its associated color map. Two common metrics derived from DTI are referred to as fractional anisotropy or FA and apparent diffusion coefficient or ADC. Figure 10.13 provides a DTI schematic depicting the relationship of FA and ADC to axon integrity and what happens with axon damage. These DTI metrics assess the microstructure of WM and are based on the characteristics of how myelin sheaths and cell membranes of WM tracts affect the movement of water molecules. Healthy axonal membranes constrain the free movement and direction of movement of water. Consequently, water molecules tend to move faster in parallel to nerve fibers rather than perpendicular to them. This characteristic, which is referred to as anisotropic diffusion and is measured by FA, is determined by the thickness of the myelin sheath and of the axons. FA ranges from 0 to 1, where 0 represents maximal isotropic diffusion (e.g., free diffusion in perfect sphere) and 1 represents maximal anisotropic diffusion, i.e., diffusion in one direction (e.g., a long cylinder of minimal diameter). Diffusion anisotropy varies across WM regions, putatively reflecting differences in fiber myelination, fiber diameter, and directionality.

The aggregate fiber tracts of an entire brain can be derived from DTI, as shown in Fig. 10.14. In TBI, DTI may demonstrate a loss of fiber tract integrity, reflected as a thinning out of the number of aggregate tracts. This is also demonstrated in

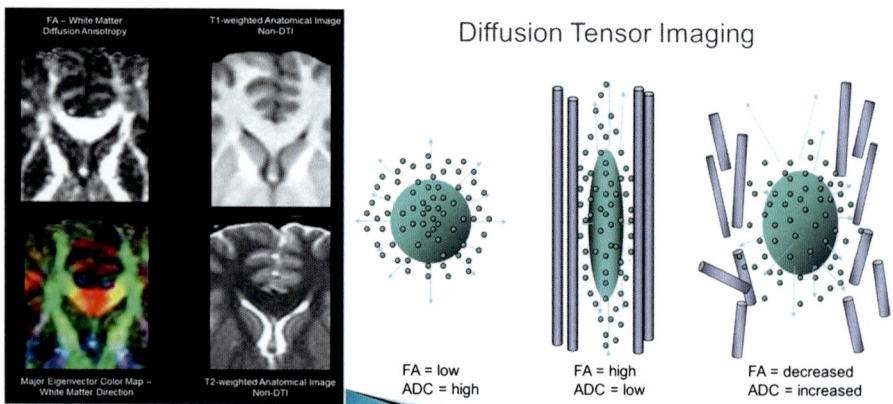

Fig. 10.13 The images on the *upper left* show the DTI acquisition image and the DTI color map (*bottom left*) in comparison to the conventional T1 and T2. The cartoon on the *right* depicts the relationship of fractional anisotropy (FA) with the apparent diffusion coefficient (ADC) showing how normal conformity of membrane anatomy constrains water diffusion; however, if membrane dissolution occurs in any fashion, such as from TBI, water is freer to move and with lack of constraint, FA elevates and ADC declines

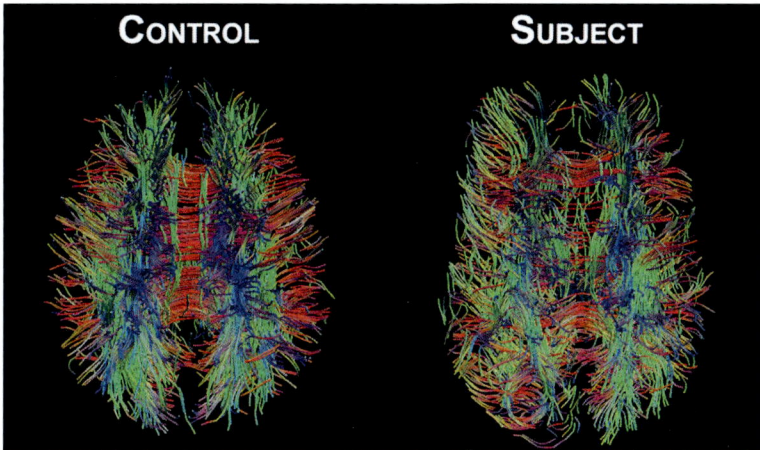

Fig. 10.14 The complexity of brain networks is readily appreciated in view whole brain DTI in a control subject and a patient with severe TBI showing reduced whole-brain network integrity. Note the WM thinning of aggregate tracts that has occurred in the case of TBI

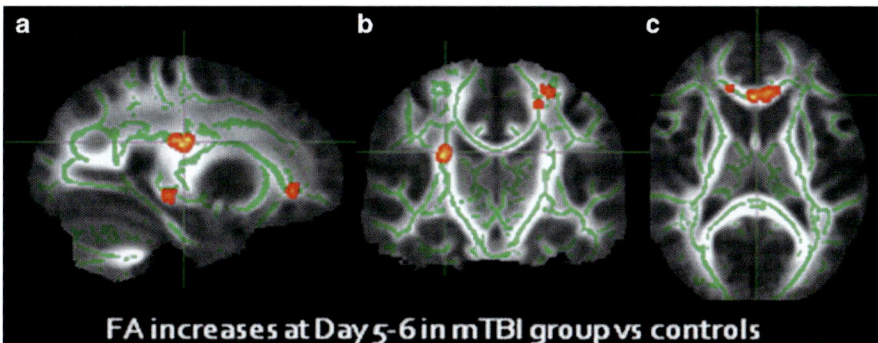

Fig. 10.15 In conjunction with the DTI demonstration of the fluctuation in fractional anisotropy (FA) and change in memory performance within the first 8 days post-injury (see Fig. 10.7), this tract-based spatial statistics output from this mTBI sample shows where there were significant regional increases in FA compared to controls. Possible interpretation of such findings is that they reflect areas of neuroinflammation. Interesting, it is at this point post-injury where some of the mTBI patients displayed their poorest performance on tasks involving memory function. (**a**) sagittal, (**b**) coronal and (**c**) axial MRI planes

Fig. 10.14, where a patient with TBI is compared to a similar aged individual with typical development. The loss of aggregate tracts in the TBI whole-brain network analysis demonstrates an overall reduction in WM connectivity. DTI methods provide various techniques to view the pathological effects of TBI within the context of WM network connectivity.

Figure 10.14 depicts the DTI findings in the individual case, but Fig. 10.15 provides an example of how group DTI findings may be presented. In this figure a technique referred to as tract-based spatial statistics is used to show where significant group differences may be observed comparing the TBI group with a matched control sample. In Fig. 10.15, the mTBI patients first described in Fig. 10.7 were compared to matched controls with the results demonstrating distinctly visible differences in FA. In this illustration it shows where significant increases in FA were observed, interpreted to be an indication of neuroinflammation. Note the statistical comparison revealed abnormalities in the anterior and posterior corpus callosum, common regions for pathology to be detected when DTI is empirically assessed in mTBI.

Trauma-induced edematous reactions in the brain compress parenchyma, which in turn, may influence water diffusion potentially detected by DTI. Using the FA metric, increases in FA beyond some normal baseline may signify edema whereas low FA may occur when axon degradation, membrane abnormalities increase water diffusion or actual degeneration has occurred, which increases extracellular water. Since TBI may induce dynamic changes over time, differences in FA over acute, subacute, and chronic time frames post-injury may differ as well. When axons degenerate, the increased space frees extracellular water in resulting in lower FA. Thus, in mTBI, low FA may reflect WM degeneration.

Heterogeneity Visible MTBI Lesions

Bigler et al. [6] examined a sample of 41 children with complicated mTBI. When assessed with MRI at least 6 months post-injury regardless of whether the residual lesion was an area of focal encephalomalacia, hemosiderin deposit or WM hyperintensity, *none* of the lesions perfectly overlapped although the majority was distributed within the frontal and temporal lobes. Just from the randomness of the lesions, this would indicate that each mTBI produced its own unique injury and with unique injury this would indicate the likelihood that mTBI sequelae would likely be rather idiosyncratic to the individual as well.

Cellular Basis of MTBI Neuropathology

Based on the position statement by the International and Interagency Initiative toward Common Data Elements for Research on Traumatic Brain Injury and Psychological Health the definition of traumatic brain injury is "… an alteration in brain function, or other evidence of brain pathology, caused by an external force [36]". External force induces brain injury via deformation of neural tissue that surpasses tolerance limits for normal displacement or strain that accompanies movement such as jumping, rapid turning of the head, simple bumps to the head, etc. So, at the most fundamental level of injury, cellular deformation disrupts anatomy and physiology sufficient to at least transiently impair function when the threshold for mTBI has been reached.

Too often, neural cells are viewed schematically as an artist's rendition of what a neural cell looks like, such as that shown in Fig. 10.16 but artistic schematics detract

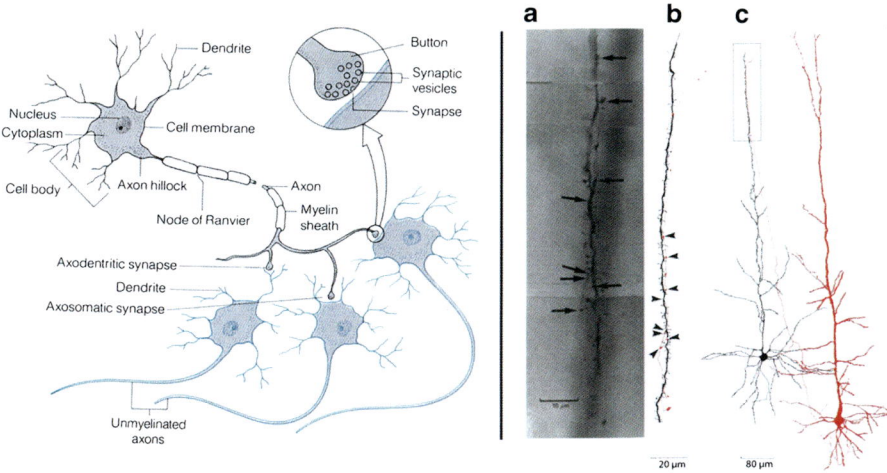

Fig. 10.16 (*Left*) The schematic of a neuron shows a hypothetical neuron with what appears to be a bulky, sturdy axon protruding from the cell body and interfacing with other neurons. However, the reality is something quite different. From: Pinel JPJ. Biopsychology. Boston: Allyn & Bacon, 1990; used with permission. (*Right*) Two cortical cells in a rat cortex that have been isolated. Note the micron level of the axon—it is infinitesimally small. Note also who the single axon intertwines the dendrite and the dendritic spines as highlighted in the photomicrograph. When thinking about TBI, one must view the potential neuropathological effects at this microscopic level. From Deuchars J, West DC, Thomson AM. Relationships between morphology and physiology of pyramid-pyramid single axon connections in rat neocortex in vitro. *J Physiol*. 1994; 478(3): 423–435; used with permission

from the true complexity and delicate nature of what really constitutes neural tissue. For example, Fig. 10.16 depicts two cortical pyramidal cells identified in the rat cerebral cortex, based on their physiological response and their appearance via electron microscopy. Note how small these structures are, note that these views are merely two-dimensional of a three-dimensional structure and note that the axon is but a few microns in thickness. Additionally note the numerous dendritic spines and how the axon intertwines with the spines.

As the definition implies, TBI occurs from some external force which, in turn must deform brain parenchyma such that a sufficient deformation of the typical shape of cellular tissue no longer lines up and/or connects as it should. Returning to Fig. 10.16, note again the complex intertwining of dendritic spines with axon segments where any misalignment would likely affect synaptic integrity. Likewise, if the axon membrane is disrupted, membrane permeability will directly impact neuronal function and propagation of axon potentials. Only one axon segment need be affected to disrupt neural transmission for the entire axon. A variety of finite elements and various methods for recreating the motion that displaces brain parenchyma that results in concussive injury have been performed, mostly using sports concussion models. For example, Viano et al. [37] showed on average in the typical sports-related concussion that the brain displaces between 4 and 8 mm in regions like the corpus callosum, midbrain, medial temporal lobe, and fornix. Viewing Fig. 10.16 from the perspective of this amount of deformation, noting that the photomicrograph depicts an axon that is about 0.1 mm in length, would reflect a massive distortion of neurons this size.

Blood vessels are just as delicate as neural tissue, especially at the capillary level. Each neuron is dependent on receiving a continuous source of glucose and oxygen with the smallest capillaries largest enough for a just single red blood cell to traverse the capillary to deliver its oxygen and glucose [3, 4]. As such, blood vessels are just as susceptible to the shear–strain biomechanics of head injury as are neurons [38].

Deformation Biomechanics

From the above discussion all deformation in mTBI must be viewed at the cellular level, but biomechanical schematics are typically presented at the whole brain level. Ropper and Gorson [39] provided a schematic of where the greatest deformations have been modeled in mTBI and this is provided in Fig. 10.17. This illustration clearly depicts the known frontotemporal regions for cortical surface compression, but also WM tracts of the upper brainstem corpus callosum and cingulum. In mTBI, as already mentioned by definition of what constitutes a TBI the WM abnormalities at the brainstem level could not represent major pathology because LOC must be brief to meet mTBI criteria. Likewise, alteration in mental status that would result in prolong posttraumatic amnesia would also disqualify someone for mTBI classification. So while subtle brainstem pathology may persist in the mTBI patient, as Heitger et al. [40] have shown, as well as frontotemporal pathology, as numerous investigators have shown, major pathologies at these levels are unlikely because if major pathology persisted in these regions during the acute phase, the individual likely would not meet criteria for mTBI. Nonetheless, what is depicted in the Fig. 10.17 from Ropper and Gorson provides a wonderful heuristic for where likely changes in mTBI will be observed in neuroimaging studies.

For example, Fig. 10.18 is from a child with mTBI from a skiing accident who sustained an mTBI. When symptoms persisted, this child, who had a negative DOI CT was scanned with MRI. The follow-up MRI revealed hemosiderin deposition in frontotemporal areas and anterior corpus callosum, as would be predicted from the schematic in Fig. 10.17.

Volumetry Findings in MTBI

As shown in Fig. 10.17, if atrophic changes associated with mTBI were to occur, they would most likely be found within those regions associated with the greatest likelihood for shear/strain and deformation injury. Indeed, several studies that have prospectively examined mTBI subjects have demonstrated this regional atrophy [41–45].

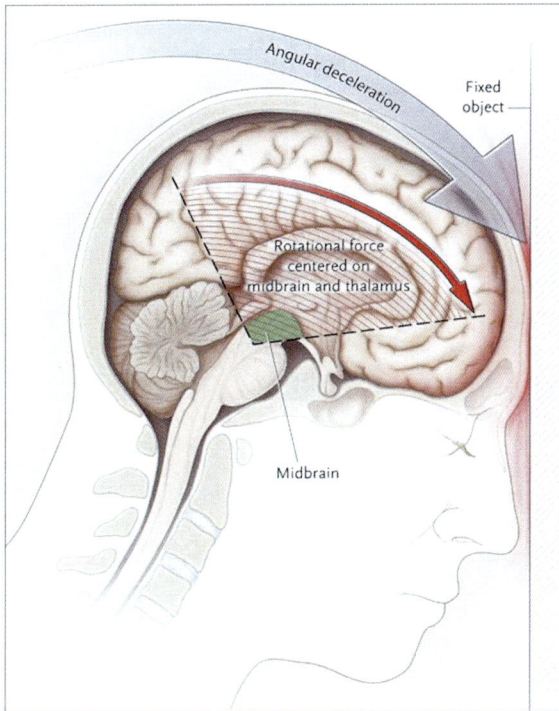

Fig. 10.17 The mechanism of concussion is outlined in this illustration. Biomechanical investigations dating back to the beginning of the twentieth century suggest that concussion results from a rotational motion of the cerebral hemispheres in the anterior–posterior plane, around the fulcrum of the fixed-in-place upper brain stem. If the neck is restrained, concussion is difficult to produce. Concussions as portrayed in movies and cartoons, in which the back of the head is struck with a blunt object and no motion is transferred to the brain, are implausible. The modern view is that there is disruption of the electrophysiological and subcellular activities of the neurons of the reticular activating system that are situated in the midbrain and diencephalic region, where the maximal rotational forces are exerted. Alternative mechanisms for concussive LOC, such as self-limited cortical seizures or a sudden increase in intracranial pressure, have also been proposed, but with limited supporting evidence. An animated version of this figure is available with the full text of the article at www.nejm.org. From Ropper AH, Gorson KC. Clinical practice. Concussion—review. *N Engl J Med.* 2007; 356(2): 166–172; used with permission

For example, Zhou et al. [42] demonstrated that by establishing a baseline in mTBI patients within the acute to early subacute time frame that when assessed with various volumetric techniques 1 year later that significant volume loss was observed in the anterior cingulum, cingulate gyrus, and scattered regions within the frontal lobes. Interestingly they observed volume loss in the cuneus and precuneus regions as well. The volume loss with the cuneus and precuneus, posterior brain regions may actually be the result of Wallerian degeneration from the more focal frontal loss disrupting long coursing frontoparietal connections particularly vulnerable to stretching and shearing effects [3, 4, 26].

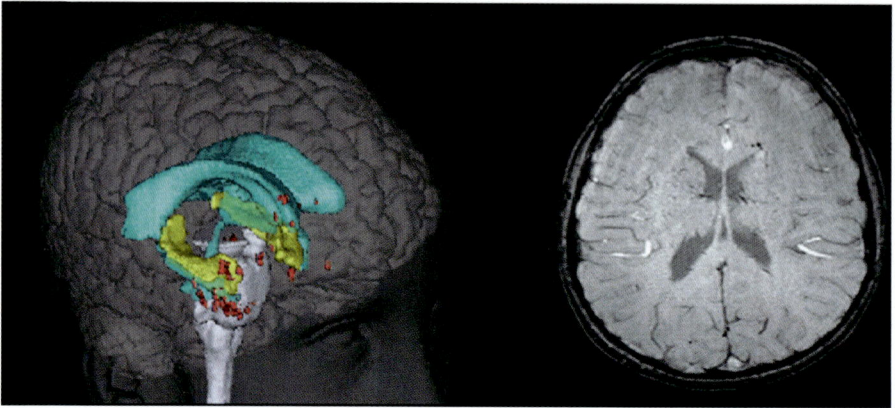

Fig. 10.18 This preadolescent child sustained an mTBI in a ski accident. When symptoms persisted MRI demonstrated multiple regions of hemosiderin deposition. Note the frontotemporal distribution and location of hemosiderin in the forceps minor region of the corpus callosum on the susceptibility weighted image on the *right*. In the three-dimensional image, the ventricle is shown in aquamarine to provide landmark points with the *red* signifying where hemosiderin was identified and the *yellow* indicates the hippocampus

Conclusion

Structural neuroimaging provides a variety of methods to detect underlying neuropathology that results from mTBI. The most common visible abnormalities are in the form of focal encephalomalacia, hemosiderin deposition, and/or WM hyperintensity. A variety of quantitative MRI methods have demonstrated techniques for the detection of underlying pathology associated with mTBI, which differ depending on the time post-injury that the scan is performed.

References

1. Yassa MA, Muftuler LT, Stark CE. Ultrahigh-resolution microstructural diffusion tensor imaging reveals perforant path degradation in aged humans in vivo. Proc Natl Acad Sci U S A. 2010;107(28):12687–91.
2. Heidemann RM, Ivanov D, Trampel R, Fasano F, Meyer H, Pfeuffer J, et al. Isotropic submillimeter fMRI in the human brain at 7 T: combining reduced field-of-view imaging and partially parallel acquisitions. Magn Reson Med. 2012;68(5):1506–16.
3. Bigler ED, Maxwell WL. Neuropathology of mild traumatic brain injury: relationship to neuroimaging findings—review. Brain Imaging Behav. 2012;6(2):108–36.
4. Bigler ED, Maxwell WL. Neuroimaging and neuropathology of TBI—review. NeuroRehabilitation. 2011;28(2):63–74.
5. Teasdale G, Jennett B. Assessment of coma and impaired consciousness. A practical scale. Lancet. 1974;2(7872):81–4.

6. Bigler ED, Abildskov TJ, Petrie J, Dennis M, Simic N, Taylor HG, et al. Heterogeneity of brain lesions in pediatric traumatic brain injury. Neuropsychology. 2013;27(4):438–51.

7. Dewitt DS, Perez-Polo R, Hulsebosch CE, Dash PK, Robertson CS. Challenges in the development of rodent models of mild traumatic brain injury. J Neurotrauma. 2013;30(9):688–701.

8. Hylin MJ, Orsi SA, Zhao J, Bockhorst K, Perez A, Moore AN, et al. Behavioral and histopathological alterations resulting from mild fluid percussion injury. J Neurotrauma. 2013;30(9): 702–15.

9. Jagoda AS. Mild traumatic brain injury: key decisions in acute management—review. Psychiatr Clin North Am. 2010;33(4):797–806.

10. Tavender EJ, Bosch M, Green S, O'Connor D, Pitt V, Phillips K, et al. Quality and consistency of guidelines for the management of mild traumatic brain injury in the emergency department. Acad Emerg Med. 2011;18(8):880–9.

11. Slobounov S, Gay M, Johnson B, Zhang K. Concussion in athletics: ongoing clinical and brain imaging research controversies—review. Brain Imaging Behav. 2012;6(2):224–43.

12. Wilde EA, Hunter BED. Pediatric traumatic brain injury: neuroimaging and neurorehabilitation outcome [Research Support, N.I.H., Extramural Review]. NeuroRehabilitation. 2012;31(3):245–60.

13. Wilde EA, Hunter JV, Bigler ED. A primer of neuroimaging analysis in neurorehabilitation outcome research—review. NeuroRehabilitation. 2012;31(3):227–42.

14. Wilde EA, Hunter JV, Bigler ED. Neuroimaging in neurorehabilitation. NeuroRehabilitation. 2012;31(3):223–6.

15. Post A, Hoshizaki B, Gilchrist MD. Finite element analysis of the effect of loading curve shape on brain injury predictors. J Biomech. 2012;45(4):679–83.

16. Statler KD, Swank S, Abildskov T, Bigler ED, White HS. Traumatic brain injury during development reduces minimal clonic seizure thresholds at maturity. Epilepsy Res. 2008;80(2–3): 163–70.

17. Bayly PV, Clayton EH, Genin GM. Quantitative imaging methods for the development and validation of brain biomechanics models [Research Support, N.I.H., Extramural Review]. Annu Rev Biomed Eng. 2012;14:369–96.

18. Feng Y, Okamoto RJ, Namani R, Genin GM, Bayly PV. Measurements of mechanical anisotropy in brain tissue and implications for transversely isotropic material models of white matter. J Mech Behav Biomed Mater. 2013;23C:117–32.

19. Kraft RH, McKee PJ, Dagro AM, Grafton ST. Combining the finite element method with structural connectome-based analysis for modeling neurotrauma: connectome neurotrauma mechanics. PLoS Comput Biol. 2012;8(8):e1002619.

20. Watanabe R, Katsuhara T, Miyazaki H, Kitagawa Y, Yasuki T. Research of the relationship of pedestrian injury to collision speed, car-type, impact location and pedestrian sizes using Human FE model (THUMS Version 4). Stapp Car Crash J. 2012;56:269–321.

21. Mao H, Elkin BS, Genthikatti VV, Morrison Iii B, Yang KH. Why is CA3 more vulnerable than CA1 in experimental models of controlled cortical impact-induced brain injury? J Neurotrauma. 2013;30(17):1521–30; Apr 4: epub ahead of print.

22. Feng Y, Clayton EH, Chang Y, Okamoto RJ, Bayly PV. Viscoelastic properties of the ferret brain measured in vivo at multiple frequencies by magnetic resonance elastography. J Biomech. 2013;46(5):863–70.

23. Prichep LS, McCrea M, Barr W, Powell M, Chabot RJ. Time course of clinical and electrophysiological recovery after sport-related concussion. J Head Trauma Rehabil. 2012;28(4):266–73; May 14: epub ahead of print.

24. Duhaime AC, Beckwith JG, Maerlender AC, McAllister TW, Crisco JJ, Duma SM, et al. Spectrum of acute clinical characteristics of diagnosed concussions in college athletes wearing instrumented helmets: clinical article. J Neurosurg. 2012;117(6):1092–9.

25. Stahel PF, Morganti-Kossmann MC, Kossmann T. The role of the complement system in traumatic brain injury—review. Brain Res Brain Res Rev. 1998;27(3):243–56.

26. Biasca N, Maxwell WL. Minor traumatic brain injury in sports: a review in order to prevent neurological sequelae—review. Prog Brain Res. 2007;161:263–91.

27. Magdesian MH, Sanchez FS, Lopez M, Thostrup P, Durisic N, Belkaid W, et al. Atomic force microscopy reveals important differences in axonal resistance to injury. Biophys J. 2012;103(3): 405–14.
28. Morrison B, Cater HL, Benham CD, Sundstrom LE. An in vitro model of traumatic brain injury utilising two-dimensional stretch of organotypic hippocampal slice cultures. J Neurosci Methods. 2006;150(2):192–201.
29. Wilde EA, McCauley SR, Barnes A, Wu TC, Chu Z, Hunter JV, et al. Serial measurement of memory and diffusion tensor imaging changes within the first week following uncomplicated mild traumatic brain injury. Brain Imaging Behav. 2012;6(2):319–28.
30. Wilde EA, McCauley SR, Hunter JV, Bigler ED, Chu Z, Wang ZJ, et al. Diffusion tensor imaging of acute mild traumatic brain injury in adolescents. Neurology. 2008;70(12):948–55.
31. Scheid R, Walther K, Guthke T, Preul C, von Cramon DY. Cognitive sequelae of diffuse axonal injury—a comparative study. Arch Neurol. 2006;63(3):418–24.
32. Scheid R, Preul C, Gruber O, Wiggins C, von Cramon DY. Diffuse axonal injury associated with chronic traumatic brain injury: evidence from T2*-weighted gradient-echo imaging at 3 T. AJNR Am J Neuroradiol. 2003;24(6):1049–56.
33. Metting Z, Rodiger LA, de Jong BM, Stewart RE, Kremer BP, van der Naalt J. Acute cerebral perfusion CT abnormalities associated with posttraumatic amnesia in mild head injury. J Neurotrauma. 2010;27(12):2183–9.
34. Metting Z, Rodiger LA, Stewart RE, Oudkerk M, De Keyser J, van der Naalt J. Perfusion computed tomography in the acute phase of mild head injury: regional dysfunction and prognostic value. Ann Neurol. 2009;66(6):809–16.
35. Smith DH, Hicks R, Povlishock JT. Therapy development for diffuse axonal injury. J Neurotrauma. 2013;30(5):307–23.
36. Menon DK, Schwab K, Wright DW, Maas AI. Position statement: definition of traumatic brain injury [Research Support, N.I.H., Extramural Research Support, Non-U.S. Gov't Research Support, U.S. Gov't, Non-P.H.S. Review]. Arch Phys Med Rehabil. 2010;91(11):1637–40.
37. Viano DC, Casson IR, Pellman EJ, Zhang L, King AI, Yang KH. Concussion in professional football: brain responses by finite element analysis: part 9—a comparative study. Neurosurgery. 2005;57(5):891–916.
38. Madri JA. Modeling the neurovascular niche: implications for recovery from CNS injury. J Physiol Pharmacol. 2009;60(4):95–104.
39. Ropper AH, Gorson KC. Clinical practice. Concussion—review. N Engl J Med. 2007;356(2): 166–72.
40. Heitger MH, Jones RD, Macleod AD, Snell DL, Frampton CM, Anderson TJ. Impaired eye movements in post-concussion syndrome indicate suboptimal brain function beyond the influence of depression, malingering or intellectual ability. Brain. 2009;132(10):2850–70.
41. Toth A, Kovacs N, Perlaki G, Orsi G, Aradi M, Komaromy H, et al. Multi-modal magnetic resonance imaging in the acute and sub-acute phase of mild traumatic brain injury: can we see the difference? J Neurotrauma. 2013;30(1):2–10.
42. Zhou Y, Kierans A, Kenul D, Ge Y, Rath J, Reaume J, et al. Mild traumatic brain injury: longitudinal regional brain volume changes. Radiology. 2013;267(3):880–90; Mar 12: epub ahead of print.
43. Ross DE, Castelvecchi C, Ochs AL. Brain MRI volumetry in a single patient with mild traumatic brain injury. Brain Inj. 2013;27(5):634–6.
44. Benson RR, Gattu R, Sewick B, Kou Z, Zakariah N, Cavanaugh JM, et al. Detection of hemorrhagic and axonal pathology in mild traumatic brain injury using advanced MRI: implications for neurorehabilitation. NeuroRehabilitation. 2012;31(3):261–79.
45. MacKenzie JD, Siddiqi F, Babb JS, Bagley LJ, Mannon LJ, Sinson GP, et al. Brain atrophy in mild or moderate traumatic brain injury: a longitudinal quantitative analysis. AJNR Am J Neuroradiol. 2002;23(9):1509–15.

Chapter 11
Metabolic Dysfunction Following Traumatic Brain Injury

David A. Hovda, Christopher C. Giza, Marvin Bergsneider,
and Paul M. Vespa

Abstract The major objective of this chapter is to provide insight on neurometabolic/
neurochemical cascade and pathophysiological processes underlying the brain
responses to biomechanical concussive forces. Specifically, I will provide you with
a brief, yet simple and straightforward notion of mild traumatic brain injury, also
known as concussion. I would like to stress that concussion: (a) is an injury to the
brain caused by biomechanical forces; it is not ischemia or stroke; (b) results in
regional and temporal cellular alteration and may produce cell death; (c) produces a
state of energy crisis and subsequent metabolic *diaschisis*; (d) changes the priorities
for fuel; and (e) can contribute to the acquisition of posttraumatic stress and more
chronic neurological degeneration related to disease. Both animal models and
human studies strongly suggest that there is *nothing "mild" about mild TBI at the
cellular level.*

Keywords Mild traumatic brain injury, metabolic diaschisis • Metabolic cascade •
Neurochemical reactions • PET

What Is so Mild About Mild Traumatic Brain Injury?

Traumatic brain injury (TBI), sometimes referred to as the "silent epidemic," has
been identified by the Centers for Disease Control and Prevention (CDC) as a major
health concern in the United States [1] and is the leading cause of disability worldwide [2]. Broken down into three grades based upon level of injury and severity,

D.A. Hovda, Ph.D. (✉) • C.C. Giza, • M. Bergsneider, • P.M. Vespa
Departments of Neurosurgery Molecular and Medical Pharmacology, UCLA Brain Injury
Research Center, David Geffen School of Medicine at UCLA, 10833 Le Conte Avenue,
18-22B Semel, Los Angeles, CA 90095-7039, USA
e-mail: dhovda@mednet.ucla.edu

S.M. Slobounov and W.J. Sebastianelli (eds.), *Concussions in Athletics:*
From Brain to Behavior, DOI 10.1007/978-1-4939-0295-8_11,
© Springer Science+Business Media New York 2014

the most common variant of TBI is the mild classification [3, 4]. Mild traumatic brain injury (mTBI), also known by its more common name concussion [5], has an annual incidence in the United States of 1.6–3.8 million cases attributed to sports [1]. Despite the staggering occurrence of sports-related concussions, these mTBIs can be the result of motor vehicle accidents or falls, and have become the dominant war-related injury seen in the military [6]. The mechanical trauma experienced during a single concussive event causes the brain to undergo forceful acceleration and deceleration [7]. This violent shaking of the malleable brain inside the hard, confined spaces of the skull is not only expressed in a linear fashion, but rotational forces associated with a concussion also apply unnecessary axonal strain, leading to diffuse axonal injury (DAI) [8, 9]. Consequently, following a concussive episode, there is a destructive pathophysiological response that initiates a complex chain of neurometabolic and neurochemical reactions.

Due to the biochemical sequelae that follow a concussion, individuals present with a constellation of symptoms that can include physical, cognitive, and emotional manifestations [3, 10]. Some of the most common clinical symptoms include headache, nausea, visual disturbances, light sensitivity, dizziness, fatigue, poor concentration, short-term memory loss, unsteady gait, and irritability [10]. These persistent symptoms from concussion can lead to post-concussive syndrome (PCS) and long-term disabilities [11]. For most sports-related concussions, there is spontaneous recovery with resolution of symptoms within 10 days post-injury [12, 13]. However, up to 15 % of individuals recovering from a concussion report symptoms for more than 1 year following insult [14].

Additionally, injury to the brain is also associated with an increased susceptibility to a number of psychiatric conditions, as well as certain neuropathologies [13, 15, 16].

Even with the multitude of signs and symptoms, alterations in the neurochemical environment, and disruption of normal neurometabolic reactions, conventional neuroimaging techniques and neuropsychological tests fail to adequately detect these alterations in the subacute phase of injury [17]. Additionally, these approaches are not always to differentiate individuals who have suffered a previous concussion from those with no history of prior head injury [18]. Making matters worse is a lack of a universally accepted definition of concussion [19] and an objective diagnostic test [20]. The lack of sensitivity and specificity of current clinical measures for concussion management is a major concern as evidenced by the mounting research demonstrating the damaging effects of cumulative concussions and sub-concussive head trauma [15, 21, 22].

Clearly, concussion is not cerebral ischemia, and it is not stroke. Rather, *concussion is a mild form of TBI*. If you try to apply the same principles in terms of treatment modalities, biomechanics, or physiology between stroke/ischemia and the TBI, this will not work. Concussion and stroke are two separate and quite different pathophysiological entities. There are, however, some overlaps. Both phenomena may result in a regional and temporal cellular alteration and may produce cell death. That means that concussion, as a mild form of TBI characteristically produces cell dysfunction. Particularly, concussion produces a regional alteration of cellular functions and some of those functions can result in cell death or axonal disconnection. As a result, concussion produces a state of energy crisis and subsequence metabolic *diaschisis*.

Biomechanics and Pathophysiology of Concussion

Throughout the years, from the early 1990s on, many people have asked me what physiologically causes a concussion. My answer is that it is an injury caused to the brain due to biomechanical forces [7]. These biomechanical forces do not have to come from a direct blow to the head, but can be the result from any forces that are translated to the head. After contact that causes translation acceleration of the head, there is a slight lag experienced by the brain which then impacts the skull. This initial contact of the brain to the skull is known as the coup, and these coup injuries often are in the frontal lobe which makes concussion hard to diagnose clinically and test for on the field. As the brain is accelerated and then recoiled, there are countre-coup injuries that are injuries away from the initial site of impact and can be shearing injuries of axons and cerebral blood vessels [23]. In addition to linear accelerations, shearing injuries can also be caused by the addition of rotational or angular forces experienced by the brain following a concussive blow, especially in the corpus callosum and structures around the third ventricle [23].

Due to the movement of the brain inside the skull that can cause stress and strain on the cellular level, as well as the impact of the brain on the interior of the skull, concussion leads to the disruption of neuronal membranes. Stretched and damaged axons swell and then separate, although most axons initially affected gradually recover with time, and for the most part the pathophysiology of concussion is thought to be neurometabolic [14]. In fact, it is speculated that these sub-concussive impacts can cause microstructural and biochemical changes in the brain similar to full blown concussive episodes just to a lesser extent [24].

Transient CNS Disorders Versus Permanent Brain Lesions: Diaschisis

The acute effects related to sports-related concussion are usually short lived [25] and for most sports-related concussions there is spontaneous recovery with resolution of symptoms within 10 days post-injury [12]. However, Rutherford et al. reported that over 50 % of the patients recovering from concussion had symptoms lasting up to 6 weeks, with 15 % of individuals reporting symptoms lasting over 1 week [25].

The idea of an energy crisis in acute phase of brain injury as related to *diaschisis* is an important issue that I would like to elaborate on in more detail. There is still confusion and controversy over what researchers mean when using the term *diaschisis*. It should be clearly understood that *every **TBI, regardless of its severity, starts out as a concussive blow***. It changes the properties and characteristics of what the brain uses for fuel and energy. For example, if someone drinks a Gatorade this afternoon, the fuel that is in that Gatorade is used in the brain in one way. If someone has a concussion this afternoon, and then uses a Gatorade, this *fuel* is used in a completely different manner. So the Gatorade that we thought was good for the physiology of the body was not the same as the Gatorade that we thought would be good for the physiology of the brain.

When trying to credit where most of today's literature about the physiology of concussion comes from, people have attributed a lot of the work primarily to me, my colleagues, and to some of my students. But if you would like to see where the first and explicit paper was published about the physiology of concussion, you have to look at the work of Earl Walker. In 1944, Dr. Walker became very interested with physiology of concussion and worked alongside with Denny Brown. In his seminal paper: "The physiological basis of concussion," Dr. Walker suggested that concussion produced a depression-like phenomenon [26]. Accordingly, *spreading depression* was called a mTBI injury. However, I fail to see what is so "mild" about mTBI.

Another important cornerstone and insight on the *diaschisis* should be attributed to Constantin von Monakow, a Swiss neurologist of Russian extraction. He worked with Broca, whom the *speech area* of the brain was famously named after, doing research in stroke patients. It is well known that people who have suffered massive strokes in the left hemisphere are *aphasic*. Aphasic patients cannot speak, though overall look normal. Dr. von Monakow treated numerous neurological patients who had strokes in the right hemispheres resulting in damage to the right part of the brain. These patients became aphasic, but they recovered over time. He described a phenomenon where the brain was not irreversibly, but rather temporarily, damaged. These stroke patients were stunned; their brain was depressed and they were dysfunctional for a period of time. Language disturbances observed in these patients with nondominant hemisphere lesions were not due to a permanent brain damage and instead resolved over a period of time. This observation inspired Dr. von Monakow to propose a clear distinction between what would be a permanent disability versus that which would be temporary neurological dysfunction. The fact that the majority of concussed individuals eventually recover over time, the concussion, as a phenomenon, may be considered as *diaschisis*. Indeed, von Monakow aimed to *distinguish between the transient central nervous system disorders due to suppression of brain activity and the deficits resulting from brain lesions that never disappear.*

The concept of *diaschisis* comes back to the idea of energy supply for the brain. It is well known that approximately 90 % of a person's energy comes from something called adenosine triphosphate or ATP that is synthesized about 522 A/s. The human body on average makes about 65 kg of ATP per day. On average, you consume about 380 l of oxygen per day. The average human works at about 100 kcal over about 116 W of power per hour. That would be comparable to a dim light bulb.

Energy Crisis After Concussive Blows

The brain contributes up to 2–4 % of the human body mass, but takes up about 20 % of the total energy demands. Most of the energy the brain consumes comes from ATP. The lack of energy supplies and the high demands for fuel in acute phase of

TBI results in energy crisis, the concept that I would like to elaborate in more detail in the following text. In order to understand the importance of the energy crisis after mTBI, I have to convince you that it takes energy to live and make the brain functional. I am also going to convince you that it takes energy and sufficient time to recover from brain injury regardless of its severity.

The most common experimental procedure to study TBI in animals is a *fluid percussion device*. This fluid percussion device is a saline filled cylinder attached to the experimental animal via a craniectomy. By then striking one end of the cylinder with a pendulum, a small amount of volume of fluid is introduced to the cranial cavity, outside of the dura. This action moves the brain a certain distance at a certain velocity. This particular procedure was developed years ago by Gurdjian and is still a valuable tool to study traumatic brain injuries in a well-controlled environment. Instead of taking the head and shaking it violently causing the brain to move, the fluid percussion device will move the brain in a systematic way inside the head. In order to understand the pathophysiological mechanisms underlying the effect of brain motion induced by fluid percussion, a special technique called cerebral microdialysis has been developed. It is a fancy term for putting a small catheter in the brain and is done both in humans and in animals. This procedure allows researchers to dialyze the extracellular space and it works the same way as if blood is dialyzed. It can also measure the concentration of neurochemical substances in the extracellular space.

Immediately after a concussion, a destructive biochemical response ensues that initiates a chain of neurometabolic and neurochemical reactions that include activation of inflammatory responses, imbalances of ion concentrations, increase in the presence of excitatory amino acids, dysregulation of neurotransmitter synthesis and release, and production of free radicals [27]. As outlined by Giza and Hovda [28], the pathophysiological response to concussion is a complex combination of changes in the brain at a vascular and cellular level. As a result from the trauma, the brain undergoes disruptions in neurochemical and neurometabolic homeostasis. This disruption via a physical tearing or shearing of the membrane itself is also compounded by the deregulation of selective ion channels.

In order to maintain normal cellular metabolism and homeostasis, the neuron relies mainly on the ATP-dependent sodium–potassium pump to restore proper membrane and equilibrium potentials. In the neuron, which undergoes repetitive depolarization and repolarization in response to excitatory and inhibitory action potentials, the sodium–potassium pump is a key regulator in cellular equilibrium. After a concussive blow, there is a large efflux of potassium out of the cell into extracellular space, as well as a large influx of calcium. This large ionic flux leads to widespread and rapid release of excitatory neurotransmitters, especially glutamate. After this large and diffuse depolarization, the brain is believed to experience the phenomenon of spreading depression. Due to the imbalance of normal neuronal ionic concentrations, the cell relies mainly on the sodium–potassium pumps to restore the imbalances.

Since the sodium–potassium pumps are not passive and require energy in the form of ATP to be driven, the cell starts a period of hypermetabolism where consumption of glucose is increased. The influx of calcium ions, can be toxic to the cell. In an attempt to avert this potentially toxic accumulation of calcium ions, the mitochondria sequester the calcium. In turn, this causes the mitochondria to become less efficient at converting glucose into ATP, creating an energy crisis and producing less ATP to drive the sodium–potassium pumps.

Following the initial period of hypermetabolism, comes a period of hypometabolism, as the cell is incapable and/or inefficient at converting glucose into ATP to run the sodium–potassium pumps to restore the ionic concentrations. This oxidative dysfunction leads to the cell turning to anaerobic respiration to meet its energy needs. This anaerobic respiration leads to the formation of lactate and then to lactic acid. As the lactic acid accumulates in the extracellular space, acidosis occurs which can break down the cellular membrane even further, thus compounding this entire cycle. As you can see this neurometabolic cascade is very damaging at the cellular level, and the main goal to restore equilibrium in the cell, which is energetically expensive, is exacerbated by the cell's inability to properly produce the required energy through mitochondrial and oxidative dysfunction. This energy crisis in turn exacerbates the cellular conditions to a state in which, if not corrected, may lead to cell death.

Where do you make the ATP that your brain needs to run the sodium–potassium pumps? Most of your ATP is made of a cell organelle called the *mitochondria*. The mitochondria are like the energy factories of the cell. You can make ATP through two different means: by anaerobic processes (does not use oxygen) or aerobic processes (does use oxygen). Not all mitochondria are the same. There are different mitochondria in neurons than there are in glia. There are different mitochondria in the cell soma than there are in the axons. Various types of mitochondria respond differently to the energy crisis created in the brain after a concussion.

In general physiology, extracellular calcium is high and intracellular calcium is low. Calcium flows into cells regularly for communication in normal cell physiology. However, too much intracellular calcium could *kill* the cell. In order to prevent cell death, the mitochondria sequester the calcium. Thus, the mitochondria essentially take up excess calcium instead of letting it reside in the cytoplasm. While the mitochondria may prevent or delay cell death by sequestering the calcium, this prevents the mitochondria from being able to have normal respiration. Along with poor respiration, excess calcium prevents the mitochondria from producing energy effectively. Essentially, after a concussion, your brain has a great need for energy (ATP), but the incoming calcium prevents your brain from producing energy, which creates an energy crisis. If the energy crisis is extreme and is unprotected, there is possibility of protease activation and cell damage. This metabolic cascade also happens in axonal injury and calcium can influx into the axons. Increasing calcium in the axons leads to axonal swelling. It is important to remember that calcium and sodium mimic each other. That same phenomenon happens in the CNS: when cells uptake sodium, they swell up. This cellular swelling is related to inflammation and myelin damage.

Thus, as the name may lead you to believe, *there is nothing "mild" about mTBI at the cellular level*. As is similar in a full blown concussive episode, repetitive subconcussive head trauma can trigger similar neurochemical and neurometabolic reactions, although often to a lesser extent [28] which may lead to long-term or chronic consequences [29].

Evaluation of Energy Crisis via Neuroimaging Tools

Magnetic resonance spectroscopy (MRS), functional magnetic resonance imaging (fMRI), diffusion tensor imaging (DTI), and positron emission tomography (PET) are among advanced neuroimaging tools currently used to evaluate the energy crisis following concussion. With current advances in neuroimaging, we can also use MRI to estimate cell death or cell damage. In addition, MRS is a useful and powerful technique that has the ability to examine brain metabolism. MRS allows for identification and quantification of cellular metabolites in vivo [30] and results not in a normal MRI image, but as a spectrum where peaks are representative of the concentrations of certain chemicals and metabolites at their resonant frequencies. MRS has been used as a noninvasive tool to help gain a better understanding of pathological conditions associated with neurological and psychological disorders [31]. Just like other advanced MRI acquisition techniques, MRS is suitable for follow-up and longitudinal neurological assessment. Due to its sensitivity to brain metabolism and the ability to quantify changes in concentrations of metabolites, MRS has promise in the evaluation of the brain following a concussion [32]. Other objective measures being developed include protein biomarkers in serum and CSF to determine the damage induced by concussive blows.

As one of the more recent advances in neuroscience and neuroimaging, fMRI has grown in popularity and become a common research tool to explore the brain function noninvasively [33]. fMRI BOLD signal is used as an index of neuronal activity as areas of the brain that require more oxygen due to activation increase their demand for oxyhemoglobin which in turn leads to higher signal intensity and less signal dephasing caused by the local field inhomogeneities associated with deoxyhemoglobin [34]. The currently accepted notion is that BOLD fMRI most likely detects secondary effects of neuronal firing due to the *hemodynamic response*, allowing *indirect* assessment of the neuronal responses to cognitive and/or sensorymotor task demands [35].

We can also use different forms of diffusion imaging to look at axonal connections and axonal injuries induced by concussive blows. Specifically, DTI is an MRI technique that exploits the molecular diffusion of water. Due to the random displacement and motion of water molecules, information about microscopic structures and tissue characteristics that are beyond the basic resolution of MRI can be obtained [36].

As is the nature of mTBI, shearing forces cause DAI and initiate a complex pathophysiological response that can alter the cellular environment and brain function [10]. DAI in the highly vulnerable white matter is known to produce microscopic lesions, myelin loss, axonal degeneration, and axonal swelling all of which can affect diffusion [8]. These damaged axons swell and separate and increased swelling in the Virchow–Robin spaces can cause damage to the white matter as well as alter diffusion characteristics [14]. Another possibility besides axonal swelling is that the release of Ca^{2+} may reduce the free space of water which in turn would reduce diffusivity [37]. The high specificity that DTI has in imaging white matter has offered promise that it may be a viable tool when assessing DAI in concussion.

PET is a nuclear imaging technique that may be used to assess glucose utilization. This technology detects pairs of gamma rays emitted indirectly by a positron-emitting radionuclide (tracer), which is introduced in the body on a biologically active molecule. If the biologically active molecule chosen for PET is flourodeoxylucose (FDG), an analogue of sugar, the concentration of tracer then is indicative of the tissue metabolic activity in terms of regional glucose uptake. FDG-PET has shown high signal acutely after TBI, followed by a variable period of glucose hypometabolism that may last days or weeks after concussion but may last longer after more severe TBI.

PET neuroimaging is based on an assumption that areas of high radioactivity are associated with brain activity. What is actually measured indirectly is the blood flow to different parts of the brain. If you stimulate the cortex, you get an increase in glucose metabolism. If you measure the same area of the cortex that you stimulated for blood flow, you will find an increase in blood flow. This phenomenon is called coupling from blood flow to metabolism. Unlike muscles, the brain does not store glucose. Instead, glucose is provided to the brain through blood flow. In fact, this is the guiding principle behind fMRI. If you stimulate part of the brain, you get an increase of blood flow to that area, which provides "fuel" in order to drive the cell activity.

In a rat model, we have also seen increased glucose utilization immediately after a concussive episode. When plotted over time, the brain at time 0 (immediately after the concussive event) showed a large increase in glucose metabolism. However, shortly after this initial increase, the brain "becomes exhausted," as evidenced by the state of metabolic depression that slowly recovers over time. This energy phenomenon is independent of the severity of the concussive episode. It should be noted that metabolic recovery over time also mimics the recovery of an animal's behavior.

Although the metabolic cascade following acute brain trauma in animal model is well documented, how can this knowledge be applied to human brain physiology? Incorporating the data obtained from PET and MRI may seem a promising approach to address this important question that has been implemented at the UCLA Brain Injury Research Center. We scanned a severe head injured patient with right frontal lobe contusion identified via anatomical MRI. We have examined collectively the oxygen metabolism, glucose metabolism, and cerebral blood flow. In normal control subjects, the intensity of neuroimages for all three measures is supposed to be proportional, a phenomenon based upon the stoichiometric relationship of glucose and oxygen for cerebral metabolism. This is also known as a "coupling effect." Similar to animal studies, we observed that traumatically injured human brain has become disrupted and uncoupled in terms of its ability to metabolize glucose and oxygen. In fact, there is evidence that the same pattern of hyperglycolysis (acute hyperglycolysis), chronic metabolic depression, and recovery can be observed in brain-injured individuals regardless of its severity.

Thus, the stoichiometric relationship of glucose and oxygen is most likely disrupted as a result of brain insult that, in fact, may lead to a by-product of lactate. Through the imaging process, we can combine the outcome of glucose and oxygen metabolism and come up with a map of the oxygen/glucose ration, a new biomarker of TBI. With a low oxygen/glucose ratio, ATP is being manufactured without oxygen (anaerobic glycolysis). On the other hand, with high oxygen/glucose ratios, the brain is burning everything it possibly can in terms of glucose, plus something else. The details of hyperglycolysis are beyond the scope of this review chapter and can be found elsewhere.

Concluding Statement

With this aforementioned information in mind, I hope that you understand that bio-mechanical forces cause a head injury. Concussions are neither cerebral ischemia nor a stroke. Concussion results in regional temporal and cellular dysfunction that may gradually recover or lead to cell death. Areas that survive produce an energy crisis and subsequent metabolic diaschisis. Also, brain cells that alter their use of "fuels" will work differently after head injury. Instead of thinking of TBI or concussion as an event that we recover from, we *should consider concussion as an ongoing disease process*. It has multiple consequences including cognitive impairment, psychological problems, socioeconomic challenges and family disruption. Many fundamental neuroscientific problems related to concussion and TBI are just now beginning to be unraveled.

References

1. Langlois JA, Rutland-Brown W, Wald MM. The epidemiology and impact of traumatic brain injury—a brief overview. J Head Trauma Rehabil. 2006;21(5):375–8.
2. Signoretti S, Pietro V, Vagnozzi R, Lazzarino G, Amorini AM, Belli A. Transient alterations of creatine, creatine phosphate, N-acetylaspartate and high-energy phosphates after mild traumatic brain injury in the rat. Mol Cell Biochem. 2009;333(1–2):269–77.
3. Bergman K, Bay E. Mild traumatic brain injury/concussion: a review for ED nurses. J Emerg Nurs. 2010;36(3):221–30.
4. Langlois JA, Rutland-Brown W, Thomas KE. The incidence of traumatic brain injury among children in the United States—differences by race. J Head Trauma Rehabil. 2005;20(3): 229–38.
5. Cantu R. Concussion classification: ongoing controversy. In: Slobounov S, Sebastianelli W, editors. Foundations of sport-related brain injuries. New York: Springer; 2006. p. 87–110.
6. Zohar O, Lavy R, Zi XM, Nelson TJ, Hongpaisan J, Pick CG, et al. PKC activator therapeutic for mild traumatic brain injury in mice. Neurobiol Dis. 2011;41(2):329–37.
7. Barkhoudarian G, Hovda DA, Giza CC. The molecular pathophysiology of concussive brain injury. Clin Sports Med. 2011;30(1):33–48.
8. Maruta J, Lee SW, Jacobs EF, Ghajar J. A unified science of concussion. Ann N Y Acad Sci. 2010;1208(1):58–66.
9. Maruta J, Suh M, Niogi SN, Mukherjee P, Ghajar J. Visual tracking synchronization as a metric for concussion screening. J Head Trauma Rehabil. 2010;25(4):293–305.
10. Bryant R, Harvey A. Postconcussive symptoms and posttraumatic stress disorder after mild traumatic brain injury. J Nerv Ment Dis. 1999;187(5):302–5.

11. Hughes D, Jackson A, Mason D, Berry E, Hollis S, Yates D. Abnormalities on magnetic resonance imaging seen acutely following mild traumatic brain injury: correlation with neuropsychological tests and delayed recovery. Neuroradiology. 2004;46(7):550–8.

12. McCrory P. Sports concussion and the risk of chronic neurological impairment. Clin J Sport Med. 2011;21(1):6–12.

13. McCrory P, Meeuwisse W, Johnston K, Dvorak J, Aubry M, Molloy M, et al. Consensus statement on concussion in sport—the 3rd international conference on concussion in sport, held in Zurich, November 2008. J Clin Neurosci. 2009;16(6):755–63.

14. Packard RC. Chronic post-traumatic headache: associations with mild traumatic brain injury, concussion, and post-concussive disorder—review. Curr Pain Headache Rep. 2008;12(1): 67–73.

15. Guskiewicz KM, McCrea M, Marshall SW, Cantu RC, Randolph C, Barr W, et al. Cumulative effects associated with recurrent concussion in collegiate football players—the NCAA concussion study. JAMA. 2003;290(19):2549–55.

16. Guskiewicz KM, Weaver NL, Padua DA, Garrett WE. Epidemiology of concussion in collegiate and high school football players. Am J Sports Med. 2000;28(5):643–50.

17. Mayer AR, Mannell MV, Ling J, Gasparovic C, Yeo RA. Functional connectivity in mild traumatic brain injury. Hum Brain Mapp. 2011;32(11):1825–35.

18. Iverson GL, Brooks BL, Lovell MR, Collins MW. No cumulative effects for one or two previous concussions. Br J Sports Med. 2006;40(1):72–5.

19. Cantu RC. Athletic concussion current understanding as of 2007. Neurosurgery. 2007;60(6): 963–4.

20. Vagnozzi R, Tavazzi B, Signoretti S, Amorini AM, Belli A, Cimatti M, et al. Temporal window of metabolic brain vulnerability to concussions: mitochondrial-related impairment—part I. Neurosurgery. 2007;61(2):379–88.

21. De Beaumont L, Brisson B, Lassonde M, Jolicoeur P. Long-term electrophysiological changes in athletes with a history of multiple concussions. Brain Inj. 2007;21(6):631–44.

22. Echemendia RJ, Cantu RC. Return to play following sports-related mild traumatic brain injury: the role for neuropsychology. Appl Neuropsychol. 2003;10(1):48–55.

23. Kirkendall D, Jordan S, Garrett W. Heading and head injuries in soccer. Sports Med. 2001;31(5):369–86.

24. Khurana VG, Kaye AH. An overview of concussion in sport—review. J Clin Neurosci. 2012;19(1):1–11.

25. Rutherford WH, Merrett JD, McDonald JR. Sequelae of concussion caused by minor head-injuries. Lancet. 1977;1(8001):1–4.

26. Walker AE. The physiological basis of concussion. J Neurosurg. 1944;1(2):103–16.

27. Wheaton P, Mathias JL, Vink R. Impact of pharmacological treatments on cognitive and behavioral outcome in the postacute stages of adult traumatic brain injury a meta-analysis—review. J Clin Psychopharmacol. 2011;31(6):745–57.

28. Giza CC, Hovda DA. The neurometabolic cascade of concussion—review. J Athl Train. 2001;36(3):228–35.

29. Jordan BD, Matser EJT, Zimmerman RD, Zazula T. Scarring and cognitive function in professional boxers. Phys Sportsmed. 1996;24(5):87–96.

30. Shekdar K, Wang DJ. Role of magnetic resonance spectroscopy in evaluation of congenital/developmental brain abnormalities. Semin Ultrasound CT MR. 2011;32(6):510–38.

31. Ross AJ, Sachdev PS. Magnetic resonance spectroscopy in cognitive research—research support, non-U.S. Gov't review. Brain Res Brain Res Rev. 2004;44(2–3):83–102.

32. Marino S, Ciurleo R, Bramanti P, Federico A, Stefano N. 1H-MR spectroscopy in traumatic brain injury. Crit Care. 2010;14(1):127–33.

33. Logothetis NK. What we can do and what we cannot do with fMRI—review. Nature. 2008;453(7197):869–78.

34. Ogawa S, Menon RS, Tank DW, Kim SG, Merkle H, Ellermann JM, et al. Functional brain mapping by blood oxygenation level-dependent contrast magnetic-resonance-imaging—a

comparison of signal characteristics with a biophysical model. Biophys J. 1993;64(3): 803–12.

35. Jueptner M, Weiller C. Review—does measurement of regional cerebral blood-flow reflect synaptic activity? Implications for PET and fMRI. Neuroimage. 1995;2(2):148–56.

36. Le Bihan D. Diffusion tensor imaging: concepts and applications. J Magn Reson Imaging. 2001;13(4):534–46.

37. Chu Z, Wilde EA, Hunter JV, McCauley SR, Bigler ED, Troyanskaya M, et al. Voxel-based analysis of diffusion tensor imaging in mild traumatic brain injury in adolescents. AJNR Am J Neuroradiol. 2010;31(2):340–6.

Chapter 12
Advanced Neuroimaging of Mild Traumatic Brain Injury

Zhifeng Kou and E. Mark Haacke

Abstract Mild traumatic brain injury (mTBI) constitutes the majority of brain trauma cases. Despite its prevalence, detection in clinical imaging remains a challenge, as does the ability to predict duration and extent of disability. Advanced magnetic resonance imaging (MRI) methods combined with improved data analytic techniques have already demonstrated the potential to meet this challenge. This chapter reviews the recent progress in detection and outcome prediction in mTBI using the latest MRI techniques, including diffusion tensor imaging (DTI) and susceptibility-weighted imaging (SWI and SWIM), among others. Several recent published reports have found that DTI is sensitive to alterations in white matter ultrastructure not revealed by conventional MRI. More specifically, DTI reveals alterations in the ultrastructure of white matter axons caused by traumatic shear and stretch, which have been shown to correlate with clinical severity indicators and neuropsychological deficits. By virtue of its excellent sensitivity to iron and deoxygenated hemoglobin, SWI/SWIM has demonstrated exquisite detection of microhemorrhages and further quantification of hemorrhage and blood oxygenation. Used together, these advanced imaging techniques have the potential to serve as a set of surrogate biomarkers which can be used in determining prognosis and will

Z. Kou, Ph.D. (✉)
Departments of Biomedical Engineering and Radiology, Wayne State University,
818 West Hancock Street, Detroit, MI 48201, USA
e-mail: zhifeng.kou@gmail.com

E.M. Haacke, Ph.D.
Department of Radiology, Wayne State University,
3990 John R Street, Detroit, MI 48201, USA
e-mail: nmrimaging@aol.com

S.M. Slobounov and W.J. Sebastianelli (eds.), *Concussions in Athletics:*
From Brain to Behavior, DOI 10.1007/978-1-4939-0295-8_12,
© Springer Science+Business Media New York 2014

likely have a major role in animal and human therapeutic trials, both to improve selection criteria of experimental subjects and to provide a number of new biomarkers for use in addition to conventional clinical and behavioral measures.

Keywords Neuroimaging • Mild TBI • SWI/SWIM-DTI

Introduction

Traumatic brain injury (TBI) affects 1.7 million Americans each year [1–3]. Most of the injuries are mild traumatic brain injury (mTBI) [4]. Today, people who might have had more severe TBI or died in motor vehicle crash (MVC) accidents suffer milder head injury, thanks to advancements in motor vehicle safety. mTBI affects over 1.2 million Americans annually. It is a major public healthcare burden, that has been overlooked for decades [1, 2]. Despite its name, the impact of mTBI on the patients and their families is not mild at all [4]. A fraction of mTBI patients typically develop a constellation of variable physical, cognitive, and emotional symptoms, collectively known as post-concussion syndrome (PCS), that significantly impact the quality of their life. The direct cost of mTBI in the United States is approximately $16.7 billion each year, which does not include the indirect costs to society and families [4–6].

The major causes of TBI are MVC accidents, falls, assaults, and sports. MVC has been thought as the major contributor to diffuse axonal injury (DAI) or traumatic axonal injury (TAI), which is more devastating than focal injury and tends to result in long-term neurocognitive sequelae [7]. Among the 1.7 million TBI patients each year, over 1.2 million (70 %) of them visit the emergency department (ED) for treatment. Among them, mild TBI accounts for over one million emergency visits per year [8]. However, most mTBI patients stay in the ED for a few hours and then are discharged home due to their negative computed tomography (CT) findings. Therefore, an ED could be the major battlefield for mTBI detection and outcome prediction.

Up to 50 % of mTBI patients develop persistent symptoms lasting 3 months and 5–15 % at 1 year [8, 9]. Meanwhile, among the 1.8 million troops who have served in Iraq and Afghanistan, it is estimated that at least 20 % of returning troops have suffered at least one concussion. This means up to 360,000 veterans may have brain injuries after discharge [10]. However, most *symptomatic* mTBI patients have normal findings on clinical CT and conventional magnetic resonance imaging (MRI) [11–13]. In addition to neuroimaging, clinical indices of severity such as the Glasgow Coma Scale (GCS) and duration of posttraumatic amnesia (PTA) are lacking in sensitivity in mTBI and are not helpful in predicting outcome [14]. In summary, using currently available clinical instruments, it is difficult to determine which mTBI patients will have prolonged or even permanent neurocognitive symptoms.

It has been recognized that TBI is not a single disease. TBI has a full spectrum of pathophysiologic conditions. From the initial biomechanical insult to neurons, axons, glia, and neural vascular system, the brain will undergo a complicated biochemical process, called secondary injury. As a result, the brain may manifest disturbed cerebral blood flow and metabolism, intracranial hemorrhage, edema, and even elevated intracranial pressure, as part of its tsunami event. Over the long run, the injured axons may suffer Wallerian degeneration, and neuronal loss manifestes as brain atrophy. There is no single "silver bullet" which captures the full spectrum of injury. However, with both hardware and pulse sequence design advances, newer MRI methods have demonstrated the ability to detect and localize with high resolution *several* of the pathologic and pathophysiologic consequences of mTBI. These advanced MR technologies include susceptibility-weighted imaging (SWI) for hemorrhage detection [15]; MR spectroscopy (MRS) for metabolite measurement [16]; diffusion-weighted and diffusion tensor imaging (DWI/DTI) for edema quantification [17] and axonal injury detection [18]; perfusion-weighted imaging (PWI) and arterial spin labeling (ASL) to measure blood flow to brain tissue [19]; and functional MRI (fMRI) to measure changes in blood oxygen level locally in response to neuronal activity [20]. Having a number of imaging biomarkers, all of which are obtained in a single scanning session (or multiple for a longitudinal study) and are sensitive to different consequence of traumatic injury, affords great advantages: (1) enhanced sensitivity; (2) ability to study interrelationships among these biomarkers and between the biomarkers and clinical/neurocognitive deficits; (3) improved clinical management resulting from more precise characterization of injuries; and (4) enhanced power of clinical interventional studies. In this chapter, we will focus on neuroimaging of traumatic vascular and axonal injury of mTBI by using two advanced MRI techniques.

Imaging Traumatic Vascular Injury

DAI or TAI has been reported as an important pathology in mild TBI. To date, limited data exists on neural vascular injury after trauma. As a matter of fact, the neural vascular system is tightly meshed into the neuronal and glial cells as well as white matter (WM) tracts. Despite the fact that only a small percentage of patients have micro-hemorrhages in mTBI, the vascular system is certainly not immune to injury during an insult to neurons/axons.

Depending on the magnitude of the insult, traumatic vascular injury (TVI) may manifest itself at different levels. During a relatively lighter impact, the tight junction of endothelia cells may undergo direct stretch and temporal opening that results in a leaky blood–brain barrier (BBB) [21–23]. As a consequence, red blood cells (RBCs) will leak into the extravascular space [24] and other central nervous system (CNS)-specific proteins will get into the blood stream, which can then be detected and used as serum-based biomarkers [25]. At this stage, the injury may not be visible on routine structural MRI scanning. When the biomechanical load at the regional level gets more severe, the damaged vascular system may suffer dis-regulated cerebral blood flow or even thrombosis, which results in reduced blood oxygenation in the venous system. In this reduced flow case, the vascular damage will manifest as prominent veins with higher contrast than regular veins on SWI images. If the vascular damage is more significant to direct rupture of vessel wall, it will cause a hemorrhagic bleeding at the local level that, if large enough, is visible on routine MRI and CT scans.

Susceptibility-Weighted Imaging of Hemorrhagic Lesions

In diagnostic radiology, intracranial hemorrhage has been sought as a biomarker of TBI. The confirmation of bleeding in mild TBI will automatically categorize a patient into "complicated mTBI," whose outcome tends to be worse than those without any intracranial bleeding and even close to moderate TBI [26]. A recent study of 135 mTBI patients, scanned at 12 days after injury, demonstrated that one or more brain contusions on structural MRI, and ≥4 foci of hemorrhagic axonal injury on MRI were each independently associated with poorer 3-month outcome [27]. Some investigators have suggested that the presence of hemorrhage in DAI is predictive of poor outcome in moderate to severe TBI [28]. SWI was developed by Haacke and colleagues [29] as a high resolution venography method. It has been used to evaluate moderate to severe TBI patients since 2003 by Tong et al. [15]. Tong and colleagues have shown that SWI is 3–6 times more sensitive than conventional T2* gradient echo imaging (GRE) for detecting suspected DAI lesions in children [15, 30]. SWI has been shown to detect tiny hemorrhages that may be the only abnormal finding that can confirm the presence of brain injury, and change management of the patient. In addition, lesion number and volume identified by SWI are negatively associated with the patients' outcome [30] and neuropsychological functions [31] in moderate to severe TBI patients.

After brain injury, the hemorrhagic bleed undergoes a temporal transformation from oxyhemoglobin to deoxyhemoglobin in the acute stage, intra- and then extracellular methemoglobin in the subacute stage, and finally hemosiderin in the chronic stage [32–34]. SWI is sensitive to deoxyhemoglobin in the acute stage as well as extracellular methemoglobin in the subacute stage, and hemosiderin in the chronic stage [32].

Therefore, positive results with SWI should provide a biomarker for hemorrhagic brain injury at any stage. However, very few studies have been reported regarding the possible role of SWI as a tool for improving detection of micro-hemorrhages and its value in prediction of a patient's outcome in mTBI. Unlike DTI, which requires complex post-processing and comparison with proper controls, SWI is readily available for radiological reading right after MRI scans. This makes SWI more likely to have a direct impact on the radiological diagnosis. As a matter of fact, many medical centers have already begun to use SWI as a prime sequence for the detection of intracranial hemorrhages in clinical radiology. Figure 12.1 demonstrates an exemplary case to show the SWI detection of brain hemorrhages in mTBI in the acute stage in comparison with the usual clinical T2* GRE.

Quantitative Susceptibility Mapping of Bleeding and Blood Oxygenation

Despite its improved sensitivity in the detection of micro-hemorrhages, SWI is still a qualitative instead of quantitative approach. Theoretically, blood products at different stages, from deoxyhemoglobin, to extracellular methemoglobin and then

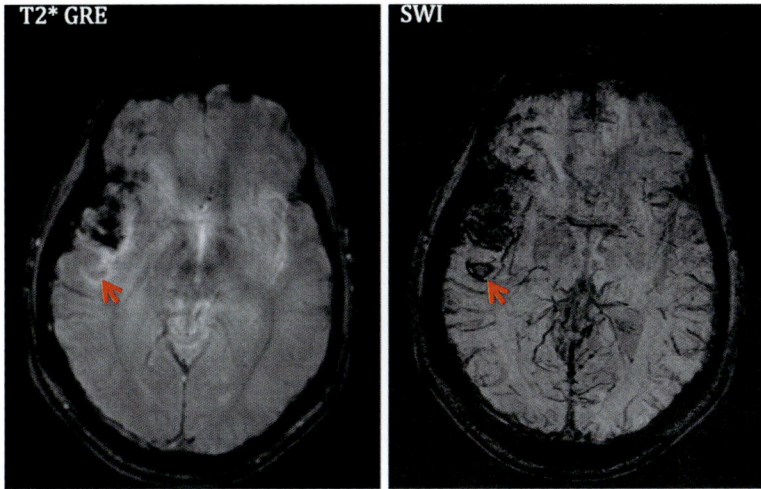

Fig. 12.1 Comparison of T2* with SWI in the detection of hemorrhagic lesions. A 45-year-old man fell down from a staircase and then visited ER with a severe headache. Both T2* GRE and SWI detected hemorrhages on the right side of the inferior temporal lobe. However, in a small area with mixed blood and edema, T2* GRE only detected edema (bright signal) and SWI detected hemorrhage (dark signal) (see *arrow*), which suggests methemoglobin at the acute stage

hemosiderin, has different susceptibilities. As a natural extension, susceptibility-weighted imaging and mapping (SWIM), also called quantitative susceptibility mapping (QSM), is the next generation of SWI development, which could quantify the susceptibility values of blood products. Ideally SWIM/QSM could have the following potential usage in mTBI:

(a) Differentiating new from old hemorrhage. Fresh blood at the acute stage of injury with deoxyhemoglobin has relatively low susceptibility, subacute blood with extracellular methemoglobin has relatively higher susceptibility, and chronic blood with hemosiderin has the highest susceptibility. Therefore, the susceptibility signal intensity may differentiate the stage of the bleeding.
(b) Improving the detection of micro-hemorrhages. One difficulty in clinical radiology is to differentiate microbleed from veins, especially at the cortical surface, where the brain is enriched with venous structure and therefore prone to bleeding. A cross section of a cortical vein or pial vein could be easily misinterpreted as a micro-hemorrhage, and a micro-hemorrhage buried in the surrounding venous structure could be easily overlooked as a vein. By using minimal intensity projection (mIP), the dark venous signal on adjacent slices can be projected onto one image to see the continuity of the venous structure. Even so, a radiologist still needs to navigate through several images to check the morphology, including the continuity of the black dots and smoothness of a potential vessel wall, to verify a vein or bleed. With the addition of SWIM, chronic bleed (hemosiderin) will likely have higher susceptibility than the surrounding veins. The high signal intensity would easily distinguish itself from the veins (see Fig. 12.2 for a chronic bleeding case).

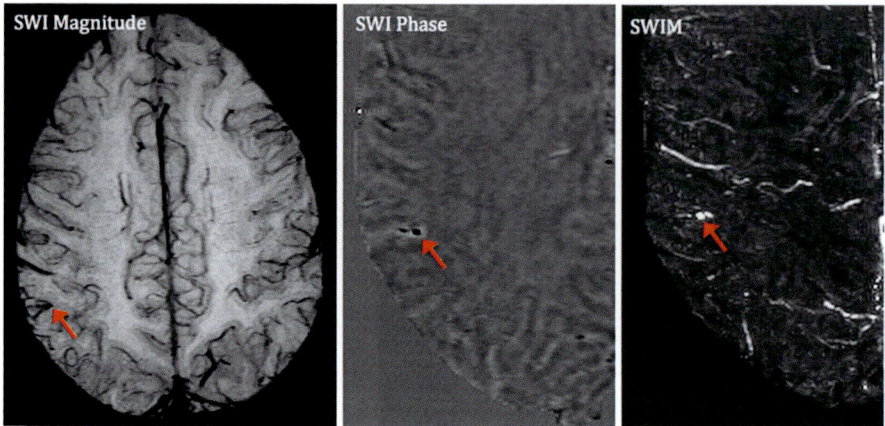

Fig. 12.2 Quantitative susceptibility mapping of chronic bleeding after mTBI. A chronic mTBI case with a microbleed embedded in a pial vein on the cortical surface. The SWI phase image demonstrates that its shape looks more like a pial vein. The SWIM result demonstrates very high susceptibility value (2,200 ppm), which is much higher than a normal vein (usually around 200 to 300). This is suggestive of chronic bleeding in the form of hemosiderin rather than a venous structure

Another challenge in clinical radiology is to differentiate hemorrhage from calcification. Empirically, calcification tends to happen in a symmetrical manner in the basal ganglia and choroid plexus in the lateral ventricles. However, it could be misinterpreted as a bleed if it is in brain parenchyma because both calcification and hemorrhage have low signal on SWI images. From the physics point of view, hemorrhage and calcification have opposite susceptibility behaviors: hemorrhage is paramagnetic and shows high signal on SWIM images in contrast with the low signal of calcification, which is diamagnetic. With SWIM, they can be easily differentiated [35].

(c) Quantifying blood oxygenation. After injury, the damaged cerebral vascular structure may present with reduced cerebral blood flow, venous stenosis, resulting from even venous thrombosis. Both animal data and recently reported clinical data identify venous thrombosis after TBI [36]. There is even an ongoing clinical trial for venous thrombolysis after TBI [36]. The reduced blood oxygenation or thrombosis will manifest as an increased susceptibility signal on SWIM images. We have developed SWIM to quantify susceptibility as a means to estimate blood oxygenation in major veins [37]. With SWIM, researchers could quantify the degree and extent of venous blood oxygenation. See Fig. 12.3 as a sample to show quantitative susceptibility signal of a transmedullary vein after blast-induced TBI.

(d) Quantify disease progression or treatment effect. The availability of a quantitative signal would allow researchers to track the progression of blood product transformation over time, which could be a biomarker for disease progression. This could be very useful for bleeding and re-bleeding cases. Chronically, the

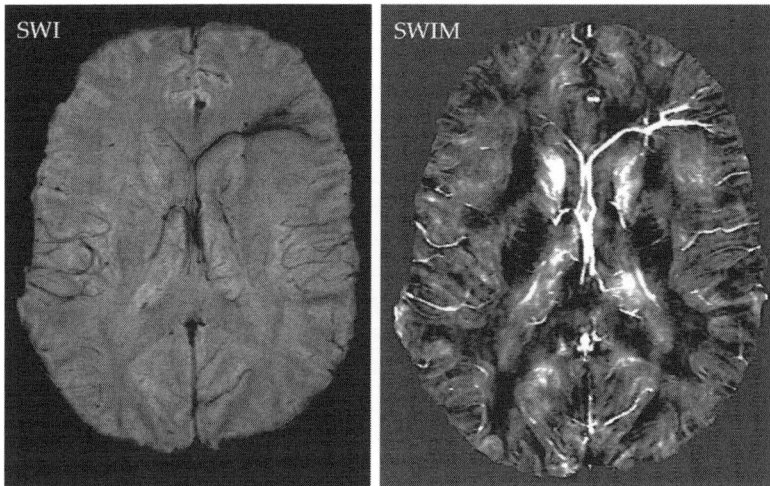

Fig. 12.3 Decreased venous blood oxygenation in septal vein after blast-induced TBI. SWI image (*left*) shows abnormal signal on left anterior septal vein but short of quantitation. SWIM (*right*) shows the decreased blood oxygenation on the vein with signal intensity linearly proportional to the concentration of deoxyhemoglobin

hemosiderin deposit after hemorrhage may stay in the brain tissue for a long time and become toxic to the brain by inducing edema [38] or hydrocephalus [39, 40]. Iron chelation drug treatment could be a treatment to remove these iron deposits and is being reported in correlation with outcome improvement in animal models of intracerebral hemorrhage [41, 42]. The availability of SWIM will certainly provide a means for in vivo assessment of iron chelation treatment.

In summary, there is still a need to investigate TVI in a large number of mTBI patients by using SWI/SWIM. This may represent a promising direction for mTBI research in the coming years.

Diffusion Tensor Imaging of Axonal Injury

Diffusion imaging sequences are sensitive to TAI secondary to stretch and shear forces. DTI measures the bulk motion of water molecular diffusion in biological tissues. It is most useful when diffusion is anisotropic, i.e., when diffusion is not equivalent in all directions, such as in skeletal muscle or axons in the white matter of the CNS. Histological studies have validated DTI's sensitivity to brain injury in both focal injury [43] and DAI [44] models. Two parameters derived from DTI, the apparent diffusion coefficient (ADC) and fractional anisotropy (FA) [45, 46], have been extensively studied in TBI. ADC is an estimate of the average *magnitude* of water movement in a voxel (regardless of direction), while FA is an index of the *directional nonuniformity*, or anisotropy, of water diffusion within a voxel.

FA has been used to detect alterations in directional diffusion resulting from tissue damage. FA in white matter is highest when fibers are long (relative to voxel dimension) and oriented uniformly (collinear) within a voxel and lowest when fibers are not collinear (e.g., "crossing fibers") or have been damaged. When axons are injured, as in acceleration/deceleration injuries (such as MVCs), diffusion anisotropy typically decreases. Loss of diffusion anisotropy is the result of a number of axonal changes after injury including: (1) increased permeability of the axonal membrane; (2) swelling of axons; (3) decreased diffusion in the axial (long axis) direction; and (4) degeneration and loss of axons in the chronic stage. In general, any pathological alteration of white matter fibers will result in FA decrease, because one or more of these axonal changes occur in disorders of white matter. Not surprisingly, most clinical studies of moderate and severe TBI have shown FA to be more sensitive than ADC to traumatic injury. On the other hand, ADC, FA, and directionally selective diffusivities (principal, intermediate, and minor components of diffusion) can help to better characterize brain injury pathologies. Trace and mean diffusivity (MD) are two other measurements similar to ADC and vary similarly. Changes in FA in association with ADC changes can differentiate the type of edema. For example, in the acute stage, decreased FA in association with increased ADC suggests vasogenic edema, while increased FA in association with decreased ADC suggests cytotoxic edema. Decreased FA in association with decreased ADC and decreased longitudinal (parallel to the long axis of the axons) water diffusivity suggests axonal transport failure as occurs in degenerative neurological diseases such as in ALS.

Regarding the location of brain lesions detected by DTI, Niogi and Mukherjee [47] summarized that the frontal association pathways, including anterior corona radiata, uncinate fasciculus, superior longitudinal fasciculus, and genu of corpus callosum (CC), are the mostly frequently injured WM structures in mTBI patients. Single subject results were not reported but it can be assumed that significant inter-individual variability for location and extent of WM injury exists due to varying injury mechanisms (and forces) and biological (neural and non-neural) differences across patients.

Imaging at Different Pathological Stages

Interestingly, despite the higher incidence of milder TBI compared with more severe TBI in western countries, there are many fewer mTBI imaging studies reported in the literature. One reason is the fact that recruitment of mTBI patients is more difficult, since they are typically outpatients. Another reason is the common conception that mTBI is a transient problem from which virtually all who are afflicted will recover fully. Therefore, some question the clinical importance of studying mTBI. Certainly, insurance reimbursement for MRI scanning of mTBI is rare and even rarer in the acute setting, so that "adding on research sequences" is not possible.

With these limitations in mind, a growing literature on DTI in TBI has begun to address the DTI findings at different stages.

Acute Stage

There are currently conflictive findings for FA and ADC in mTBI at the acute stage. Chu et al. [48] and Wilde et al. [49, 50] from Baylor College of Medicine scanned 10–12 adolescents with mTBI within 6 days of injury and reported *increased FA*, *reduced ADC*, and *reduced radial (short axis) diffusivity* in WM regions and the left thalamus. Similarly, Bazarian et al. [51] studied six mTBI patients within 72 h and reported *increased FA* in the posterior CC and *reduced ADC* in the anterior limb of the internal capsule (IC). Similar to Chu et al. [48] and Wilde et al. [49, 50], Mayer et al. [52] studied 22 mTBI patients within 12 days of injury and reported *increased FA* and *reduced radial* diffusivity in the CC and left hemisphere tracts.

Inglese et al. [53], in contradiction to Chu et al. [48], Wilde et al. [49, 50], Bazarian et al. [51], and Mayer et al. [52], found *reduced FA* in the splenium of CC and posterior limb of IC in 20 mTBI patients imaged up to 10 days after injury (mean = 4 days). Manually drawn regions of interest were used to assess the genu and splenium of the CC, the centrum semiovale, and the posterior limb IC bilaterally. In the same line as Inglese et al., Arfanakis and colleagues [54] studied a handful of mTBI patients at the acute stage and reported FA decrease in major WM tracts.

Most recent data on sports injury further reported that DTI FA changes could be bidirectional, which means the coexistence of both *increased* and *decreased FA* in different locations of the same brain [55]. Kou et al. also demonstrated this bidirectional change of FA in mTBI patients in the acute setting (within 24 h after injury) [56].

Subacute Stage

Many studies reported *reduced FA* and/or *increased diffusivity*, i.e., ADC, trace or mean diffusivity (MD), at this stage. Messé et al. [57] studied 23 mTBI patients at the subacute stage and found significantly *increased MD* in mTBI patients with poor outcome [57]. Lipton et al. [58] scanned 20 mTBI patients in the subacute stage and demonstrated *reduced FA* and *increased MD* in frontal subcortical WM. Miles et al. [59] studied 17 acute and subacute mTBI patients and found *reduced FA* and *increased MD*. All of these studies at the subacute stage reported a similar profile of DTI measures except for different locations of injury.

Chronic Stage

Three studies report either *reduced FA* or *increased diffusivity* or both and one study reported *increased FA* at this stage. Cubon et al. [60] studied ten collegiate athletes with concussion at the chronic stage and found *increased MD* in left WM tracts, internal capsule, and thalamic acoustic radiations. Lo et al. studied ten mTBI patients and reported *reduced FA* and *increased ADC* in the left genu of the CC and *increased FA* in internal capsule bilaterally [61]. Niogi et al. [62] studied 43 chronic mTBI patients and reported *reduced FA* in a large number of WM tracts. In contrast, Michael Lipton et al. [63] reported bidirectional changes (both increase and decrease) of FA in chronic mTBI patients.

All DTI studies of moderate to severe TBI patients [18, 64–66] and most sub-acute/chronic mTBI patients [53, 62, 67–69] report *increased FA* which are correlated with clinical or neuropsychological measures. However, the seemingly contradictory findings in mTBI in the acute stage do not fit this pattern. It has been suggested that *decreased FA* may reflect vasogenic edema at the acute stage. In contrast, *increased FA acutely* may reflect cytotoxic edema [50], which would shunt extracellular fluid into swollen cells. This could have the effect of reducing inter-axonal free water and therefore increasing anisotropy. The bidirectional changes of FA in recent studies further suggest the coexistence of both types of edema and clinical data could be much more complicated than we thought [55, 56].

Longitudinal Studies

Only a few investigators have followed FA over time in the *same* patients. Sidaros et al. [70] studied 23 severe TBI patients at 8 weeks and again at 12 months and found that partial recovery of initially *decreased FA* values in the internal capsule and centrum semiovale predicted a favorable outcome. Kumar et al. [71] studied 16 moderate to severe TBI patients at 2 weeks or less, 6 months, and 2 years and found persistently reduced FA except in the genu of the corpus callosum where there was partial normalization by 2 years. Recently, two studies by Mayer et al. [52] and Rutgers et al. [68] reported that a normalizing FA may reflect recovery. This evidence suggests that a systematic investigation of a large number of mTBI patients at acute, subacute, and chronic stages is warranted to reveal the evolution of pathophysiology in mTBI.

Correlation Between DTI-Derived WM Injury Topography and Neuropsychological Deficits

Mild TBI patients often develop a constellation of physical, cognitive, and emotional symptoms that are collectively known as PCS. In terms of neurocognitive symptoms, there are four key domains implicated in chronic neuropsychological impairment after mTBI. These domains include: (1) higher-order attention, (2) executive function, (3) episodic memory, and (4) speed of information processing. To date, several studies have demonstrated typical mTBI cognitive profiles and association with DTI findings. Niogi and Mukherjee summarized the topographic and neurocognitive deficits [47].

Damage to the frontal WM has been reported to be associated with impaired executive function. Lipton et al. [58] studied 20 acute to subacute patients and reported that reduced FA in WM of dorsolateral prefrontal cortex (DLPRC) is correlated with worse executive function.

Frontal WM injury is also associated with attention deficit. Niogi et al. [72] reported that reduced FA in the left anterior corona radiata is correlated with attention control in chronic mild TBI patients.

Injury at the temporal WM tracts or cingulum bundle may cause memory problems. Niogi et al. reported that reduced FA in the uncinate fasciculus correlated with memory performance [72]. Wu et al. [49] reported that an FA measure of left cingulum bundle correlated with delayed recall.

Injury of the callosal fibers has been reported to be associated with PCS scores. Wilde et al. [50] studied ten adolescent mTBI patients in the acute stage and reported that increased FA and decreased ADC and MD in corpus callosum is correlated with patients' PCS score. Bazarian et al. [51] studied six mild TBI patients in the acute stage and reported a lower mean trace in the left anterior IC and a higher FA in the posterior CC. FA values correlated with patients' 72 h PCS score and visual motor speed and impulse control.

The overall burden or extent of WM injury is associated with both speed of information processing and overall functional outcome. Niogi et al. [62] studied 34 subacute to chronic mTBI patients and reported that FA decreased in several WM regions, including anterior corona radiata, uncinate fasciculus, CC genu, and cingulum bundle. They demonstrated that the number of damaged WM regions is correlated with patient's reaction time. Miles et al. [59] studied 17 mTBI patients at the acute stage and followed them up to 6 months after injury. They reported that, at the acute stage, the increased mean diffusivity (MD) in the central semiovale, the genu and splenium of CC, and the posterior limb of IC tended to correlate with a patient's response speed at 6 months after injury. Regarding the overall outcome, Messé et al. [57] divided mTBI patients into two outcome groups: poor outcome (PO) vs. good outcome (GO). PO patients showed significantly higher mean diffusivity (MD) values than both controls and GO patients in the corpus callosum, the right anterior thalamic radiations, the superior longitudinal fasciculus, the inferior longitudinal fasciculus, and the fronto-occipital fasciculus bilaterally.

Interestingly, injury or reduced blood supply in the thalamus, which is the relay station of neuronal pathways, may cause a constellation of symptoms in the speed of information processing, memory, verbal, and executive function. Grossman et al. studied 22 subacute to chronic mTBI patients by using diffusion kurtosis imaging, which is a more advanced form of diffusion analysis, and demonstrated that overall cognitive impairment is associated with the diffusion measurement in the thalamus and internal capsule [73]. This work is along the same line of a perfusion study by the same group, which demonstrated that reduced blood flow in the thalamus correlated with patient's overall neurocognitive function [74]. See Fig. 12.4 as an example of axonal injury. In summary, significant progress has been made by researchers in recent years regarding the prognostic value of DTI in

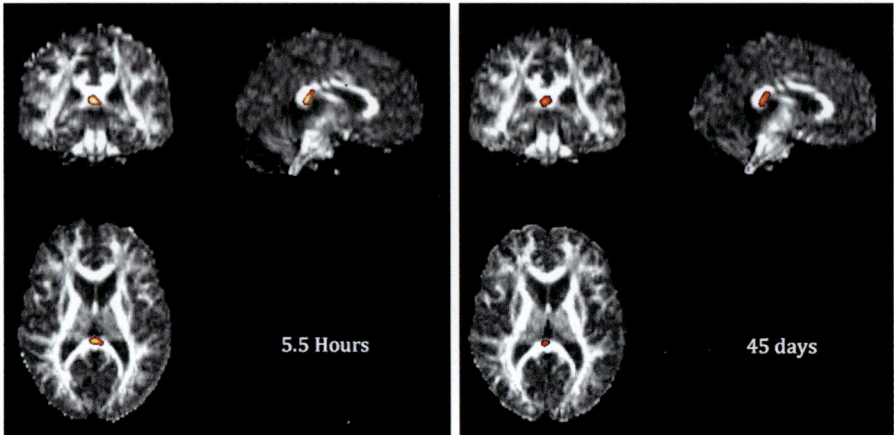

Fig. 12.4 DTI analysis of an mTBI patient scanned on the day of injury (5.5 h after injury) and 6 weeks later. A 31-year-old male fell 10 ft. off a ladder striking the back of his head with brief loss of consciousness and confusion. The patient developed persistent mild cognitive symptoms after 6 weeks of injury. Note the same location of reduced FA in left corona radiata. Global WM FA mean was within normal

the form of FA for mTBI patients' neurocognitive outcome. However, more and more evidence suggests that a tensor model may not be the ideal approach to the complicated pathophysiological process in TBI. Particularly, despite its high sensitivity, DTI suffers low specificity to trauma. Numerous medical reasons could cause water diffusivity changes and lead to changed FA; examples include neurodegenerative diseases, stroke, cancer, multiple sclerosis, hypertension, and diabetes, to name a few. Any preexisting conditions in the brain could affect the diffusivity and FA changes. Conflicting data on FA changes at the acute stage suggest that the field needs a better approach to characterizing the injury pathology than the current DTI model. This approach should be more specific to a TBI pathological process. It could be used to evaluate the neural basis of patients' injury to recovery process in longitudinal studies over a large number of patients.

Deliver the Impact to mTBI Care

Despite the fact that the emergency department ED sees the majority of mTBI patients [75], most of them stay in the ED for only a few hours and then are discharged home. After that, most patients fail to be followed up. The acute stage, within 24 h after injury, is therefore the critical time point for imaging to deliver a real impact to patient care [76]. Either improved detection or outcome prediction will greatly help emergency physicians to better determine referral pattern or management plans for the patient and family. However, most of the mTBI patients at the acute stage do not get an MRI scan due to the high cost and improper imaging techniques. To date, very few studies are designed to target this critical time point.

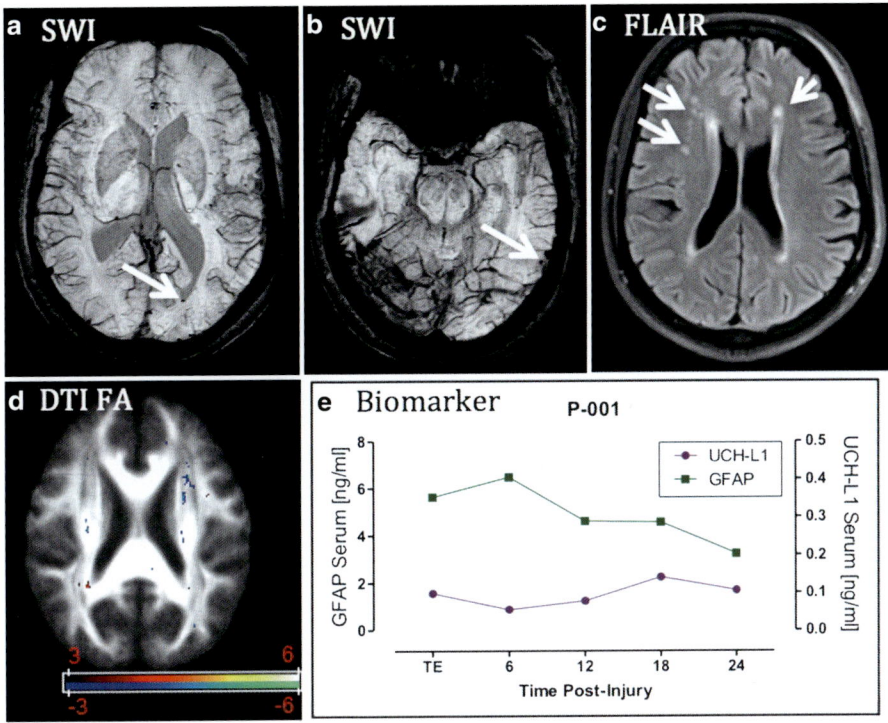

Fig. 12.5 MRI and biomarker profile in a patient with intraventricular hemorrhage missed by CT. Panels (**a**) and (**b**) are SWI images at different locations of the brain showing intraventricular blood and left lingual gyrus blood product (see *arrows*); panel (**c**) is FLAIR image showing nonspecific white matter hyper-intensities (see *arrows*); panel (**d**) is DTI FA map showing the coexistence of voxels with increased and decreased FA measures (*red color* means FA decrease and *blue color* FA increase in comparison with controls, $t > 3$ for t-test); and panel (**e**) is blood biomarker temporal profile, which exhibits extraordinarily high GFAP levels over time in comparison with controls (median 0.004, interquartile range 0.004–0.015). Despite being missed by CT, the patient's case was still detected by both blood biomarker and MRI

There is an urgent need for a comprehensive use of advanced MRI techniques to evaluate patients across all stages of injury. In the future, the availability of MR magnets in EDs and reduced costs for MRI scanning will make acute stage imaging possible. However, to determine who will get MRI scan in ED will be another question due to the cost. In addition, to avoid the high cost of scanning patients who are unlikely to have findings, serum blood biomarkers could provide an excellent screening tool to determine imaging criteria. Kou was the first one reporting a complementary use of both MRI and blood biomarkers [56, 77]. His pilot study data suggest that mTBI patients with intracranial hemorrhage on SWI have significantly higher glial fibrillary acidic protein (GFAP) levels than those without hemorrhage, implying that GFAP could serve as a screening tool for intracranial hemorrhage. See Fig. 12.5 as an example. This might represent an important future direction for mTBI clinical diagnosis.

Conclusions

Taken together, MRI has demonstrated superior capabilities over CT in the detection of subtle changes in the brain after mTBI. As an advanced MRI technique, DTI can detect white matter abnormalities that are unseen in structural MRI and further correlate with the patients' specific domain of neuropsychological symptoms. SWIM can improve the detection and quantification of traumatic hemorrhage and blood oxygenation after vascular injury. In the future, these advanced MRI techniques should be used in a comprehensive way in a large cohort of patients to provide a panoramic view of brain pathologies. MRI investigations during the acute stage, within 24 h after injury, will most likely impact emergency medicine, which is at the forefront of mTBI care. Furthermore the use of serum biomarkers may help identify patients who need advanced MRI imaging in the acute setting.

Acknowledgement Supported by grants from the Department of Defense (PI: EM Haacke) and International Society for Magnetic Resonance in Medicine (PI: Zhifeng Kou).

References

1. Kay T. Neuropsychological treatment of mild traumatic brain injury. J Head Trauma Rehabil. 1993;8:74–85.
2. National Institutes of Health. NIH consensus development panel on rehabilitation of persons with traumatic brain injury. JAMA. 1999;282:974–83.
3. Faul M, Xu L, Wald MM, Coronado VG. Traumatic brain injury in the United States: emergency department visits, hospitalizations, and deaths. Atlanta, GA: Centers for Disease Control and Prevention, National Center for Injury Prevention and Control; 2010.
4. CDC. Report to congress on mild traumatic brain injury in the United States: steps to prevent a serious public health problem. Atlanta, GA: Centers for Disease Control and Prevention, National Center for Injury Prevention and Control; 2003.
5. Bazarian JJ, McClung J, Shah MN, Cheng YT, Flesher W, Kraus J. Mild traumatic brain injury in the United States, 1998–2000. Brain Inj. 2005;19(2):85–91.
6. Ruff R. Two decades of advances in understanding of mild traumatic brain injury. J Head Trauma Rehabil. 2005;20(1):5–18.
7. Gennarelli TA. Mechanisms of brain injury. J Emerg Med. 1993;11:5–11.
8. Bazarian JJ, Wong T, Harris M, et al. Epidemiology and predictors of post-concussive syndrome after minor head injury in an emergency population. Brain Inj. 1999;13:173–89.
9. Alves W, Macciocchi SN, Barth JT. Postconcussive symptoms after uncomplicated mild head injury. J Head Trauma Rehabil. 1993;8(3):48–59.
10. Warden D. Military TBI, during the Iraq and Afghanistan wars. J Head Trauma Rehabil. 2006;21(5):398–402.
11. Belanger HG, Vanderploeg RD, Curtiss G, Warden DL. Recent neuroimaging techniques in mild traumatic brain injury. J Neuropsychiatry Clin Neurosci. 2007;19(1):5–20.
12. National Academy of Neuropsychology. Mild traumatic brain injury—an online course. Denver, CO: National Academy of Neuropsychology; 2002.
13. Teasdale E, Hadley DM. Imaging the injury. In: Reilly P, Bullock R, editors. Head injury. London: Chapman & Hall; 1997. p. 167–207.

14. Tellier A, Della Malva LC, Cwinn A, Grahovac S, Morrish W, Brennan-Barnes M. Mild head injury: a misnomer. Brain Inj. 1999;13:463–75.
15. Tong KA, Ashwal S, Holshouser BA, Shutter LA, Herigault G, Haacke EM, Kido D. Hemorrhagic shearing lesions in children and adolescents with posttraumatic diffuse axonal injury: improved detection and initial results. Radiology. 2003;27(2):332–9.
16. Holshouser BA, Tong KA, Ashwal S, Oyoyo U, Ghamsary M, Saunders D, Shutter L. Prospective longitudinal proton magnetic resonance spectroscopy imaging in adult traumatic brain injury. J Magn Reson Imaging. 2006;24:33–40.
17. Marmarou A, Signoretti S, Fatouros PP, Portella G, Aygok GA, Bullock MR. Predominance of cellular edema in traumatic brain swelling in patients with severe head injuries. J Neurosurg. 2006;104(5):720–30.
18. Benson RR, Meda SA, Vasudevan S, Kou Z, Govindarajan KA, et al. Global white matter analysis of diffusion tensor images is predictive of injury severity in TBI. J Neurotrauma. 2007;24(3):446–59.
19. Kim J, Whyte J, Patel S, Avants B, Europa E, et al. Resting cerebral blood flow alterations in chronic traumatic brain injury: an arterial spin labeling perfusion FMRI study. J Neurotrauma. 2010;27(8):1399–411.
20. McAllister TW, Saykin AJ, Flashman LA, Sparling MB, Johnson SC, Guerin SJ, Mamourian AC, Weaver JB, Yanofsky N. Brain activation during working memory 1 month after mild traumatic brain injury: a functional MRI study. Neurology. 1999;53(6):1300–8.
21. Rinder L, Olsson Y. Studies on vascular permeability changes in experimental brain concussion, part 2. Duration of altered permeability. Acta Neuropathol. 1968;11:201–9.
22. Povlishock JT, Kontos HA, Rosenblum WI, et al. A scanning electron microscope analysis of the intraparenchymal brain vasculature following experimental hypertension. Acta Neuropathol. 1980;51:203–12.
23. Povlishock JT, Kontos HA. The pathophysiology of pial and intraparenchymal vascular dysfunction. In: Grossman RG, Gildenberg PL, editors. Head injury, basic and clinical aspects. New York: Raven; 1982. p. 15–30.
24. Maxwell WL, Irvine A, Adams JH, et al. Response of cerebral microvasculature to brain injury. J Pathol. 1988;155:327–35.
25. Manley GT, Diaz-Arrastia R, Brophy M, Engel D, Goodman C, et al. Common data elements for traumatic brain injury: recommendations from the biospecimens and biomarkers working group. Arch Phys Med Rehabil. 2010;9(11):1667–72.
26. Williams DH, Levin HS, Eisenberg HM. Mild head injury classification. Neurosurgery. 1990;217(3):442–8.
27. Yuh EL, Mukherjee P, Lingsma HF, Yue JK, Ferguson AR, Gordon WA, et al. Magnetic resonance imaging improves 3-month outcome prediction in mild traumatic brain injury. Ann Neurol. 2013;73(2):224–35.
28. Paterakis K, Karantanas AH, Komnos A, Volikas Z. Outcome of patients with diffuse axonal injury: the significance and prognostic value of MRI in the acute phase. J Trauma. 2000;49:1071–5.
29. Reichenbach JR, Venkatesan R, Schillinger DJ, Kido DK, Haacke EM. Small vessels in the human brain: MR venography with deoxyhemoglobin as an intrinsic contrast agent. Radiology. 1997;204:272–7.
30. Tong KA, Ashwal S, Holshouser BA, Nickerson JP, Wall CJ, et al. Diffuse axonal injury in children: clinical correlation with hemorrhagic lesions. Ann Neurol. 2004;56:36–50.
31. Babikian T, Freier MC, Tong KA, Nickerson JP, Wall CJ, et al. Susceptibility weighted imaging: neuropsychologic outcome and pediatric head injury. Pediatr Neurol. 2005;33(3):184–94.
32. Kou Z, Benson RR, Haacke EM. Susceptibility weighted imaging in traumatic brain injury. In: Gillard J, Waldman A, Barker P, editors. Clinical MR neuroimaging. 2nd ed. Cambridge, MA: Cambridge University Press; 2010.

33. Thulborn KR, Sorensen AG, Kowall NW, McKee A, Lai A, et al. The role of ferritin and hemosiderin in the MR appearance of cerebral hemorrhage: a histopathologic biochemical study in rats. AJNR Am J Neuroradiol. 1990;11:291–7.
34. Bradley WG. MR appearance of hemorrhage in the brain. Radiology. 1993;189:15–26.
35. Schweser F, Deistung A, Lehr BW, Reichenbach JR. Differentiation between diamagnetic and paramagnetic cerebral lesions based on magnetic susceptibility mapping. Med Phys. 2010;37(10):5165–78.
36. Jamjoom AA, Jamjoom AB. Safety and efficacy of early pharmacological thromboprophylaxis in traumatic brain injury: systematic review and meta-analysis. J Neurotrauma. 2013;30(7):503–11.
37. Haacke EM, Tang J, Neelavalli J, Cheng YCN. Susceptibility mapping as a means to visualize veins and quantify oxygen saturation. J Magn Reson Imaging. 2010;32:663–76.
38. Dong M, Xi G, Keep RF, Hua Y. Role of iron in brain lipocalin 2 upregulation after intracerebral hemorrhage in rats. Brain Res. 2013;1505:86–92.
39. Okubo S, Strahle J, Keep RF, Hua Y, Xi G. Subarachnoid hemorrhage-induced hydrocephalus in rats. Stroke. 2013;44(2):547–50.
40. Wang L, Xi G, Keep RF, Hua Y. Iron enhances the neurotoxicity of amyloid β. Transl Stroke Res. 2012;3(1):107–13.
41. Okubo S, Xi G, Keep RF, Muraszko KM, Hua Y. Cerebral hemorrhage, brain edema, and heme oxygenase-1 expression after experimental traumatic brain injury. Acta Neurochir Suppl. 2013;118:83–7.
42. Keep RF, Hua Y, Xi G. Intracerebral haemorrhage: mechanisms of injury and therapeutic targets. Lancet Neurol. 2012;11(8):720–31.
43. Mac Donald CL, Dikranian K, Song SK, Bayly PV, Holtzman DM, Brody DL. Detection of traumatic axonal injury with diffusion tensor imaging in a mouse model of traumatic brain injury. Exp Neurol. 2007;205(2007):116–31.
44. Kou Z, Shen Y, Zakaria N, Kallakuri S, Cavanaugh JM, et al. Correlation of fractional anisotropy with histology for diffuse axonal injury in a rat model. Joint annual meeting ISMRM-ESMRMB, Berlin, Germany, 19–25 May 2007.
45. Shimony JS, McKinstry RC, Akbudak E, Aronovitz JA, Snyder AZ, et al. Quantitative diffusion-tensor anisotropy brain MR imaging: normative human data and anatomic analysis. Radiology. 1999;212:770–84.
46. Conturo TE, McKinstry RC, Akbudak E, Robinson BH. Encoding of anisotropic diffusion with tetrahedral gradients: a general mathematical diffusion formalism and experimental results. Magn Reson Med. 1996;35:399–412.
47. Niogi SN, Mukherjee P. Diffusion tensor imaging of mild traumatic brain injury. J Head Trauma Rehabil. 2010;25(4):241–55.
48. Chu Z, Wilde EA, Hunter JV, McCauley SR, Bigler ED, et al. Voxel-based analysis of diffusion tensor imaging in mild traumatic brain injury in adolescents. AJNR Am J Neuroradiol. 2010;31(2):340–6.
49. Wu TC, Wilde EA, Bigler ED, Yallampalli R, McCauley SR, et al. Evaluating the relationship between memory functioning and cingulum bundles in acute mild traumatic brain injury using diffusion tensor imaging. J Neurotrauma. 2010;27(2):303–7.
50. Wilde EA, McCauley SR, Hunter JV, Bigler ED, Chu Z, et al. Diffusion tensor imaging of acute mild traumatic brain injury in adolescents. Neurology. 2008;70(12):948–55.
51. Bazarian JJ, Zhong J, Blyth B, Zhu T, Kavcic V, Peterson D. Diffusion tensor imaging detects clinically important axonal damage after mild traumatic brain injury: a pilot study. J Neurotrauma. 2007;24(9):1447–59.
52. Mayer AR, Ling J, Mannell MV, Gasparovic C, Phillips JP, et al. A prospective diffusion tensor imaging study in mild traumatic brain injury. Neurology. 2010;74(8):643–50.
53. Inglese M, Makani S, Johnson G, Cohen BA, Silver JA, et al. Diffuse axonal injury in mild traumatic brain injury: a diffusion tensor imaging study. J Neurosurg. 2005;103:298–303.
54. Arfanakis K, Haughton VM, Carew JD, Rogers BP, Dempsey RJ, Meyerand ME. Diffusion tensor MR imaging in diffuse axonal injury. AJNR Am J Neuroradiol. 2002;23:794–802.

55. Bazarian JJ, Zhu T, Blyth B, Borrino A, Zhong J. Subject-specific changes in brain white matter on diffusion tensor imaging after sports-related concussion. Magn Reson Imaging. 2012;30(2):171–80.
56. Zhifeng K, Kobeissy F, Welch R, O'Neil B, Woodard J, et al. Combining biochemical and imaging markers to improve diagnosis and characterization of mild traumatic brain injury in the acute setting: results from a pilot study. PLoS One. 2013;8(11):e80296. doi: 10.1371/journal.pone.0080296.
57. Messé A, Caplain S, Paradot G, Garrigue D, Mineo JF, et al. Diffusion tensor imaging and white matter lesions at the subacute stage in mild traumatic brain injury with persistent neurobehavioral impairment. Hum Brain Mapp. 2011;32(6):999–1011.
58. Lipton ML, Gulko E, Zimmerman ME, Friedman BW, Kim M, et al. Diffusion-tensor imaging implicates prefrontal axonal injury in executive function impairment following very mild traumatic brain injury. Radiology. 2009;252(3):816–24.
59. Miles L, Grossman RI, Johnson G, Babb JS, Diller L, Inglese M. Short-term DTI predictors of cognitive dysfunction in mild traumatic brain injury. Brain Inj. 2008;22(2):115–22.
60. Cubon VA, Putukian M, Boyer C, Dettwiler A. A diffusion tensor imaging study on the white matter skeleton in individuals with sports-related concussion. J Neurotrauma. 2011;28(2):189–201.
61. Lo C, Shifteh K, Gold T, Bello JA, Lipton ML. Diffusion tensor imaging abnormalities in patients with mild traumatic brain injury and neurocognitive impairment. J Comput Assist Tomogr. 2009;33(2):293–7.
62. Niogi SN, Mukherjee P, Ghajar J, Johnson C, Kolster RA, et al. Extent of microstructural white matter injury in postconcussive syndrome correlates with impaired cognitive reaction time: a 3T diffusion tensor imaging study of mild traumatic brain injury. AJNR Am J Neuroradiol. 2008;29(5):967–73.
63. Lipton ML, Kim N, Park YK, Hulkower MB, Gardin TM, et al. Robust detection of traumatic axonal injury in individual mild traumatic brain injury patients: intersubject variation, change over time and bidirectional changes in anisotropy. Brain Imaging Behav. 2012;6(2):329–42.
64. Newcombe VF, Williams GB, Nortje J, Bradley PG, Harding SG, et al. Analysis of acute traumatic axonal injury using diffusion tensor imaging. Br J Neurosurg. 2007;21(4):340–8.
65. Levin HS, Wilde EA, Chu Z, Yallampalli R, Hanten GR, et al. Diffusion tensor imaging in relation to cognitive and functional outcome of traumatic brain injury in children. J Head Trauma Rehabil. 2008;23(4):197–208.
66. Kou Z, Gattu R, Benson RR, Raz N, Haacke EM, editor. Region of interest analysis of DTI FA histogram differentiates mild traumatic brain injury from controls. Proceedings of international society for magnetic resonance in medicine, Toronto, Canada; 2008.
67. Wozniak JR, Krach L, Ward E, Mueller BA, Muetzel R, et al. Neurocognitive and neuroimaging correlates of pediatric traumatic brain injury: a diffusion tensor imaging (DTI) study. Arch Clin Neuropsychol. 2007;22(5):555–68.
68. Rutgers DR, Fillard P, Paradot G, Tadié M, Lasjaunias P, Ducreux D. Diffusion tensor imaging characteristics of the corpus callosum in mild, moderate, and severe traumatic brain injury. AJNR Am J Neuroradiol. 2008;29(9):1730–5.
69. Kraus MF, Susmaras T, Caughlin BP, Walker CJ, Sweeney JA, Little DM. White matter integrity and cognition in chronic traumatic brain injury: a diffusion tensor imaging study. Brain. 2007;130:2508–19.
70. Sidaros A, Engberg AW, Sidaros K, Liptrot MG, Herning M, et al. Diffusion tensor imaging during recovery from severe traumatic brain injury and relation to clinical outcome: a longitudinal study. Brain. 2008;131(2):559–72.
71. Kumar R, Saksena S, Husain M, Srivastava A, Rathore RK, et al. Serial changes in diffusion tensor imaging metrics of corpus callosum in moderate traumatic brain injury patients and their correlation with neuropsychometric tests: a 2-year follow-up study. J Head Trauma Rehabil. 2010;25(1):31–42.

72. Niogi SN, Mukherjee P, Ghajar J, Johnson CE, Kolster R, et al. Structural dissociation of attentional control and memory in adults with and without mild traumatic brain injury. Brain. 2008;131(12):3209–21.
73. Grossman EJ, Ge Y, Jensen JH, Babb JS, Miles L, et al. Thalamus and cognitive impairment in mild traumatic brain injury: a diffusional kurtosis imaging study. J Neurotrauma. 2011;29:2318–27.
74. Ge Y, Patel MB, Chen Q, Grossman EJ, Zhang K, et al. Assessment of thalamic perfusion in patients with mild traumatic brain injury by true FISP arterial spin labelling MR imaging at 3T. Brain Inj. 2009;23(7):666–74.
75. Bazarian JJ, McClung J, Cheng YT, Flesher W, Schneider SM. Emergency department management of mild traumatic brain injury in the USA. Emerg Med J. 2005;22:473–7.
76. Jagoda AS, Bazarian JJ, Bruns Jr JJ, Cantrill SV, Gean AD, et al. Clinical policy: neuroimaging and decisionmaking in adult mild traumatic brain injury in the acute setting. Ann Emerg Med. 2008;52(6):714–48.
77. Kou Z, VandeVord P. Traumatic white matter injury and glial activation. Glia, 2014. Accepted.

Chapter 13
Biomarkers for Concussion

Linda Papa

Abstract Diagnostic and prognostic tools for risk stratification of concussion patients are limited in the early stages of injury in the acute setting. Unlike other organ-based diseases where rapid diagnosis employing biomarkers from blood tests is clinically essential to guide diagnosis and treatment, such as for myocardial ischemia or kidney and liver dysfunction, there are no rapid, definitive diagnostic tests for traumatic brain injury (TBI). Research in the field of TBI biomarkers has increased exponentially over the last 20 years with most of the publications on the topic of TBI biomarkers occurring in the last 10 years. Accordingly, studies assessing biomarkers in TBI have looked at a number of potential markers that could lend diagnostic and, prognostic, as well as therapeutic information. Despite the large number of published studies, there is still a lack of any FDA-approved biomarkers for clinical use in adults and children.

Developments in the field of proteomics, along with improved laboratory techniques, have led to the discovery and rapid detection of new biomarkers not previously available. Proteomic research has recently developed due to advances in protein separation, identification, and quantification technologies that only became available in the last decade. Some proteins are highly expressed in the cerebrospinal fluid following a TBI. However, this does not necessarily translate into availability in peripheral blood. With the increasing sensitivity of analytical tools for biomarker detection, measurement of biomarkers in peripheral blood has also improved.

L. Papa, M.D., C.M., M.Sc. (✉)
Department of Emergency Medicine, Orlando Regional Medical Center,
86 West Underwood (S-200), Orlando, FL 32806, USA

University of Central Florida College of Medicine, Orlando, FL, USA

University of Florida College of Medicine, Gainesville, FL, USA

Florida State University College of Medicine, Tallahassee, FL, USA
e-mail: lpstat@aol.com

S.M. Slobounov and W.J. Sebastianelli (eds.), *Concussions in Athletics:*
From Brain to Behavior, DOI 10.1007/978-1-4939-0295-8_13,
© Springer Science+Business Media New York 2014

In an effort to prevent chronic traumatic encephalopathy (CTE) and long-term consequences of concussion/mild TBI, early diagnostic and prognostic tools are becoming increasingly important, particularly in sports injuries and in military personnel where concussions/mild TBI are common occurrences. The studies conducted on biofluid biomarkers for mild TBI to date show great promise. Should serum biomarkers for TBI be validated and become widely available, they could have many roles. They could help with clinical decision making by clarifying injury severity and help monitor progression of injury and/or recovery. Biomarkers could have a role in managing patients at high risk of repeated injury and could be incorporated into guidelines for return to duty, work, or sports activities.

This chapter will discuss the current literature on biofluid biomarkers for concussion/mild TBI, address gaps in research, and discuss their future role.

Keywords Biomarkers • Blood • Serum • Cerebrospinal fluid • Concussion • Mild TBI • Head injury • S100β[beta] • GFAP • NSE • UCH-L1 • SBDP150 • SBDP145 • Tau • MBP • Neurofilament proteins • Proteomics • Diagnosis • Prognosis • Risk stratification • Detection • Pathophysiology • Monitoring • Biochemical markers

Introduction

Concussion is also known as mild traumatic brain injury (TBI) and is an unfortunately common occurrence in athletes of all ages. Diagnosis of concussion acutely depends on a variety of measures including neurological examination, neuropsychological evaluation, and neuroimaging. Neuroimaging techniques such as computed tomographic (CT) scanning and magnetic resonance imaging (MRI) are used to provide objective information. However, CT scanning has low sensitivity to diffuse brain damage and confers exposure to radiation. MRI can provide information on the extent of diffuse injuries but its widespread application is restricted by cost, availability, and its yet undefined role in management of these patients [1, 2]. Early and tailored management of athletes following a concussion can provide them with the best opportunity to avoid further injury.

The term "mild TBI" is really a misnomer. Individuals with mild TBI or concussion are acutely at risk for bleeding and axonal injury [3, 4] and can suffer impairment of physical, cognitive, and psychosocial functioning [5–9] long term. Repeated episodes of mild TBI can lead to chronic traumatic encephalopathy (CTE), a term used to describe clinical changes in cognition, mood, personality, behavior, and/or movement occurring years following concussion [10, 11]. With the growing incidence of CTE among athletes, strategies that reduce the risk of becoming injured need to be developed and diagnostic tools that could identify injuries earlier need to be explored.

The degree of brain injury depends on the primary mechanism/magnitude of injury, secondary insults, and the patient's genetic and molecular response. Following the initial injury, cellular responses and neurochemical and metabolic cascades contribute to secondary injury [12, 13]. There are two aspects to injury caused by TBI:

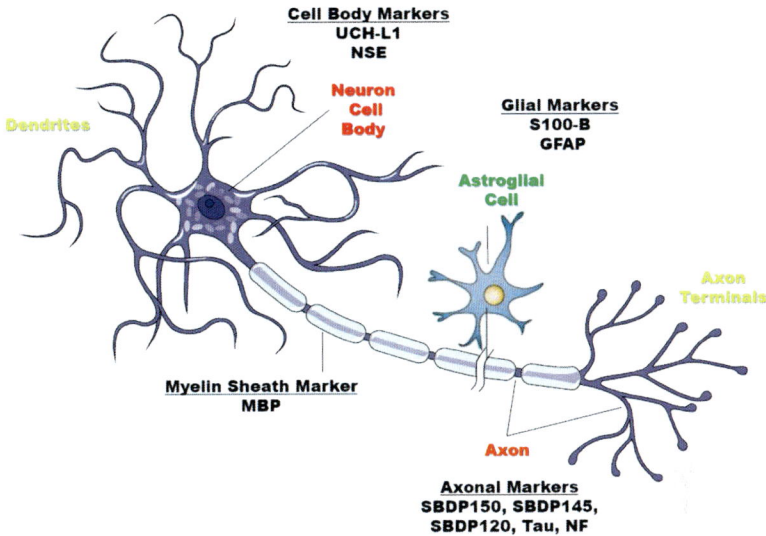

Fig. 13.1 This figure describes the neuroanatomical locations of the blood-based biomarkers that will be reviewed

the damage caused by the initial impact or insult, and that which may subsequently evolve over the ensuing hours and days, referred to as secondary insults. Secondary insults can be mediated through physiologic events which decrease supply of oxygen and energy to the brain tissue or through a cascade of cytotoxic events. These events are mediated by many molecular and cellular processes [14, 15].

Developments in the field of proteomics along with improved laboratory techniques have led to the discovery and rapid detection of new biomarkers not previously available. Proteomic research has recently developed due to advances in protein separation, identification, and quantification technologies that only became available in the last decade. Some proteins are highly expressed in the cerebrospinal fluid (CSF) following a TBI. However, this does not necessarily translate into availability in peripheral blood. With the increasing sensitivity of analytical tools for biomarker detection, measurement of biomarkers in peripheral blood has also improved.

This chapter will discuss the current literature on biomarkers for concussion or mild TBI in the athlete, address gaps in research, and discuss the role of serum biomarkers. Figure 13.1 describes the neuroanatomical locations of the biomarkers that will be reviewed.

Need for Serum Biomarkers for Concussion

Diagnostic and prognostic tools for risk stratification of concussion patients are limited in the early stages of injury in the acute setting. Unlike other organ-based diseases where rapid diagnosis employing biomarkers from blood tests is clinically essential to guide diagnosis and treatment, such as for myocardial ischemia or kidney and liver dysfunction, there are no rapid, definitive diagnostic tests for TBI. Research in the field of TBI biomarkers has increased exponentially over the last 20 years [16, 17], with most of the publications on the topic of TBI biomarkers occurring in the last 10 years [18]. Accordingly, studies assessing biomarkers in TBI have looked at a number of potential markers that could lend diagnostic and, prognostic, as well as therapeutic information. Despite the large number of published studies, there is still a lack of any FDA-approved biomarkers for clinical use in adults and children [17, 18]. Properties that should be considered when evaluating a biomarker for clinical application include the following: does the biomarker: (1) demonstrate a high sensitivity and specificity for brain injury; (2) stratify patients by severity of injury; (3) have a rapid appearance in accessible biological fluid; (4) provide information about injury mechanisms; (5) have well defined biokinetic properties; (6) monitor progress of disease and response to treatment; and (7) predict functional outcome [17, 19].

Biofluid Biomarkers of Astroglial Injury

S100β[Beta]

S100β[beta] is the major low affinity calcium binding protein in astrocytes [20] that helps to regulate intracellular levels of calcium and is considered a marker of astrocyte injury or death. It can also be found in non-neural cells such as adipocytes, chondrocytes, and melanoma cells [21, 22]. S100β[beta] is one of the most extensively studied biomarkers [23–33] and elevation of S100β[beta] levels in serum has been associated with increased incidence of post-concussive syndrome and impaired cognition [34, 35]. Other studies have reported that serum levels of S-100β[beta] are associated with MRI abnormalities and with neuropsychological examination disturbances after mild TBI [36, 37]. A number of studies have found significant correlations between elevated serum levels of S100β[beta] and CT abnormalities [38–40]. It has been suggested that adding the measurement of S100β[beta] concentration to clinical decision tools for mild TBI patients could potentially reduce the number of CT scans by 30 % [40]. Other investigators have failed to detect associations between S100β[beta] and CT abnormalities [41–44].

Amateur boxers have slightly elevated levels of S100β[beta] in CSF samples obtained by lumbar puncture after a bout [45]. In a study of S100β[beta] in basketball and hockey players by Stalnacke et al. in 2003, there was a significant correlation between the change in S100β[beta] (postgame–pregame values) and jumps in basketball players ($r=0.706$, $p=0.002$). In one ice hockey player who experienced concussion during play, S100β[beta] was increased more than for the other players [46]. The same investigators conducted a study of soccer players and found that changes in S100β[beta] concentrations (postgame minus pregame values) were statistically correlated to the number of headers ($r=0.428$, $p=0.02$) and to the number of other trauma events ($r=0.453$, $p=0.02$) [47]. Although S100β[beta] remains promising as an adjunctive marker, its utility in the setting of multiple trauma remains controversial because it also increases in trauma patients without head injuries and therefore be considered nonspecific to TBI [48–51].

Glial Fibrillary Acid Protein

Glial fibrillary acidic protein (GFAP) is a monomeric intermediate protein found in astroglial skeleton that was first isolated by Eng et al. in 1971 [52]. GFAP is found in white and gray brain matter and is strongly upregulated during astrogliosis [53]. Current evidence indicates that serum GFAP might be a useful marker for various types of brain damage from neurodegenerative disorders [54, 55] and stroke [56], to severe TBI [51, 57–61]. In 2010, Vos et al. described serum-increased GFAP profile in severe and moderate TBI with GCS <12 and found an association with unfavorable outcome at 6 months [32]. More recently, Metting et al. found GFAP to be elevated in patients with axonal injury on MRI in patients with mild TBI at 3 months post-injury, but it was not predictive of global outcome at 6 months [62]. In a study by Papa et al. in 2012, GFAP was detectable in serum less than 1 h after a concussion and was able to distinguish concussion patients from other trauma patients (without head injury) who had orthopedic injuries or who were in motor vehicle crashes [63]. In this same study, serum GFAP was significantly higher in mild TBI patients with intracranial lesions on CT compared to those without lesions and predicted patients who required neurosurgical intervention [63]. Similarly, Metting et al. demonstrated that serum GFAP was increased in patients with an abnormal CT after mild TBI. These studies suggest that GFAP has a good specificity for brain injury acutely after injury.

In amateur boxers, GFAP has also been found to be elevated in CSF samples obtained by lumbar puncture after a bout [45, 64]. Neselius et al. examined the CSF of 30 Olympic boxers and 25 non-boxing matched controls at 1–6 days after a bout and after a rest period (>14 days). Both GFAP and S100β[beta] concentrations were significantly increased after boxing as compared to controls. However, GFAP concentrations remained elevated after the rest period but S100β[beta] did not. It was suggested that the presence of GFAP after the rest period indicated ongoing degeneration.

Biofluid Biomarkers of Neuronal Injury

Neuron-Specific Enolase

Neuron-specific enolase (NSE) is one of the five isozymes of the glycolytic enzyme enolase found in central and peripheral neuronal cell bodies and it has been shown to be elevated following cell injury [65]. NSE is also present in erythrocytes and endocrine cells and has a biological half-life of 48 h [66]. This protein is passively released into the extracellular space only under pathological conditions during cell destruction. Several reports on serum NSE measurements of mild TBI have been published [65, 67–70]. Many of these studies either utilized inadequate control groups or concluded that serum NSE had limited utility as a marker of neuronal damage. Early increased levels of NSE and MBP concentrations have been correlated with outcome in children, particularly those under 4 years of age [71–74]. A limitation of NSE is the occurrence of false-positive results in the setting of hemolysis [75, 76].

Stalnacke et al. obtained blood samples from 44 female soccer players before and after a competitive game and found that both S100β and NSE were increased after the game. NSE was not related to the number of headers and other trauma events but S100β was [77].

Ubiquitin C-Terminal Hydrolase (UCH-L1)

A promising candidate biomarker for TBI currently under investigation is ubiquitin C-terminal hydrolase-L1 (UCH-L1). UCH-L1 was previously used as a histological marker for neurons due to its high abundance and specific expression in neurons [78]. This protein is involved in the addition and removal of ubiquitin from proteins that are destined for metabolism [79]. It has an important role in the removal of excessive, oxidized, or misfolded proteins during both normal and pathological conditions in neurons [80]. Clinical studies in humans with severe TBI have confirmed, using ELISA analysis, that the UCH-L1 protein is significantly elevated in human CSF [81, 82], is detectable very early after injury, and remains significantly elevated for at least 1 week post-injury [82]. Further studies in severe TBI patients have revealed a very good correlation between CSF and serum levels [83]. Increases in serum UCH-L1 have also been found in children with moderate and severe TBI [84]. Most recently, UCH-L1 was detected in the serum of mild and moderate traumatic brain injury (MMTBI) patients within an hour of injury [85]. Serum levels of UCH-L1 discriminated concussion patients from uninjured and non-head-injured trauma control patients who had orthopedic injuries or motor vehicle trauma without head injury. Most notable was that levels were significantly higher in those with intracranial lesions on CT than those without lesions, as well as those eventually requiring neurosurgical intervention [85].

Biofluid Biomarkers of Axonal Injury

Alpha-II-Spectrin Breakdown Products

Alpha-II-spectrin (280 kDa) is the major structural component of the cortical membrane cytoskeleton and is particularly abundant in axons and presynaptic terminals [86, 87]. It is also a major substrate for both calpain and caspase-3 cysteine proteases [88, 89]. A hallmark feature of apoptosis and necrosis is an early cleavage of several cellular proteins by activated caspases and calpains. A signature of caspase-3 and calpain-2 activation is cleavage of several common proteins such as cytoskeletal α[alpha]II-spectrin [90, 91]. Levels of spectrin breakdown products (SBDPs) have been reported in CSF from adults with severe TBI and they have shown a significant relationship with severity of injury and clinical outcome [92–98]. The time course of calpain-mediated SBDP150 and SBDP145 (markers of necrosis) differs from that of caspase-3-mediated SBDP120 (marker of apoptosis). Average SBDP values measured in CSF early after injury have been shown to correlate with severity of injury, CT scan findings, and outcome at 6 months postinjury [99].

Serum SBDP145 has also been measured in serum in children with TBI. Levels were significantly greater in subjects with moderate and severe TBI than in controls and were correlated with dichotomized GOS at 6 months. This correlation did not hold true for mild TBI. More recently, however, serum levels of SBDP150 have been examined in patients with mild TBI and have shown significant association with acute measures of injury severity, such as GCS score, intracranial injuries on CT, and neurosurgical intervention [100]. In this study, serum SBDP150 levels were much higher in patients with mild TBI/concussion than in other trauma patients who did not have a head injury [100].

TAU Protein

Following a concussion, axons appear to be most susceptible to damage. Two promising biofluid biomarkers localized in the axons are tau protein and neurofilament protein. A supposedly cleaved form of tau, c-tau, has been investigated as a potential biomarker of CNS injury. Tau is preferentially localized in the axon and tau lesions are apparently related to axonal disruption [101, 102]. CSF levels of c-tau were significantly elevated in TBI patients as compared to control patients and these levels correlated with clinical outcome [103, 104]. Though levels of c-tau were also elevated in plasma from patients with severe TBI, there was no correlation between plasma levels and clinical outcome [105]. Total tau protein is highly expressed in thin, nonmyelinated axons of cortical interneurons [106], thus may be indicative of axonal damage in grey matter neurons. It has been found to be correlated with severity of injury in severe TBI [107–110]. Ost et al. found that total tau measured in CSF on days 2–3 post-injury discriminated between TBI and controls (normal pressure hydrocephalus) and also between good and bad outcome at 1 year per dichotomized GOS score [109]. However, total tau was not detected in serum throughout the study. In a study by Zetterberg et al. in amateur boxers, levels of total tau in CSF from lumbar puncture within 10 days of a bout were elevated in both boxers who had received many hits (>15) or high-impact hits to the head, as well as in boxers who reported few hits.

Neurofilaments

Neurofilaments are heteropolymeric components of the neuron cytoskeleton that consist of a 68 kDa light neurofilament subunit (NF-L) backbone with either 160 kDa medium (NF-M) or 200 kDa heavy subunit (NF-H) side-arms [111]. Following TBI, calcium influx into the cell contributes to a cascade of events that activates calcineurin, a calcium-dependent phosphatase that dephosphorylates neurofilament side-arms, presumably contributing to axonal injury [112]. Phosphorylated NF-H has been found to be elevated in the CSF of adult patients with severe TBI as compared to controls [81]. Similarly, hyperphosphorylated NF-H has also been correlated with severity of brain injury in children [113]. In a study by Zurek et al. NF-H levels taken on the second to fourth days remained significantly higher in patients with poor outcomes in comparison to patients with good outcomes. Additionally, NF-H was significantly higher in those children with diffuse axonal injury on initial CT scan [113].

NF-L has also been shown to be elevated in amateur boxers with mild TBI following a bout when measured in CSF after lumbar puncture [45, 64]. The levels were associated with the number of hits to the head, as well as subjective and objective estimates of the intensity of the fight.

Conclusion

In an effort to prevent CTE and long-term consequences of concussion/mild TBI, early diagnostic and prognostic tools are becoming increasingly important, particularly in athletes and in military personnel, where concussions/mild TBI are common occurrences. The studies conducted on biofluid biomarkers for mild TBI to date show great promise. Should serum biomarkers for TBI be validated and become widely available, they could have many roles. They could help with clinical decision making by clarifying injury severity and help monitor progression of injury and/or recovery. Biomarkers could have a role in managing patients at high risk of repeated injury and could be incorporated into guidelines for return to duty, work, or sports activities.

As a final thought, we must continue the exploration and validation of biomarkers for TBI, especially mild TBI. Ideally, biomarkers would provide information on the pathophysiology of injury, improve stratification, assist in the monitoring of injury progression, monitor response to treatment, and predict functional outcome. Despite the heterogeneity of TBI, there is a unique opportunity to use the insight offered by biochemical markers to shed light on the complexities of this injury process. The development of a clinical tool to help healthcare providers manage TBI patients more effectively and improve patient care is the ultimate goal.

References

1. Kesler EA. APECT, MR and quantitative MR imaging: correlates with neuropsycholgical. Brain Inj. 2000;14:851–7.
2. Jagoda AS, Bazarian JJ, Bruns Jr JJ, Cantrill SV, Gean AD, Howard PK, et al. Clinical policy: neuroimaging and decisionmaking in adult mild traumatic brain injury in the acute setting. Ann Emerg Med. 2008;52(6):714–48.
3. Benson RR, Gattu R, Sewick B, Kou Z, Zakariah N, Cavanaugh JM, et al. Detection of hemorrhagic and axonal pathology in mild traumatic brain injury using advanced MRI: implications for neurorehabilitation. NeuroRehabilitation. 2013;31(3):261–79.
4. Govind V, Gold S, Kaliannan K, Saigal G, Falcone S, Arheart KL, et al. Whole-brain proton MR spectroscopic imaging of mild-to-moderate traumatic brain injury and correlation with neuropsychological deficits. J Neurotrauma. 2010;27(3):483–96.
5. Millis SR, Rosenthal M, Novack TA, Sherer M, Nick TG, Kreutzer JS, et al. Long-term neuropsychological outcome after traumatic brain injury. J Head Trauma Rehabil. 2001;16(4):343–55.
6. Alves W, Macciocchi S, Barth JT. Postconcussive symptoms after uncomplicated mild head injury. J Head Trauma Rehabil. 1993;8(3):48–59.
7. Rimel RW, Giordani B, Barth JT, Boll TJ, Jane JA. Disability caused by minor head injury. Neurosurgery. 1981;9(3):221–8.
8. Alexander MP. Mild traumatic brain injury: pathophysiology, natural history, and clinical management. Neurology. 1995;45(7):1253–60.
9. Barth JT, Macciocchi SN, Giordani B, Rimel R, Jane JA, Boll TJ. Neuropsychological sequelae of minor head injury. Neurosurgery. 1983;13(5):529–33.
10. Gavett BE, Stern RA, McKee AC. Chronic traumatic encephalopathy: a potential late effect of sport-related concussive and subconcussive head trauma. Clin Sports Med. 2011;30(1):179–88, xi.
11. Gavett BE, Cantu RC, Shenton M, Lin AP, Nowinski CJ, McKee AC, et al. Clinical appraisal of chronic traumatic encephalopathy: current perspectives and future directions. Curr Opin Neurol. 2012;24(6):525–31.
12. Graham DI, Adams JH, Nicoll JA, Maxwell WL, Gennarelli TA. The nature, distribution and causes of traumatic brain injury. Brain Pathol. 1995;5(4):397–406.
13. Graham DI, Horsburgh K, Nicoll JA, Teasdale GM. Apolipoprotein E and the response of the brain to injury. Acta Neurochir Suppl. 1999;73:89–92.
14. Povlishock JT, Katz DI. Update of neuropathology and neurological recovery after traumatic brain injury. J Head Trauma Rehabil. 2005;20(1):76–94.
15. Povlishock JT. Traumatically induced axonal injury: pathogenesis and pathobiological implications. Brain Pathol. 1992;2(1):1–12.
16. Kochanek PM, Berger RP, Bayr H, Wagner AK, Jenkins LW, Clark RS. Biomarkers of primary and evolving damage in traumatic and ischemic brain injury: diagnosis, prognosis, probing mechanisms, and therapeutic decision making. Curr Opin Crit Care. 2008;14(2):135–41.
17. Papa L. Exploring the role of biomarkers for the diagnosis and management of traumatic brain injury patients. In: Man TK, Flores RJ, editors. Proteomics—human diseases and protein functions. 1st ed. Rijeka, Croatia: InTech Open Access Publisher; 2012.
18. Papa L, Ramia MM, Kelly JM, Burks SS, Pawlowicz A, Berger RP. Systematic review of clinical research on biomarkers for pediatric traumatic brain injury. J Neurotrauma. 2013;30(5):324–38.
19. Papa L, Robinson G, Oli M, Pineda J, Demery J, Brophy G, et al. Use of biomarkers for diagnosis and management of traumatic brain injury patients. Expert Opin Med Diagn. 2008;2(8):937–45.

20. Xiong H, Liang WL, Wu XR. [Pathophysiological alterations in cultured astrocytes exposed to hypoxia/reoxygenation]. Sheng Li Ke Xue Jin Zhan. 2000;31(3):217–21.
21. Zimmer DB, Cornwall EH, Landar A, Song W. The S100 protein family: history, function, and expression. Brain Res Bull. 1995;37(4):417–29.
22. Olsson B, Zetterberg H, Hampel H, Blennow K. Biomarker-based dissection of neurodegenerative diseases. Prog Neurobiol. 2011;95(4):520–34.
23. Missler U. S-100 protein and neuron-specific enolase concentrations in blood as indicators of infarction volume and prognosis in acute ischemic stroke. Stroke. 1997;28:1956–60.
24. Ytrebø LM, Nedredal GI, Korvald C, Holm Nielsen OJ, Ingebrigtsen T, et al. Renal elimination of protein S-100beta in pigs with acute encephalopathy. Scand J Clin Lab Invest. 2001;61:217–25.
25. Jonsson HJP, Hoglund P, Alling C, Blomquist S. The elimination of S-100b and renal function after cardiac surgery. J Cardiothorac Vasc Anesth. 2000;14:698–701.
26. Usui AKK, Abe T, Murase M, Tanaka M, Takeuchi E. S-100ao protein in blood and urine during open-heart surgery. Clin Chem. 1989;35:1942–4.
27. Raabe A, Grolms C, Seifert V. Serum markers of brain damage and outcome prediction in patients after severe head injury. Br J Neurosurg. 1999;13(1):56–9.
28. Haimoto H, Hosoda S, Kato K. Differential distribution of immunoreactive S100-a and S100-b proteins in normal nonnervous human tissues. Lab Invest. 1987;57:489–98.
29. Woertgen C, Rothoerl RD, Holzschuh M, Metz C, Brawanski A. Comparison of serial S-100 and NSE serum measurements after severe head injury. Acta Neurochir (Wien). 1997;139(12):1161–4; discussion 1165.
30. Romner B, Ingebrigtsen T, Kongstad P, Borgesen SE. Traumatic brain damage: serum S-100 protein measurements related to neuroradiological findings. J Neurotrauma. 2000;17(8):641–7.
31. Korfias S, Stranjalis G, Boviatsis E, Psachoulia C, Jullien G, Gregson B, et al. Serum S-100B protein monitoring in patients with severe traumatic brain injury. Intensive Care Med. 2007;33(2):255–60.
32. Vos PE, Jacobs B, Andriessen TM, Lamers KJ, Borm GF, Beems T, et al. GFAP and S100B are biomarkers of traumatic brain injury: an observational cohort study. Neurology. 2010;75(20):1786–93.
33. Berger RP, Pierce MC, Wisniewski SR, Adelson PD, Kochanek PM. Serum S100B concentrations are increased after closed head injury in children: a preliminary study. J Neurotrauma. 2002;19(11):1405–9.
34. Ingebrigtsen T, Romner B. Management of minor head injuries in hospitals in Norway. Acta Neurol Scand. 1997;95(1):51–5.
35. Waterloo K, Ingebrigtsen T, Romner B. Neuropsychological function in patients with increased serum levels of protein S-100 after minor head injury. Acta Neurochir (Wien). 1997;139(1):26–31; discussion 31–2.
36. Ingebrigtsen T, Romner B. Serial S-100 protein serum measurements related to early magnetic resonance imaging after minor head injury. Case report. J Neurosurg. 1996;85(5):945–8.
37. Ingebrigtsen T, Waterloo K, Jacobsen EA, Langbakk B, Romner B. Traumatic brain damage in minor head injury: relation of serum S-100 protein measurements to magnetic resonance imaging and neurobehavioral outcome. Neurosurgery. 1999;45(3):468–75; discussion 75–6.
38. Ingebrigtsen T, Romner B, Marup-Jensen S, Dons M, Lundqvist C, Bellner J, et al. The clinical value of serum S-100 protein measurements in minor head injury: a Scandinavian multicentre study. Brain Inj. 2000;14(12):1047–55.
39. Muller K, Townend W, Biasca N, Unden J, Waterloo K, Romner B, et al. S100B serum level predicts computed tomography findings after minor head injury. J Trauma. 2007;62(6):1452–6.
40. Biberthaler P, Linsenmeier U, Pfeifer KJ, Kroetz M, Mussack T, Kanz KG, et al. Serum S-100B concentration provides additional information for the indication of computed tomography in patients after minor head injury: a prospective multicenter study. Shock. 2006;25(5):446–53.

41. Phillips JP, Jones HM, Hitchcock R, Adama N, Thompson RJ. Radioimmunoassay of serum creatine kinase BB as index of brain damage after head injury. Br Med J. 1980;281 (6243):777–9.
42. Rothoerl RD, Woertgen C, Holzschuh M, Metz C, Brawanski A. S-100 serum levels after minor and major head injury. J Trauma. 1998;45(4):765–7.
43. Piazza O, Storti MP, Cotena S, Stoppa F, Perrotta D, Esposito G, et al. S100B is not a reliable prognostic index in paediatric TBI. Pediatr Neurosurg. 2007;43(4):258–64.
44. Bechtel K, Frasure S, Marshall C, Dziura J, Simpson C. Relationship of serum S100B levels and intracranial injury in children with closed head trauma. Pediatrics. 2009;124(4): e697–704.
45. Neselius S, Brisby H, Theodorsson A, Blennow K, Zetterberg H, Marcusson J. CSF-biomarkers in Olympic boxing: diagnosis and effects of repetitive head trauma. PLoS One. 2012;7(4):e33606.
46. Stalnacke BM, Tegner Y, Sojka P. Playing ice hockey and basketball increases serum levels of S-100B in elite players: a pilot study. Clin J Sport Med. 2003;13(5):292–302.
47. Stalnacke BM, Tegner Y, Sojka P. Playing soccer increases serum concentrations of the biochemical markers of brain damage S-100B and neuron-specific enolase in elite players: a pilot study. Brain Inj. 2004;18(9):899–909.
48. Rothoerl RD, Woertgen C. High serum S100B levels for trauma patients without head injuries. Neurosurgery. 2001;49(6):1490–1; author reply 2–3.
49. Romner B, Ingebrigtsen T. High serum S100B levels for trauma patients without head injuries. Neurosurgery. 2001;49(6):1490; author reply 2–3.
50. Anderson RE, Hansson LO, Nilsson O, Dijlai-Merzoug R, Settergen G. High serum S100B levels for trauma patients without head injuries. Neurosurgery. 2001;49(5):1272–3.
51. Pelinka LE, Kroepfl A, Schmidhammer R, Krenn M, Buchinger W, Redl H, et al. Glial fibrillary acidic protein in serum after traumatic brain injury and multiple trauma. J Trauma. 2004;57(5):1006–12.
52. Eng LF, Vanderhaeghen JJ, Bignami A, Gerstl B. An acidic protein isolated from fibrous astrocytes. Brain Res. 1971;28(2):351–4.
53. Duchen LW. General pathology of neurons and neuroglia. In: Adams JA, Corsellis JAN, Duchen LW, editors. Greenfield's neuropathology. London: Edward Arnold; 1984. p. 1–52.
54. Baydas G, Nedzvetskii VS, Tuzcu M, Yasar A, Kirichenko SV. Increase of glial fibrillary acidic protein and S-100B in hippocampus and cortex of diabetic rats: effects of vitamin E. Eur J Pharmacol. 2003;462(1–3):67–71.
55. Mouser PE, Head E, Ha KH, Rohn TT. Caspase-mediated cleavage of glial fibrillary acidic protein within degenerating astrocytes of the Alzheimer's disease brain. Am J Pathol. 2006;168(3):936–46.
56. Herrmann M, Vos P, Wunderlich MT, de Bruijn CH, Lamers KJ. Release of glial tissue-specific proteins after acute stroke: a comparative analysis of serum concentrations of protein S-100B and glial fibrillary acidic protein. Stroke. 2000;31(11):2670–7.
57. Missler U, Wiesmann M, Wittmann G, Magerkurth O, Hagenstrom H. Measurement of glial fibrillary acidic protein in human blood: analytical method and preliminary clinical results. Clin Chem. 1999;45(1):138–41.
58. Pelinka LE, Kroepfl A, Leixnering M, Buchinger W, Raabe A, Redl H. GFAP versus S100B in serum after traumatic brain injury: relationship to brain damage and outcome. J Neurotrauma. 2004;21(11):1553–61.
59. van Geel WJ, de Reus HP, Nijzing H, Verbeek MM, Vos PE, Lamers KJ. Measurement of glial fibrillary acidic protein in blood: an analytical method. Clin Chim Acta. 2002; 326(1–2):151–4.
60. Nylen K, Ost M, Csajbok LZ, Nilsson I, Blennow K, Nellgard B, et al. Increased serum-GFAP in patients with severe traumatic brain injury is related to outcome. J Neurol Sci. 2006;240(1–2):85–91.
61. Mondello S, Papa L, Buki A, Bullock R, Czeiter E, Tortella F, et al. Neuronal and glial markers are differently associated with computed tomography findings and outcome in patients with severe traumatic brain injury: a case control study. Crit Care. 2011;15(3):R156.

62. Metting Z, Wilczak N, Rodiger LA, Schaaf JM, van der Naalt J. GFAP and S100B in the acute phase of mild traumatic brain injury. Neurology. 2012;78(18):1428–33.
63. Papa L, Lewis LM, Falk JL, Zhang Z, Silvestri S, Giordano P, et al. Elevated levels of serum glial fibrillary acidic protein breakdown products in mild and moderate traumatic brain injury are associated with intracranial lesions and neurosurgical intervention. Ann Emerg Med. 2012;59(6):471–83.
64. Zetterberg H, Hietala MA, Jonsson M, Andreasen N, Styrud E, Karlsson I, et al. Neurochemical aftermath of amateur boxing. Arch Neurol. 2006;63(9):1277–80.
65. Skogseid IM, Nordby HK, Urdal P, Paus E, Lilleaas F. Increased serum creatine kinase BB and neuron specific enolase following head injury indicates brain damage. Acta Neurochir (Wien). 1992;115(3–4):106–11.
66. Schmechel D, Marangos PJ, Brightman M. Neurone-specific enolase is a molecular marker for peripheral and central neuroendocrine cells. Nature. 1978;276(5690):834–6.
67. Ergun R, Bostanci U, Akdemir G, Beskonakli E, Kaptanoglu E, Gursoy F, et al. Prognostic value of serum neuron-specific enolase levels after head injury. Neurol Res. 1998; 20(5):418–20.
68. Yamazaki Y, Yada K, Morii S, Kitahara T, Ohwada T. Diagnostic significance of serum neuron-specific enolase and myelin basic protein assay in patients with acute head injury. Surg Neurol. 1995;43(3):267–70; discussion 70–1.
69. Ross SA, Cunningham RT, Johnston CF, Rowlands BJ. Neuron-specific enolase as an aid to outcome prediction in head injury. Br J Neurosurg. 1996;10(5):471–6.
70. Fridriksson T, Kini N, Walsh-Kelly C, Hennes H. Serum neuron-specific enolase as a predictor of intracranial lesions in children with head trauma: a pilot study. Acad Emerg Med. 2000;7(7):816–20.
71. Berger RP, Adelson PD, Pierce MC, Dulani T, Cassidy LD, Kochanek PM. Serum neuron-specific enolase, S100B, and myelin basic protein concentrations after inflicted and noninflicted traumatic brain injury in children. J Neurosurg. 2005;103(1 Suppl):61–8.
72. Berger RP, Beers SR, Richichi R, Wiesman D, Adelson PD. Serum biomarker concentrations and outcome after pediatric traumatic brain injury. J Neurotrauma. 2007;24(12):1793–801.
73. Varma S, Janesko KL, Wisniewski SR, Bayir H, Adelson PD, Thomas NJ, et al. F2-isoprostane and neuron-specific enolase in cerebrospinal fluid after severe traumatic brain injury in infants and children. J Neurotrauma. 2003;20(8):781–6.
74. Bandyopadhyay S, Hennes H, Gorelick MH, Wells RG, Walsh-Kelly CM. Serum neuron-specific enolase as a predictor of short-term outcome in children with closed traumatic brain injury. Acad Emerg Med. 2005;12(8):732–8.
75. Johnsson P, Blomquist S, Luhrs C, Malmkvist G, Alling C, Solem JO, et al. Neuron-specific enolase increases in plasma during and immediately after extracorporeal circulation. Ann Thorac Surg. 2000;69(3):750–4.
76. Ramont L, Thoannes H, Volondat A, Chastang F, Millet MC, Maquart FX. Effects of hemolysis and storage condition on neuron-specific enolase (NSE) in cerebrospinal fluid and serum: implications in clinical practice. Clin Chem Lab Med. 2005;43(11):1215–7.
77. Stalnacke BM, Ohlsson A, Tegner Y, Sojka P. Serum concentrations of two biochemical markers of brain tissue damage S-100B and neurone specific enolase are increased in elite female soccer players after a competitive game. Br J Sports Med. 2006;40(4):313–6.
78. Jackson P, Thompson RJ. The demonstration of new human brain-specific proteins by high-resolution two-dimensional polyacrylamide gel electrophoresis. J Neurol Sci. 1981;49(3):429–38.
79. Tongaonkar P, Chen L, Lambertson D, Ko B, Madura K. Evidence for an interaction between ubiquitin-conjugating enzymes and the 26S proteasome. Mol Cell Biol. 2000; 20(13):4691–8.
80. Gong B, Leznik E. The role of ubiquitin C-terminal hydrolase L1 in neurodegenerative disorders. Drug News Perspect. 2007;20(6):365–70.
81. Siman R, Toraskar N, Dang A, McNeil E, McGarvey M, Plaum J, et al. A panel of neuron-enriched proteins as markers for traumatic brain injury in humans. J Neurotrauma. 2009;26(11):1867–77.

82. Papa L, Akinyi L, Liu MC, Pineda JA, Tepas III JJ, Oli MW, et al. Ubiquitin C-terminal hydrolase is a novel biomarker in humans for severe traumatic brain injury. Crit Care Med. 2010;38(1):138–44.
83. Brophy G, Mondello S, Papa L, Robicsek S, Gabrielli A, Tepas Iii J, et al. Biokinetic analysis of ubiquitin C-terminal hydrolase-L1 (Uch-L1) in severe traumatic brain injury patient bio-fluids. J Neurotrauma. 2011;28(6):861–70.
84. Berger RP, Hayes RL, Richichi R, Beers SR, Wang KK. Serum concentrations of ubiquitin C-terminal hydrolase-L1 and alphaII-spectrin breakdown product 145 kDa correlate with outcome after pediatric TBI. J Neurotrauma. 2012;29(1):162–7.
85. Papa L, Lewis LM, Silvestri S, Falk JL, Giordano P, Brophy GM, et al. Serum levels of ubiquitin C-terminal hydrolase distinguish mild traumatic brain injury from trauma controls and are elevated in mild and moderate traumatic brain injury patients with intracranial lesions and neurosurgical intervention. J Trauma Acute Care Surg. 2012;72(5):1335–44.
86. Goodman SR, Zimmer WE, Clark MB, Zagon IS, Barker JE, Bloom ML. Brain spectrin: of mice and men. Brain Res Bull. 1995;36(6):593–606.
87. Riederer BM, Zagon IS, Goodman SR. Brain spectrin(240/235) and brain spectrin(240/235E): two distinct spectrin subtypes with different locations within mammalian neural cells. J Cell Biol. 1986;102(6):2088–97.
88. Wang KK, Posmantur R, Nath R, McGinnis K, Whitton M, Talanian RV, et al. Simultaneous degradation of alphaII- and betaII-spectrin by caspase 3 (CPP32) in apoptotic cells. J Biol Chem. 1998;273(35):22490–7.
89. McGinn MJ, Kelley BJ, Akinyi L, Oli MW, Liu MC, Hayes RL, et al. Biochemical, structural, and biomarker evidence for calpain-mediated cytoskeletal change after diffuse brain injury uncomplicated by contusion. J Neuropathol Exp Neurol. 2009;68(3):241–9.
90. Pike BR, Flint J, Dave JR, Lu XC, Wang KK, Tortella FC, et al. Accumulation of calpain and caspase-3 proteolytic fragments of brain-derived alphaII-spectrin in cerebral spinal fluid after middle cerebral artery occlusion in rats. J Cereb Blood Flow Metab. 2004;24(1):98–106.
91. Ringger NC, O'Steen BE, Brabham JG, Silver X, Pineda J, Wang KK, et al. A novel marker for traumatic brain injury: CSF alphaII-spectrin breakdown product levels. J Neurotrauma. 2004;21(10):1443–56.
92. Cardali S, Maugeri R. Detection of alphaII-spectrin and breakdown products in humans after severe traumatic brain injury. J Neurosurg Sci. 2006;50(2):25–31.
93. Pineda JA, Lewis SB, Valadka AB, Papa L, Hannay HJ, Heaton SC, et al. Clinical significance of alphaII-spectrin breakdown products in cerebrospinal fluid after severe traumatic brain injury. J Neurotrauma. 2007;24(2):354–66.
94. Papa L, D'Avella D, Aguennouz M, Angileri FF, de Divitiis O, Germano A, et al. Detection of alpha-II spectrin and breakdown products in humans after severe traumatic brain injury [abstract]. Acad Emerg Med. 2004;11(5):515–16.
95. Papa L, Lewis SB, Heaton S, Demery JA, Tepas JJ III, Wang KKW, et al. Predicting early outcome using alpha-II spectrin breakdown products in human CSF after severe traumatic brain injury [abstract]. Acad Emerg Med. 2006;13(5 Suppl 1):S39–40.
96. Papa L, Pineda J, Wang KKW, Lewis SB, Demery JA, Heaton S, et al. Levels of alpha-II spectrin breakdown products in human CSF and outcome after severe traumatic brain injury [abstract]. Acad Emerg Med. 2005;12(5 Suppl 1):139–40.
97. Farkas O, Polgar B, Szekeres-Bartho J, Doczi T, Povlishock JT, Buki A. Spectrin breakdown products in the cerebrospinal fluid in severe head injury—preliminary observations. Acta Neurochir (Wien). 2005;147(8):855–61.
98. Mondello S, Robicsek SA, Gabrielli A, Brophy GM, Papa L, Tepas J, et al. AlphaII-spectrin breakdown products (SBDPs): diagnosis and outcome in severe traumatic brain injury patients. J Neurotrauma. 2010;27(7):1203–13.
99. Brophy GM, Pineda JA, Papa L, Lewis SB, Valadka AB, Hannay HJ, et al. AlphaII-spectrin breakdown product cerebrospinal fluid exposure metrics suggest differences in cellular injury mechanisms after severe traumatic brain injury. J Neurotrauma. 2009;26(4):471–9.
100. Papa L, Wang KW, Brophy GM, Demery JA, Silvestri S, Giordano P, et al. Serum levels of spectrin breakdown product 150 (SBDP150) distinguish mild traumatic brain injury from

trauma and uninjured controls and predict intracranial injuries on CT and neurosurgical intervention. J Neurotrauma. 2012;29(Abstract Suppl):A28.

101. Kosik KS, Finch EA. MAP2 and tau segregate into dendritic and axonal domains after the elaboration of morphologically distinct neurites: an immunocytochemical study of cultured rat cerebrum. J Neurosci. 1987;7(10):3142–53.

102. Higuchi M, Lee VM, Trojanowski JQ. Tau and axonopathy in neurodegenerative disorders. Neuromolecular Med. 2002;2(2):131–50.

103. Shaw GJ, Jauch EC, Zemlan FP. Serum cleaved tau protein levels and clinical outcome in adult patients with closed head injury. Ann Emerg Med. 2002;39(3):254–7.

104. Zemlan FP, Jauch EC, Mulchahey JJ, Gabbita SP, Rosenberg WS, Speciale SG, et al. C-tau biomarker of neuronal damage in severe brain injured patients: association with elevated intracranial pressure and clinical outcome. Brain Res. 2002;947(1):131–9.

105. Chatfield DA, Zemlan FP, Day DJ, Menon DK. Discordant temporal patterns of S100beta and cleaved tau protein elevation after head injury: a pilot study. Br J Neurosurg. 2002;16(5):471–6.

106. Trojanowski JQ, Schuck T, Schmidt ML, Lee VM. Distribution of tau proteins in the normal human central and peripheral nervous system. J Histochem Cytochem. 1989;37(2):209–15.

107. Franz G, Beer R, Kampfl A, Engelhardt K, Schmutzhard E, Ulmer H, et al. Amyloid beta 1-42 and tau in cerebrospinal fluid after severe traumatic brain injury. Neurology. 2003;60(9):1457–61.

108. Marklund N, Blennow K, Zetterberg H, Ronne-Engstrom E, Enblad P, Hillered L. Monitoring of brain interstitial total tau and beta amyloid proteins by microdialysis in patients with traumatic brain injury. J Neurosurg. 2009;110(6):1227–37.

109. Ost M, Nylen K, Csajbok L, Ohrfelt AO, Tullberg M, Wikkelso C, et al. Initial CSF total tau correlates with 1-year outcome in patients with traumatic brain injury. Neurology. 2006;67(9):1600–4.

110. Sjogren M, Blomberg M, Jonsson M, Wahlund LO, Edman A, Lind K, et al. Neurofilament protein in cerebrospinal fluid: a marker of white matter changes. J Neurosci Res. 2001;66(3):510–6.

111. Julien JP, Mushynski WE. Neurofilaments in health and disease. Prog Nucleic Acid Res Mol Biol. 1998;61:1–23.

112. Buki A, Povlishock JT. All roads lead to disconnection?—Traumatic axonal injury revisited. Acta Neurochir (Wien). 2006;148(2):181–93; discussion 93–4.

113. Zurek J, Bartlova L, Fedora M. Hyperphosphorylated neurofilament NF-H as a predictor of mortality after brain injury in children. Brain Inj. 2012;25(2):221–6.

Chapter 14
Functional Magnetic Resonance Imaging in Mild Traumatic Brain Injury

Andrew R. Mayer and Patrick S.F. Bellgowan

Abstract Patients with concussion (mild traumatic brain injury (mTBI)) frequently complain of both cognitive and emotional disturbances in the days to weeks after their injury, with a percentage of patients (5–20 %) remaining chronically symptomatic. Relative to other static neuroimaging techniques, functional MRI (fMRI) offers great promise for elucidating the underlying neuropathology associated with dynamic processes such as higher-order cognition. Not surprisingly, the majority of mTBI studies have focused on working memory and attention, with results suggesting a complex relationship between cognitive load/attentional demand and functional activation. More recently researchers have used functional connectivity analyses to investigate how injury may affect intrinsic neuronal activation. Several groups have reported that connectivity within the default-mode network is disrupted following injury, which may also contribute to patient reports of increased distractibility. The general benefits and drawbacks of the two methods (evoked versus connectivity studies) are discussed in the context of the injury literature. Mood disturbances are also prevalent following concussion, but fewer studies (evoked or connectivity) have been conducted to investigate the integrity of the emotional processing network. Finally, fMRI can also be used as a surrogate biomarker of

A.R. Mayer, Ph.D. (✉)
Department of Cognitive Neuroscience, The Mind Research Network/Lovelace Biomedical and Environmental Research Institute, 1101 Yale Blvd NE, Albuquerque, NM 87106, USA

Department of Neurology, University of New Mexico School of Medicine, Albuquerque, NM, USA

Department of Psychology, University of New Mexico, Albuquerque, NM, USA
e-mail: amayer@mrn.org

P.S.F. Bellgowan, Ph.D.
Faculty of Community Medicine, The University of Tulsa, Laureate Institute for Brain Research, 6655 South Yale Avenue, Tulsa, OK 74104, USA
e-mail: pbellgowan@laureateinstitute.org

S.M. Slobounov and W.J. Sebastianelli (eds.), *Concussions in Athletics: From Brain to Behavior*, DOI 10.1007/978-1-4939-0295-8_14,
© Springer Science+Business Media New York 2014

pharmacological and cognitive rehabilitation treatment efficacy, although only preliminary work has been conducted in this area to date. The chapter also discusses the methodological challenges of performing and evaluating fMRI research with brain-injured patients, including clinical heterogeneity in patient selection criteria and variations in scan time post-injury. Finally, the chapter concludes with a discussion of the physiological underpinnings of the blood oxygen level-dependent (BOLD) response and the many ways in which trauma can affect this complex signal. We conclude that the fMRI signal represents a complex filter through which researchers can more directly measure the physiological correlates of concussive symptoms, an important goal for this burgeoning field.

Keywords Mild traumatic brain injury • Functional magnetic resonance imaging • Evoked activation • Functional connectivity • Confounds • Physiological basis

Introduction

Mild traumatic brain injury (mTBI) remains a poorly understood clinical phenomenon, despite lifetime incidence rates between 110 and 550 per 100,000 individuals [1]. This is primarily a result of the variable definitions of mTBI [2], which are entirely determined by clinical observations and self-reported symptomatology rather than objective markers. Findings from standard clinical neuroimaging sequences (CT scans; T_1 and T_2 weighted images) are typically negative for the majority of patients [3, 4], leading to a proliferation of studies that have attempted to define more objective imaging biomarkers of mTBI [5, 6]. Since the seminal studies of McAllister et al. [7, 8], there has been great interest in using functional magnetic resonance imaging (fMRI) to study mTBI given its ability to perform in vivo measurements during demanding cognitive tasks [9] and, more recently, to characterize intrinsic neuronal activity [10–12].

Single episode mTBI is characterized by subtle neurobehavioral deficits within the first few weeks of injury that typically resolve spontaneously within 3–6 months of injury in approximately 80–95 % of patients [5, 13–16]. Recent evidence suggests that the cumulative effects of multiple mTBIs result in a fourfold increase in neurodegenerative diseases [17] and a unique neuropathological syndrome involving tauopathies in periventricular spaces/deep cortical sulci with an overrepresentation of frontal and medial temporal pathology [18, 19]. Thus, although considerable challenges remain [20], mTBI offers a unique opportunity for examining both transient and permanent disruptions in cognitive and emotional functioning in human injury models. The chapter first provides a review of mTBI research using both evoked paradigms as well as functional connectivity, which have more recently been used to study the effects of brain trauma. Next, we focus on the considerable methodological challenges of performing fMRI research with brain-injured patients. Finally, a review of the physiological underpinnings of the blood oxygen level-dependent (BOLD) response, which represents a complex filter through which researchers attempt to noninvasively capture the effects of neuronal injury, is also provided.

Review of Current Findings from the Literature

fMRI offers great promise for elucidating the underlying neuropathology associated with neurobehavioral sequelae following mTBI, especially when used in conjunction with tasks that dynamically tap into higher-order cognitive functioning [5, 21]. The seminal fMRI studies on mTBI focused on working memory paradigms, with results suggesting a complex relationship between cognitive load and functional activation. In a series of studies on semi-acute (within 1 month of injury) mTBI patients, McAllister et al. [7, 8] reported hyperactivation in right dorsolateral prefrontal cortex (DLPFC) and lateral parietal regions for mTBI patients compared to healthy controls (HC) for moderate processing loads (1-back to 2-back conditions), but hypoactivation for the lower loads (0-back to 1-back conditions). Additional studies by McAllister and colleagues indicated that mTBI patients exhibited frontoparietal hyperactivation in the 1-back to 2-back condition, but hypoactivation going from 2-back to 3-back. Other groups have reported a positive correlation between self-report measures of symptom severity and increased activation both within the working memory network (e.g., dorsolateral and ventrolateral prefrontal cortex) and other regions, suggesting potential compensatory activation [22]. Using both fMRI and event-related potentials, Gosselin reported that mTBI patients had decreased BOLD signal changes in the left and right mid-dorsolateral prefrontal cortex (which correlated with symptom severity), the putamen, the body of the caudate nucleus, and the right thalamus, coupled with a reduced N350 ERP amplitude [23]. Others have not observed significant differences between a relatively large cohort of mTBI patients ($N=43$) and HC ($N=20$) on a similar n-back task, instead finding that length of post-traumatic amnesia (PTA) was related to hippocampal deactivation (0-back > 2-back) [24].

Demonstrating many of the methodological and interpretive challenges involved in imaging mTBI patients, results from fMRI studies of working memory using concussed athletes have been also been conflicting. In contrast to McAllister's findings of hyperactivation in the right DLPFC, athletes with persistent post-concussive symptoms (PCS) imaged while performing both verbal and visual design working memory tasks show hypoactivation of the right DLPFC [25, 26]. Chen et al. [25] also report both hypo- and hyperactivation in the left prefrontal cortex that was not related to PCS severity and, in general, more diffuse activation patterns in the PCS athlete group. Longitudinal imaging of one patient at 6 months with PCS symptoms and later at 9 months without PCS symptoms provided evidence for a negative correlation between right DLPFC activation and symptom severity but not between DLPFC activation and symptom duration. The correlation between PCS symptom severity and bilateral DLPFC hypoactivation was further supported using a whole brain analysis comparing nine low and nine high PCS severity patients in a verbal working memory task [27]. Importantly, multiple methodological differences exist between the McAllister findings and those of Chen and colleagues including auditory versus visual working memory, athletes versus emergency room patients, time–post-injury, and operational definitions of symptom severity.

There are additional examples of hyperactivation measured with fMRI during task. Using a pre- vs. post-injury design, Jantzen et al. showed hyperactivation of frontal regions post-injury even in the absence of cognitive performance differences [28] suggestive of a compensatory mechanism. The degree of abnormal activation (hyperactivation) may be indicative of a prolonged recovery profile in athletes, particularly when accompanied by more sparse and diffuse activation patterns [29]. Finally, recent fMRI data suggest that significant neuropathological changes can be missed if the focus of sports-related head injuries remains only on diagnosed concussions. Based on the high frequency of American-rules football-offensive lineman in postmortem neuropathological cases [18], it was proposed that sub-concussive hits also contribute to the development of chronic traumatic encephalopathy (CTE). To investigate the effects of sub-concussive hits, Talavage and colleagues scanned high school football athletes pre- and postseason with embedded sensors in the helmet to tally the number of head hits throughout the season. Results demonstrated that prolonged exposure to sub-concussive hits resulted in hypoactivation within left middle and superior temporal gyri, left middle occipital gyrus, and bilateral cerebellum during an n-back working memory task [30]. Interestingly, Talavage also showed that this pattern of decreased activity correlated with poorer working memory performance in non-concussed high school football players.

Several groups have also examined attentional and memory functioning following mTBI. Smits et al. reported increased activation within the anterior cingulate gyrus, inferior frontal gyrus, insula, and posterior parietal areas during attention tasks with an increased incidence of post-concussive symptoms [22]. Previous results from our lab have indicated hypoactivation within several deep cortical, cerebellar, and subcortical sites during an auditory attention task in independent adult [31] and pediatric mTBI [32] cohorts, with within-group comparisons also indicating decreased cortical activation for mTBI patients during more attentionally demanding conditions [31]. Similarly, we have also seen decreased cortical activation during within-subject comparisons in mTBI relative to HC during a multimodal numeric Stroop task in conjunction with aberrant task-induced deactivation within the default-mode network (DMN) [33]. Witt and colleagues used a three-stimulus (standard, target, and novel stimuli) auditory oddball paradigm with low attentional demand [34]. An ROI analysis suggested that mTBI patients exhibited less activity in right DLPFC compared to HC while detecting target stimuli. In addition, during detection of novel stimuli, patients exhibited decreased activation in areas in the DMN and increased in right superior and inferior parietal areas. Finally, Slobounov and colleagues reported increased volumes of activity for recently concussed athletes within the DLPFC, parietal cortex, and hippocampus on a spatial memory task relative to non-concussed HC [35].

The effects of treatment on BOLD activity following mTBI have also recently been explored. McAllister and colleagues examined whether pharmacological challenges to the dopaminergic system may explain some of these brain abnormalities in working memory circuitry following mTBI. The authors reported that whereas HC performance improved during the n-back task following the administration of bromocriptine, compared to placebo, mTBI patients did not show any behavioral improvement [36]. Moreover, HC in both drug conditions had higher activation in areas involved in working memory relative to patients, whereas mTBI patients on bromocriptine instead had higher activation in areas outside this working memory network. A similar complex pattern of activation was observed within the working memory circuitry when mTBI patients were placed on guanfacine, which indirectly affects dopamine transmission [37]. mTBI patients have also exhibited both increased and decreased activations following cognitive rehabilitation therapy on visually guided saccades and reading comprehension tasks in a relatively small sample of patients [38]. Although these findings are all in their preliminary stages, it suggests that BOLD-based activity may offer a mechanism for noninvasively measuring how treatment affects disrupted neurophysiology following mTBI.

In addition to evoked studies of BOLD activity, researchers are increasingly turning to measures of functional connectivity (fcMRI) to examine neuronal health following mTBI. Connectivity studies are based on intrinsic neuronal fluctuations that synchronously occur over spatially distributed networks in both humans and animals [39]. The majority (60–80 %) of the brain's energy resources is expended to maintain homeostasis [40, 41], and intrinsic neuronal activity likely contributes to this heavy metabolic load. Previous research indicates changes in baseline metabolism following TBI [42] as well as abnormal slow-wave electrophysiological activity during passive mental activity [43–45], providing the biological relevance for fcMRI as a biomarker of mTBI.

These intrinsic fluctuations in neuronal activity tend to alias to low frequency fluctuations (0.01–0.10 Hz) in BOLD signal, and therefore can be measured on any MRI scanner with a conventional echo-planar sequence. During these resting state scans, participants are simply asked to either fixate on a visual stimulus or close their eyes for a relatively brief period of time (approximately 5 min). As such, resting state paradigms have been criticized based on the general lack of control over participant's mental activities and the inability to specify what cognitive tasks the participant actually performed in the scanner [46]. Similarly, mTBI participants do not perform difficult cognitive tasks during resting state scans, which are of greater clinical interest given that patients tend to report more difficulties under these conditions in everyday life [5, 21]. Finally, noise has a more direct influence on the correlation coefficient in fcMRI relative to evoked signals [47], which can further complicate interpretation of group-wise results.

However, resting state scans also have several advantages over more traditional evoked studies and may eliminate several potential confounds associated with cognitive tasks. Foremost, using a relatively simple task (i.e., passively maintaining fixation), it is possible to probe the neuronal integrity of the multiple sensory, motor, and cognitive networks that exist in the human brain. Specifically, Smith and colleagues demonstrated that intrinsic neuronal activity measured from 36 participants was organized into distinct networks that mirror activity evoked across a variety (30,000 archival data sets) of cognitive challenges [48]. Second, eliminating the complex requirements for presenting sensory stimuli and monitoring motor responses (e.g., interfacing with a computer, projecting stimuli, special nonferrous motor response devices) renders fcMRI more readily available for performing clinical scans.

Third, the passive nature of resting state scans (eyes closed or maintaining fixation) reduces some of the confounds associated with evoked studies due to lack of effort, effects of pain, and fatigue. Fourth, in the presence of task-based behavioral differences, it is difficult to disambiguate whether differences in BOLD-related activity directly result from behavioral performance differences, alterations in neurophysiology, or some combination of effects. Similarly, interpretation of evoked data is also frequently complicated by learning and/or practice effects, which are minimal during a passive task. Finally, as has already been demonstrated by several research groups [49–51], fcMRI can be used across the entire TBI spectrum (e.g., mildest injury to minimally conscious patients).

To date, the majority of connectivity studies following TBI have focused on activation in the DMN. The primary nodes of the DMN include the rostral anterior cingulate gyrus (rACC), posterior cingulate gyrus (PCC), superior temporal/supramarginal gyrus (SMG), and ventromedial prefrontal cortex, with the rACC and PCC serving as central hubs [52]. The DMN is believed to mediate a variety of mental activities such as episodic memory review and future-oriented thought processes that occur during periods of unconstrained mental activity [53]. DMN activity parametrically varies with task difficulty [54] and is predictive of attentional lapses during cognitively demanding tasks [55, 56]. In addition, DMN BOLD signals are negatively (i.e., anticorrelated) correlated with activity in the lateral prefrontal cortex and inferior parietal lobes [57], suggesting that the two networks may act in conjunction to produce states of high (decreased DMN activity) or low (increased DMN activity) attentiveness to external events.

Early fcMRI studies focused on severely injured [58] or minimally conscious [49–51] TBI patients, with most studies reporting decreased DMN connectivity (but see [59]). In the semi-acute phase of mTBI, reduced connectivity has been reported within the DMN using a seed-based approach, with increased connectivity between the rACC and ventrolateral prefrontal cortex [11]. These abnormalities in DMN connectivity remained relatively stable approximately 4 months post-injury. Another study utilized independent component analysis (ICA) to examine DMN connectivity, reporting reduced connectivity in the posterior hubs (PCC and SMG) of the DMN in conjunction with increased connectivity within the ventromedial prefrontal cortex [60]. Similarly, Johnson and colleagues reported generally reduced connections across multiple nodes of the DMN in recently concussed athletes relative to HC, as well as a larger departure from typical DMN connectivity as a function of the number of previous mTBI episodes [10]. However, a subsequent study by the same group did not find any significant differences within DMN connectivity unless a physical stress challenge was presented to recently concussed athletes [61].

Others have reported disrupted interhemispheric fcMRI in the visual cortex, hippocampus, and DLPFC during task-based connectivity analyses [62], as well as decreased symmetry of connectivity based on thalamic seeds [63]. Another group also used ICA to investigate fcMRI [12], reporting decreased functional connectivity within the motor-striatal network and increased connectivity in the right frontoparietal network. Finally, Stevens and colleagues reported disrupted (both increased and decreased) connectivity in 30 semi-acutely injured mTBI patients across 12 different sensory and cognitive networks [64]. On the basis of these studies, fcMRI appears to be well poised for interrogating connectivity within all major structures and networks of the brain following mTBI.

Overarching Issues in FMRI Research Following mTBI

As alluded to in the preceding paragraphs, there are several potential confounds that need to be carefully considered when performing and evaluating fMRI studies of mTBI. Some of the more common clinical confounds include injury-related pain (orthopedic), fatigue, poor effort, cognitive deficits, and the presence of other prescribed medications (e.g., narcotics or sedatives) that may alter neurovascular coupling [65–67]. Some of the nonspecific somatic confounds (e.g., pain and fatigue) and medication issues can be reduced or eliminated by recruiting orthopedically injured patients as control subjects, as has previously been done in the clinical literature [68, 69]. Confounds that can be controlled through careful experimental design include reducing heterogeneity in terms of both injury severity and post-injury scan time. For example, patients who are only dazed following a blow to the head, patients who are unconscious for up to 30 min, and patients with large subdural hematomas can all be classified as having suffered from mTBI under current nosology [2]. However, the symptoms and recovery trajectories of these patients are likely to be very different [70, 71].

Developing methods for improving the nosology of mTBI and understanding of symptom trajectory will be critical for coalescing disparate neuroimaging findings. The temporal dynamics of mTBI has been elucidated using animal models, demonstrating a complex, multifaceted, and time-varying pathology that characterizes mTBI in the minutes to weeks following injury [72]. However, inclusion criteria for previous studies in human mTBI have ranged from days to years post-injury, with some studies focusing on chronically symptomatic patients. Several meta-analyses have documented that the majority of single-episode mTBI patients are expected to recover spontaneously from a neurobehavioral perspective within a few weeks to a few months post-injury [5, 13–16]. Understanding why a percentage of single episode mTBI patients remain chronically symptomatic is critical for the field. However, this cohort represents a subset of the larger mTBI population and findings from this sample may not generalize. Thus, while it is important to recognize the heterogeneity and chaos associated with mTBI [20], it is also important to foster studies based on homogeneous samples in clearly defined time-windows (acute, subacute, or chronic post-injury stages).

It is notable that mTBI patients who meet strict inclusion criteria (homogeneous in both injury severity and scan-time post-injury) are challenging to enroll, and fMRI data is financially costly to accumulate. The combination of these factors has resulted in another methodological challenge: namely, the utilization of low sample sizes despite the inherently low signal-to-noise ratio of fMRI [73]. Specifically, the majority of fMRI studies following mTBI have been reported with sample sizes just at or below commonly accepted recommendations. As a result, it is likely that these studies may be underpowered, suffering from low positive predictive power and providing poor estimates of the true effect size [74]. Therefore, conflicting findings from previously discussed working memory studies following mTBI may be the result of simple methodological differences (described above) and/or a result of the small sample sizes employed across the various studies. Importantly, fMRI studies of other cognitions (e.g., attentional and memory deficits) are not exempt from this critique, but independent replication attempts of these findings have been fewer. To combat the problem of small sample sizes, funding agencies have recently developed standard clinical definitions, common data elements, and informational platforms for creating community-wide data sharing initiatives (e.g., Federal Interagency Traumatic Brain Injury Research; FITBIR). These efforts should accelerate research in this critical area by permitting the pooling of data for meta-analyses.

A third methodological consideration relates to the self-reporting of symptoms. Importantly, symptom self-report may vary as a function of sample with sports-related populations underreporting neurobehavioral symptoms to return to play [75–77] whereas other mTBI populations may over-report symptoms [78, 79], especially in the presence of potential financial compensation. Multiple sociological barriers may account for the underreporting of concussive symptoms ranging from lack of education regarding the seriousness of concussion (parents, players, and coaches), hesitancy to report symptoms that do not result in significant pain, desire not to be removed from play, and stigmatization of concussion as a non-real injury [77, 80]. The peer pressure to continue play and not report injury is particularly important in vulnerable populations such as children who may not comprehend and underestimate the risks involved in continued participation, and in low socioeconomic areas where participation is perceived as a path to future benefit [81]. Additional pressures are on the coaching staffs who may feel pressured to win and underestimate the risk of returning a player to the field prematurely. Unfortunately, the rate of underreporting of concussion symptoms in high school football has been reported to be as high as 53 % [82].

Regardless of the sociological factors, underreporting of symptoms can lead to premature "return to play" decisions and put players at risk for exacerbated outcomes related to the occurrence of multiple sports-related concussions [83–86]. Repeat concussions (concussions occurring within the same sports season) increase the risk of long-term cognitive and psychiatric dysregulation by 1.5–3-fold relative to those with a single concussive incident [87]. A study of nearly 3,000 concussions in NCAA athletes clearly demonstrates that an initial concussion dramatically increases that player's risk of a repeat concussion [87, 88]. Athletes with a history of concussion are also more likely to report more baseline symptoms than are those with no history of concussion [85]. The increased risks of neuropathological incidence and behavioral decline associated with repeat concussions has been modeled in piglets and shows a worse neuropathological and neurobehavioral outcome for injuries that occur in temporal proximity [89]. Importantly, neuronal recovery may lag behind the recovery of behavioral and cognitive symptoms, emphasizing the need for objective biomarkers of when it is truly safe to return to play.

Psychiatric Sequelae and mTBI

Among the more challenging outcome measures to operationalize are psychiatric sequelae of TBI. Episodes of major depression are the most commonly diagnosed neuropsychiatric complication in TBI, regardless of injury severity [90–93]. The incidence of concussed high school and collegiate athletes reporting anxiety, depression, and irritability is reported to be range between 17 and 46 % [68, 94–96], whereas basal rates of self-reported mood disorders in collegiate athletes is equal to or slightly less (15–30 %) than the typical collegiate students [97–99]. Unfortunately, affective dysregulation resulting from sports-related concussion, at all ages, can linger for years in those diagnosed with post-concussion syndrome [100–105]. In pediatric and adolescent populations, TBI increases both rates of long-term depression and anxiety, dependent upon the lesion laterality and age at time of injury [106–108]. In addition, younger athletes reporting concussion-related mood sequelae have more prolonged depressive episodes [109, 110].

Understanding and assessing the basis of mood dysregulation following mTBI is complicated by the possibility of having three potentially coexisting, yet distinct etiological mechanisms for depressed mood following mTBI. First, predisposition for mood disorder, including family history of mood disorders, has been shown to be a strong factor in the presence and severity of post-concussive depression [90, 111–113]. Second, psychiatric sequelae may result from the indirect effects of TBI secondary to psychosocial and psychosomatic consequences of the injury (somatoform depression). These include decreased the ability to perform at a job, poor social functioning, perceived stigma of a non-visible injury and depression secondary to other injuries or losses (e.g., deceased spouse) sustained during the traumatic incident [90, 91, 114–116].

A final primary etiological path for psychiatric sequelae is a biologically based disruption of the emotional processing neural network. Potential pathologies include direct damage to the network nodes and/or damage to white-matter connections within emotional processing networks. Secondary events such as neuroinflammation may also contribute by inducing "sickness behavior" [117–119], and are believed to be critically involved in CTE and post-concussive disorder [120, 121]. Further support for a pathophysiological mechanism of the depressive mood state following concussion is supported by the neuroinflammatory model of post-concussive state that mechanistically mimics the inflammatory model of major depressive disorder. Bellgowan and colleagues [122] demonstrated increased levels of the inflammatory marker IL-1B negatively correlate with connectivity within the subgenual ACC and other regions of the medial emotional network [123]. Regardless of the etiology, all processes result in negative affect that increases stress and interferes with the hypothalamic-pituitary-adrenal (HPA) axis [124–126], resulting in further dysregulation of emotional processing networks [127, 128].

The increased incidence of mood disturbances observed in retired boxers and professional football players with a history of concussion provides prognostic evidence for the neuropathological etiology of concussion-related mood dysregulation [18, 19].

Of particular concern in those that have been diagnosed with CTE is the high rate of suicidality [18, 129, 130]. Suicide rates for concussed persons who are at risk for mood disorder or have a diagnostic history of mood disorder are also significantly elevated [131, 132]. Though the mood disturbances reported in retired players and diagnosed CTE cases were obtained retrospectively and lack prior psychiatric history, others [84] have demonstrated that the later life diagnosis of clinical depression is correlated with concussion history [84].

fMRI Physiology and Trauma

The exact linkage between neuronal transmission and resultant hemodynamic activity (neurovascular coupling) remains an active area of investigation. During intrinsic activity (at rest), a tight coupling exists between the cerebral metabolic rate of glucose (CMR_{glu}), the cerebral metabolic rate of oxygen ($CMRO_2$) and cerebral blood flow (CBF) to maintain homeostasis [133]. Following excitatory neuronal transmission, energy (glucose) is required to reverse ionic influx and excess glutamate needs to be rapidly removed from the synaptic cleft [134–136]. Excess glutamate is taken up by astrocytes and converted to glutamine, nitric oxide is released co-temporally by neurons and vasoactive agents are released by astrocytes [134], all of which likely contribute to vasodilation and a concomitant increase in CBF. Importantly, there is a decoupling between CBF and oxidative metabolism [137] following neuronal activation, which leads to an excess in oxygenated blood, a decrease in the ratio of deoxyhemoglobin relative to oxyhemoglobin, and a subsequent increase in signal.

As such, it has long been recognized that the BOLD response represents an amalgamation of signals derived from the ratio of oxy- to deoxyhemoglobin (primary), CBF, and cerebral blood volume (CBV) [73, 138, 139]. The shape of the BOLD response is also complex in nature, with the canonical hemodynamic response function (HRF) consisting of two primary components, a positive signal change that peaks approximately 4–6 s post-stimulus onset, and a post-stimulus undershoot (PSU) that peaks 6–10 s after the stimulus ends [138, 140]. As previously discussed, the positive phase of the BOLD response has been associated with an increase in CBF, and subsequent change in the ratio of oxy- to deoxyhemoglobin intravascularly [138]. The biophysical origins of the PSU remain more controversial. An early model attributed the PSU to temporal delays between when CBF (earlier response) and CBV (delayed response) returned to baseline levels [138, 141]. However, more recent work suggests that the duration of the PSU extends beyond even when CBV returns to baseline [142], leading others to suggest that increased metabolic demands ($CMRO_2$) following cellular signaling may contribute to the PSU [142, 143].

Thus, there are several different individual mechanisms as well as combinatory effects by which head trauma can alter the different phases of the BOLD response. Foremost, trauma can result in frank neuronal (e.g., alterations in synchronous neuronal activity) dysfunction, causing downstream effects on BOLD-based activity by changing the amount of glutamate in the synaptic cleft and the energetic needs of cells following neurotransmission [73, 134]. Direct support for this hypothesis comes from reports of neuronal loss in animal models of fluid percussion injury [144] and abnormal cell signaling [145]. Indirect support for this hypothesis comes from findings of altered concentrations of glutamate and glutamine in the semi-acute stage of mTBI during magnetic resonance spectroscopy [146–148] as well as through more invasive measures during more severe injury models [149–152].

TBI has also been shown to directly reduce both CBF and metabolism, both of which would affect the BOLD response. CBF and transit time are reduced in human models of severe TBI [153], as well as cerebral perfusion [154]. Metabolic failure following TBI occurs even in the presence of normal perfusion [155], with an initial decoupling between CBF and CMR_{glu}, followed by a generally reduced cerebral metabolism [72, 154]. Animal models suggest that alterations in CBF and CMR_{glu} may be the most long-lasting physiological deficits of concussion [72], and thus the BOLD response should also be similarly affected for a longer duration following injury. Trauma may also directly affect the structural integrity of the microvasculature. Animal studies based on the fluid percussion model indicate a semi-acute reduction in capillary number and diameter both at the injury site and distally [156], with other studies suggesting that TBI also results in neurogenic damage within the perivascular nerve network [157]. Hemosiderin depositions, secondary to microhemorrhages and inflammation, have also been noted in the autopsy report of an mTBI patient who died 7 months post-injury [158].

At present, it would be unfeasible to draw conclusions about the relative importance of these different mechanisms as they pertain to previously reported finding of hypo- and hyperactivation in clinical samples of mTBI [9, 31]. Animal models of injury frequently make recordings during the baseline state (e.g., anesthetized animals), which is known to produce differential dynamics between BOLD constituents (e.g., CBF, $CMRO_2$, and CMR_{glu}) relative to more dynamic states (evoked activity). Several papers have recently examined fcMRI in animal models of neuronal injury [159, 160], with other studies [161] reducing/eliminating anesthesia protocols that can alter the neuronal response and/or neurovascular coupling. Future animal studies that specifically examine how mTBI affects both intrinsic and evoked BOLD-related activity will greatly improve our knowledge of the true bench-to-bedside capabilities of this technique in a more controlled environment.

Similarly, multimodal neuroimaging techniques can be used in conjunction with standard BOLD imaging techniques to potentially isolate physiological changes associated with neuropathophysiology. For example, spectroscopy can be used in conjunction with fMRI to get more direct measures of the level of excitatory neurotransmitters and measures of cellular energetics and death [146, 148, 162, 163]. Matthews and colleagues used combined DTI and fMRI methods to understand differences in amygdala activation to emotional faces in concussed Operation Enduring Freedom and Iraqi Freedom veterans with and without depressive symptoms [164]. fMRI results demonstrated abnormal amygdala activity in veterans with depressive symptoms that was associated with lower fractional anisotropy (FA) in several white matter tracts, suggesting that functional disruption may be the direct results of structural pathology in white matter tracts. Similarly, we have examined the relationship between functional connectivity and FA within white matter tracts that connect the DMN and frontal areas during the semi-acute and more chronic stages of mTBI [11]. Finally, electroencephalography (EEG) and magnetoencephalography (MEG) both provide a more direct measure of neuronal activity at much higher temporal resolution [23, 43, 165, 166], eliminating some of the interpretative problems associated with fMRI. Importantly, EEG and fMRI can be acquired simultaneously within the scanner environment [167, 168], providing an unheralded access into brain pathology following mTBI that affords both high spatial and temporal fidelity.

As previously discussed, fMRI signals are critically linked to CBF, and the dysregulation of autonomic control of neurovascular coupling remains a challenge for future neuroimaging studies of mTBI. Arterial spin labeling measures of CBF have also been used to calibrate the BOLD signal [169, 170], although the measurements must be made in a quantitative fashion. Hypercapnic normalization is another frequently used technique that is achieved through the administration of CO_2, a voluntary breathhold scan or more regularized breathing [171, 172]. This method assumes that hypercapnia has a limited effect on neural activity and oxygen metabolism and thus primarily measures CBF [173, 174]. Previous results suggest that the hypercapnia method accounts for variability in subject vasculature and physiology differences during task performance, as well as changes in magnetic field strength [175–177]. A primary limitation of the method is that it requires the subjects to calmly hold their breath during an EPI acquisition and/or the administration of CO_2, both of which may increase the rate of anxiety in participants and subsequently affect subject motion.

fMRI Analyses

The final section of the chapter discusses several analytic considerations for performing fMRI research following mTBI. First, in spite of the known complexity of the BOLD response, previous research in both mild and more severe forms of TBI has typically estimated only a single parameter (typically a beta coefficient) by convolving an assumed canonical HRF (e.g., a gamma variate or a double gamma variate function) with known experimental conditions (e.g., onset of a particular trial) to derive a predictor function (e.g., regressor). Importantly, this assumes that the different phases of the hemodynamic response (positive phase and PSU) and their relationship to each other are largely unaffected by mTBI. To date, only a single study has explicitly examined the HRF in more severe TBI [178] reporting that although basic visual stimuli were associated with an increased volume of activation in the TBI group, there were no differences in the basic shape of the HRF.

More fMRI studies are needed in both human and animal models that explicitly compare the different aspects of the HRF as well as their individual sensitivity and specificity.

Investigators have also traditionally utilized region of interest (ROI) or voxel-wise analyses to directly compare the BOLD response between mTBI patients and healthy controls. However, both of these analytic methods are based on the implicit assumption that heterogeneous initial injury conditions (e.g., patients in a motor vehicle accidents versus patients who experienced a blow to the left temple) results in a homogenous (i.e., high degree of spatial overlap) pattern of grey matter abnormalities that would survive group-wise statistics. Although lesions tend to be more common in the diencephalon, mid-brain, limbic circuit, and prefrontal cortex [6, 179], the basic premise of the spatial homogeneity assumption is likely to be flawed. Therefore, it is increasingly being recognized that novel approaches for classifying heterogeneous lesion locations are necessary for performing mTBI imaging research [180–182]. For example, in diffusion tensor imaging studies of white matter injuries, variations on normative (i.e., z-scores) transformations [181–185] or bootstrapping [186] have been utilized to identify voxel-wise abnormalities on a patient-by-patient basis. While the logical appeal of these newer approaches is clearly superior, the underlying assumptions are likely to be dependent on the statistical properties of the data (e.g., sample size, distribution properties, and normalcy) and have not been thoroughly vetted in the context of typical neuroimaging data [180]. To our knowledge, these novel approaches have not yet been applied to BOLD imaging data to determine regions of anomalous activity on an individual subject level.

Conclusions

In summary, fMRI provides researchers with the ability to noninvasively measure the functional integrity of neuronal circuitry in both animal and human models of mTBI at relatively high spatial resolution. The ability to dynamically measure brain function during higher-order cognitive and emotive tasks represents a clear advantage relative to other imaging techniques that are only capable of measuring structural integrity (e.g., susceptibility weighted imaging, DTI). Moreover, unlike other functional techniques, fMRI is equally capable of probing deep grey structures as well as cortex. However, the dynamic nature of the BOLD signal also makes it more susceptible to nonspecific effects of trauma (e.g., pain, fatigue), behavioral performance, effort on testing, and normal day-to-day variations in human behavior. Moreover, the BOLD signal represents an indirect measure of neuronal activity that results from a complex mixture of many underlying physiological processes, all of which can be affected by trauma. Thus, clearly identifying the one, two, or multiple mechanistic causes of an "abnormal" BOLD signal will not be feasible when this technique is used in isolation.

References

 1. Faul M, Xu L, Wald MM, Coronado VG. Traumatic brain injury in the United States: emergency department visits, hospitalizations, and deaths. Atlanta, GA: CDC; 2010.
 2. Ruff RM, Iverson GL, Barth JT, Bush SS, Broshek DK. Recommendations for diagnosing a mild traumatic brain injury: a National Academy of Neuropsychology education paper. Arch Clin Neuropsychol. 2009;24(1):3–10.
 3. Hughes DG, Jackson A, Mason DL, Berry E, Hollis S, Yates DW. Abnormalities on magnetic resonance imaging seen acutely following mild traumatic brain injury: correlation with neuropsychological tests and delayed recovery. Neuroradiology. 2004;46(7):550–8.
 4. Iverson GL. Complicated vs uncomplicated mild traumatic brain injury: acute neuropsychological outcome. Brain Inj. 2006;20(13–14):1335–44.
 5. Belanger HG, Vanderploeg RD, Curtiss G, Warden DL. Recent neuroimaging techniques in mild traumatic brain injury. J Neuropsychiatry Clin Neurosci. 2007;19(1):5–20.
 6. Bigler ED, Maxwell WL. Neuropathology of mild traumatic brain injury: relationship to neuroimaging findings. Brain Imaging Behav. 2012;6(2):108–36.
 7. McAllister TW, Saykin AJ, Flashman LA, Sparling MB, Johnson SC, Guerin SJ, et al. Brain activation during working memory 1 month after mild traumatic brain injury: a functional MRI study. Neurology. 1999;53(6):1300–8.
 8. McAllister TW, Sparling MB, Flashman LA, Guerin SJ, Mamourian AC, Saykin AJ. Differential working memory load effects after mild traumatic brain injury. Neuroimage. 2001;14(5):1004–12.
 9. McDonald BC, Saykin AJ, McAllister TW. Functional MRI of mild traumatic brain injury (mTBI): progress and perspectives from the first decade of studies. Brain Imaging Behav. 2012;6(2):193–207.
10. Johnson B, Zhang K, Gay M, Horovitz S, Hallett M, Sebastianelli W, et al. Alteration of brain default network in subacute phase of injury in concussed individuals: resting-state fMRI study. Neuroimage. 2012;59(1):511–8.
11. Mayer AR, Mannell MV, Ling J, Gasparovic C, Yeo RA. Functional connectivity in mild traumatic brain injury. Hum Brain Mapp. 2011;32(11):1825–35.
12. Shumskaya E, Andriessen TM, Norris DG, Vos PE. Abnormal whole-brain functional networks in homogeneous acute mild traumatic brain injury. Neurology. 2012;79(2):175–82.
13. Belanger HG, Curtiss G, Demery JA, Lebowitz BK, Vanderploeg RD. Factors moderating neuropsychological outcomes following mild traumatic brain injury: a meta-analysis. J Int Neuropsychol Soc. 2005;11(3):215–27.
14. Bigler ED. Neuropsychology and clinical neuroscience of persistent post-concussive syndrome. J Int Neuropsychol Soc. 2008;14(1):1–22.
15. Iverson GL. Outcome from mild traumatic brain injury. Curr Opin Psychiatry. 2005;18(3):301–17.
16. Schretlen DJ, Shapiro AM. A quantitative review of the effects of traumatic brain injury on cognitive functioning. Int Rev Psychiatry. 2003;15(4):341–9.
17. Lehman EJ, Hein MJ, Baron SL, Gersic CM. Neurodegenerative causes of death among retired National Football League players. Neurology. 2012;79(19):1970–4.
18. McKee AC, Cantu RC, Nowinski CJ, Hedley-Whyte ET, Gavett BE, Budson AE, et al. Chronic traumatic encephalopathy in athletes: progressive tauopathy after repetitive head injury. J Neuropathol Exp Neurol. 2009;68(7):709–35.
19. McKee AC, Stein TD, Nowinski CJ, Stern RA, Daneshvar DH, Alvarez VE, et al. The spectrum of disease in chronic traumatic encephalopathy. Brain. 2012;136(Pt 1):43–64.
20. Rosenbaum SB, Lipton ML. Embracing chaos: the scope and importance of clinical and pathological heterogeneity in mTBI. Brain Imaging Behav. 2012;6(2):255–82.
21. McAllister TW, Flashman LA, McDonald BC, Saykin AJ. Mechanisms of working memory dysfunction after mild and moderate TBI: evidence from functional MRI and neurogenetics. J Neurotrauma. 2006;23(10):1450–67.

22. Smits M, Dippel DW, Houston GC, Wielopolski PA, Koudstaal PJ, Hunink MG, et al. Postconcussion syndrome after minor head injury: brain activation of working memory and attention. Hum Brain Mapp. 2009;30(9):2789–803.
23. Gosselin N, Bottari C, Chen JK, Petrides M, Tinawi S, de Guise E, et al. Electrophysiology and functional MRI in post-acute mild traumatic brain injury. J Neurotrauma. 2011;28(3): 329–41.
24. Stulemeijer M, Vos PE, van der Werf S, Van DG, Rijpkema M, Fernandez G. How mild traumatic brain injury may affect declarative memory performance in the post-acute stage. J Neurotrauma. 2010;27(9):1585–95.
25. Chen JK, Johnston KM, Frey S, Petrides M, Worsley K, Ptito A. Functional abnormalities in symptomatic concussed athletes: an fMRI study. Neuroimage. 2004;22(1):68–82.
26. Chen JK, Johnston KM, Collie A, McCrory P, Ptito A. A validation of the post concussion symptom scale in the assessment of complex concussion using cognitive testing and functional MRI. J Neurol Neurosurg Psychiatry. 2007;78(11):1231–8.
27. Chen JK, Johnston KM, Petrides M, Ptito A. Neural substrates of symptoms of depression following concussion in male athletes with persisting postconcussion symptoms. Arch Gen Psychiatry. 2008;65(1):81–9.
28. Jantzen KJ, Anderson B, Steinberg FL, Kelso JA. A prospective functional MR imaging study of mild traumatic brain injury in college football players. AJNR Am J Neuroradiol. 2004;25(5):738–45.
29. Lovell MR, Pardini JE, Welling J, Collins MW, Bakal J, Lazar N, et al. Functional brain abnormalities are related to clinical recovery and time to return-to-play in athletes. Neurosurgery. 2007;61(2):352–9.
30. Talavage TM, Nauman E, Breedlove EL, Yoruk U, Dye AE, Morigaki K, et al. Functionally-detected cognitive impairment in high school football players without clinically-diagnosed concussion. J Neurotrauma. E-publication April 2013.
31. Mayer AR, Mannell MV, Ling J, Elgie R, Gasparovic C, Phillips JP, et al. Auditory orienting and inhibition of return in mild traumatic brain injury: a FMRI study. Hum Brain Mapp. 2009;30(12):4152–66.
32. Yang Z, Yeo R, Pena A, Ling J, Klimaj S, Campbell R, et al. A fMRI study of auditory orienting and inhibition of return in pediatric mild traumatic brain injury. J Neurotrauma. 2012;26(12): 2124–36.
33. Mayer AR, Yang Z, Yeo RA, Pena A, Ling JM, Mannell MV, et al. A functional MRI study of multimodal selective attention following mild traumatic brain injury. Brain Imaging Behav. 2012;6(2):343–54.
34. Witt ST, Lovejoy DW, Pearlson GD, Stevens MC. Decreased prefrontal cortex activity in mild traumatic brain injury during performance of an auditory oddball task. Brain Imaging Behav. 2010;4(3–4):232–47.
35. Slobounov SM, Zhang K, Pennell D, Ray W, Johnson B, Sebastianelli W. Functional abnormalities in normally appearing athletes following mild traumatic brain injury: a functional MRI study. Exp Brain Res. 2010;202(2):341–54.
36. McAllister TW, Flashman LA, McDonald BC, Ferrell RB, Tosteson TD, Yanofsky NN, et al. Dopaminergic challenge with bromocriptine one month after mild traumatic brain injury: altered working memory and BOLD response. J Neuropsychiatry Clin Neurosci. 2011;23(3): 277–86.
37. McAllister TW, McDonald BC, Flashman LA, Ferrell RB, Tosteson TD, Yanofsky NN, et al. Alpha-2 adrenergic challenge with guanfacine one month after mild traumatic brain injury: altered working memory and BOLD response. Int J Psychophysiol. 2011;82(1):107–14.
38. Laatsch LK, Thulborn KR, Krisky CM, Shobat DM, Sweeney JA. Investigating the neurobiological basis of cognitive rehabilitation therapy with fMRI. Brain Inj. 2004;18(10):957–74.
39. Raichle ME, Mintun MA. Brain work and brain imaging. Annu Rev Neurosci. 2006;29: 449–76.
40. Hyder F, Patel AB, Gjedde A, Rothman DL, Behar KL, Shulman RG. Neuronal-glial glucose oxidation and glutamatergic-GABAergic function. J Cereb Blood Flow Metab. 2006;26(7): 865–77.

264   A.R. Mayer and P.S.F. Bellgowan

41. Mangia S, Giove F, Tkac I, Logothetis NK, Henry PG, Olman CA, et al. Metabolic and hemodynamic events after changes in neuronal activity: current hypotheses, theoretical predictions and in vivo NMR experimental findings. J Cereb Blood Flow Metab. 2009;29(3):441–63.
42. Barkhoudarian G, Hovda DA, Giza CC. The molecular pathophysiology of concussive brain injury. Clin Sports Med. 2011;30(1):33–348.
43. Huang M, Theilmann RJ, Robb A, Angeles A, Nichols S, Drake A, et al. Integrated imaging approach with MEG and DTI to detect mild traumatic brain injury in military and civilian patients. J Neurotrauma. 2009;26(8):1213–26.
44. Huang MX, Nichols S, Robb A, Angeles A, Drake A, Holland M, et al. An automatic MEG low-frequency source imaging approach for detecting injuries in mild and moderate TBI patients with blast and non-blast causes. Neuroimage. 2012;61(4):1067–82.
45. Lewine J, Davis J, Sloan J, Kodituwakku P, Orrison WJ. Neuromagnetic assessment of pathophysiologic brain activity induced by minor head. AJNR Am J Neuroradiol. 1999;20(5): 857–66.
46. Morcom AM, Fletcher PC. Does the brain have a baseline? Why we should be resisting a rest. Neuroimage. 2007;37(4):1073–82.
47. Saad ZS, Gotts SJ, Murphy K, Chen G, Jo HJ, Martin A, et al. Trouble at rest: how correlation patterns and group differences become distorted after global signal regression. Brain Connect. 2012;2(1):25–32.
48. Smith SM, Fox PT, Miller KL, Glahn DC, Fox PM, Mackay CE, et al. Correspondence of the brain's functional architecture during activation and rest. Proc Natl Acad Sci USA. 2009; 106(31):13040–5.
49. Boly M, Phillips C, Tshibanda L, Vanhaudenhuyse A, Schabus M, Dang-Vu TT, et al. Intrinsic brain activity in altered states of consciousness: how conscious is the default mode of brain function? Ann N Y Acad Sci. 2008;1129:119–29.
50. Boly M, Tshibanda L, Vanhaudenhuyse A, Noirhomme Q, Schnakers C, Ledoux D, et al. Functional connectivity in the default network during resting state is preserved in a vegetative but not in a brain dead patient. Hum Brain Mapp. 2009;30(8):2393–400.
51. Vanhaudenhuyse A, Noirhomme Q, Tshibanda LJ, Bruno MA, Boveroux P, Schnakers C, et al. Default network connectivity reflects the level of consciousness in non-communicative brain-damaged patients. Brain. 2010;133(1):161–71.
52. Buckner RL, Andrews-Hanna J, Schacter D. The brain's default network: anatomy, function, and relevance to disease. Ann N Y Acad Sci. 2008;1124:1–38.
53. Andrews-Hanna JR, Reidler JS, Sepulcre J, Poulin R, Buckner RL. Functional-anatomic fractionation of the brain's default network. Neuron. 2010;65(4):550–62.
54. Binder JR, Frost JA, Hammeke TA, Bellgowan PS, Rao SM, Cox RW. Conceptual processing during the conscious resting state: a functional MRI study. J Cogn Neurosci. 1999;11(1):80–95.
55. Eichele T, Debener S, Calhoun VD, Specht K, Engel AK, Hugdahl K, et al. Prediction of human errors by maladaptive changes in event-related brain networks. Proc Natl Acad Sci USA. 2008;105(16):6173–8.
56. Weissman DH, Roberts KC, Visscher KM, Woldorff MG. The neural bases of momentary lapses in attention. Nat Neurosci. 2006;9(7):971–8.
57. Fox MD, Snyder AZ, Vincent JL, Corbetta M, Van E, Raichle ME. The human brain is intrinsically organized into dynamic, anticorrelated functional networks. Proc Natl Acad Sci USA. 2005;102(27):9673–8.
58. Nakamura T, Hillary FG, Biswal BB. Resting network plasticity following brain injury. PLoS One. 2009;4(12):e8220.
59. Bonnelle V, Leech R, Kinnunen KM, Ham TE, Beckmann CF, De Boissezon X, et al. Default mode network connectivity predicts sustained attention deficits after traumatic brain injury. J Neurosci. 2011;31(38):13442–51.
60. Zhou Y, Milham MP, Lui YW, Miles L, Reaume J, Sodickson DK, et al. Default-mode network disruption in mild traumatic brain injury. Radiology. 2012;265(3):882–92.
61. Zhang K, Johnson B, Gay M, Horovitz SG, Hallett M, Sebastianelli W, et al. Default mode network in concussed individuals in response to the YMCA physical stress test. J Neurotrauma. 2012;29(5):756–65.

62. Slobounov SM, Gay M, Zhang K, Johnson B, Pennell D, Sebastianelli W, et al. Alteration of brain functional network at rest and in response to YMCA physical stress test in concussed athletes: RsFMRI study. Neuroimage. 2011;55(4):1716–27.
63. Tang L, Ge Y, Sodickson DK, Miles L, Zhou Y, Reaume J, et al. Thalamic resting-state functional networks: disruption in patients with mild traumatic brain injury. Radiology. 2011;260(3):831–40.
64. Stevens MC, Lovejoy D, Kim J, Oakes H, Kureshi I, Witt ST. Multiple resting state network functional connectivity abnormalities in mild traumatic brain injury. Brain Imaging Behav. 2012;6(2):293–318.
65. Sperling R, Greve D, Dale A, Killiany R, Holmes J, Rosas HD, et al. Functional MRI detection of pharmacologically induced memory impairment. Proc Natl Acad Sci USA. 2002;99(1):455–60.
66. Vollm B, Richardson P, McKie S, Elliott R, Deakin JF, Anderson IM. Serotonergic modulation of neuronal responses to behavioural inhibition and reinforcing stimuli: an fMRI study in healthy volunteers. Eur J Neurosci. 2006;23(2):552–60.
67. Wagner G, Koch K, Schachtzabel C, Sobanski T, Reichenbach JR, Sauer H, et al. Differential effects of serotonergic and noradrenergic antidepressants on brain activity during a cognitive control task and neurofunctional prediction of treatment outcome in patients with depression. J Psychiatry Neurosci. 2010;35(4):247–57.
68. Hutchison M, Mainwaring LM, Comper P, Richards DW, Bisschop SM. Differential emotional responses of varsity athletes to concussion and musculoskeletal injuries. Clin J Sport Med. 2009;19(1):13–9.
69. Hutchison M, Comper P, Mainwaring L, Richards D. The influence of musculoskeletal injury on cognition: implications for concussion research. Am J Sports Med. 2011;39(11):2331–7.
70. Lee H, Wintermark M, Gean AD, Ghajar J, Manley GT, Mukherjee P. Focal lesions in acute mild traumatic brain injury and neurocognitive outcome: CT versus 3T MRI. J Neurotrauma. 2008;25(9):1049–56.
71. Kashluba S, Hanks RA, Casey JE, Millis SR. Neuropsychologic and functional outcome after complicated mild traumatic brain injury. Arch Phys Med Rehabil. 2008;89(5):904–11.
72. Giza CC, Hovda DA. The neurometabolic cascade of concussion. J Athl Train. 2001;36(3):228–35.
73. Logothetis NK. What we can do and what we cannot do with fMRI. Nature. 2008;453(7197):869–78.
74. Desmond JE, Glover GH. Estimating sample size in functional MRI (fMRI) neuroimaging studies: statistical power analyses. J Neurosci Methods. 2002;118(2):115–28.
75. Booher MA, Wisniewski J, Smith BW, Sigurdsson A. Comparison of reporting systems to determine concussion incidence in NCAA Division I collegiate football. Clin J Sport Med. 2003;13(2):93–5.
76. Echemendia RJ, Cantu RC. Return to play following sports-related mild traumatic brain injury: the role for neuropsychology. Appl Neuropsychol. 2003;10(1):48–55.
77. Greenwald RM, Chu JJ, Beckwith JG, Crisco JJ. A proposed method to reduce underreporting of brain injury in sports. Clin J Sport Med. 2012;22(2):83–5.
78. Bianchini KJ, Curtis KL, Greve KW. Compensation and malingering in traumatic brain injury: a dose–response relationship? Clin Neuropsychol. 2006;20(4):831–47.
79. Greve KW, Bianchini KJ, Doane BM. Classification accuracy of the test of memory malingering in traumatic brain injury: results of a known-groups analysis. J Clin Exp Neuropsychol. 2006;28(7):1176–90.
80. Chrisman SP, Quitiquit C, Rivara FP. Qualitative study of barriers to concussive symptom reporting in high school athletics. J Adolesc Health. 2013;52(3):330–5.
81. Gilbert F, Johnson LS. The impact of American tackle football-related concussion in youth athletes. AJOB Neurosci. 2011;2(4):48–59.
82. McCrea M, Hammeke T, Olsen G, Leo P, Guskiewicz K. Unreported concussion in high school football players: implications for prevention. Clin J Sport Med. 2004;14(1):13–7.

83. Guskiewicz KM, Marshall SW, Bailes J, McCrea M, Cantu RC, Randolph C, et al. Association between recurrent concussion and late-life cognitive impairment in retired professional football players. Neurosurgery. 2005;57(4):719–26.
84. Guskiewicz KM, Marshall SW, Bailes J, McCrea M, Harding Jr HP, Matthews A, et al. Recurrent concussion and risk of depression in retired professional football players. Med Sci Sports Exerc. 2007;39(6):903–9.
85. Harmon KG, Drezner JA, Gammons M, Guskiewicz KM, Halstead M, Herring SA, et al. American Medical Society for Sports Medicine position statement: concussion in sport. Br J Sports Med. 2013;47(1):15–26.
86. McCrory P, Meeuwisse WH, Aubry M, Cantu B, Dvorak J, Echemendia RJ, et al. Consensus statement on concussion in sport: the 4th International Conference on Concussion in Sport held in Zurich, November 2012. Br J Sports Med. 2013;47(5):250–8.
87. Guskiewicz KM, McCrea M, Marshall SW, Cantu RC, Randolph C, Barr W, et al. Cumulative effects associated with recurrent concussion in collegiate football players: the NCAA Concussion Study. JAMA. 2003;290(19):2549–55.
88. McCrea M, Guskiewicz KM, Marshall SW, Barr W, Randolph C, Cantu RC, et al. Acute effects and recovery time following concussion in collegiate football players: the NCAA Concussion Study. JAMA. 2003;290(19):2556–63.
89. Friess SH, Ichord RN, Ralston J, Ryall K, Helfaer MA, Smith C, et al. Repeated traumatic brain injury affects composite cognitive function in piglets. J Neurotrauma. 2009;10:1111–21.
90. Dikmen SS, Bombardier CH, Machamer JE, Fann JR, Temkin NR. Natural history of depression in traumatic brain injury. Arch Phys Med Rehabil. 2004;85(9):1457–64.
91. Jorge RE, Robinson RG, Starkstein SE, Arndt SV. Depression and anxiety following traumatic brain injury. J Neuropsychiatry Clin Neurosci. 1993;5(4):469–74.
92. Koponen S, Taiminen T, Portin R, Himanen L, Isoniemi H, Heinonen H, et al. Axis I and II psychiatric disorders after traumatic brain injury: a 30-year follow-up study. Am J Psychiatry. 2002;159(8):1315–21.
93. Kreutzer JS, Seel RT, Gourley E. The prevalence and symptom rates of depression after traumatic brain injury: a comprehensive examination. Brain Inj. 2001;15(7):563–76.
94. Covassin T, Elbin III RJ, Larson E, Kontos AP. Sex and age differences in depression and baseline sport-related concussion neurocognitive performance and symptoms. Clin J Sport Med. 2012;22(2):98–104.
95. Kontos AP, Covassin T, Elbin RJ, Parker T. Depression and neurocognitive performance after concussion among male and female high school and collegiate athletes. Arch Phys Med Rehabil. 2012;93(10):1751–6.
96. Schaal K, Tafflet M, Nassif H, Thibault V, Pichard C, Alcotte M, et al. Psychological balance in high level athletes: gender-based differences and sport-specific patterns. PLoS One. 2011;6(5):e19007.
97. American College of Health Association. American College Health Association-National College Health Assessment II: Reference Group Executive Summary Fall 2011. Hanover, MD: American College Health Association; 2012.
98. Donohue B, Covassin T, Lancer K, Dickens Y, Miller A, Hash A, et al. Examination of psychiatric symptoms in student athletes. J Gen Psychol. 2004;131(1):29–35.
99. Eisenberg D, Gollust SE, Golberstein E, Hefner JL. Prevalence and correlates of depression, anxiety, and suicidality among university students. Am J Orthopsychiatry. 2007;77(4):534–42.
100. Ackery A, Provvidenza C, Tator CH. Concussion in hockey: compliance with return to play advice and follow-up status. Can J Neurol Sci. 2009;36(2):207–12.
101. Hoge CW, McGurk D, Thomas JL, Cox AL, Engel CC, Castro CA. Mild traumatic brain injury in U.S. soldiers returning from Iraq. N Engl J Med. 2008;358(5):453–63.
102. Konrad C, Geburek AJ, Rist F, Blumenroth H, Fischer B, Husstedt I, et al. Long-term cognitive and emotional consequences of mild traumatic brain injury. Psychol Med. 2011;41(6):1197–211.

103. Lange RT, Iverson GL, Rose A. Post-concussion symptom reporting and the "good-old-days" bias following mild traumatic brain injury. Arch Clin Neuropsychol. 2010;25(5):442–50.
104. Mittenberg W, Strauman S. Diagnosis of mild head injury and the postconcussion syndrome. J Head Trauma Rehabil. 2000;15(2):783–91.
105. Yang CC, Hua MS, Tu YK, Huang SJ. Early clinical characteristics of patients with persistent post-concussion symptoms: a prospective study. Brain Inj. 2009;23(4):299–306.
106. Max JE, Keatley E, Wilde EA, Bigler ED, Levin HS, Schachar RJ, et al. Anxiety disorders in children and adolescents in the first six months after traumatic brain injury. J Neuropsychiatry Clin Neurosci. 2011;23(1):29–39.
107. Max JE, Keatley E, Wilde EA, Bigler ED, Schachar RJ, Saunders AE, et al. Depression in children and adolescents in the first 6 months after traumatic brain injury. Int J Dev Neurosci. 2012;30(3):239–45.
108. Yeates KO, Kaizar E, Rusin J, Bangert B, Dietrich A, Nuss K, et al. Reliable change in post-concussive symptoms and its functional consequences among children with mild traumatic brain injury. Arch Pediatr Adolesc Med. 2012;166(7):615–22.
109. Field M, Collins MW, Lovell MR, Maroon J. Does age play a role in recovery from sports-related concussion? A comparison of high school and collegiate athletes. J Pediatr. 2003;142(5):546–53.
110. McCrory P, Johnston K, Meeuwisse W, Aubry M, Cantu R, Dvorak J, et al. Summary and agreement statement of the 2nd International Conference on Concussion in Sport, Prague 2004. Br J Sports Med. 2005;39(4):196–204.
111. Bombardier CH, Fann JR, Temkin NR, Esselman PC, Barber J, Dikmen SS. Rates of major depressive disorder and clinical outcomes following traumatic brain injury. JAMA. 2010;303(19): 1938–45.
112. Cicerone KD, Kalmar K. Does premorbid depression influence post-concussive symptoms and neuropsychological functioning? Brain Inj. 1997;11(9):643–8.
113. Clarke LA, Genat RC, Anderson JF. Long-term cognitive complaint and post-concussive symptoms following mild traumatic brain injury: the role of cognitive and affective factors. Brain Inj. 2012;26(3):298–307.
114. Alderfer BS, Arciniegas DB, Silver JM. Treatment of depression following traumatic brain injury. J Head Trauma Rehabil. 2005;20(6):544–62.
115. Bay E, Kirsch N, Gillespie B. Chronic stress conditions do explain posttraumatic brain injury depression. Res Theory Nurs Pract. 2004;18(2–3):213–28.
116. Pagulayan KF, Hoffman JM, Temkin NR, Machamer JE, Dikmen SS. Functional limitations and depression after traumatic brain injury: examination of the temporal relationship. Arch Phys Med Rehabil. 2008;89(10):1887–92.
117. Dantzer R. Cytokine-induced sickness behavior: mechanisms and implications. Ann N Y Acad Sci. 2001;933:222–34.
118. Dantzer R, O'Connor JC, Lawson MA, Kelley KW. Inflammation-associated depression: from serotonin to kynurenine. Psychoneuroendocrinology. 2011;36(3):426–36.
119. Dantzer R. Depression and inflammation: an intricate relationship. Biol Psychiatry. 2012;71(1):4–5.
120. Blaylock RL, Maroon J. Immunoexcitotoxicity as a central mechanism in chronic traumatic encephalopathy—a unifying hypothesis. Surg Neurol Int. 2011;2:107.
121. Patterson ZR, Holahan MR. Understanding the neuroinflammatory response following concussion to develop treatment strategies. Front Cell Neurosci. 2012;6:58.
122. Bellgowan P, Singh R, Kuplicki R, Taylor A, Polanski D, Allen T, et al. Global functional connectivity in the visceromotor network is negatively correlated with IL-1ß serum levels in concussed athletes. J Neurotrauma. 2012;29(10):58.
123. Price JL, Drevets WC. Neural circuits underlying the pathophysiology of mood disorders. Trends Cogn Sci. 2012;16(1):61–71.
124. Holsboer F, Lauer CJ, Schreiber W, Krieg JC. Altered hypothalamic-pituitary-adrenocortical regulation in healthy subjects at high familial risk for affective disorders. Neuroendocrinology. 1995;62(4):340–7.

125. Urry HL, van Reekum CM, Johnstone T, Kalin NH, Thurow ME, Schaefer HS, et al. Amygdala and ventromedial prefrontal cortex are inversely coupled during regulation of negative affect and predict the diurnal pattern of cortisol secretion among older adults. J Neurosci. 2006;26(16):4415–25.
126. Watson D, Pennebaker JW. Health complaints, stress, and distress: exploring the central role of negative affectivity. Psychol Rev. 1989;96(2):234–54.
127. Erickson K, Drevets W, Schulkin J. Glucocorticoid regulation of diverse cognitive functions in normal and pathological emotional states. Neurosci Biobehav Rev. 2003;27(3):233–46.
128. Johnson EO, Kamilaris TC, Chrousos GP, Gold PW. Mechanisms of stress: a dynamic overview of hormonal and behavioral homeostasis. Neurosci Biobehav Rev. 1992;16(2):115–30.
129. Gavett BE, Stern RA, McKee AC. Chronic traumatic encephalopathy: a potential late effect of sport-related concussive and subconcussive head trauma. Clin Sports Med. 2011;30(1): 179–88.
130. Gavett BE, Cantu RC, Shenton M, Lin AP, Nowinski CJ, McKee AC, et al. Clinical appraisal of chronic traumatic encephalopathy: current perspectives and future directions. Curr Opin Neurol. 2011;24(6):525–31.
131. Barnes SM, Walter KH, Chard KM. Does a history of mild traumatic brain injury increase suicide risk in veterans with PTSD? Rehabil Psychol. 2012;57(1):18–26.
132. Teasdale TW, Engberg AW. Suicide after traumatic brain injury: a population study. J Neurol Neurosurg Psychiatry. 2001;71(4):436–40.
133. Sokoloff L, Reivich M, Kennedy C, Des Rosiers MH, Patlak CS, Pettigrew KD, et al. The [14C]deoxyglucose method for the measurement of local cerebral glucose utilization: theory, procedure, and normal values in the conscious and anesthetized albino rat. J Neurochem. 1977;28(5):897–916.
134. Attwell D, Buchan AM, Charpak S, Lauritzen M, Macvicar BA, Newman EA. Glial and neuronal control of brain blood flow. Nature. 2010;468(7321):232–43.
135. Logothetis NK, Wandell BA. Interpreting the BOLD signal. Annu Rev Physiol. 2004;66: 735–69.
136. Mangia S, Tkac I, Gruetter R, Van de Moortele PF, Maraviglia B, Ugurbil K. Sustained neuronal activation raises oxidative metabolism to a new steady-state level: evidence from 1H NMR spectroscopy in the human visual cortex. J Cereb Blood Flow Metab. 2007;27(5):1055–63.
137. Fox PT, Raichle ME. Focal physiological uncoupling of cerebral blood flow and oxidative metabolism during somatosensory stimulation in human subjects. Proc Natl Acad Sci USA. 1986;83(4):1140–4.
138. Buxton RB, Uludag K, Dubowitz DJ, Liu TT. Modeling the hemodynamic response to brain activation. Neuroimage. 2004;23(1):S220–33.
139. Shen Q, Ren H, Duong TQ. CBF, BOLD, CBV, and CMRO(2) fMRI signal temporal dynamics at 500-msec resolution. J Magn Reson Imaging. 2008;27(3):599–606.
140. Cohen M. Parametric analysis of fMRI data using linear systems methods. Neuroimage. 1997;6(2):93–103.
141. Buxton RB, Wong EC, Frank LR. Dynamics of blood flow and oxygenation changes during brain activation: the balloon model. Magn Reson Med. 1998;39(6):855–64.
142. Lu H, Golay X, Pekar JJ, van Zijl PC. Sustained poststimulus elevation in cerebral oxygen utilization after vascular recovery. J Cereb Blood Flow Metab. 2004;24(7):764–70.
143. Schroeter ML, Kupka T, Mildner T, Uludag K, von Cramon DY. Investigating the post-stimulus undershoot of the BOLD signal—a simultaneous fMRI and fNIRS study. Neuroimage. 2006;30(2):349–58.
144. Lowenstein DH, Thomas MJ, Smith DH, McIntosh TK. Selective vulnerability of dentate hilar neurons following traumatic brain injury: a potential mechanistic link between head trauma and disorders of the hippocampus. J Neurosci. 1992;12(12):4846–53.
145. Alwis DS, Yan EB, Morganti-Kossmann MC, Rajan R. Sensory cortex underpinnings of traumatic brain injury deficits. PLoS One. 2012;7(12):e52169.
146. Henry LC, Tremblay S, Leclerc S, Khiat A, Boulanger Y, Ellemberg D, et al. Metabolic changes in concussed American football players during the acute and chronic post-injury phases. BMC Neurol. 2011;11:105.

147. Gasparovic C, Yeo R, Mannell M, Ling J, Elgie R, Phillips J, et al. Neurometabolite concentrations in gray and white matter in mild traumatic brain injury: a 1H magnetic resonance spectroscopy study. J Neurotrauma. 2009;26(10):1635–43.

148. Yeo RA, Gasparovic C, Merideth F, Ruhl D, Doezema D, Mayer AR. A longitudinal proton magnetic resonance spectroscopy study of mild traumatic brain injury. J Neurotrauma. 2011;28(1):1–11.

149. Di X, Gordon J, Bullock R. Fluid percussion brain injury exacerbates glutamate-induced focal damage in the rat. J Neurotrauma. 1999;16(3):195–201.

150. Globus MY, Alonso O, Dietrich WD, Busto R, Ginsberg MD. Glutamate release and free radical production following brain injury: effects of posttraumatic hypothermia. J Neurochem. 1995;65(4):1704–11.

151. Hartley CE, Varma M, Fischer JP, Riccardi R, Strauss JA, Shah S, et al. Neuroprotective effects of erythropoietin on acute metabolic and pathological changes in experimentally induced neurotrauma. J Neurosurg. 2008;109(4):708–14.

152. Palmer AM, Marion DW, Botscheller ML, Swedlow PE, Styren SD, DeKosky ST. Traumatic brain injury-induced excitotoxicity assessed in a controlled cortical impact model. J Neurochem. 1993;61(6):2015–24.

153. Hillary FG, Biswal B. The influence of neuropathology on the FMRI signal: a measurement of brain or vein? Clin Neuropsychol. 2007;21(1):58–72.

154. Soustiel JF, Sviri GE. Monitoring of cerebral metabolism: non-ischemic impairment of oxidative metabolism following severe traumatic brain injury. Neurol Res. 2007;29(7):654–60.

155. Vespa PM, O'Phelan K, McArthur D, Miller C, Eliseo M, Hirt D, et al. Pericontusional brain tissue exhibits persistent elevation of lactate/pyruvate ratio independent of cerebral perfusion pressure. Crit Care Med. 2007;35(4):1153–60.

156. Park E, Bell JD, Siddiq IP, Baker AJ. An analysis of regional microvascular loss and recovery following two grades of fluid percussion trauma: a role for hypoxia-inducible factors in traumatic brain injury. J Cereb Blood Flow Metab. 2009;29(3):575–84.

157. Ueda Y, Walker SA, Povlishock JT. Perivascular nerve damage in the cerebral circulation following traumatic brain injury. Acta Neuropathol. 2006;112(1):85–94.

158. Bigler ED. Neuropsychological results and neuropathological findings at autopsy in a case of mild traumatic brain injury. J Int Neuropsychol Soc. 2004;10(5):794–806.

159. Heffernan ME, Huang W, Sicard KM, Bratane BT, Zhang N, Fisher M, et al. Multi-modal approach for investigating brain and behavior changes in an animal model of traumatic brain injury. J Neurotrauma. 2013;30(11):1007–12.

160. Pawela CP, Biswal BB, Hudetz AG, Li R, Jones SR, Cho YR, et al. Interhemispheric neuroplasticity following limb deafferentation detected by resting-state functional connectivity magnetic resonance imaging (fcMRI) and functional magnetic resonance imaging (fMRI). Neuroimage. 2010;49(3):2467–78.

161. Liang Z, King J, Zhang N. Uncovering intrinsic connectional architecture of functional networks in awake rat brain. J Neurosci. 2011;31(10):3776–83.

162. Govind V, Gold S, Kaliannan K, Saigal G, Falcone S, Arheart KL, et al. Whole-brain proton MR spectroscopic imaging of mild-to-moderate traumatic brain injury and correlation with neuropsychological deficits. J Neurotrauma. 2010;27(3):483–96.

163. Vagnozzi R, Signoretti S, Cristofori L, Alessandrini F, Floris R, Isgro E, et al. Assessment of metabolic brain damage and recovery following mild traumatic brain injury: a multicentre, proton magnetic resonance spectroscopic study in concussed patients. Brain. 2010;133(11): 3232–42.

164. Matthews SC, Strigo IA, Simmons AN, O'Connell RM, Reinhardt LE, Moseley SA. A multimodal imaging study in U.S. veterans of operations Iraqi and enduring freedom with and without major depression after blast-related concussion. Neuroimage. 2011;54(1):69–75.

165. Lewine JD, Davis JT, Bugler ED, Thoma R, Hill D, Funke M, et al. Objective documentation of traumatic brain injury subsequent to mild head trauma: multimodal brain imaging with MEG, SPECT, and MRI. J Head Trauma Rehabil. 2007;22(3):141–55.

166. Slobounov S, Cao C, Sebastianelli W. Differential effect of first versus second concussive episodes on wavelet information quality of EEG. Clin Neurophysiol. 2009;120(5):862–7.

167. Laufs H, Holt JL, Elfont R, Krams M, Paul JS, Krakow K, et al. Where the BOLD signal goes when alpha EEG leaves. Neuroimage. 2006;31(4):1408–18.
168. Yuan H, Zotev V, Phillips R, Drevets WC, Bodurka J. Spatiotemporal dynamics of the brain at rest—exploring EEG microstates as electrophysiological signatures of BOLD resting state networks. Neuroimage. 2012;60(4):2062–72.
169. Liau J, Liu TT. Inter-subject variability in hypercapnic normalization of the BOLD fMRI response. Neuroimage. 2009;45(2):420–30.
170. Stefanovic B, Warnking JM, Pike GB. Hemodynamic and metabolic responses to neuronal inhibition. Neuroimage. 2004;22(2):771–8.
171. Bandettini PA, Wong EC. A hypercapnia-based normalization method for improved spatial localization of human brain activation with fMRI. NMR Biomed. 1997;10(4–5):197–203.
172. Thomason ME, Glover GH. Controlled inspiration depth reduces variance in breath-holding-induced BOLD signal. Neuroimage. 2008;39(1):206–14.
173. Sicard KM, Duong TQ. Effects of hypoxia, hyperoxia, and hypercapnia on baseline and stimulus-evoked BOLD, CBF, and $CMRO_2$ in spontaneously breathing animals. Neuroimage. 2005;25(3):850–8.
174. Zappe AC, Uludag K, Oeltermann A, Ugurbil K, Logothetis NK. The influence of moderate hypercapnia on neural activity in the anesthetized nonhuman primate. Cereb Cortex. 2008;18(11):2666–73.
175. Biswal BB, Kannurpatti SS, Rypma B. Hemodynamic scaling of fMRI-BOLD signal: validation of low-frequency spectral amplitude as a scalability factor. Magn Reson Imaging. 2007;25(10):1358–69.
176. Cohen ER, Rostrup E, Sidaros K, Lund TE, Paulson OB, Ugurbil K, et al. Hypercapnic normalization of BOLD fMRI: comparison across field strengths and pulse sequences. Neuroimage. 2004;23(2):613–24.
177. Thomason ME, Foland LC, Glover GH. Calibration of BOLD fMRI using breath holding reduces group variance during a cognitive task. Hum Brain Mapp. 2007;28(1):59–68.
178. Palmer HS, Garzon B, Xu J, Berntsen EM, Skandsen T, Haberg AK. Reduced fractional anisotropy does not change the shape of the hemodynamic response in survivors of severe traumatic brain injury. J Neurotrauma. 2010;27(5):853–62.
179. McAllister TW, Stein MB. Effects of psychological and biomechanical trauma on brain and behavior. Ann N Y Acad Sci. 2010;1208:46–57.
180. Kim N, Branch CA, Kim M, Lipton ML. Whole brain approaches for identification of microstructural abnormalities in individual patients: comparison of techniques applied to mild traumatic brain injury. PLoS One. 2013;8(3):e59382.
181. Ling JM, Pena A, Yeo RA, Merideth FL, Klimaj S, Gasparovic C, et al. Biomarkers of increased diffusion anisotropy in semi-acute mild traumatic brain injury: a longitudinal perspective. Brain. 2012;135(4):1281–92.
182. Lipton ML, Kim N, Park YK, Hulkower MB, Gardin TM, Shifteh K, et al. Robust detection of traumatic axonal injury in individual mild traumatic brain injury patients: intersubject variation, change over time and bidirectional changes in anisotropy. Brain Imaging Behav. 2012;6(2):329–42.
183. Davenport ND, Lim KO, Armstrong MT, Sponheim SR. Diffuse and spatially variable white matter disruptions are associated with blast-related mild traumatic brain injury. Neuroimage. 2012;59(3):2017–24.
184. Jorge RE, Acion L, White T, Tordesillas-Gutierrez D, Pierson R, Crespo-Facorro B, et al. White matter abnormalities in veterans with mild traumatic brain injury. Am J Psychiatry. 2012;169(12):1284–91.
185. Mayer AR, Ling JM, Yang Z, Pena A, Yeo RA, Klimaj S. Diffusion abnormalities in pediatric mild traumatic brain injury. J Neurosci. 2012;32(50):17961–9.
186. Bazarian JJ, Zhu T, Blyth B, Borrino A, Zhong J. Subject-specific changes in brain white matter on diffusion tensor imaging after sports-related concussion. Magn Reson Imaging. 2012;30(2):171–80.

Part IV
Pediatric Sport-Related Concussions

Chapter 15
Predicting Postconcussive Symptoms After Mild Traumatic Brain Injury in Children and Adolescents

Keith Owen Yeates

Abstract The vast majority of traumatic brain injuries (TBI) in children are of mild severity. A small but significant proportion of children with mild TBI experience persistent postconcussive symptoms (PCS), with negative consequences for their broader and longer-term psychosocial functioning. A key issue for clinical management is how to predict which children with mild TBI will go on to display persistent PCS. This chapter reviews the existing literature regarding the prediction of PCS following mild TBI in children and adolescents, considering both injury-related and non-injury-related factors as possible prognostic indicators. The chapter summarizes conceptual and methodological issues that arise in research on the prediction of the outcomes of mild TBI. The chapter concludes with suggestions for future research, the long-term goal of which is to develop evidence-based decision rules that facilitate the identification of children at risk for poor outcomes after mild TBI.

Keywords Mild traumatic brain injury • Concussion • Pediatric • Outcomes • Diagnosis • Methodology

Introduction

Mild traumatic brain injuries (TBI) are a common occurrence in children and adolescents. Annually, as many as 700,000 youth ages 0–19 in the United States sustain TBI that require hospital-based medical care, and the large majority of these injuries are mild in severity [1, 2]. The total number of youth sustaining mild

---

K.O. Yeates, Ph.D. (✉)
Section of Pediatric Psychology and Neuropsychology, Department of Psychology,
Nationwide Children's Hospital, Columbus, OH, USA

Department of Pediatrics, The Ohio State University, Columbus, OH, USA
e-mail: Keith.yeates@nationwidechildrens.org

S.M. Slobounov and W.J. Sebastianelli (eds.), *Concussions in Athletics:*
From Brain to Behavior, DOI 10.1007/978-1-4939-0295-8_15,
© Springer Science+Business Media New York 2014

TBI each year is likely to be far higher, because many mild TBI are cared for outside of hospital settings [3] and even more likely never receive any formal medical attention [4]. Thus, mild TBI is a major public health problem in children and adolescents.

Hospitalization rates for children with mild TBI have declined markedly in recent decades [5], and health care providers in emergency medicine and other outpatient settings need guidance to make informed decisions regarding the assessment and management of mild TBI in children [6–8]. Research is therefore imperative to identify children who are at risk for negative outcomes [9]. In recent years, the National Institutes of Health (NIH), Centers for Disease Control and Prevention, and World Health Organization (WHO) have all called for additional research on the outcomes of pediatric mild TBI, to help shape its diagnosis and management [10–12].

The outcomes of mild TBI in children and adolescents have been controversial [13, 14]. Although some systematic reviews have suggested that mild TBI have few short- or long-term effects [15–18], a growing body of literature indicates that post-concussive symptoms (PCS) occur more often after mild TBI than after injuries not involving the head or among healthy children [19–28]. PCS include a range of somatic (e.g., headache, dizziness), cognitive (e.g., inattention, forgetfulness), and affective (e.g., irritability, disinhibition) symptoms commonly reported after mild TBI, albeit not specific to that condition. Group differences in PCS tend to be most pronounced shortly after injury and to resolve over time [19, 22, 24, 29]; however, a small but significant proportion of children with mild TBI experience persistent PCS, with negative consequences for their broader and longer-term psychosocial functioning [27, 28, 30–32].

A key issue for the purposes of clinical management is how to predict which children with mild TBI will go on to display persistent PCS [33]. This chapter begins by describing a model for predicting PCS following mild TBI in children and adolescents mild TBI. It then reviews the existing literature regarding the prediction of PCS, examining both injury-related and non-injury-related factors as possible prognostic indicators. The chapter next summarizes conceptual and methodological issues that arise in research on the prediction of the outcomes of mild TBI, and concludes with suggestions for future research directions. The long-term goal of the chapter is to foster the development of evidence-based decision rules to facilitate the identification of children at risk for poor outcomes after mild TBI.

A Model for PCS

Figure 15.1 portrays a conceptual model for predicting PCS following mild TBI in youth. The model draws on existing theories regarding children's adaptation to illness, including the Disability-Stress-Coping Model [34] and the Transactional Stress and Coping Model [35], as well models of adaptation specific to mild TBI [36, 37]. The model presumes that the occurrence of PCS following mild TBI will

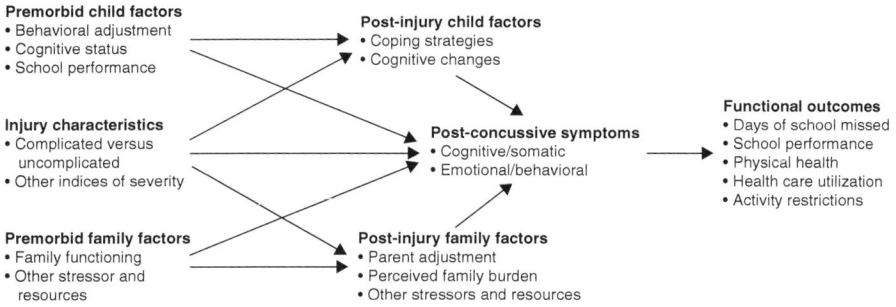

Fig. 15.1 Model for study of postconcussive symptoms in children with mild traumatic brain injury. Reprinted with permission from Yeates and Taylor, 2005, *Pediatric Rehabilitation*, Vol. 8, p. 12. © 2005 by Informa Medical and Pharmaceutical Science Journals

depend on the combined influences of premorbid child and family functioning, the nature of the injury, the extent to which the injury results in deficits in cognitive functioning, post-injury child and parent coping and adjustment, and the additional stresses and resources that affect children and families. The model also assumes that the influences of these factors can be both direct and indirect. For example, changes in brain structure or function associated with mild TBI may give rise to PCS directly because of the effect of brain impairment on behavior, but they also may result in PCS indirectly because of their effects on children's cognitive functioning or ability to cope with stress, which in turn increase the risk of PCS.

The relationship between various risk factors and PCS is assumed to vary as a function of time since injury [38]. Shortly after an injury, the onset of PCS is more likely to depend on premorbid child and family factors, injury characteristics, and post-injury cognitive performance. The likelihood that PCS will persist over time may depend more on children's and parents' post-injury coping and adjustment, as well as on the other stressors and resources in their lives. Premorbid factors, injury characteristics, and post-injury cognitive deficits may be relevant to both acute and chronic symptoms. However, the relative influence of post-injury child and parent reactions and other stressors and resources may be larger for chronic symptoms. In other words, the ways in which children and their parents react to the acute disruptions associated with mild TBI is likely to be a significant determinant of the persistence of PCS.

The relationship between various child and family factors and PCS also is assumed to vary as a function of symptom type. Cognitive and somatic symptoms may be influenced by the child's premorbid cognitive status, injury characteristics, and the effects of any acute brain insult. For instance, fatigue, headache, inattention, and forgetfulness are symptoms that may be more likely to arise directly as a result of brain impairment associated with mild TBI. In contrast, emotional and behavioral symptoms, such as depression or aggression, may be more likely to reflect children's and parents' premorbid adjustment, their coping following the injury, and the effects of other stressors and resources.

Predictors of PCS

Relatively little research has examined the prediction of PCS in children after mild TBI [33]. The research varies in methodological quality, with only a few studies involving prospective recruitment of representative samples of children with mild TBI and appropriate control groups who are then followed longitudinally. Few studies have examined both injury and non-injury factors as potential predictors of PCS, much less compared to their relative contributions at different times post-injury [38]. The following sections summarize existing research about the predictors of PCS.

Injury Factors

A variety of injury factors have been considered as potential predictors of PCS. One is the occurrence of previous concussions or mild TBI. Although an early study of a national birth cohort suggested that multiple concussions did not result in specific cognitive deficits [39], subsequent studies of sports concussions found evidence for cumulative effects [40]. In a recent study, children with a history of previous concussion, especially recent or multiple concussions, demonstrated more protracted symptoms after mild TBI than did children without previous concussion [41].

Various indices of injury severity have also been studied as potential predictors of PCS. Acute clinical signs and symptoms that have been shown to be associated with an increased risk of PCS include loss of consciousness [19, 24, 26–28, 42], posttraumatic amnesia [22, 42], and headache [43]. The presence of intracranial abnormalities on acute neuroimaging has also been associated with increased PCS [24, 26–28, 44]. Several indirect proxies for injury severity have also been associated with an increased likelihood of PCS, including hospital admission [24, 43, 45], high-speed mechanism of injury [24], and the presence of associated injuries not involving the head [24, 38].

Non-injury Factors

Among various non-injury factors, pre-injury symptoms consistently account for the most variance in PCS [38, 46]. Pre-injury symptoms are typically assessed retrospectively after injury, except in sports concussion research where pre-injury baselines are possible, and so may be subject to bias. However, retrospective ratings of pre-injury symptoms do not differ for children with mild TBI versus those with orthopedic injuries [38], suggesting that bias is likely minimal if the ratings are obtained shortly after the injury occurs. More generally, pre-injury learning and behavior problems also increase the risk of PCS [22].

Children's cognitive abilities may also be related to PCS after mild TBI. Although neurocognitive deficits typically resolve within a few weeks after mild TBI [15–18], neuropsychological testing can be used to identify children who show acute decrements in their cognitive functioning and those who have low cognitive reserve capacity, and both types of children may be at risk for PCS. Cognitive ability has been shown to be a significant moderator of PCS, such that children of lower cognitive ability with a mild TBI associated with abnormalities on neuroimaging are especially prone to PCS [47]. Children's coping skills also can help account for PCS. Children with mild TBI are at greater risk for PCS relative to children with orthopedic injuries if they rely on avoidance or wishful thinking to cope with their injuries as compared to other coping strategies [48].

Demographic factors such as age and sex may also help account for PCS. The relationship of age to PCS has not been entirely consistent. Some studies have found greater PCS among adolescents than younger children [19, 43], while others have found evidence of more PCS among younger as compared to older children [24]. Differences in results across studies may reflect whether PCS were assessed by self-report or by parent ratings; adolescents tend to report more PCS than younger children, but parents may report more PCS for younger than older children. Few studies have specifically examined whether age moderates the effects of mild TBI on PCS; one showed evidence for larger group differences (mild TBI versus orthopedic injury) for PCS among younger versus older children [24]. Sex has been a more consistent predictor of PCS, such that girls typically report more symptoms than boys [24, 43], although differences in PCS between children with mild TBI and those with orthopedic injuries do not appear to be more pronounced for girls than boys [24].

A variety of environmental factors may also account for PCS. For instance, family socioeconomic status has been negatively correlated with greater self-reports of PCS in at least one study [24], and parent psychological distress is positively correlated with PCS [46, 49]. Somewhat surprisingly, families that were higher functioning and had more environmental resources were more likely to demonstrate somatic PCS following mild TBI than those from poorer functioning homes with fewer resources [27, 28]. This finding runs counter to previous research among children with severe TBI showing that the effects of TBI are exacerbated in the context of poorer premorbid family functioning [50].

Relative Contributions of Injury Versus Non-injury Factors

Few studies have directly compared injury versus non-injury factors as predictors of PCS. In one study [19], family functioning and parent adjustment did not account for differences in PCS as a function of injury severity, although the specific contributions of the former variables were not estimated statistically. More recently, a study of 186 children with mild TBI and 99 with mild orthopedic injuries [38] examined the prediction of PCS at four occasions during the first year post-injury from: (1) demographic variables; (2) premorbid child factors; (3) family factors;

and (4) injury factors (mild TBI, with or without loss of consciousness and with or without associated injuries, versus orthopedic injuries). Injury factors predicted parent and child ratings of PCS but showed a decreasing contribution over time. Demographic variables consistently predicted symptom ratings across time. Pre morbid child factors, especially retrospective ratings of premorbid symptoms, accounted for the most variance in PCS. Family factors, particularly parent adjustment, consistently predicted parent, but not child, ratings of PCS. The findings suggest that mild TBI predicts increased PCS in the first months following injury, but shows a decreasing contribution over time. In contrast, non-injury factors are more consistently related to PCS.

Research Issues

Definition of Mild TBI

A variety of methodological shortcomings have characterized previous research on mild TBI [51]. One of the major limitations involves the definition of mild TBI, which has varied substantially across studies, along with associated inclusion/exclusion criteria [33, 52]. Most studies have defined mild TBI based on Glasgow Coma Scale scores ranging from 13 to 15 [53], but they have been inconsistent in applying other criteria, such as presence or duration of unconsciousness or posttraumatic amnesia. Some studies have not clearly defined both the lower and upper limits of severity of mild TBI, which can range from brief alterations in mental status without loss of consciousness to more severe signs and symptoms, including loss of consciousness, posttraumatic amnesia, transient neurological abnormalities, and positive neuroimaging findings. Issues of definition and classification are especially problematic in studies of infants and younger children, for whom traditional measures of injury severity such as the Glasgow Coma Scale may not be valid [54].

Some previous studies have excluded children whose injuries are accompanied by positive findings on neuroimaging. These practices have engendered potentially erroneous conclusions about the outcomes of mild TBI. The WHO Collaborating Centre Task Force on Mild Traumatic Brain Injury [16] cited two studies to justify their conclusion that PCS in children are usually transient and largely resolve within 2–3 months of the injury. However, both studies excluded children with neuroimaging abnormalities, despite the inclusion of such abnormalities in the Task Force's operational definition of mild TBI.

Outcome Measurement

The measurement of PCS has typically been limited to questionnaires and rating scales, usually completed only by parents. Parent–child agreement regarding postconcussive symptoms is significant but modest [55, 56], suggesting that both child and parents reports should be explored in studies of mild TBI. Only parent ratings may be available for infants and younger children, but the validity of ratings in that age range warrants further investigation. The reporting of postconcussive symptoms may also depend on the format for symptom reporting. For example, in adults, rating scales elicit reports of more symptoms than do open-ended structured interviews [57, 58].

Previous studies have also frequently treated PCS as if they occur along a single dimension. However, research indicates that PCS in children with mild TBI are multidimensional, with a clear distinction between somatic and cognitive symptoms [59]. The dimensions of PCS not only can be distinguished psychometrically, but also follow distinct trajectories following mild TBI [24]. They also appear to be distinct from other kinds of symptoms, such as those associated with posttraumatic stress disorder [60, 61].

Assessment of Risk Factors

The assessment of risk factors that predict outcomes following mild TBI has been problematic. Most studies have not adequately characterized the severity of children's injuries. Children with mild TBI are often treated as a homogenous group, without regard to whether factors such as loss of consciousness or abnormalities on neuroimaging increase the risk of negative outcomes. Advanced neuroimaging techniques, such as susceptibility-weighted and diffusion tensor imaging, may also provide a more sensitive assessment of injury severity in mild TBI [62–65].

Research also needs to incorporate measures of non-injury-related risk factors as possible predictors. In many cases, children with premorbid learning or behavior problems are omitted from studies, although they may be at particular risk for persistent postconcussive symptoms [33]. As noted earlier, a variety of non-injury factors are likely relevant to the prediction of PCS, and may moderate its occurrence after mild TBI, including children's premorbid cognitive ability and coping skills [47], demographic factors and socioeconomic status [24], and parent and family functioning [27, 28, 46, 49].

Alternative Explanations

Previous research has rarely considered a variety of potential alternative explanations for persistent PCS, including children's effort or motivation, pain, and symptom exaggeration. Performance on effort testing has been shown to account for substantial variance in cognitive test performance among children with mild TBI [66], although effort did not account for group differences in PCS in another study [23]. Pain has not been examined, but is a common consequence of TBI and may contribute to poor cognitive test performance and also exacerbate related symptom complaints [67]. Finally, some children or parents may be prone to symptom exaggeration, perhaps because of the lay expectations associated with mild TBI [68]. Research that incorporates indices of symptom exaggeration may help to determine whether reports of PCS after mild TBI are influenced by such expectations.

Timing of Outcome Assessment

Research on mild TBI has often been cross-sectional and focused on relatively short-term outcomes. This problem is compounded in some studies by retrospective recruitment of participants from among clinical referrals or hospital admissions, creating a significant ascertainment bias. Prospective and longitudinal studies of unselected samples are needed to examine how the relationship of risk factors to PCS varies post-injury [22, 38]. The timing of assessments is particularly critical in longitudinal studies [69]. Acute post-injury assessments are often desirable, not only to document the immediate effects of mild TBI, but also to obtain retrospective measures of children's premorbid symptoms as soon as possible after the injury, and thereby increase the validity of parent recall. The timing of subsequent assessments will be based in part on the expected course of recovery following mild TBI. Given that research suggests that PCS resolve in 2–3 months in many cases of mild TBI [19, 26], more frequent assessment during the first few months post-injury may be warranted. However, longer-term assessments will be needed to determine whether PCS result in significant ongoing impairment in children's social or academic functioning.

Prediction of Individual Outcomes

Studies of mild TBI have focused on outcomes at a group level, in part because most common statistical techniques yield results that are based on group averages. Thus, most analyses are variable-centered and reflect only group trends [70]. In clinical practice, however, we want to know whether mild TBI is likely to be followed by persistent PCS in a particular patient. One way to focus on individual outcomes is to divide groups into subgroups based on certain characteristics and then determine if outcomes are different for persons in different subgroups. Parsing a sample of children with mild TBI into those with versus those without loss of consciousness exemplifies this approach [24]. A second approach is to identify individuals with a given outcome, such as persistent PCS, and then determine the risk factors linked to this outcome [42]. An advantage of the latter, person-centered method is that it permits the researcher to identify combinations of risk factors associated with the outcome.

Growth curve modeling permits the investigation of change at an individual level in relation to multiple risk factors [24, 71]. Mixture modeling, in contrast, is used to

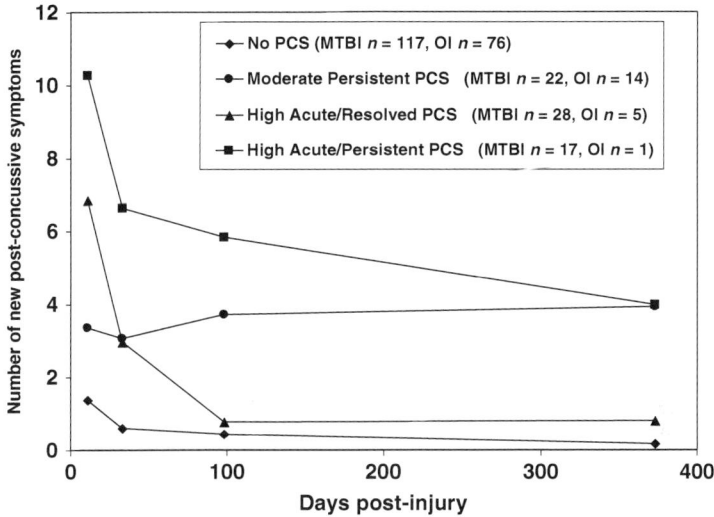

Fig. 15.2 Illustration of developmental trajectory analysis of postconcussive symptoms in children with mild TBI (mTBI) or orthopedic injuries (OI). Four latent groups were identified on the basis of the number of new postconcussive symptoms reported at four occasions post-injury, irrespective of whether participants were in the mTBI or OI group. Modified with permission from Yeates et al., 2009, from *Pediatrics*, Vol. 123, p. 738. © 2009 by American Academy of Pediatrics

empirically identify latent classes of individuals based on different developmental trajectories [72]. Figure 15.2 provides an example of this approach; it shows developmental trajectories of PCS in children with mild TBI and orthopedic injuries [26]. In this study, children with mild TBI were more likely than those with orthopedic injuries to demonstrate trajectories involving high acute levels of PCS. Moreover, children with mild TBI whose acute clinical presentation reflected more severe injury were especially likely to demonstrate such trajectories, in contrast to those with mild TBI with less severe acute presentations. Analyses of reliable change also can be used to identify individual children who display unusually large increases in PCS compared to pre-injury estimates and to study the risk factors associated with such increases [73]. For instance, Fig. 15.3 is drawn from a study of reliable change in PCS after mild TBI. The figure shows the proportion of children with mild TBI showing reliable increases in somatic symptoms as a function of loss consciousness or abnormalities on magnetic resonance imaging, as compared to children with orthopedic injuries [27, 28].

Building Prognostic Models and Decision Rules

In the long run, prognostic models and decision rules are needed that can predict which children with mild TBI will demonstrate significant PCS. To be clinically useful, research on outcome prediction needs to incorporate a variety of

Fig. 15.3 Probability of
reliable change in somatic
symptoms as a function of
group membership. Children
with mild TBI are divided
into those (**a**) with and
without LOC and (**b**) with
and without abnormalities on
MRI. Modified with
permission from Yeates et al.,
2012, from *Archives of
Pediatrics & Adolescent
Medicine*, Vol. 166, p. 618.
© 2012 by American
Medical Association

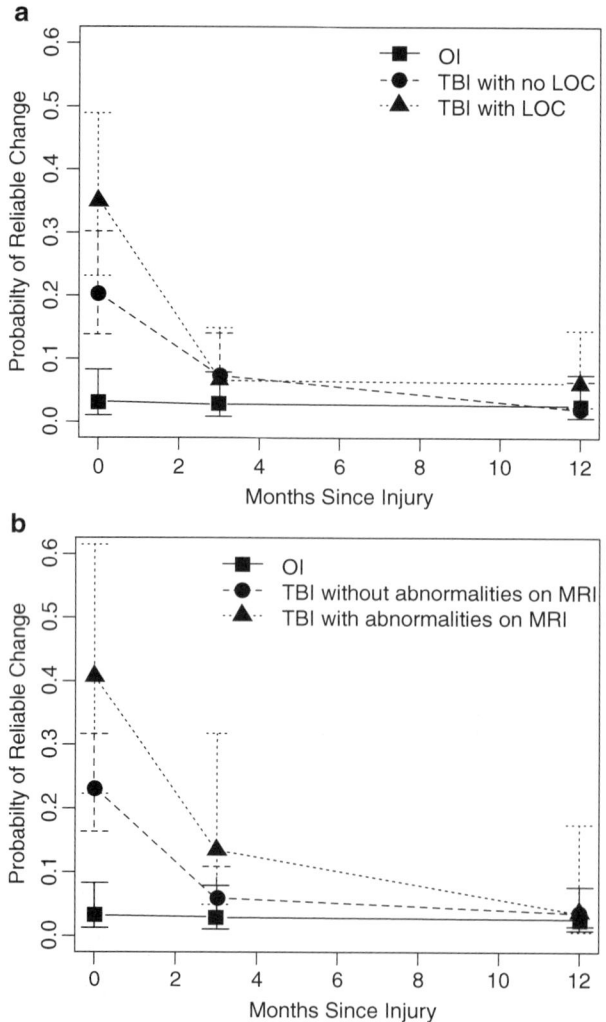

methodological improvements [74]. Sample sizes need to be relatively large (ideally
>500), both to reflect the inherent heterogeneity of mild TBI and to be representa-
tive of the broader population. The selection of predictors should be plausible, based
on previous research and expert opinion; the number of predictors should be kept
reasonably small, to avoid overfitting of models. Both outcomes and predictors need
to be defined precisely, measured with good reliability, and readily obtainable.
Statistical models need to be based on valid approaches to managing missing data
and on appropriate data analysis techniques for the selection of predictors and estimation of prognostic effects. Models also need to be validated both internally (e.g.,
bootstrapping) and externally, using different patient samples. Model performance
needs to be assessed using sensible and interpretable measures that assess both

model calibration (i.e., agreement between observed outcome frequencies and predicted probabilities) and discrimination of those with versus without persistent PCS. The results of modeling should be presented in a readily applicable format.

Future Directions

Future research on predicting PCS after mild TBI in children should acknowledge the likely contributions of multiple biological, psychological, and environmental influences on outcomes. At a biological level, genetic factors may play an important role. The apolipoprotein E gene has not been found to predict PCS after mild TBI in children [75], but many other candidate genes should be examined [76]. Research at a biological level may also yield more sensitive and precise measures of brain injury that may be related to outcomes. For instance, various biomarkers are being considered as possible indicators of underlying brain injury in mild TBI [77]. Advanced neuroimaging techniques may also provide a more sensitive assessment of injury severity in mild TBI [62]. At a psychological level, future research may lead to more sensitive measures of cognitive functioning in mild TBI. Computerized testing has the advantage of being able to assess reaction time, which has been shown to be sensitive to concussion [78]. More research is needed to determine if early post-injury cognitive deficits predict persistent PCS. Finally, at an environmental level, further research is needed to clarify which aspects of the family and broader social environment are related to the occurrence of PCS following mild TBI in children [27, 28, 38].

A key long-term goal for research on the outcomes of mild TBI is to develop prognostic models that incorporate developmental considerations and allow for individual variability in the importance of different risk factors. Ideally, such models will enable health care providers to provide parents and children with evidence-based information regarding the effects of mild TBI and to identify those children who are most at risk for demonstrating negative outcomes. Health care providers can then target at-risk children and their families for appropriate management [79].

Acknowledgment This manuscript has not been published previously either electronically or in print. The work was supported by grants HD44099 and HD39834 from the National Institutes of Health to the author.

References

1. Bazarian JJ, McClung J, Shah MN, Cheng YT, Flesher W, Kraus J. Mild traumatic brain injury in the United States, 1998–2000. Brain Inj. 2005;19:85–91.
2. Faul M, Xu L, Wald MM, Coronado VG. Traumatic brain injury in the United States: emergency department visits, hospitalizations and deaths 2002–2006. Atlanta, GA: Centers for Disease Control and Prevention, National Center for Injury Prevention and Control; 2010.

3. Collins CL, Pommering TL, Yeates KO, Andridge R, Coronado VG, et al. Clinical presentation patterns and settings for pediatric traumatic brain injury. Paper under review; 2013.
4. Sosin DM, Sniezek JE, Thurman DJ. Incidence of mild and moderate brain injury in the United States, 1991. Brain Inj. 1996;10:47–54.
5. Bowman SM, Bird TM, Aitken ME, Tilford JM. Trends in hospitalizations associated with pediatric traumatic brain injuries. Pediatrics. 2008;122:988–93.
6. Kamerling SN, Lutz N, Posner JC, Vanore M. Mild traumatic brain injury in children: practice guidelines for emergency department and hospitalized patients. Pediatr Emerg Care. 2003;19:431–40.
7. Lumba AK, Schnadower D, Joseph MM. Evidence-based assessment of pediatric mild traumatic brain injury. Pediatr Emerg Med Pract. 2011;8:1–20.
8. Scorza KA, Raleigh MF, O'Connor FG. Current concepts in concussion: evaluation and management. Am Fam Physician. 2012;85:123–32.
9. Rosenbaum SB, Lipton ML. Embracing chaos: the scope and importance of clinical and pathological heterogeneity in mTBI. Brain Imaging Behav. 2012;6:255–82.
10. Carroll LJ, Cassidy JD, Holm L, Kraus J, Coronado VG. Methodological issues and research recommendations for mild traumatic brain injury: the WHO Collaborating Centre Task Force on Mild Traumatic Brain Injury. J Rehabil Med. 2004;43(Suppl):113–25.
11. National Center for Injury Prevention and Control. Report to congress on mild traumatic brain injury in the United States: steps to prevent a serious public health problem. Atlanta, GA: Centers for Disease Control and Prevention; 2003.
12. NIH Consensus Panel on Rehabilitation of Persons with Traumatic Brain Injury. Rehabilitation of persons with traumatic brain injury. JAMA. 1999;282:974–83.
13. McKinlay A. Controversies and outcomes associated with mild traumatic brain injury in childhood and adolescence. Child Care Health Dev. 2009;36:3–21.
14. Yeates KO. Mild traumatic brain injury and postconcussive symptoms in children and adolescents. J Int Neuropsychol Soc. 2010;16:953–60.
15. Babikian T, Asarnow R. Neurocognitive outcomes and recovery after pediatric TBI: meta-analytic review of the literature. Neuropsychology. 2009;23:283–96.
16. Carroll LJ, Cassidy JD, Peloso PM, Borg J, von Holst H, et al. Prognosis for mild traumatic brain injury: results of the WHO Collaborating Centre Task Force on Mild Traumatic Brain Injury. J Rehabil Med. 2004;43(Suppl):84–105.
17. Satz P. Mild head injury in children and adolescents. Curr Dir Psychol Sci. 2001;10:106–9.
18. Satz P, Zaucha K, McCleary C, Light R, Asarnow R. Mild head injury in children and adolescents: a review of studies (1970–1995). Psychol Bull. 1997;122:107–31.
19. Barlow KM, Crawford S, Stevenson A, Sandhu SS, Belanger F, Dewey D. Epidemiology of postconcussion syndrome in pediatric mild traumatic brain injury. Pediatrics. 2010;126: e374–81.
20. Hawley CA. Reported problems and their resolution following mild, moderate, and severe traumatic brain injury amongst children and adolescents in the UK. Brain Inj. 2003;17: 105–29.
21. Mittenberg W, Wittner MS, Miller LJ. Post-concussion syndrome occurs in children. Neuropsychology. 1997;11:447–52.
22. Ponsford J, Willmott C, Rothwell A, Cameron P, Ayton G, et al. Cognitive and behavioral outcomes following mild traumatic head injury in children. J Head Trauma Rehabil. 1999;14: 360–72.
23. Sroufe NS, Fuller DS, West BT, Singal BM, Warschausky SA, Maio RF. Postconcussive symptoms and neurocognitive function after mild traumatic brain injury in children. Pediatrics. 2010;125:e1331–9.
24. Taylor HG, Dietrich A, Nuss K, Wright M, Rusin J, et al. Post-concussive symptoms in children with mild traumatic brain injury. Neuropsychology. 2010;24:148–59.
25. Yeates KO, Luria J, Bartkowski H, Rusin J, Martin L, Bigler ED. Post-concussive symptoms in children with mild closed-head injuries. J Head Trauma Rehabil. 1999;14:337–50.

26. Yeates KO, Taylor HG, Rusin J, Bangert B, Dietrich A, et al. Longitudinal trajectories of post-concussive symptoms in children with mild traumatic brain injuries and their relationship to acute clinical status. Pediatrics. 2009;123:735–43.
27. Yeates KO, Taylor HG, Rusin J, Bangert B, Dietrich A, et al. Premorbid child and family functioning as predictors of post-concussive symptoms in children with mild traumatic brain injuries. Int J Dev Neurosci. 2012;30:231–7.
28. Yeates KO, Kaizar E, Rusin J, Bangert B, Dietrich A, et al. Reliable change in post-concussive symptoms and its functional consequences among children with mild traumatic brain injury. Arch Pediatr Adolesc Med. 2012;166:585–684.
29. Nacajauskaite O, Endziniene M, Jureniene K, Schrader H. The validity of post-concussion syndrome in children: a controlled historical cohort study. Brain Dev. 2006;28:507–14.
30. McKinlay A, Dalrymple-Alford JC, Horwood LJ, Fergusson DM. Long term psychosocial outcomes after mild head injury in early childhood. J Neurol Neurosurg Psychiatry. 2002; 73:281–8.
31. Moran LM, Taylor HG, Rusin J, Bangert B, Dietrich A, Nuss KE, Wright M, Minich N, Yeates KO. Quality of life in pediatric mild traumatic brain injury and its relationship to post-concussive symptoms. J Pediatr Psychol. 2012;37:736–44.
32. Overweg-Plandsoen WCG, Kodde A, van Straaten M, van der Linden EAM, Neyens LGJ, et al. Mild closed head injury in children compared to traumatic fractured bone; neurobehavioural sequelae in daily life 2 years after the accident. Eur J Pediatr. 1999;158:249–52.
33. Zemek RL, Farion KJ, Sampson M, McGahern C. Prognosticators of persistent symptoms following pediatric concussion: a systematic review. JAMA Pediatr. 2013;167:259–65.
34. Wallander JL, Varni JW. Adjustment in children with chronic physical disorders: programmatic research on a disability-stress-coping model. In: La Greca AM, Siegal L, Wallander JL, Walker CE, editors. Stress and coping with pediatric conditions. New York: Guilford Press; 1992. p. 279–98.
35. Thompson RJ, Gil KM, Keith BR, Gustafson KE, George LK, Kinney TR. Psychological adjustment of children with sickle cell disease: stability and change over a 10-month period. J Consult Clin Psychol. 1994;62:856–60.
36. Kay T, Newman B, Cavallo M, Ezrachi O, Resnik M. Toward a neuropsychological model of functional disability after mild traumatic brain injury. Neuropsychology. 1992;6:371–84.
37. Wood RL. Understanding the 'miserable minority': a diathesis-stress paradigm for post-concussional syndrome. Brain Inj. 2004;18:1135–53.
38. McNally KA, Bangert B, Dietrich A, Nuss K, Rusin J, et al. Injury versus non-injury factors as predictors of post-concussive symptoms following mild traumatic brain injury in children. Neuropsychology. 2013;27:1–12.
39. Bijur PE, Haslum M, Golding J. Cognitive outcomes of multiple head injuries in children. J Dev Behav Pediatr. 1996;17:143–8.
40. Collins MW, Lowell MR, Iverson GL, Cantu RC, Maroon JC, Field M. Cumulative effects of concussion in high school athletes. Neurosurgery. 2002;51:1175–81.
41. Eisenberg MA, Andrea J, Meehan W, Mannix R. Time interval between concussions and symptom duration. Pediatrics. 2013;132:1–10.
42. McCrea M, Guskiewicz K, Randolph C, Barr WB, Hammeke TA, et al. Incidence, clinical course, and predictors of prolonged recovery time following sports-related concussion in high school and college athletes. J Int Neuropsychol Soc. 2012;18:1–12.
43. Babcock L, Byczkowski T, Wade SL, Ho M, Mookerjee S, Bazarian JJ. Predicting postconcussion syndrome after mild traumatic brain injury in children and adolescents who present to the emergency department. JAMA Pediatr. 2013;167:156–61.
44. Levin HS, Hanten G, Roberson G, Li X, Ewing-Cobbs L, et al. Prediction of cognitive sequelae based on abnormal computed tomography findings in children following mild traumatic brain injury. J Neurosurg Pediatr. 2008;1:461–70.
45. McKinlay A, Grace RC, Horwood LJ, Fergusson DM, MacFarlane MR. Long-term behavioural outcomes of pre-school mild traumatic brain injury. Child Care Health Dev. 2010;36: 22–30.

46. Ollson KA, Lloyd OT, Lebrocque RM, McKinlay L, Anderson VA, Kennardy JA. Predictors of post-concussion symptoms at 6 and 18 months following mild traumatic brain injury. Brain Inj. 2013;27:145–57.

47. Fay TB, Yeates KO, Taylor HG, Bangert B, Dietrich A, et al. Cognitive reserve as a moderator of postconcussive symptoms in children with complicated and uncomplicated mild traumatic brain injury. J Int Neuropsychol Soc. 2009;16:94–105.

48. Woodrome SE, Yeates KO, Taylor HG, Rusin J, Bangert B, et al. Coping strategies as a predictor of post-concussive symptoms in children with mild traumatic brain injury versus mild orthopedic injury. J Int Neuropsychol Soc. 2011;17:317–26.

49. Ganesalingam K, Yeates KO, Ginn MS, Taylor HG, Dietrich A, et al. Family burden and parental distress following mild traumatic brain injury in children and its relationship to post-concussive symptoms. J Pediatr Psychol. 2008;33:621–9.

50. Yeates KO, Taylor HG, Drotar D, Wade SL, Klein S, et al. Pre-injury family environment as a determinant of recovery from traumatic brain injuries in school-age children. J Int Neuropsychol Soc. 1997;3:617–30.

51. Dikmen SS, Levin HS. Methodological issues in the study of mild head injury. J Head Trauma Rehabil. 1993;8:30–7.

52. Williams DH, Levin HS, Eisenberg HM. Mild head injury classification. Neurosurgery. 1990;27:422–8.

53. Teasdale G, Jennett B. Assessment of coma and impaired consciousness: a practical scale. Lancet. 1974;2:81–4.

54. Durham SR, Clancy RR, Leuthardt E, Sun P, Kamerling S, et al. CHOP Infant Coma Scale ('Infant Face Scale'): a novel coma scale for children less than 2 years of age. J Neurotrauma. 2000;17:729–37.

55. Gioia GA, Schneider JC, Vaughan CG, Isquith PK. Which symptom assessments and approaches are uniquely appropriate for paediatric concussion? Br J Sports Med. 2009; 43(Suppl):i13–22.

56. Hajek CA, Yeates KO, Taylor HG, Bangert B, Dietrich A, et al. Agreement between parents and children on ratings of postconcussive symptoms following mild traumatic brain injury. Child Neuropsychol. 2011;17:17–33.

57. Iverson GL, Brooks BL, Ashton VL, Lange RT. Interview versus questionnaire symptom reporting in people with the postconcussion syndrome. J Head Trauma Rehabil. 2010; 25:23–30.

58. Nolin P, Villemure R, Heroux L. Determining long-term symptoms following mild traumatic brain injury: method of interview affects self-report. Brain Inj. 2006;20:1147–54.

59. Ayr LK, Yeates KO, Taylor HG, Browne M. Dimensions of post-concussive symptoms in children with mild traumatic brain injuries. J Int Neuropsychol Soc. 2009;15:19–30.

60. Bryant RA, Harvey AG. Post-concussive symptoms and posttraumatic stress disorder after mild traumatic brain injury. J Nerv Ment Dis. 1999;187:302–5.

61. Hajek CA, Yeates KO, Taylor HG, Bangert B, Dietrich A, et al. Relationships among postconcussive symptoms and symptoms of PTSD in children following mild traumatic brain injury. Brain Inj. 2010;24:100–9.

62. Ashwal S, Tong KA, Bartnik-Olson B, Holshouser BA. Neuroimaging. In: Kirkwood MW, Yeates KO, editors. Mild traumatic brain injury in children and adolescents: from basic science to clinical management. New York: Guilford Press; 2012. p. 162–95.

63. Beauchamp MH, Ditchfield M, Babl FE, Kean M, Catroppa C, Yeates KO, Anderson V. Detecting traumatic brain lesions in children: CT vs MRI vs susceptibility weighted imaging (SWI). J Neurotrauma. 2011;28:915–27.

64. Chu Z, Wilde EA, Hunter JV, McCauley SR, Bigler ED, et al. Voxel-based analysis of diffusion tensor imaging in mild traumatic brain injury in adolescents. AJNR Am J Neuroradiol. 2010;31:340–6.

65. Wilde EA, McCauley SR, Hunger JV, Bigler ED, Levin HS. Diffusion tensor imaging of acute mild traumatic brain injury in adolescents. Neurology. 2008;70:948–55.

66. Kirkwood M, Yeates KO, Randolph C, Kirk J. The implications of symptom validity test failure for ability-based test performance in a pediatric sample. Psychol Assess. 2012;24: 36–45.

67. Nampiaparampil DE. Prevalence of chronic pain after traumatic brain injury: a systematic review. JAMA. 2008;300:711–9.

68. Mittenberg W, DiGiulio DV, Perrin S, Bass AE. Symptoms following mild head injury: expectation as aetiology. J Neurol Neurosurg Psychiatry. 1992;55:200–4.

69. Taylor HG, Alden J. Age-related differences in outcome following childhood brain injury: an introduction and overview. J Int Neuropsychol Soc. 1997;3:555–67.

70. Laursen B, Hoff E. Person-centered and variable-centered approaches to longitudinal data. Merrill Palmer Q (Wayne State Univ Press). 2006;52:377–89.

71. Francis DJ, Fletcher JM, Stuebing KK, Davidson KC, Thompson NM. Analysis of change: modeling individual growth. J Consult Clin Psychol. 1991;59:27–37.

72. Nagin DS. Group-based modeling of development. Cambridge, MA: Harvard University Press; 2005.

73. McCrea M, Barr WB, Guskiewicz K, Randolph C, Marshall SW, et al. Standard regression-based methods for measuring recovery after sport-related concussion. J Int Neuropsychol Soc. 2005;11:58–69.

74. Mushkudiani NA, Hukkelhoven CWPM, Hernandez AV, Murray GD, Choi SC, et al. A systematic review finds methodological improvements necessary for prognostic models in determining traumatic brain injury outcomes. J Clin Epidemiol. 2008;61:331–43.

75. Moran LM, Taylor HG, Ganesalingam K, Gastier-Foster JM, Frick J, et al. Apolipoprotein E4 as a predictor of outcomes in pediatric mild traumatic brain injury. J Neurotrauma. 2009;26: 1489–95.

76. Jordan BD. Genetic influences on outcome following traumatic brain injury. Neurochem Res. 2007;32:905–15.

77. Berger RP, Zuckerbraun N. Biochemical markers. In: Kirkwood MW, Yeates KO, editors. Mild traumatic brain injury in children and adolescents: from basic science to clinical management. New York: Guilford Press; 2012. p. 145–61.

78. Iverson GL, Brooks BL, Collins MW, Lovell MR. Tracking neuropsychological recovery following concussion in sport. Brain Inj. 2006;20:245–52.

79. Kirkwood MW, Yeates KO, Taylor HG, Randolph C, McCrea M, Anderson VA. Management of pediatric mild traumatic brain injury: a neuropsychological review from injury through recovery. Clin Neuropsychol. 2008;22:769–800.

Chapter 16
Long-Term Effects of Pediatric Mild Traumatic Brain Injury

Rimma Danov

Abstract There is a growing amount of research confirming that many cognitive, behavioral, and emotional symptoms may persist for months after a mild traumatic brain injury (TBI), or a concussion. Studies that have detected long-term impairments include various neuropsychological tests and rating scales, as well as metabolic and radiological findings, all of which support the hypothesis that some individuals experience persistent disruption of the integrity of the neural fiber and metabolic balance, which lead to the disruption of cerebral functioning even after a mild TBI. As a result, a subgroup of concussed individuals continues to suffer from various mood changes, behavioral disturbances, concentration and memory problems, and other functional impairments.

When we are investigating a mild TBI in children, we need to consider not only the short-term cognitive, behavioral, and emotional impairments that they experience for the first weeks and months post TBI, but also the long-term consequences of metabolic and structural neurological changes that may cause a profound and protracted effect on child's brain development. While some children show a remarkable recovery from a concussion, others continue to suffer from the emotional, behavioral, and cognitive dysfunction, which prevents them from acquiring and developing more complex, higher-order skills in the first few years after the injury.

Such disruption of the developmental process produces more than just a suboptimal adaptation to the changing environment; it also brings out new challenges that children face as they grow and are expected to acquire and demonstrate new, advanced level skills, as projected for their peer group. Functional milestones for different age groups are different, and may include a stronger impulse control, the

R. Danov, Ph.D. (✉)
Dr. Danov Neuropsychologist PC, 9511 Shore Road, Suite C, Brooklyn, NY 11209, USA

Pennsylvania State University, State College, PA, USA
e-mail: DrDanov@NeuropsychNYC.com

S.M. Slobounov and W.J. Sebastianelli (eds.), *Concussions in Athletics:*
From Brain to Behavior, DOI 10.1007/978-1-4939-0295-8_16,
© Springer Science+Business Media New York 2014

ability to read social cues, specific math skills, better sustained focus, and the ability to organize one's thoughts or information details, to name a few. Thus, some effects of a pediatric concussion are not easily observed after the brain injury, yet they contribute to protracted academic, cognitive, and interpersonal struggles.

Keywords TBI • Pediatric brain injury • Concussion • Attention • Memory • Child development • Social–emotional skills • Academic performance • Behavioral regulation • Executive dysfunction • Neuropsychological assessment • Neuroimaging

Introduction

While there might be some discrepancy in the reported rates of pediatric brain injury among numerous published studies, the average rate is approximately 180 per 100,000 head injuries per year in children under 15 years of age [1]. Sixteen percent of children under 10 years of age sustain at least one traumatic brain injury (TBI) [2]. Most of these head injuries are mild. According to the National Pediatric Trauma Registry, 76 % of pediatric brain injuries are mild, 10 % are moderate, and 15 % are severe [3]. Given these staggering rates, brain injury presents a significant health risk to children and even the mild form of brain injury may sometimes create significant obstacles in children's lives at home and in school.

The most recent consensus statement regarding a concussion, or a mild TBI, is that while it may cause neuropathological changes, they are largely associated with functional deficits rather than structural abnormalities, wherein the latter are traditionally detected by neuroimaging [4]. Thus, thousands of children every year sustain mild head injuries and experience various neuropathological changes that greatly affect their academic, behavioral, emotional, and cognitive functioning. While the majority of children with mild TBI recover within the first few weeks or months, a subgroup of these children continue to suffer from persistent cognitive and emotional deficits that compromise their academic performance, social interactions, and emotional stability.

The actual number of children with mild TBI, who experience long-term functional deficits, varies from author to author. Kraus [1] showed that only 10 % of children with closed head injury experienced moderate disability. Bruce and Schut [5] concluded that approximately 50 % of children continue to experience some form of long-term cognitive deficits post TBI. Other authors have determined that 11 % of children in their research sample displayed symptoms 3 months after a mild brain injury and 2.3 % of this sample continued to display cognitive and emotional symptoms 1 year later [6]. Thus, while researchers utilize various outcome measures of post-TBI symptoms and focus on different age groups, which likely generates the diversity in rates and severity of functional dysfunction and neuropsychological symptoms, one fact remains clear: a lot of children sustain relatively mild head injuries and appear seemingly well after the first few months post

TBI, when pain, scrapes and bumps disappear, but some of them continue to suffer from disturbing cognitive and emotional symptoms.

Even if only 2–10 % of children with a mild brain injury are struggling to learn in school, appropriately interact with peers and adults, and keep up with the increasing social and academic demands, it is important to advance our understanding of a mild TBI in order to help these children. So far, our current knowledge about structural and metabolic changes that occur at different points of time after a mild brain injury point to the need to reassess, intervene, and address the long-term post-TBI deficits at different points of time, in addition to most immediate post-injury care. Such protracted cognitive, emotional, and behavioral difficulties should be addressed as soon as they arise, even if they become pronounced some time after the injury, so that these children can receive the needed treatment and finally return to their normal developmental trajectory.

Short-Term Versus Long-Term Post-concussion Symptoms

Common short-term cognitive symptoms of pediatric brain injury, such as impaired attention, processing speed, visual perception, working memory, motor functioning, emotional lability, and hyperactivity, have been observed and documented by numerous studies over the years [7–9]. It appears that these symptoms may affect virtually all areas of functioning in children. For instance, in addition to having trouble sustaining focus, quickly and accurately processing new information, and retaining new facts, concussed children tend to have fewer friends and experience poor social skills and increased emotional lability [10–12]. Their family relationships may be compromised as well [13] and their academic performance is likely to decline [14, 15].

Moreover, Wozniak et al. [16] showed that traumatic injury to the white matter in the supracallosal region is specifically related to overt behavioral deficits, such as hyperactivity, aggression, and attention deficit. In this study, while children with mild and moderate brain injury did not differ from controls in general intelligence scores, their sustained focus and behavioral and emotional regulation were impaired when assessed 6–12 months after the brain injury. This finding is very important in the understanding of post-TBI functioning and performance, as it illustrates that, unlike the core intellectual abilities, which remain largely resilient to a mild white matter trauma, regulatory functions and efficiency skills are much more susceptible to impairment. This is a critical aspect of post-TBI life, as regulatory functions and efficiency skills are essential functions that allow one to utilize core intellectual abilities while completing academic tasks, listening to and following daily directions, and navigating social conflicts and relationships.

As our understanding of a mild TBI expands, we see that many children may quickly recover from the external head trauma and return to school, but some of them remain irritable, easily angered, hyperactive, and fidgety and have difficulty sustaining focus, effectively planning and organizing their activities and study material, adequately capturing and processing new concepts and rules, retaining new facts and retrieving information they have recently learned. They may also omit and misread social cues and display inappropriate reactions to daily stressors and changes in their environment. As we know, cognitive skills, academic abilities, and emotional stability are closely intertwined in many educational and social activities that children engage on a daily basis. Thus, it is difficult to separate where poor focus and retention problems end and irritability and frustration begin, when a child fails to listen to and follow directions, inhibit impulses, and sustain his focus to solve a math problem and, instead, fidgets and talks in class and disrupts his classmates. As a result, while these children have seemingly recovered from their mild head injury that they might have sustained on a playground or while playing sports, their entire life, including behaviors, relationships, and academic performance, come under assault of residual cognitive deficits and mood changes that cause ongoing disruption and anguish.

Over the past decades, we have learned a lot about the immediate head injury symptoms that children may experience during the first days and weeks post TBI. While immediate symptoms of a mild brain injury in children have been extensively documented, more recent research studies focus on identifying long-term cognitive symptoms, such as memory impairment that persists in some children 2 years post TBI [17]. Barlow and her colleagues [6] investigated mild brain injury in children and showed that 11 % of children displayed post-concussion symptoms 3 months after their injury and 1 year later these symptoms were still seen in 2.3 % of injured children. These studies helped us develop a better understanding of how and why some children's recovery patterns differ from the majority of their peers, who have also sustained a mild TBI, and how persistent post-injury symptoms alter their normal developmental trajectory.

We can glean answers to these questions from the unique developmental processes that take place in a growing child's brain. Children's brains differ significantly from the adult brain and it is not just by virtue of being less mature or less capable. There are multiple developmental processes that are constantly changing the matrix of a child's brain, making it more or less sensitive to various brain insults, treatment efforts, and environmental changes and stressors. Some of those developmental factors include ongoing myelination, sensitivity to oxidative stress, higher water content, open sutures, and brain plasticity [18, 19]. In fact, it is believed that maturation of white matter continues until approximately 30 years of age, as summarized by Maxwell [19]. Since the brain development is such a fluid process, any insult to the growing brain at any specific time would technically produce a different outcome because the brain was at a different state of development, with certain developmental goals already accomplished and certain developmental goals still at various stages of completion.

Over the past two decades, several authors have suggested that the damage caused by a traumatic injury to a developing brain can interfere with such processes as neuronal myelination and frontal lobe maturation [20, 21]. Indeed, during childhood and adolescence, a child's brain is constantly undergoing a major construction of complex cortical networks, making it possible for the child to utilize self-regulation of emotions and behavior, sustain focus on lengthy assignments, organize his belongings and activities, and reflect on, compare, and associate various concepts. It is a complex, multidimensional scaffolding process that would be suspended and/or interrupted if some aspects of it are damaged and cannot, at least for some period of time, play their role in advancing the higher-order skills and supporting the associated cerebral functions. Levin [22] specifically questioned whether diffuse injury, which often occurs in mild brain injury cases, disrupts the development of networks that support higher-order cognitive functions in childhood.

Thus, if a mild cerebral insult produces diffuse injury, it may not be always detected by the traditional neuroimaging studies [4]. Yet, it still sets off a disruption of the ongoing myelination and maturation of white matter in a child's brain. How long can this disruption last for before it generates long lasting effects on the cognitive, academic, and emotional maturity of a child? If some skill development is suspended for some time after the mild TBI, how does it affect the development of associated skills and how long does it take for the specific skill expansion, or evolution, to catch up with its original developmental goal?

Cognitive Impairment and Structural Abnormalities

In the past decades, numerous research findings have provided tremendous advances in understanding the short-term and long-term effects of focal brain damage on cognitive functioning. For example, studies that used neuropsychological measures of cognitive abilities and MRI results have determined that extrafrontal and temporal lesion volume predicted memory deficits as late as 1 year after the brain injury [23]. Also, Power and colleagues [24] have concluded that combined frontal and extrafrontal lesions predicted attention deficit 5 years after TBI, while the severity of individual frontal lesions were not predictive of attentional function.

However, if a mild TBI produces mainly diffuse white matter injury, which is not always detected by the traditional MRI scans, how can we illuminate the disruption of a complex web of constantly evolving cortical networks and its protracted effect over time on a child's functioning at home and in school? Such interruption in the maturation of white matter of a child's brain may not only delay the advancement of the existing skills but also delay the acquisition of more complex abilities. Indeed, in a growing child's brain which undergoes rapid restructuring and layering of cognitive and emotional skills, a delay in maturation of lower-level abilities may significantly disrupt the scaffolding of higher-level abilities. While this hypothesis is not entirely new, recent studies investigating mild TBI have offered more support as they have found persistent cognitive impairments, as measured by neuropsychological tests, that correlate with metabolic disruptions and structural impairments in the brain.

It has been noted that conventional MRI can measure small lesions or hemorrhages and MRI findings correlate with neuropsychological and psychiatric outcome, but MRI may also underestimate diffuse axonal injury that is frequently seen in mild TBI [16]. While traditional MRI studies are not always able to detect structural impairment in mild brain injury cases [4], a newer neuroimaging technique, diffusion tensor imaging (DTI), offers a much more precise method of measuring post-concussion changes that occur in the white matter and contribute to persistent post-concussion symptoms and functional impairment months after the mild TBI.

DTI study measures the integrity of the white matter fibers via diffusion of water molecules [25]. If some axons are damaged and myelin sheath has diminished, the inter-axonal water volume increases. Therefore, DTI can detect injured axons and destroyed myelin even in mild TBI by measuring the integrity of white matter fibers; such axonal injury was observed months after the brain injury [16]. This is a new advancement in the detection of neuronal injury over the traditional MRI scan, which is not able to "see" such minor brain damage. In addition to being able to detect minor, yet important changes in white matter shortly after the brain injury, DTI allows the detection of long-term axonal injuries. For example, Bendlin and colleagues [26] described long-term impairments of white matter, as seen in DTI studies, 1 year after the injury. Her group detected specific axonal injury via fractional anisotropy and mean diffusivity reduction that was much greater than normal white matter changes expected in age-matched peers.

Thus, DTI technique allows us to detect some structural abnormalities in concussed individuals that were not visible on traditional neuroimaging studies, but those abnormalities remained for months or more post TBI. While these structural abnormalities might be minor, they are not inconsequential and do contribute to significant functional impairment that disturbs a brain injured person's ability to complete daily chores, learn new information, and effectively interact with and adapt to his environment. In the recent years, such functional dysfunction, which is traditionally measured by neuropsychological tests, was found to correlate with structural abnormalities, as detected by DTI, further supporting the idea that even a mild brain injury may produce long-term cognitive functional impairments in some individuals.

For example, Wozniak and colleagues [16] showed that decreased cortical white matter fractional anisotropy, as measured by DTI, is associated with impaired neurocognitive test scores, mainly with executive functioning and motor speed neuropsychological measures (tests and rating scales) 6–12 months after the injury. This study has shown that children with mild and moderate brain injury had lower fractional anisotropy in three white matter regions—inferior frontal, superior frontal, and supracallosal regions. When DTI study results were compared to neuropsychological test results, fractional anisotropy in frontal and supracallosal regions correlated with neuropsychological test scores on measures of executive functioning, while fractional anisotropy in supracallosal region correlated with test scores measuring motor speed, and supracallosal fractional anisotropy correlated with behavioral ratings. This group concluded that greater impairment of white matter in the frontal lobe was associated with functional deficits, as reflected in low scores on specific neuropsychological measures (the Tower of London and the reports and ratings of daily behaviors on the Behavior Rating Inventory of Executive Function), which measure executive functions such as planning, impulse control, sustained focus, self-monitoring, and other aspects of executive, or frontal lobe functions. Thus, while the detected axonal damage was minimal, children with mild and moderate brain injury in this study demonstrated measurable cognitive and behavioral deficits. Such findings of objective neuropsychological tools, in combination with advanced technology, further solidify the notion that diffuse axonal injury can cause persistent disruption in a child's daily functioning. Knowing this, we can help children and their families effectively cope with and remediate multiple changes in cognition, academics, and behavior.

Cognitive Impairment and Metabolic Alterations

Further support for the notion of post-concussion functional disruption comes from research studies that focused on metabolic abnormalities secondary to TBI. Different neurochemical concentrations reflect different neuropathological processes that occur at different stages of life and post-injury period. Some of these metabolic changes, which have been detected from infancy to up to 16 years of age, are involved in the normal course of development and contribute to the development of various cognitive and emotional abilities [27].

Recent studies have shown that posttraumatic metabolic changes may signal the presence of axonal injury that is not always easily identified. For example, lower N-acetyl aspartate (NAA) concentration may reflect neuronal and axonal damage, which is consistent with diffuse axonal injury but not seen on traditional MRI studies [28]. Researchers have also detected specific changes in NAA and cholines (Cho) levels in mild and severe pediatric TBI cases, with Cho levels decreasing in the first year after the brain injury; in severe TBI cases decreased Cho levels may reflect neuronal death and cerebral atrophy [29, 30]. Cholines, such as glycerol-phosphocholine and phosphocholine, are markers of cell membrane synthesis and repair, while NAA is a marker of neuronal and axonal functioning. Thus, any posttraumatic changes in the brain cell metabolic concentrations signal the disruption of the cell integrity and functioning. Interestingly, NAA concentration changes post TBI are associated not only with axonal loss due to various trauma mechanisms, but also with milder forms of axonal injury, such as axonal swelling, stretching, and myelin damage.

The influence of metabolic changes in the growing child's brain on everyday functioning is undeniable. As brain injury triggers a chain reaction of certain metabolic changes in a child's brain, it disrupts the normal ratio of metabolic concentrations that is necessary for optimal functioning in school and at home. Specifically, Chertkoff Walz and his colleagues [29] have determined that higher metabolic concentration is associated with better academic skills and social competence. They also showed positive correlation between Cho levels and spatial, spelling, and pragmatic language abilities.

Thus, a growing body of research leads us to believe that even a mild brain injury may cause an ongoing disruption of the normative developmental changes in the brain's metabolism, which, in turn, compromises the integrity of a child's neuropsychological functioning, as reflected in cognitive difficulties, declining academic performance, and social–emotional problems that disrupt the lives of some children after a mild TBI.

Post-concussion Recovery and Assessment Challenges

Recovery from a mild brain injury is also laced with peculiarities that are specific to a growing child's brain. Several researchers have concluded that some aspects of a child's brain, such as plasticity and functional reorganization, are helpful in recovery from a focal brain injury but not from a diffuse brain injury [31, 32]. White matter at different stages of development may respond differently to the traumatic process and if some higher-level skills, such as social comprehension, sustained and divided attention, impulse inhibition, or complex reasoning, did not have a chance to develop before the onset of TBI, concussed children may experience slowed maturation of these skills in the following months. In fact, Gerrard-Morris and colleagues [33] showed that deficits in pragmatic language emerged some 12 months after the brain injury, while Anderson and colleagues [34] showed that memory problems did not emerge in young children until 1 year after the brain injury. These long-term effects may be different for children in different age groups, but it is important to know that if some children are too young to demonstrate full-fledged abilities involving social communication (pragmatic language) or certain aspects of memory, their cognitive impairment and social deficits may not be acknowledged, measured, and remediated following their mild brain injury.

Levin and Hanten [35] have pointed out that executive system in children is undergoing such significant and rapid changes that greatly complicate the study of the effects of brain injury on pediatric executive system. As a result, children who sustained a brain injury, specifically frontal lobe injury, at a younger age, when organization, impulse control, self-regulation, and other frontal lobe functions have not developed and matured yet, may not demonstrate executive system deficits until much later in life. Thus, we may not appreciate the extent of the brain injury until after the child has recovered from all external and overt physical and cognitive symptoms.

Moreover, the age of onset of TBI and the severity of injury are not the only variables affecting the outcome of pediatric TBI, as different brain functions may suffer different long-term post-concussion effects. One study investigated the variability in dysexecutive symptom expression in children post TBI, specifically looking at focal versus diffuse brain injury and the extent of frontal lobe involvement and the effect of pre-injury functioning [36]. This research group has determined that children who sustained a concussion at a younger age are more vulnerable to executive skill impairment and long-term deficits. In fact, when concussed children were assessed 2 years post injury, 14–50 % of them performed below grade level in math. Other authors have also showed that the development of arithmetic skills is most vulnerable to the effects of TBI, while their samples' word recognition was relatively unchanged [37]. Their finding is not surprising, as math is an academic achievement ability that builds upon such cognitive skills as sustained focus, sequencing, planning, spatial reasoning, planning, and organization—the same cognitive abilities that are often impaired by a concussion.

In addition, it was determined that attention control and literacy mature by approximately 8 years of age, while goal setting and arithmetic skills mature by approximately 12 years [36]. Thus, if some children sustain a brain injury before 8 or 12 years of age, they may experience protracted post-TBI deficits, including the delay in maturation of attention control, literacy, goal setting, and arithmetic skills, which were not so obvious shortly after their brain injury.

Now, when a student scores low on a math test, experiences difficulty in reasoning and developing a multi-step plan for a science project, or has trouble sustaining focus on lengthy standardized tests, teachers and parents do not immediately connect these academic problems with a concussion that took place last summer or during winter break. Thus, concussed children may end up following a dwindling road of poor academic performance and conflicts with peers and adults, while their caretakers and educators are not recognizing these problems as long-term symptoms of a mild brain injury; hence, they do not proactively monitor concussed children for possible academic and cognitive problems in order to address them at the earliest point of time and in their mildest form, which is easier to remediate.

School work is the major responsibility of a child and it requires a child to utilize all of his cognitive and socio-emotional resources. Academic activities depend on the executive skills, as students are required to reason and apply appropriate rules and formulas, sustain focus for prolonged period of time, organize their assignments, plan their study and test preparation activities, extract essential elements from a reading material, compare and contrast facts, and perform many other executive functions. Social interactions also heavily depend on executive skills, as children are required to monitor their environment and behavior, regulate their emotional reactions and behavioral actions in accordance with social norms, inhibit impulses to act and talk when necessary, etc. These are all very important abilities that allow children to establish and maintain appropriate and rewarding relationships with peers and adults, behave and regulate their mood and attention so that they can learn in class, adapt and apply their new knowledge and skills to ever-changing life circumstances.

If some protracted post-TBI deficits do not come to the surface until months later, children who sustained mild brain injury during their summer vacation may be viewed as fully recovered when they start their new academic year in September. It is possible that we do not consider a concussion as a precipitating factor when some children start experiencing pragmatic language deficits, aggression, hyperactivity, frequent conflicts, and social interaction problems months after their concussion, as at that point their brain injury incident is so far removed that parents and teachers may believe that these problems are not related to a brain injury. Of course, a thorough neuropsychological assessment is required in such cases to rule out developmental disorders that also involve pragmatic language deficits and social interaction problems, such as Asperger's disorder and pervasive developmental disorder. Neuropsychological assessment and academic achievement testing are also needed to rule out specific pre-TBI learning disabilities involving math, reading, and writing in children who display declining academic performance post TBI. In essence, neuropsychological evaluation becomes an essential tool in bringing all these different pieces of a puzzle together in order to sort out preexisting conditions, protracted post-TBI symptoms, and normally developing brain functions. It is a complicated task, but certainly worth attempting for the sake of satisfying a child's life.

Neuropsychologists who specialize in the assessment of children and developmental disorders possess a unique expertise to evaluate functional integrity of a child's brain immediately after the brain injury and at a later time, when some children might be experiencing long-term effects of a brain injury that prevent them from adequately adapting to changing academic, cognitive, and social demands of their peer group and the environment. Hence, the timeline for monitoring concussed children should include at least 12 months post brain injury. Subsequent neuropsychological assessments can be performed at 24 months post-TBI mark if prior evaluation detected any lingering cognitive, emotional, or behavioral deficits. If no such deficits were detected at the 24 months mark post brain injury, concussed children can be discharged from a neuropsychological care. Any later follow-up is suggested if the children display any newfound difficulties in social, emotional, academic, or general cognitive functioning, such as difficulty reading social cues, negotiating conflicts, inhibiting impulses at age appropriate level, or developing higher-order reasoning, academic, and comprehension skills.

Neuropsychological measures provide objective, structured symptom assessment and ecologically valid functional description of executive (i.e., organization, emotional regulation, self-monitoring of performance and behavior, social judgment, goal directed behavior, problem solving, abstraction, impulse control), memory, motor, language, attention, speed, information processing, and emotional and behavioral abilities relative to a child's age norm, which is critical in post-injury return to school, home life, sports, and social settings. The wealth of objective data gathered during the neuropsychological assessment allows neuropsychologists to track the developmental trajectory of cognitive and behavioral skills, the foundation of a more targeted, individualized treatment and create an intervention plan before cognitive, academic, and behavioral problems that have worsened and higher-order cognitive skills have failed to develop.

Conclusion

The wealth of the existing research knowledge, supported by the ever-developing technology that helps us to detect even minor effects of the brain injury, allows more precise investigation of concussion diagnosis and short-term and long-term symptomatology. It also prompts us to consider recovery patterns and the developmental level of a child's individual skill sets, which may or may not have matured at the time of the injury. We know now that brain injury may retard the development of any cognitive or emotional abilities while they are at their "budding" stage and that impairment becomes more apparent at a later time, when a child fails to acquire, mature, and demonstrate more advanced skills.

Some children, who sustained a concussion and returned to classrooms, appear to have fully recovered yet may still experience cognitive, emotional, and behavioral problems at a later time because those particular skills were not required or utilized at the age when they sustained a concussion; hence, their impairment was not "visible." However, as the social and academic demands increase with time, some children who sustained a mild brain injury may fail to adapt to the changing environment because they did not fully develop and acquire higher-order skills that support a steady learning curve and make a successful adaptation possible. This hypothesis resonates with findings that showed that behavioral and emotional problems, including impulsivity, aggressive behaviors, and frequent mood changes, increase with time after the TBI, while physical and cognitive complaints decrease [38].

Of course, the long-term concussion effects on child brain development are dependent on many important factors, such as the child's age at the time of concussion, pre-concussion level of cognitive, behavioral, and emotional development, and the resources available to children to help them recover from concussion and catch up on developmental milestones. Since such a multitude of variables are involved, research studies may produce varying results based on the different characteristics of pediatric samples and measurement tools involved. We do not have a precise matrix of all these factors yet, but future pediatric concussion research may help us construct a concussion evaluation and recovery model that would include protracted effects of a mild TBI and, hence, allow us identify the child's trajectory of recovery from a concussion and his future development of specific cognitive, emotional, and behavioral skills.

The treatment of such long-term effects of concussions would depend on the type and severity of their symptoms and would need to be tailored to individual characteristics of these children and their environment. While frequent repetitive neuropsychological testing would not be necessary, occasional neuropsychological assessments of concussed children would produce important information about their overall cognitive, emotional, and behavioral development, including their adjustment to changing peer environment and academic demands. Thus, useful guidelines can be generated for concussed children's parents, teachers, school psychologists, and caretakers as to which cognitive, emotional, or behavioral weaknesses exist in a child's neuropsychological profile and how to reduce them (e.g., social skills and communication skills group therapy to improve reasoning, pragmatic language, and social interactions).

And the final thought, any children who were unfortunate enough to experience the long-term effects of a mild brain injury could be detected before their post-concussion symptoms have seriously interfered with their academic performance and peer relationships and limited their future educational and career advancement.

Adopting more proactive approach to identifying such weaknesses in children with mild TBI should certainly yield better functioning and happier children who can truly state that they have survived a brain injury and successfully developed their cognitive, emotional, and behavioral skills up to par with their age-matched peers.

References

1. Kraus JF. Epidemiological features of brain injury in children: occurrence, children at risk, causes and manner of injury, severity, and outcomes. In: Broman SH, Michel ME, editors. Traumatic head injury in children. New York: Oxford University Press; 1995. p. 22–39.
2. Langlois JA, Rutland-Brown W, Thomas KE. Traumatic brain injury in the United States: emergency department visits, hospitalizations, and deaths. Atlanta, GA: Centers for Disease Control and Prevention, National Center for Injury Prevention and Control; 2006. http://www.cdc.gov/ncipc/pub-res/tbi_in_us_04/tbi_ed
3. Lescohier I, DiScala C. Blunt trauma in children: causes and outcomes of head versus intracranial injury. Pediatrics. 1993;91:721–5.
4. McCrory P, Meeuwisse WH, Aubry M, Cantu B, Dvorak J, Echemendia RJ, et al. Consensus statement on concussion in sport: the 4th international conference on concussion in sport held in Zurich, November 2012. Br J Sports Med. 2013;47:250–8.
5. Bruce DA, Schut L. Concussion and contusion following pediatric head trauma. In: McLaurin RL, editor. Pediatric neurosurgery: surgery of the developing system; 1982.
6. Barlow KM, Crawford S, Stevenson A, Sandhu SS, Belanger F, Dewey D. Epidemiology of post-concussion syndrome in pediatric mild traumatic brain injury. Pediatrics. 2010;126(2):374–81.
7. Matz PG. Classification diagnosis, and management of mild traumatic brain injury: a major problem presenting in a minor way. Semin Neurosurg. 2003;14(2):125–30.
8. Tremont G, Mittenberg W, Miller LJ. Acute intellectual effects of pediatric head trauma. Child Neuropsychol. 1999;5:104–14.
9. Schaffer D. Behavioral sequelae of serious head injury in children and adolescents: the British studies. In: Broman SH, Michel ME, editors. Traumatic head injury in children. New York: Oxford University Press; 1995. p. 55–69.
10. Prigatano GP, Gupta S. Friends after traumatic brain injury in children. J Head Trauma Rehabil. 2006;21(6):505–13.
11. Janusz JA, Kirkwood MW, Yeates KO, Taylor HG. Social problem-solving skills in children with traumatic brain injury: long-term outcomes and predictions of social competence. Child Neuropsychol. 2002;8:179–94.
12. Ganesalingam K, Sanson A, Anderson V, Yeates KO. Self-regulation and social behavioral functioning following childhood traumatic brain injury. J Int Neuropsychol Soc. 2006;12:609–21.
13. Hawley CA. Reported problems and their resolution following mild, moderate, and severe traumatic brain injury amongst children and adolescents in the UK. Brain Inj. 2003;17(2):105–29.
14. Hawley CA, Ward AB, Magnay AR, Long J. Children's brain injury: a postal follow-up of 525 children from one health region in UK. Brain Inj. 2002;16:969–85.
15. Hooper SR, Alexander J, Moore D, Sasser HC, Laurent S, King J, et al. Caregiver reports of common symptoms in children following traumatic brain injury. NeuroRehabilitation. 2004;19:175–89.
16. Wozniak J, Krach L, Ward E, Mueller BA, Muetzel R, Schnoebelen S, Kiragu A, Lim KO. Neurocognitive and neuroimaging correlates of pediatric traumatic brain injury: a diffusion tensor imaging (DTI) study. Arch Clin Neuropsychol. 2007;22(5):555–68.

17. Levin HS, Hanten G, Zhang L, Swank PR, Ewing-Cobbs L, Dennis M. Changes in working memory after traumatic brain injury in children. Neuropsychology. 2004;18(2):240–7.
18. Bauer R, Fritz H. Pathophysiology of traumatic injury in the developing brain: an introduction and short update. Exp Toxicol Pathol. 2004;56:65–73.
19. Maxwell WL. Traumatic brain injury in the neonate, child and adolescent human: an overview of pathology. Int J Dev Neurosci. 2012;30(3):167–83.
20. Ewing-Cobbs L, Prasad MR, Swank P, Kramer L, Cox CS, Fletcher JM, et al. Arrested development and disrupted callosal microstructure following pediatric traumatic brain injury in children: relation to neurobehavioral outcomes. Neuroimage. 2008;42:1305–15.
21. Thatcher RW. Maturation of the human frontal lobes, physiological evidence for staging. Dev Neuropsychol. 1991;7:397–419.
22. Levin HS. Neuroplasticity following non-penetrating traumatic brain injury. Brain Inj. 2003;17(8):665–74.
23. Salorio CF, Slomine BS, Grados MA, Vasa RA, Christensen JR, Gerring J. Neuroanatomic correlates of CVLT-C performance following pediatric traumatic brain injury. J Int Neuropsychol Soc. 2005;11(6):686–96.
24. Power T, Catroppa C, Coleman L, Ditchfield M, Anderson V. Do lesion sites and severity predict deficits in attentional control after preschool traumatic brain injury (TBI)? Brain Inj. 2007;21:279–92.
25. Basser PJ, Jones DK. Diffusion-tensor MRI: theory, experimental design and data analysis—a technical review. NMR Biomed. 2002;15(7–8):456–67.
26. Bendlin BB, Ries ML, Lazar M, Alexander AL, Dempsey RJ, Rowley HA, et al. Longitudinal changes in patients with traumatic brain injury assessed with diffusion-tensor and volumetric imaging. Neuroimage. 2008;42:503–14.
27. van der Knapp M, van der Grond J, van Rijen P. Age-dependent changes in localized proton and phosphorus MR spectroscopy of the brain. Radiology. 1990;176:509–15.
28. Holshouser BA, Tong KA, Ashwal S. Proton MR spectroscopic imaging depicts diffuse axonal injury in children with traumatic brain injury. AJNR Am J Neuroradiol. 2005;26:1276–85.
29. Chertkoff Walz N, Cecil KM, Wade SL, Michaud LJ. Late proton magnetic resonance spectroscopy following traumatic brain injury during early childhood: relationship with neurobehavioral outcomes. J Neurotrauma. 2008;25:94–103.
30. Parry L, Shores A, Rae C, Kemp A, Waugh M, Chaseling R, Joy P. An investigation of neuronal integrity in severe pediatric traumatic brain injury. Child Neuropsychol. 2004;10(4):248–61.
31. Anderson VA, Morse SA, Catroppa C, Haritou F, Rosenfeld JV. Thirty month outcome from early childhood head injury: a prospective analysis of neurobehavioral recovery. Brain. 2004;127:2608–20.
32. Sauskauer SJ, Huisman TAGM. Neuroimaging in pediatric traumatic brain injury: current and future predictors of functional outcome. Dev Disabil Res Rev. 2009;15:117–23.
33. Gerrard-Morris A, Taylor G, Yeates KO, Chertkoff Walz N, Stacin T, Minich N, et al. Cognitive development after traumatic brain injury in young children. J Int Neuropsychol Soc. 2009;16:157–68.
34. Anderson VA, Catropa C, Rosenfeld J, Haritou F, Morse SA. Recovery of memory function following traumatic brain injury in pre-school children. Brain Inj. 2000;14:679–92.
35. Levin HS, Hanten G. Executive functions after traumatic brain injury in children. Pediatr Neurol. 2005;33(2):79–93.
36. Anderson V, Catroppa C. Recovery of executive skills following pediatric traumatic brain injury (TBI): a 2 year follow-up. Brain Inj. 2005;19(6):459–70.
37. Ewing-Cobbs L, Fletcher JM, Levin HS, Iovino L, Miner ME. Academic achievement and academic placement following traumatic brain injury in children and adolescents: a two-year longitudinal study. J Clin Exp Neuropsychol. 1998;20:769–81.
38. Yeates KO, Taylor HG, Drotar D, Wade S, Stacin T. Neurobehavioral symptoms in childhood closed-head injuries: changes in prevalence and correlates during the first year post-injury. J Pediatr Psychol. 2001;26:79–91.

Chapter 17
Neuropsychological Assessment of Sports-Related Concussion: Pediatric Challenges

Mark R. Lovell

Abstract Many factors are important regarding the neural integration of psychological assessment into the overall picture of concussion management. A whole team of experts are required to manage concussions properly, including neuropsychological testing and at times brain imaging. First, I will share my perspective on neuropsychological assessment and how it fits into the overall paradigm of how we manage concussions. Secondly, I will present a little history on that subject. Lastly, a case will be presented that is relatable to many real life concussion cases. My primary focus in this chapter will be pediatric concussion which is the most puzzling issue of concussive injury.

Keywords Concussion • Neuropsychology • Pediatric concussion • Second impact syndrome

Introduction

There has been a huge amount of publicity over the last 5 years regarding concussion, due to increased recognition of head injury at the NFL level. Some of the work that Dr. Constantine has done has increased recognition of sports-related concussion in the media. This work has led to many legislative changes, including big changes in the Pennsylvania state law. Despite the fact that there is a long way to go, all of this has led to improved safety standards and we are moving in the right direction. However, there are some challenges with respect to pediatric concussions.

M.R. Lovell, Ph.D. (✉)
ImPact, LLC, 2000 Technology Drive, Suite 150, Pittsburgh, PA 15219, USA

Department of Neurological Surgery, University of Pittsburgh, Pittsburgh, PA, USA
e-mail: mlovell@Impacttest.com

S.M. Slobounov and W.J. Sebastianelli (eds.), *Concussions in Athletics:*
From Brain to Behavior, DOI 10.1007/978-1-4939-0295-8_17,
© Springer Science+Business Media New York 2014

It is understood that athletes cannot be trusted to explain what is wrong with them. So, often times, a fundamental problem of dealing with this injury can be the players concealing their symptoms. Athletes often lie about their symptoms, not only at the professional level but also at all ages. This may include younger children who will not say if they have a headache because if they admit to the headache, they will not be able to attend the following game.

This concealment starts at an early age and culminates in professional sports. An USA Today article published on Dale Earnhardt describes the common issue of the athlete being the last person to admit that something is wrong with him or her. In motor sports especially this is a problem because a driver may be inches apart from another driver's wheel going 220 mph. Some of the other drivers do not want to be on the track with someone who has a concussion. To put it mildly, the diagnosis can be tricky, and the misdiagnosis of injury is very common. For example, labs can elaborate a disease but diagnosing a concussion is more like trying to interpret the moods of an Irish setter that this presents an enormous challenge.

The reason that I got into management of concussions over 25 years ago was because of this dilemma of having people who were understood to be injured, but would not admit that they were injured and to find technology that could prove this. Initially, I started at the NFL level with the Pittsburg Steelers, but our major concern now is obviously with children since they are a precious commodity. Most concussions occur in children, and even though a very small number of child athletes make it to the college or professional level, almost everybody plays sports as a kid. Their exposures/risk of concussion is therefore higher and it has been found that their brains are more vulnerable than adults. Some of the work that Dr. Cantu and others have done over the years solidifies that brain injuries can seriously interfere with a child's development leading to serious problems in school. Dr. Joy discussed that children will often deny their symptoms, even after they are educated on what symptoms to look for and how to report them. It is important to always be cognizant of this fact.

There is also the issue of second impact syndrome [1], which is a very disturbing rare condition that many people believe is something we need to be careful about in children. There are a number of videos showing kids playing tackle football. First of all, there can be a long discussion about whether or not kids should be playing tackle football and ramming into another child at high speeds since he probably does not have the strength to hold his head erect. But, this happens all the time. I work a lot in these sports in Pennsylvania and particularly in western Pennsylvania in the Pittsburg area. In this area, people start playing tackle football at age 6. Now when I was a kid, it was age 8 and philosophically, I have a problem with that. For example in baseball, kids in t-ball are learning skills on how to hit off the tee. But for kids this age in football, they get thrown into situations where they can have a significant impact on their health. This is why working with children is so important for the sake of their safety as well as for their physical and psychological well-being.

From the standpoint of being a neuropsychologist, these are some of the symptoms that have been found in athletes, specifically high school and college athletes.

Other researchers have done similar studies and have found pretty much the same thing [2]. Headaches are always the number one symptom seen in most of the concussion studies. Symptoms of feeling slowed down/sluggishness, difficulty concentrating, fogginess, and memory dysfunction have to do with the cognitive systems in the brain. This area specifically is where neuropsychological assessment is particularly useful because these symptoms are things that athletes are not very good at reporting or being aware of. This cries out for a tool that can help manage the cognitive aspects of injury. Setting the research bias aside, the symptoms that athletes are likely to have in terms of these four general systems must be thought about. This was done by factor analysis and what is observed is that the system constellations hanging together have more of the migraine type of symptoms.

There is certainly the cognitive aspect and the issues with sleep [3]. Sleep indeed is a big issue in both concussed athletes and military personnel and can fall into a neuropsychiatric category. It is believed that cognitive and sleep problems are very firmly related to changes that take place in the brain following injury. This leads us to begin thinking about treatments for concussion. Not surprisingly, the most common recommendation to concussed patients is sleep and rest.

Recovery After Concussion

The recovery process is not a simple matter and has been formally studied for years with lack of success. There was a general thought in the scientific community that people get better from concussions on their own in 3–10 days. Earlier guidelines were based on those timelines and assumptions. Soon, it was discovered that theory did not work very well and that the recovery time is actually much longer than previously understood, particularly in children. Dr. Joy discussed this idea in a study that Dr. Micky Collins and I did years ago. A number of high school football players in western Pennsylvania were very carefully monitored over time. It should be noted that we had good connections with the athletic trainers in charge of concussed athletes so it was known when these athletes were getting better. Surprisingly at 3 weeks, there was still a significant amount of athletes who were not back to normal. Clinically, about 15–20 % of our high school athletes do not get better for months. This is a big issue because these athletes end up being treated with medication and completing Cyber School or home-based school because they cannot tolerate the school environment anymore. This became such a big issue in our clinic in Pittsburg that we had to hire a full time rehabilitation doctor PMR specialist to deal with the influx of patients who needed ongoing management of their injuries. Overall, it is a complicated injury; therefore, sophisticated treatment modalities should be implemented in a clinical practice.

There are other risk factors that are associated with prolonged recovery and age is becoming increasingly more relevant with young athletes. Having a history of migraines or a family history of migraines tends to be a factor in our clinical practice associated with recovery. Both Dr. Guskiewicz and our research team have published information about how learning disabilities and repetitive concussions are related. There is growing scientific evidence regarding the long-term consequence of concussive injury in the pediatric population. There is also growing literature that looks at gender. Specifically, there is still controversy in the literature as to whether males or females recover faster after concussion. There is evidence from our lab and other labs that female athletes tend to have a bigger problem with concussions than male athletes and may often take longer to recover. There are obviously specific factors associated with poor recovery that we are still not aware of.

There is a protocol at UPMC for management of concussion and I will break it down completely, not just how neurological assessment fits into it. A very large athletic training system is affiliated with us in Pittsburg, including over 90 certified athletic trainers working directly with us in high schools. This has allowed for many research opportunities because of the expertise that is out on the fields for the games. Athletic trainers are constantly looking for symptoms on the sidelines. At least, the trainers should do a neurological examination and some type of brief cognitive assessment to see what they're dealing with. It is also emphasized that trainers should keep an eye on the athletes even if they passed the initial screening. Often, one might have to go back and do another evaluation to see if the athlete is more confused as these injuries can evolve over time. *Once an athlete is identified as being injured, the athlete should definitely not go back to sports participation.* The saying that came from the Vienna conference, "When in doubt, sit them out," is a good edict in protecting kids from further injury.

Dr. Gioia mentioned that there are different tools out there to test for ability to return to participation. This tool is just another example from Dick's Sporting Goods. It is a massive educational program that in the last 2 years has combined with ImPact. National spokesmen, Drone Battus, and Drew Breese, have really done a lot in trying to get the word out. In their stores they have a relatively simple educational tool that has a quiz built into it about concussion, which is free and can be downloaded onto iTunes. There are other programs out there, including the CAT tool, and other iTunes applications that all provide information about initial screening on-field assessment of the individual. These easy-to-use apps should be taken advantage of by sideline and on-field management care. After the athletes are injured, they often go to see their pediatrician or they go to the emergency room. By the time the children come into the clinic, it is usually several days after the injury, which is actually beneficial because the children should not be subjected to a lot of psychological testing the day of their injury as it will make them sick. Our evaluation includes a clinical interview, vestibular screening, balance evaluation, and neuropsychological evaluation. Children come in with their parents so more information can be obtained about the injury. A visual exam is extremely useful in trying to determine what is going on with the children and to determine if the children can return to school. If they are having problems focusing their eyes or have blurred vision, they will get headaches. After the initial visit, we want the patients to walk out the door with a plan in terms of: What are we going to do this week in school? Do I need to take several days off? Do they need accommodations so their teacher doesn't make them take a math test that day when they have a splitting headache?

All of these things are important to take into account. Now that the state law has changed, concussion experts have a responsibility to assist the schools in caring for the patient's needs.

Brief Walk Through Testing

We examine athletes for abnormal eye movements, dizziness or blurriness, and balance-vestibular dysfunctions. We also examine for convergence which is often abnormal after a concussion. A balance examination is also completed and a balance therapist uses the BESS protocol to collect data on each athlete. Dr. Guskiewicz has done a lot of work in this area and deserves a lot of credit for bringing this to our attention over the years.

Baseline testing has become a very useful technique for documenting changes in concussion patients. Baseline testing is often used in the NFL and NHL. Changes in player performance can be observed. Our concussion program uses preseason testing and compares these results to information gathered immediately after the player is injured. Follow-up testing is done as needed to ensure a proper timeline for the athlete returning to play. This model is used very commonly today and the technology used has evolved.

Looking Back on Concussion Management

The history of and development of different approaches to neuropsychological testing began in the 1980s with Jeff Barth. He examined many universities with baseline testing programs already established. Originally, the study was done to look at the recovery from a mild or traumatic brain injury and was done by hand. Dr. Lovell began redesigning this method to involve computers as it allowed researchers to measure various neurocognitive variable and reaction times very accurately.

A study done has shown the effectiveness of the neuropsychological tests. Two hundred high school students in the Pittsburg, Pennsylvania area, were given baseline tests. After they were injured, they were given a functional MRI (fMRI). The athletes were clinically followed during the time they were not allowed to participate and when the students stated they felt normal again, another fMRI was done. Comparing the pre- and post-injury scans and using a standard memory test, MBAT, it was found that the athletes with fMRI hyperactivation (as evidenced by BOLD signal in the dorsolateral and prefrontal cortex, which are areas involved in thinking, memory, and judgment) took twice as long to recover than those with no pattern of high BOLD activation. This study proved that the cognitive tests show the same results as the fMRI. During hyperactivation, the brain needs more nutrition and blood flow to an area while completing a task. To return to participation, athletes had to show no symptoms, normal cognitive behavior, and no abnormalities in their scans.

Of this group of athletes, 25 % were back to participation in 15 days and 50 % were back in 26 days. Some participants never returned to activity and still remain symptomatic.

Concussion Treatment

One of the big issues in concussion treatment is how to manage players with concussions and how to assess their symptoms. Athletes often lie about their symptoms and there have been some studies that show that up to 50 % of athletes experience concussion symptoms per year, but only 10 % will admit to having an injury. According to an ESPN survey, many high school athletes stated that they would not admit to having concussion symptoms, even after being educated on the consequences of returning to play too early. Another interesting study was done with college athletes at the University of Pittsburg who were diagnosed with concussions. Four days after their injury, players were examined and placed into two groups: those that said they were uninjured and those who admitted to still having symptoms. The group of athletes who claimed they were uninjured showed interesting results. The uninjured group performed the best on the tests while the symptomatic group performed the worst on memory tests. Athletes that claimed they were uninjured showed mixed results leading researchers to not allow the judgment of the athlete to determine return to play.

Another study done asked the patient and their parents "what percentage of back to normal do you feel you are" every time the patient came into the clinic. They were asked to rate themselves on a scale of 0–100 % with 100 % feeling as good as before the injury and 0 % being dead. The correlation of how they performed on cognitive testing and how it related to their self-diagnosed symptom scale was computed. There was a fairly high correlation in terms of the symptoms, which was expected because they are being asked about their symptoms in two different forms. What was a little shocking was that it was expected that they would have been much more in tune with their cognitive processes than they were here. When the parents were asked to rate their children on how they were doing in terms of cognitive functioning on that scale, the parents did better, especially the mothers. Fathers generally said to put their child back into action. This simple experiment showed that athletes are well attuned to their level of cognitive functioning and pay attention to symptoms like headaches and dizziness, but are not in tune with their actual cognitive functioning.

Case Study

The results of this experiment are not a desirable outcome. For example, one 15-year-old sophomore shows typical issues in diagnosing and treating concussions. This boy was an honors student and the starting quarterback and had a normal family medical history with only a history of migraines on the maternal side. He received two concussions but did not report any symptoms and continued playing. After his concussions, he did not seek help until the end of the football season, and even then his symptoms were not picked up. His first concussion was received when he was tackled to the ground, yet he continued to play. A few weeks later, he sustained his second concussion when he was clipped, causing his head to spin around. He continued to play the rest of the season however his level of play declined. The athlete stated that "after the first hit, I had blurriness, dizziness, etc. ... a little difficulty making calls and plays, but not really all that obvious" and that his symptoms worsened as the season continued. His school grades also started to drop and he became more irritable and grouchy. When he was finally seen, he presented with bad headaches, dizziness, and short-term memory difficulties. His baseline neuropsychological testing showed that he was at the 90th percentile in terms of reaction time, visual and motor speed 95th percentile, visual and memory 80th percentile, and verbal memory 68th percentile; all the expected scores given his academic background. After the season, and significantly after his injury, all of his scores dropped, even the simple verbal memory one. His visual memory was at 36th percentile, but his reaction time plummeted to 1st percentile.

Doctors told the athlete to slow down and not push himself in school. The child did not slow down so his symptoms did not improve, shown by his low scores. He eventually had to leave school to rest and see a PMR physician. Because his injury was missed and the child did not report it, his concussion became very severe. The child eventually became 100 % asymptomatic and was taken off of medication. He was able to resume full physical and cognitive exertion and his grades improved.

Conclusion

One of the controversies surrounding cognitive testing is *when* to do it. Unless it is completely necessary, "torturing" athletes with testing when they are still having a lot of symptoms can be postponed. There is also the issue of what age to begin baseline testing. If a child is playing a contact sport, baseline testing becomes a good idea. The outcomes can be improved by having a comprehensive concussion program that includes neuropsychological testing. With the tools available today, including new medications, progress is being made into developing more effective tools for diagnosing and treating concussions. Surely, we are on the right track regarding the management of sports-related concussion. With the collective efforts of medical practitioners, athletic trainers, and brain researches, we will be able soon to significantly improve diagnostic protocols, prognosticate more accurately the consequences of concussion, and, most importantly, improve the safety of our children participating in sports.

References

1. Cantu R. Second impact syndrome. Clinics in Sports Medicine, 1998;18(1):37–44.
2. McCrory P, Johnston K, Meeuwisse W, Audry M, Cantu R, Dvorak J, et al. Summary and agreement statement of the 2nd international conference on concussion in sport, Prague 2004. Br J Sport Med. 2005;39–196–204.
3. Smith-Seemiller L, Fow N, Franzen M. Presence of post-concussion syndrome symptoms in patients with chronic pain vs. mild traumatic brain injury. Brain Injury, 2003;17(3):196–206.

Part V
Clinical Management and Rehabilitation of Concussions

Chapter 18
Management of Collegiate Sport-Related Concussions

Steven P. Broglio and Kevin M. Guskiewicz

Abstract The identification and evaluation of sport-related concussion are key components of the concussion management process. Integral to this process is a well thought out and rehearsed emergency action plan and concussion management policy that outlines how each injury will be handled. The on-field and follow-up evaluations should be systematically approached and executed to ensure the thorough assessment of neurocognitive functioning, postural control, and athlete-reported symptoms. Each of these domains should be considered in conjunction with the clinical exam when making the injury diagnosis and eventual return to play decision.

Keywords Mild traumatic brain injury • Symptom assessment • Balance and postural control • Neurocognitive function • Emergency action plan

Introduction

The difference between a good and bad outcome when managing sport-related concussion often comes down to a careful, well thought out management plan. In most cases, the sideline assessment serves as a triage for determining if an injury such as a concussion has occurred and if so, establishes a benchmark for determining if a more serious and potentially catastrophic condition could be developing.

S.P. Broglio, Ph.D., A.T.C. (✉)
NeuroSport Research Laboratory, School of Kinesiology, University of Michigan,
401 Washtenaw Avenue, Ann Arbor, MI 48109, USA
e-mail: broglio@umich.edu

K.M. Guskiewicz, Ph.D., A.T.C.
College of Arts and Sciences, University of North Carolina at Chapel Hill,
Chapel Hill, NC 27599, USA
e-mail: gus@email.unc.edu

S.M. Slobounov and W.J. Sebastianelli (eds.), *Concussions in Athletics:*
From Brain to Behavior, DOI 10.1007/978-1-4939-0295-8_18,
© Springer Science+Business Media New York 2014

Given its description as "a complex pathophysiological process affecting the brain, induced by traumatic biomechanical forces" [1], concussion has the potential to evolve into something far more serious if signs and symptoms go undetected or are ignored. While these events are rare in the context of sport, they are a real possibility with every injury.

Concussions can occur in all sport settings, including men's and women's and contact and non-contact events. Regardless of the setting, sports medicine clinicians must be prepared to manage these complex and somewhat misunderstood injuries, which have been labeled as a "hidden epidemic" by the Centers for Disease Control and Prevention. Developing and instituting a concussion policy and management protocol constitutes the first step in properly treating the athlete suspected of sustaining a concussion, which should be backed by proper planning and practice of the on-field management strategy.

Much of the inherent complexity in evaluating athletes suspected of sustaining a concussion lies in the broad spectrum of outcomes associated with the injury. Knowing your athlete and his or her medical background, concussion history, and ability and willingness to provide information about his or her condition can minimize the challenges of the injury evaluation. Research has shown that previous history of concussive injuries [2], learning disabilities [3], age [4], and sex [5] can alter the risk of concussion and in some cases the outcomes following injury. To further complicate matters, no definitive diagnostic tool is available for concussion at this time. Standard computed tomography (CT) or magnetic resonance imaging (MRI) is insensitive to the functional deficits observed following concussion. Functional MRI (fMRI), diffusion tensor imaging (DTI), single photon emission computed tomography (SPECT), and magnetic resonance spectroscopy (MRS) are showing promise, but their widespread use as a diagnostic tool has not yet been substantiated. Several objective clinical measures (e.g., neurocognitive and balance tests) are recommended to support the clinical examination, and their use can aid in making the concussion diagnosis, but the clinical examination remains the gold standard for evaluation and diagnosis [6].

Emergency Action Planning and Establishing a Concussion Policy

Before the first preseason practice, the sports medicine clinician in-charge of on-field injury management should make sure to have an *emergency action plan* in place. In addition to concussive injuries, this plan should incorporate strategies to address other potentially catastrophic conditions (Table 18.1). When developing the concussion management component of the plan, the clinician should develop both a *concussion policy* and a *concussion protocol*. The concussion protocol outlines the clinical tests that will be used for assessments and a graduated return to play progression.

The policy, however, is put in place preseason and outlines the concussion management steps and includes roles and responsibilities of the sports medicine team. The policy should at the very least consider four components: (1) preseason

Table 18.1 General guidelines for developing emergency action plans

1. Establish roles—adapt to specific team/sport/venue, may be best to have more than one person assigned to each role in case of absence/turnover
   - Immediate care of the athlete
     - Typically physician, ATC, first responder but also those trained in basic life support
   - Activation of emergency medical system
     - Could be school administrator, anyone
   - Emergency equipment retrieval
     - Could be student assistant, coach, anyone
   - Direction of EMS to scene
     - Could be administrator, coach, student assistant, anyone
2. Communication
   - Primary method
     - May be fixed (landline) or mobile (cellular phone, radio)
     - List all key personnel and all phones associated with this person
   - Back-up method
     - Often a landline
   - Test prior to event
     - Cell phone/radio reception can vary, batteries charged, landline working
     - Make sure communication methods are accessible (identify and post location, are there locks or other barriers, change available for pay-phone)
   - Activation of EMS
     - Identify contact numbers (911, ambulance, police, fire, hospital, poison control, suicide hotline)
     - Prepare script (caller name/location/phone number, nature of emergency, number of victims and their condition, what treatment initiated, specific directions to scene)
     - Post both of the above near communication devices, other visible locations in venue, and circulate to appropriate personnel
   - Student emergency information
     - Critical medical information (conditions, medications, allergies)
     - Emergency contact information (parent/guardian)
     - Accessible (keep with athletic trainer for example)
3. Emergency equipment
   - For example, automated external defibrillators, bag-valve mask, spine board, splints
   - Personnel trained in advance on proper use
   - Must be accessible (identify and post location, within acceptable distance for each venue, are there locks or other barriers)
   - Proper condition and maintenance
     - Document inspection (log book)
4. Emergency transportation
   - Ambulance on site for high risk events (know difference between basic life support and advanced life support vehicles/personnel)
     - Designated location
     - Clear route for exiting venue
   - When ambulance not on site
     - Entrance to venue clearly marked and accessible
     - Identify parking/loading point and confirm area is clear
   - Coordinate ahead of time with local emergency medical services

(continued)

Table 18.1 (continued)

5. Additional considerations
• Must be venue-specific (football field, gymnasium, etc.)
• Put plan in writing
• Involve all appropriate personnel (administrators, coaches, sports medicine, EMS)
– Development
– Approval with signatures
• Post the plan in visible areas of each venue and distribute
• Review plan at least annually
• Rehearse plan at least annually
• Document
– Events of emergency situation
– Evaluation of response
– Rehearsal, training, equipment maintenance
Specific considerations for *head and neck injury*
• Athletic trainer/first responder should be prepared to remove the face-mask from a football helmet in order to access a victim's airway without moving the cervical spine
• Sports medicine team should communicate ahead of time with local EMS
– Agree upon C-spine immobilization techniques (e.g., leave helmet and shoulder pads on for football players)
– Type of immobilization equipment available on site and from EMS
• Athletes and coaches should be trained not to move victims

planning and baseline testing, (2) on-field/sideline evaluation, (3) removal from play, and (4) graduated return to play progression. While the focus of this chapter is on the sideline exam and removal from play, the planning component is very important. It is during the preseason planning that the roles and responsibilities of the sports medicine team are clarified. For example, the concussion protocol should ensure clarity and an understanding regarding:

• Who will be responsible for the on-field response?
• Who will conduct the emergency assessment and handle communication if advanced help is needed?
• Who will observe the athlete on the sideline following injury?
• Who will make the diagnosis, especially in the absence of a physician?
• Who will communicate the diagnosis and prognosis with the parents and coaches?

Additionally, preseason planning should include drills and planning for sporting events both at the home venue and away events. In both of these situations, it is important to assess the availability of emergency medical responders and the location of any trauma centers.

The sports medicine team should also develop and enact a plan for educating all relevant personnel about concussion. Regardless of the setting, the athletes, coaches, and medical personnel must be educated about concussion and should read and sign a statement confirming that they understand the signs and symptoms of a concussion, and understand their responsibility to report a suspected concussion to the team's medical staff (Table 18.2). The program should also discuss the potential long-term consequences of concussion and the expectations for safe play.

Table 18.2 Student-athlete concussion statement

□ I understand that it is my responsibility to report all injuries and illnesses to my athletic trainer and/or team physician.

□ I have read and understand the *Concussion Fact Sheet.*

After reading the *Concussion Fact Sheet*, I am aware of the following information:

_____ A concussion is a brain injury, which I am responsible for reporting to my team physician or athletic trainer.

_____ A concussion can affect my ability to perform everyday activities, including reaction time, balance, sleep, and classroom performance.

_____ I realize I cannot see a concussion, but I might notice some symptoms right away. Other symptoms can show up hours or days later.

_____ If I suspect a teammate has a concussion, I am responsible for reporting the injury to my team physician or athletic trainer.

_____ I will not return to play in a game or practice if I have received a blow to the head or body that results in concussion-related symptoms.

_____ Following concussion the brain needs time to heal. I understand that I am much more likely to have a repeat concussion if I return to play before symptoms resolve.

_____ In rare cases, repeat concussions can cause permanent brain damage, and even death.

_____ I have read and understand the signs and symptoms presented on the *Concussion Fact Sheet.*

_____   _____
Signature of Student-Athlete   Date

_____
Printed name of Student-Athlete

Ideally, the concussion policy and protocol will include a preseason baseline evaluation that includes a clinical exam that evaluates concussion-related symptoms, and an evaluation of neurostatus and neurocognitive function, and balance. The most commonly used neurocognitive tests assess a range of brain behaviors including memory, concentration, information processing, executive function, and reaction time. In some instances additional resources and health care professionals may be needed to administer and interpret these tests.

Injury Identification

The most perplexing portion of the concussion assessment process is injury identification. In many settings, athletic trainers represent the front line of defense in protecting concussed athletes from returning to a game or practice and placing themselves at risk for further injury. Athletic trainers have the advantage of knowing the personalities and habits of their athletes which affords them the opportunity to rapidly identify alterations that would lead one to suspect a concussion has occurred. As only 10 % of all injuries involve loss of consciousness [7] and over 50 % of injuries are thought to go unreported [8] the sports medicine professional has historically had to rely on overt signs and symptoms or athlete self-report. Recent technological advances, however, are offering the promise of real-time injury identification using helmet-based accelerometers that communicate with sideline computers or other wireless devices.

The intent of telemetered accelerometers was to identify a variable or a set of variables that, if met, would serve as diagnostic criteria for concussion. Despite numerous publications on high school [9–14] and collegiate [15–22] football athletes, no research team has successfully integrated any single or combination of variables that can identify concussed athletes with a clinically acceptable level of diagnostic accuracy.

Concussive injuries aside, the majority of impacts resulting from football participation are relatively mild. For example, in a mixed sample of collegiate and high school football players, 79 % of all impacts fall below 30 g of acceleration [9] and with college-only data the magnitude of impact increases as the frequency of impacts decreases. That is, Duma reported that 89 % of impacts were less than 60 g [19] while Brolinson found that 97.5 % of impacts were less than 75 g [23]. Impacts resulting in acceleration values in excess of 75 g are rare with less than 2 % exceeding 80.6 g and only 1 % exceeding 99.2 g [9]. Interestingly, collegiate athletes sustain a greater number of high magnitude impacts when compared to high school level athletes [24]. This intuitively suggests that collegiate athletes are at greater risk for concussion, yet the epidemiological data do not support this assumption. Indeed, the incidence of concussion appears to be about the same across both levels of play with 3.6–5.6 % [7, 25] of high school and 4.8–6.3 % of collegiate football athletes [2, 7] sustaining concussions on an annual basis. As the literature indicates that larger magnitude impacts are occurring at the collegiate level with comparable concussion rates as high school athletes, it is possible that college players may be more likely to hide concussive symptoms from medical professionals [8, 26] or they have an injury threshold that differs from the adolescent athlete.

Much of the biomechanical research surrounding concussion has focused on identifying a concussion threshold using biomechanical variables. Several papers have described a case-by-case evaluation of the biomechanical properties of concussion captured by the HIT System [9, 19, 23]. The aggregate data, however, provides a better view of the concussion thresholds of collegiate athletes. An analysis of 13 collegiate concussions made no attempt to use biomechanical variables for injury prediction, but reported the mean linear acceleration of the injuries to be 102.8 g, angular acceleration of 5,311.6 rad/s/s, and 12 of the 13 injuries occurred when the athlete was struck at the front, side, or top of the helmet. There was a significant range in the impact magnitudes that resulted in concussion (60.5–168.7 g and 163.4–8,994.4 rad/s/s) [20]. Greenwald and colleagues later applied a principal component analysis to a mixed set of collegiate and high school concussions [18]. The novel equation, referred to as HITsp, weights linear acceleration, rotational acceleration, Head Injury Criterion, Gadd Severity Index, and impact location to indicate a 75 % injury risk when in excess of 63. By comparison, a classification and regression tree analysis (CART) was applied to more than 50,000 high school level impacts, which included 13 concussive episodes. Concussions resulted from a spectrum of impact magnitudes with linear accelerations ranging from 74.0 to 146.0 g and angular accelerations from 5,582.6 to 9,515.6 rad/s/s. Ultimately, decision points for predicting concussion were made when the resultant angular acceleration exceeded 5,582 rad/s/s, linear acceleration exceeded 96.1 g, and the impact occurred to the front, side, and top of the helmet [14].

When viewing the aggregate concussion data, high school and collegiate athletes appear to have comparable injury thresholds. The notable difference, however, lies in the greater number of high magnitude impacts sustained by collegiate athletes while maintaining a similar injury incidence rate. Collegiate athletes may have a greater tolerance to these impacts, but the reasons for this are not entirely clear. It is possible that the additional year or two of cerebral development [27] may play a protective role or it may be that those that are more susceptible to injury are filtered out and not able to compete at higher levels of play. Other factors that are not measurable with biomechanical variables may also play a role. For example, anatomical differences in the dura, cerebral vascularization, or cranial topography may all influence injury tolerance. As such, while biomechanical systems have contributed significantly to our understanding of head impacts and concussion mechanics, they are not diagnostic. At best, these tools can be used to identify those that have sustained a large magnitude impact that would warrant a clinical evaluation on the sideline or in the athletic training room.

The On-Field/Sideline Assessment

Primary Survey

With injury identification continuing to be the rate limiting step in the assessment process, knowing the athlete and his or her normal disposition is critical. Many athletes will hide symptoms of a concussion because they do not want to be removed from participation or let down their coach and teammates [8, 26]. In most cases, the athlete will show no outwardly visible signs of concussion. In the event an athlete is rendered unconscious, the clinician should also suspect a cervical spine injury when approaching him or her on the playing field. Following a determination of level of consciousness, the primary survey should include an assessment of the athlete's airway, breathing, and circulation while maintaining the cervical spine in a neutral position. Once the athlete regains consciousness and more severe injuries (e.g., cervical spine or cranial fracture) have been ruled out, the athlete can be moved to the sideline for further evaluation. If the athlete remains in an unconscious state, he or she should be transported immediately to the nearest medical facility for further evaluation. The clinician should also consider transport to a medical facility if the athlete's condition deteriorates during the evaluation process or displays signs or symptoms associated with spine or skull fracture, or severe bleeding.

Secondary Survey

During the sideline secondary survey, the clinician can draw from the preseason baseline scores to aid in making the diagnosis. The highly variable nature of concussion calls for an individualized approach to injury management [1] and warrants the use of baseline assessments for each athlete during an uninjured state. Regardless of the specific tests employed, the evaluation should include measures of concussion-related symptoms, balance, and neurocognitive function [28]. Each of these will be addressed in detail below. When evaluating an athlete following a suspected concussive blow, the pre-morbid data can be used to objectively identify post-injury change that will support the decision derived from the clinical examination.

The sideline assessment for concussion should follow a standardized protocol that involves the use of a seven-step process including: *history, observation, palpation, special tests, range of motion tests, strength tests,* and *functional tests.* In many instances the clinician will have witnessed the concussive blow and has already established a mechanism of injury. However, if this is not possible, the athlete, teammates, coaches, or other personnel may provide beneficial information [29]. Obtaining a *history,* through detailed questioning of the athlete about the injury, will provide pertinent information relative to the injury. First, a level of consciousness can be established by talking with the athlete. If the athlete is not alert enough to understand the questions or is passing in and out of consciousness, he or she should be transported to a medical facility for further evaluation. Second, the clinician can ascertain if the athlete is suffering from retrograde or anterograde amnesia. To establish the presence or absence of retrograde amnesia, injury history questions should start at the time of concussion and work backwards. For example, the clinician may ask: Do you remember being hit? Do you recall the play you were running? What team are we playing against? What did you eat for breakfast or lunch? Conversely, the assessment of anterograde amnesia should begin with questions surrounding events following the concussion, such as: who was the first person you saw on the field? or who brought you to the sideline? Providing the athlete with

Graded Symptom Checklist (GSC)

Symptom	Time of injury	2-3 Hours postinjury	24 Hours postinjury	48 Hours postinjury	72 Hours postinjury
Blurred vision					
Dizziness					
Drowsiness					
Excess sleep					
Easily distracted					
Fatigue					
Feel "in a fog"					
Feel "slowed down"					
Headache					
Inappropriate emotions					
Irritability					
Loss of consciousness					
Loss or orientation					
Memory problems					
Nausea					
Nervousness					
Personality change					
Poor balance/coordination					
Poor concentration					
Ringing in ears					
Sadness					
Seeing stars					
Sensitivity to light					
Sensitivity to noise					
Sleep disturbance					
Vacant stare/glassy eyed					
Vomiting					

NOTE: The GSC should be used not only for the initial evaluation but for each subsequent follow-up assessment until all signs and symptoms have cleared at rest and during physical exertion. In lieu of simply checking each symptom present, the ATC can ask the athlete to grade or score the severity of the symptom on a scale of 0-6, where 0=not present, 1=mild, 3=moderate, and 6=most severe.

Fig. 18.1 The Graded Symptom Checklist (GCS)

three unrelated words to recall at a later time (10–15 min intervals) is also useful for assessing anterograde amnesia.

The sideline history evaluation should then follow with a series of questions addressing the presence or absence of a variety of concussion-related symptoms, and the severity of any symptoms. Several consensus groups have recommended the use of a graded symptom checklist for tracking the number, type, and severity of symptoms during serial assessments. The National Athletic Trainers' Association's Position Statement of Concussion Management recommends the use of a 22-item symptom checklist (Fig. 18.1) [28], although a number of similar assessment tools are available [30–32].

These symptom scales use a Likert rating of severity that allows for an aggregate symptom severity score that can be used to track the severity over time. The presentation of symptoms will vary widely between concussed athletes, but some symptoms are reported to appear more often than others. For instance, headache has been reported in up to 83 % of concussed athletes, while dizziness (65 %) and confusion (57 %) may also appear, but less frequently [2, 7, 33, 34]. The clinician should recognize that some athletes removed from the field of play may report symptoms of dehydration and not concussive injury [35]. Thus, the presence of symptoms in the absence of an insult to the head or torso may indicate dehydration rather than concussion. Regardless of which signs and symptoms appear, the endorsement of any symptom related to a concussion is sufficient to withhold an athlete from returning to play [29].

Observation and *palpation* of the athlete can be completed throughout the injury evaluation process as the clinician interacts with the athlete. Attention should be paid to variance in the athlete's speech pattern from the norm with difficulty finding or saying the correct words when responding to questions (i.e., aphasia) [36]. The clinician should also check equivalency of pupil size, their reaction to light, and the fluidity of eye movement in multiple directions (i.e., nystagmus). Further, an evaluation of pulse and blood pressure should be completed to rule out a life-threatening condition. A high pulse pressure (i.e., systolic minus diastolic >70 mmHg) immediately following exercise is a common result of increased stroke volume [37], but should be restored within 10 min. If the pulse pressure remains high and is combined with a pulse rate that is substantially lower than expected following physical exertion, the athlete may be suffering from increased intracranial pressure [38]. A clinical examination that reveals abnormalities in any of these areas suggests the injury is more significant than concussion and warrants immediate transport and examination at a medical facility. The cervical spine and facial bones should also be palpated to rule out fractures or other trauma to these areas which may be associated with high acceleration impacts to the head.

Special tests used to evaluate for concussion on the sideline should consist of an evaluation of neurostatus, balance, and cranial nerve integrity. While a variety of tests and questions have been recommended, traditional questions of orientation such as "where are you?" and "what is your name?" have been found to be insensitive to the effects of concussion [39, 40]. Alternatively, the Standardized Assessment of Concussion (SAC) was developed as a quick and reliable mental status exam for use on the sideline [40]. Different from more comprehensive pen and paper or computer-based neurocognitive assessments, the SAC does not require specific training in neuropsychology for the purposes of administration or interpretation [41]. These characteristics make it ideal for the practicing athletic trainer who can administer the test in 6–8 min on the sideline.

The SAC consists of five sections that evaluate the areas of Orientation, Immediate Memory, Concentration, and Delayed Recall (Fig. 18.2). A brief screening has also been included to rule out gross neurological deficiencies. Performance on each of the cognitive domains is summed for a total possible score of 30. The most accurate post-morbid assessment is completed when the post-injury score is compared to a preseason baseline assessment. Multiple versions of the SAC are available to reduce potential practice effects associated with multiple test administrations.

Standardized Assessment of Concussion (SAC)

1) ORIENTATION:

Month: _____   0   1
Date: _____   0   1
Day of week: _____   0   1
Year: _____   0   1
Time (within 1 hr.): _____   0   1

Orientation Total Score _____ /   5

2) IMMEDIATE MEMORY: (all 3 trials are completed regardless of score on trial 1 & 2; total score equals sum across all 3 trials)

List	Trial 1	Trial 2	Trial 3
Word 1	0 1	0 1	0 1
Word 2	0 1	0 1	0 1
Word 3	0 1	0 1	0 1
Word 4	0 1	0 1	0 1
Word 5	0 1	0 1	0 1
Total			

Immediate Memory Total Score ____ / 15

(Note: Subject is not informed of Delayed Recall testing of memory)

NEUROLOGICAL SCREENING:

Loss of Consciousness: (occurrence, duration)

Pre- & Post-traumatic Amnesia: (recollection of events pre- and post-injury)

Strength:

Sensation:

Coordination:

3) CONCENTRATION:

Digits Backward (If correct, go to next string length. If incorrect, read trial 2. Stop after incorrect on both trials)

4-9-3	6-2-9	_____ 0 1
3-8-1-4	3-2-7-9	_____ 0 1
6-2-9-7-1	1-5-2-8-6	_____ 0 1
7-1-8-4-6-2	5-3-9-1-4-8	_____ 0 1

Months in reverse order : (entire sequence correct for 1 point)
Dec-Nov-Oct-Sep-Aug-Jul
Jun-May-Apr-Mar-Feb-Jan _____ 0   1

Concentration Total Score _____ / 5

EXERTIONAL MANEUVERS
(when appropriate)
5 jumping jacks   5 push-ups
5 sit-ups   5 knee bends

4) DELAYED RECALL

Word 1   0   1
Word 2   0   1
Word 3   0   1
Word 4   0   1
Word 5   0   1

Delayed Recall Total Score _____/   5

Summary of Total Scores :

Orientation	_____/	5
Immediate Memory	_____/	15
Concentration	_____/	5
Delayed Recall	_____/	5

Overall Total Score _____ / 30

McCrea, Kelly & Randolph, 2000

Fig. 18.2 The Standardized Assessment of Concussion (SAC)

Performance decrements of one point or more are consistent with impaired cognitive functioning following concussion. Specifically, when administered immediately following injury, a 94 % sensitivity and 76 % specificity are obtained when a one-point drop in test performance is used as a cut-off for concussion [42]. A follow-up investigation yielded similar sensitivity (80 %) and specificity (91 %) results when both concussed and control athletes were evaluated at similar time points following injury [43].

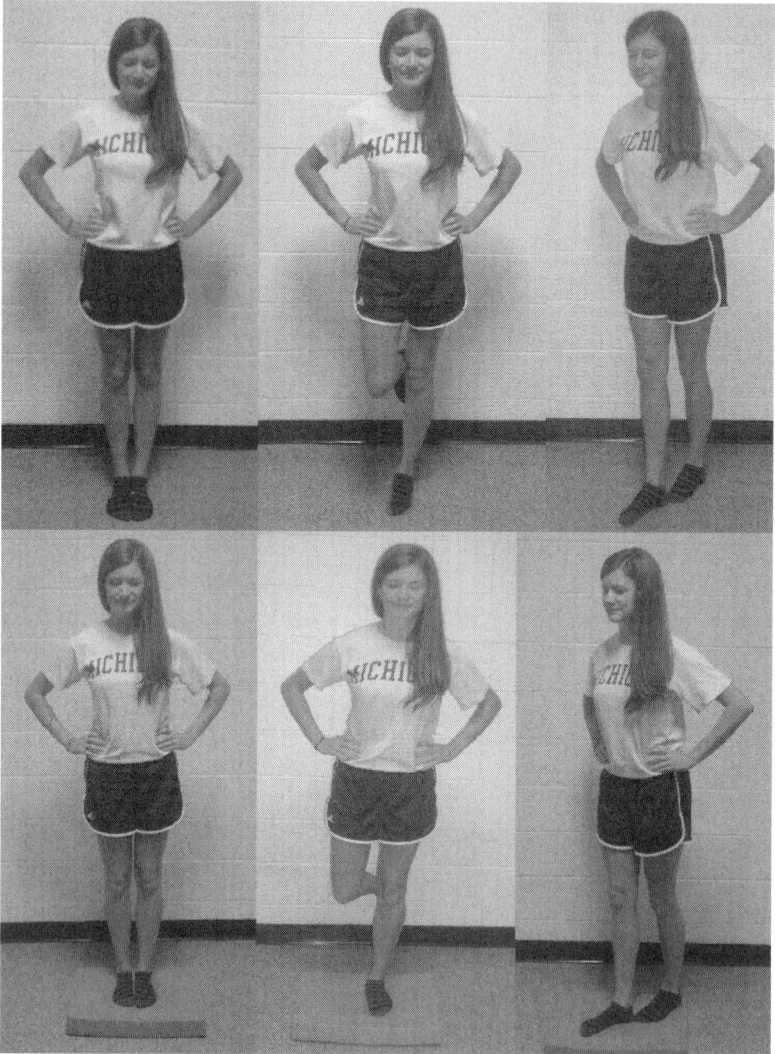

Fig. 18.3 Stances for the Balance Error Scoring System (BESS)

One of the hallmark signs of concussion is a decreased ability to maintain balance. Concussed individuals will commonly show increased postural sway following injury and the degree of sway will often increase when the eyes are closed, removing the visual referencing. Assessments of sway, such as the Romberg test, have been used [44], but are limited by the subjective nature of post-injury interpretation. The Balance Error Scoring System (BESS) was developed as an objective postural control measure that can be implemented on the sideline [45]. The BESS test is conducted under six different stance conditions (Fig. 18.3): on a firm surface the athlete stands in a double leg stance, single leg stance, and heel-to-toe tandem stance.

Table 18.3 Balance Error Scoring System (BESS) countable errors

Errors
Hands lifted off the iliac crests
Opening eyes
Step, stumble, or fall
Moving the hip into more than 30° of flexion or extension
Lifting the forefoot or heel
Remaining out of the testing position for more than 5 s

The same three stances are repeated on a compliant foam surface such as an Airex balance pad (Alcan Airex AG, Switzerland). Each stance is evaluated for 20 s and the athlete places his or her hands on the hips with the eyes closed. During the trials the clinician counts the number of errors committed by the athlete (Table 18.3) with a higher number of errors representing suppressed balance. An increase of three errors or more over the baseline score has been suggested as a significant change indicative of a balance impairment [46] with a sensitivity to concussion reported at 34 % and the specificity at 91 % [43].

Similar to the SAC assessment, an individualized approach to interpreting the post-injury BESS scores provides the clinician with the most accurate information. Thus, comparing the post-concussion assessment to the athlete's baseline assessment is recommended. To obtain the most accurate results, certain factors should be noted. For example, application of an external ankle support (e.g., taping or bracing) has been shown to influence BESS scores [47]. Thus, when evaluating athletes on the sideline, it may be necessary to remove any ankle support that was not present at the time of baseline testing. Further, Wilkins et al. [48] noted a decrease in BESS performance when individuals were subjected to a 20 min fatigue protocol. Athletes removed from a competition for an injury evaluation are likely experiencing some level of fatigue, necessitating some rest (13–20 min) prior to testing [49, 50].

Clinically meaningful deficits suggestive of neurological impairment have been debated. However, as a general rule, an impact to the head with an accompanying increased symptom score, decreased SAC score (1 or more point) [42], or increased BESS score (3 or more points) [46] warrants removal from further participation. Current practice guidelines set forth by the National Collegiate Athletic Association and several position and consensus groups [1, 51, 52] mandate that no player return to participation on the same day with a diagnosed concussion. Research supports this recommendation, as athletes have a higher likelihood of delayed symptom onset when returning to play on the same day compared to those withheld following the concussion [2]. Likewise, concussed athletes whose symptoms resolve within 25 min of injury have demonstrated impaired neurocognitive function 36 h following the injury [53].

Although complete disruption of one or more cranial nerves is rare in the sporting context, the clinician should also be cognizant that one or more of the cranial nerves may be affected as a result of the concussive blow. The assessment of many cranial nerves is imbedded throughout the concussion assessment (e.g., CN II during the visual testing and VIII during the BESS test), but the integrity of the remaining nerves should be appraised as part of the sideline clinical assessment. A cranial nerve assessment revealing functional decrements may also indicate a more severe injury causing increased intracranial pressure and warrants a timely assessment at a medical facility.

While the graded symptom checklist, SAC, and BESS have been discussed as options for special tests, other sideline assessment measures such as the Sideline Concussion Assessment Tool (i.e., SCAT3) [1] have been proposed for a multifaceted sideline assessment tool to assess symptoms, cognitive function, and balance. This assessment tool also includes additional questions for the evaluation of more severe brain injuries and orientation. The SCAT3 has shown promise, but to date it is limited by undefined psychometric properties and a lack of scientific studies validating its utility for concussion diagnosis and recovery.

Should the symptom report, BESS, and SAC scores all appear normal, the clinician should continue with an evaluation of *cervical range of motion* (*ROM*) and *strength testing*. An examination of ROM for flexion, extension, and rotation in both directions should be conducted both actively and passively. Similarly, manual muscle testing in the same directions should be performed. If limitations are noted in either ROM or muscle strength the athlete should be withheld for further evaluation. Limitations in these areas may place the athlete at risk for further injury by restricting his or her ability to protect the head from impacts secondary to oncoming opponents.

Functional testing marks the final step in the sideline concussion assessment, but should not be confused with same day return to play decision making. Rather, functional testing should only be completed if the athlete has performed at or above the baseline level of evaluation for symptoms, balance, and cognitive function and there are no other contraindications appearing during the clinical examination. The goal of functional testing is to elicit symptoms that may present under the physical demands that the athlete might face after a return to play. A progressive approach to the physical activity should be taken with the clinician asking if concussion-related symptoms have been elicited before moving to the next step. Simple tasks such as a Valsava maneuver, push-ups, and sit-ups should be performed first. This may be followed by jogging and short sprints. In the final step the athlete should be able to complete a series of sport-specific activities at an intensity necessitated by the level of play. The clinician should ask the athlete at each progression to see if concussion-related symptoms have emerged. If the athlete indicates symptoms have resulted from exertion, then he or she should not be returned to participation or progressed to the next step in the graduated return to play progression. If no symptoms emerge and all other tests demonstrate normal findings, the athlete has likely not sustained a concussion and may be considered for a return to play.

Conclusion

The evolution of sport-related concussion has placed an emphasis on concussion education, awareness, and prevention and brought technology and objective testing methods to the forefront of concussion management. Perhaps the greatest influence clinicians can have in preventing these injuries and a catastrophic outcome is to educate athletes and coaches about the dangers of playing while still symptomatic following a concussion. Second is the implementation of a well-established concussion policy and emergency action plan. Contemporary methods of concussion assessment, involving the use of symptom checklists, neurocognitive testing, and postural stability testing, are indicated for any athlete suspected of having sustained a concussion and research has shown the utility of these when incorporated into a systematic sideline assessment. Following a primary survey, the clinician should garner an injury history and observe and palpate the athlete for indications of more severe trauma. Special tests for mental status and postural control, along with reports of concussion-related symptoms, can provide the objective information that supports the clinical exam. Throughout the evaluation process the clinician should inquire about the development, the presence and intensity, or return of concussion-related symptoms. In no instance should an athlete be returned to play if he or she reports any symptoms consistent with concussion, substantiating the dictum "when in doubt, sit them out" [54].

References

1. McCrory P, Meeuwisse WH, Aubry M, et al. Consensus statement on concussion in sport: the 4th international conference on concussion in sport held in Zurich, November 2012. Br J Sports Med. 2013;47:250–8.
2. Guskiewicz KM, McCrea M, Marshall SW, et al. Cumulative effects associated with recurrent concussion in collegiate football players: the NCAA concussion study. JAMA. 2003;290: 2549–55.
3. Collins MW, Grindel SH, Lovell MR, et al. Relationship between concussion and neuropsychological performance in college football players. JAMA. 1999;282:964–70.
4. Field M, Collins MW, Lovell MR, Maroon JC. Does age play a role in recovery from sports-related concussion? A comparison of high school and collegiate athletes. J Pediatr. 2003;142: 546–53.
5. Covassin T, Elbin RJ, Harris W, Parker T, Kontos A. The role of age and sex in symptoms, neurocognitive performance, and postural stability in athletes after concussion. Am J Sports Med. 2012;40(6):1303–12.
6. Grindel SH, Lovell MR, Collins MW. The assessment of sport-related concussion: the evidence behind neuropsychological testing and management. Clin J Sport Med. 2001;11:134–43.
7. Guskiewicz KM, Weaver NL, Padua DA, Garrett WE. Epidemiology of concussion in collegiate and high school football players. Am J Sports Med. 2000;28:643–50.
8. McCrea M, Hammeke T, Olsen G, Leo P, Guskiewicz K. Unreported concussion in high school football players: implications for prevention. Clin J Sport Med. 2004;14:13–7.
9. Schnebel B, Gwin JT, Anderson S, Gatlin R. In vivo study of head impacts in football: a comparison of National Collegiate Athletic Association Division I versus high school impacts. Neurosurgery. 2007;60:490–5.
10. Broglio SP, Eckner JT, Surma T, Kutcher JS. Post-concussion cognitive declines and symptomatology are not related to concussion biomechanics in high school football players. J Neurotrauma. 2011;28:2061–8.
11. Broglio SP, Eckner JT, Martini D, Sosnoff JJ, Kutcher JS, Randolph C. Cumulative head impact burden in high school football. J Neurotrauma. 2011;28:2069–78.
12. Eckner JT, Sabin MN, Kutcher JS, Broglio SP. No evidence for a cumulative impact effect on concussion injury threshold. J Neurotrauma. 2011;28:2079–90.

13. Broglio SP, Swartz EE, Crisco JJ, Cantu RC. In vivo biomechanical measurements of a football player's C6 spine fracture. N Engl J Med. 2011;365:279–81.
14. Broglio SP, Schnebel B, Sosnoff JJ, et al. Biomechanical properties of concussions in high school football. Med Sci Sports Exerc. 2010;42:2064–71.
15. Crisco JJ, Wilcox BJ, Machan JT, McAllister TW, Duhaime AC, Duma SM, Rowson S, Beckwith JG, Chu JJ, Greenwald RM. Magnitude of head impact exposures in individual collegiate football players. J Appl Biomech. 2012;28(2):174–83.
16. Crisco JJ, Wilcox BJ, Beckwith JG, et al. Head impact exposure in collegiate football players. J Biomech. 2011;44:2673–8.
17. Crisco JJ, Fiore R, Beckwith JG, et al. Frequency and location of head impact exposures in individual collegiate football players. J Athl Train. 2010;45:549–59.
18. Greenwald RM, Gwin JT, Chu JJ, Crisco JJ. Head impact severity measures for evaluating mild traumatic brain injury risk exposure. Neurosurgery. 2008;62:789–98.
19. Duma SM, Manoogian SJ, Bussone WR, et al. Analysis of real-time head accelerations in collegiate football players. Clin J Sport Med. 2005;15:3–8.
20. Guskiewicz KM, Mihalik JP, Shankar V, et al. Measurement of head impacts in collegiate football players: relationship between head impact biomechanics and acute clinical outcome after concussion. Neurosurgery. 2007;61:1244–52.
21. McCaffrey MA, Mihalik JP, Crowell DH, Shields EW, Guskiewicz KM. Measurement of head impacts in collegiate football players: clinical measures of concussion after high- and low-magnitude impacts. Neurosurgery. 2007;61:1236–43.
22. Mihalik JP, Bell DR, Marshall SW, Guskiewicz KM. Measurement of head impacts in collegiate football players: an investigation of positional and event-type differences. Neurosurgery. 2007;61:1229–35.
23. Brolinson PG, Manoogian S, McNeely D, Goforth M, Greenwald R, Duma S. Analysis of linear head accelerations from collegiate football impacts. Curr Sports Med Rep. 2006;5:23–8.
24. Broglio SP, Surma T, Ashton-Miller JA. High school and collegiate football athlete concussions: a biomechanical review. Ann Biomed Eng. 2012;40:37–46.
25. Powell JW, Barber-Foss KD. Traumatic brain injury in high school athletes. JAMA. 1999;282:958–63.
26. Sefton JM, Pirog K, Capitao A, Harackiewicz D, Cordova ML. An examination of factors that influence knowledge and reporting of mild brain injuries in collegiate football [abstract]. J Athl Train. 2004;39:S52–3.
27. Giedd JN, Blumenthal J, Jefferies NO, et al. Brain development during childhood and adolescence: a longitudinal MRI study. Nat Neurosci. 1999;2:861–3.
28. Guskiewicz KM, Bruce SL, Cantu RC, et al. National athletic trainers' association position statement: management of sport-related concussion. J Athl Train. 2004;29:280–97.
29. Broglio SP, Guskiewicz KM. Concussion in sport: the sideline assessment. Sports Health. 2009;1:361–9.
30. Piland SG, Motl RW, Ferrara MS, Peterson CL. Evidence for the factorial and construct validity of a self-report concussion symptoms scale. J Athl Train. 2003;38:104–12.
31. Lovell MR, Collins MW. Neuropsychological assessment of the college football player. J Head Trauma Rehabil. 1998;13:9–26.
32. Potter S, Leigh E, Wade D, Fleminger S. The Rivermead Post Concussion Symptoms Questionnaire: a confirmatory factor analysis. J Neurol. 2006;253:1603–14.
33. Delaney JS, Lacroix VJ, Leclerc S, Johnston KM. Concussions among university football and soccer players. Clin J Sport Med. 2002;12:331–8.
34. McCrory PR, Ariens M, Berkovic SF. The nature and duration of acute concussive symptoms in Australian football. Clin J Sport Med. 2000;10:235–8.
35. Patel AV, Mihalik JP, Notebaert AJ, Guskiewicz KM, Prentice WE. Neuropsychological performance, postural stability, and symptoms after dehydration. J Athl Train. 2007;42:66–75.
36. Ropper AH, Gorson KC. Clinical practice: concussion. N Engl J Med. 2007;356:166–72.

37. Dart AM, Kingwell BA. Pulse pressure—a review of mechanisms and clinical relevance. J Am Coll Cardiol. 2001;37:975–84.
38. Sanders MJ, McKenna K. Head and facial trauma. In: Mosby's paramedic textbook. 2nd ed. St. Louis, MO: Mosby; 2001. p. 624–51.
39. Maddocks DL, Dicker GD, Saling MM. The assessment of orientation following concussion in athletes. Clin J Sport Med. 1995;5:32–5.
40. McCrea M, Kelly JP, Kluge J, Ackley B, Randolph C. Standardized assessment of concussion in football players. Neurology. 1997;48:586–8.
41. McCrea M. Standardized mental status assessment of sports concussion. Clin J Sport Med. 2001;11:176–81.
42. Barr WB, McCrea M. Sensitivity and specificity of standardized neurocognitive testing immediately following sports concussion. J Int Neuropsychol Soc. 2001;7:693–702.
43. McCrea M, Barr WB, Guskiewicz KM, et al. Standard regression-based methods for measuring recovery after sport-related concussion. J Int Neuropsychol Soc. 2005;11:58–69.
44. Romberg MH. A manual of the nervous disease of man. London: Sydenham Society; 1853.
45. Riemann BL, Guskiewicz KM, Shields EW. Relationship between clinical and forceplate measures of postural stability. J Sport Rehabil. 1999;8:71–82.
46. Valovich McLeod TC, Barr WB, McCrea M, Guskiewicz KM. Psychometric and measurement properties of concussion assessment tools in youth sports. J Athl Train. 2006;41:399–408.
47. Broglio SP, Monk A, Sopiarz K, Cooper ER. The influence of ankle support on postural control. J Sci Med Sport. 2009;12:388–92.
48. Wilkins JC, Valovich TC, Perrin DH, Gansneder BM. Performance on the Balance Error Scoring System decreases after fatigue. J Athl Train. 2004;39:156–61.
49. Susco TM, Valovich McLeod TC, Gansneder BM, Shultz SJ. Balance recovers within 20 minutes after exertion as measured by the Balance Error Scoring System. J Athl Train. 2004;39:241–6.
50. Fox ZG, Mihalik JP, Blackburn JT, Battaglini CL, Guskiewicz KM. Return of postural control to baseline after anaerobic and aerobic exercise protocols. J Athl Train. 2008;43:456–63.
51. Giza CC, Kutcher JS, Ashwal S, et al. Summary of evidence-based guideline update: evaluation and management of concussion in sports: report of the Guideline Development Subcommittee of the American Academy of Neurology. Neurology. 2013;80(24):2250–7.
52. Herring SA, Cantu RC, Guskiewicz KM, et al. Concussion (mild traumatic brain injury) and the team physician: a consensus statement—2011 update. Med Sci Sports Exerc. 2011;43:2412–22.
53. Lovell MR, Collins MW, Iverson GL, Johnston K, Bradley JP. Grade 1 or "ding" concussions in high school athletes. Am J Sports Med. 2004;32:47–54.
54. Cantu RC. Athletic concussion: current understanding as of 2007. Neurosurgery. 2007;60:963–4.

Chapter 19
Sports-Related Subconcussive Head Trauma

Brian D. Johnson

Abstract There is a growing concern in clinical practice regarding the immediate and long-term effects of multiple and frequent subconcussive blows in athletes participating in full contact sports. The effects of repetitive subconcussive head trauma, occurring in full contact sports, on brain structural, functional, and metabolic integrity has not been sufficiently investigated. It is yet to be determined whether these multiple subconcussive blows induce transient alterations in the brain or long-term deficits. Animal, neuropsychological, biomechanical, neuroimaging, and postmortem studies have all been used to study subconcussive head trauma. However, there is no consistency throughout the literature about whether or not subconcussive impacts have detrimental effects. More recent studies highlighting the prevalence of certain neurological etiologies, like chronic traumatic encephalopathy associated with a history of repetitive concussive and subconcussive head trauma, highlights the need for future research into this area of research.

Keywords Subconcussive • Concussion • Mild traumatic brain injury (mTBI) • Multiple impacts • Head trauma

B.D. Johnson, Ph.D., M.S., R.T.(MR)(N) (✉)
Department of Kinesiology, Pennsylvania State University,
24 Rec Hall, University Park, PA 16802, USA

The Pennsylvania State University Center for Sports Concussion
Research and Service, University Park, PA, USA
e-mail: bdj5039@psu.edu

S.M. Slobounov and W.J. Sebastianelli (eds.), *Concussions in Athletics:*
From Brain to Behavior, DOI 10.1007/978-1-4939-0295-8_19,
© Springer Science+Business Media New York 2014

Introduction

Recently, concussion and subconcussive head trauma have garnered a lot of attention, not only in the scientific and medical communities, but in the public as well. Widespread media coverage and several high profile cases have brought in to question the damaging and long-term effects of sports-related traumatic brain injury (TBI) [1]. Specifically, there has been a broad range of neurodegenerative diseases and processes that include postconcussion syndrome, posttraumatic stress disorder, cognitive impairment, chronic traumatic encephalopathy (CTE), and *dementia pugilistica* that have been linked to repetitive sports-related head injury of any kind [2]. Referred to as the "silent epidemic," as many of the physical, cognitive, behavioral, and emotional symptoms go unrecognized, TBI is not only a major health concern in the United States [3] but is the leading cause of disability worldwide [4].

There is a growing concern in clinical practice regarding the immediate and long-term effects of multiple and frequent subconcussive blows in athletes participating in full contact sports. These effects, in terms of neurocognitive, behavioral, and underlying neural substrates have not been sufficiently studied. In particular, concern is growing about the effect of subconcussive impacts to the head and how it may adversely affect cerebral functions [5–7].

Subconcussive blows are below the threshold to cause a concussion [8] and do not result in a clinically identifiable concussion signs or symptoms [5–7]. Despite this lack of any concussion-related signs and symptoms, subconcussive head impacts should in no way be taken likely. Animal and human studies have shown that even though these subconcussive blows do not result in apparent behavioral alterations they can cause damage to the central nervous system [2, 9]. Moreover, these impacts that are below the threshold to induce a concussion still have the potential to transfer a high degree of linear and rotational acceleration forces to the brain [10]. Unlike concussions, subconcussive blows go undiagnosed and are not assessed by medical professionals during the course of a game, resulting in exposure to a staggering number of these impacts over a season and a career [1, 11]. Furthermore, postmortem studies have identified that repeated subconcussive impacts may have an accumulative effect [8]. It has been hypothesized that these frequent and repetitive subconcussive impacts exacerbate the cognitive aging process by reducing the cognitive reserve at an accelerated rate and lead to altered neuronal biology that may not present itself till later in life [12]. Recent studies have eluded that brain injury does not only come from concussive episodes but also the accrual of these subconcussive blows [13] can cause pathophysiological changes in the brain [14]. However, similar to the research focused on concussion and mild traumatic brain injury (mTBI), the current literature on subconcussive head trauma is limited and the studies that are available seem to raise more questions than they answer [15].

Animal Models of Subconcussive Head Trauma

It has been known since the late nineteenth century that repeated mild blows to the head in animal experiments could be lethal even though there was no evidence of structural brain damage [16]. Initial animal models probing the difference between a single versus multiple concussive and subconcussive insults revealed that following a single subconcussive blow there were no behavioral and histologic changes, yet repetitive subconcussive head trauma resulted in permanent injury [17]. In an early experiment looking at concussion in the rat, it was noted that following sub-concussive blows, the animals showed signs of "posttraumatic amnesia" [18]. Additionally, Govons et al. [18] reported that subconcussive blows produced con-vulsions in some of the rats, altered activity for 24 h, and that the impact caused the animal to be momentarily stunned. Additionally, subconcussive head trauma has shown to decrease the polarizability of the cerebrum although not to the extent of a full concussive blow [19]. Tedeschi [16] reported that repetitive subconcussive blows received over a short duration in a rat model elicited a higher incidence of ill effects. Furthermore, postmortem examination of these rats revealed widespread evidence of neuronal injury, myelin loss, and glial proliferation. Other studies of subconcussive head trauma have reported neuropsychological changes and ionic fluctuations and have been hypothesized to leave the brain more vulnerable to a repeated injury [20]. In a recent animal study investigating the effects of subconcus-sive head trauma induced by a mild lateral fluid percussion, Shultz et al. [8] found that such an injury caused acute neuroinflammation despite any significant axonal injury, or cognitive, emotional, or sensorimotor alterations. Specifically, they docu-mented a short-term increase in microglia, macrophages, and reactive astrogliosis which returned to normal at a 4-week follow-up.

Acute neuroinflammation has also been documented in other animal and human studies of TBI. Repetitive mTBI, similar to neuroinflammation may have cumula-tive effects leading to neurodegeneration [8] and linked to behavioral impairments after TBI [21]. Conversely it has been thought that neuroinflammation may have a neuroprotective quality [22] and the brain may be better protected following an initial TBI [23]. Complementary to this notion of neuroprotection, it has also been reported that by gradually increasing the amount of brain injury, animals could tol-erate trauma that would otherwise kill normal animals. This so-called trauma resis-tance was attributed to a stabilization of metabolic processes [24] and this idea of preconditioning has been detailed in cerebral ischemia [25]. Fujita et al. [26] reported that subthreshold head trauma did not cause axonal or vascular changes in the rat, even with repetitive blows. Although postmortem studies have identified that repeated subconcussive head trauma may have an accumulative effect and lead to neurodegenerative diseases [8], Slemmer and Weber [25], using a mechanical stretch to simulate an mTBI in hippocampal cell cultures, found that when the tissue was preconditioned they observed a significant decrease in S-100β indicating a positive effect of glial preconditioning. Moreover, Allen et al. [23] reported a rat model of repetitive mTBI preconditioning served to preserve motor function following a severe TBI and also elicited activation of secondary sites in the brain that may aide in recovery. Whether or not this response to repetitive insult is beneficial or detrimental is yet to be determined and is not only limited to animal research. In a recent human study looking at serum nerve growth factor (NGF) and brain-derived neurotrophic factor (BDNF) levels in soccer players following a session of headers, Bamac et al. [27] reported increased NGF and BDNF from baseline levels. This increase was attributed to the microtrauma caused by the subconcussive impacts from heading the ball. However, this increase is ambiguous as elevated NGF levels could be a sign of neuroprotective or destructive processes in the brain. These studies give evidence that subconcussive blows to the head can cause injury and should not be overlooked as trifle.

Biomechanical Studies of Subconcussive Head Trauma

Compared to the literature on sports-related concussion, biomechanical studies solely focusing on subconcussive head trauma are scarce, and if any data is presented, it usually limited to the quantification of the number of impacts. Although this not to say that researchers have not tried, and biomechanical studies have shown that significant amount of forces are transmitted to deep midbrain and brainstem structures even in less severe head injury that does not result in concussion or loss of consciousness [28]. Biomechanical studies report that the forces like momentum and energy transfer associated with heading the soccer ball are far less than those found in football, boxing, hockey, and other full contact sports [29]. With the advent of new technologies, like the Head Impact Telemetry System (HITS) that has been employed in football helmets, tracking the number and quantification of forces at impact has become more feasible. In a recent study Broglio et al. [10] used the HITS to measure and record head impacts in 95 high school football players over a 4-year period of time. The results of this study highlighted the number of blows to the head an athlete is exposed to over the course of a season as well as the high degree of linear and rotational accelerations forces sustained during these impacts. Probably the most shocking data to come out of these studies are the sheer quantity of subconcussive impacts endured of the course of a season, let alone an athlete's career. This number can be upwards of thousands of subconcussive impacts during the course of a single season [1], with one study using accelerometers in football helmets reporting players sustaining over 1,400 subconcussive blows over the course of a season [30]. Consequently, a recent laboratory study of football helmets found that current varsity helmets are less protective to their older leather helmet counterparts when it comes to subconcussive blows [31].

These subconcussive hits are not only relegated to the contact sports that immediately come to mind when we think of concussion like football, ice-hockey, and rugby. Soccer is a contact sport and chronic traumatic brain injury (CTBI) has been well documented in the literature [32]. During an average game, a soccer player heads the ball 6–12 times which is estimated to be over 5,000 headers for a 15-year career [9, 29]. However, most of the documented cases of concussion in soccer occur due to the players head contacting another player's head, the ground, or the goal post, not from purposeful heading [33]. However, repeated subconcussive blows that are incurred from heading the soccer ball account for many clinical symptoms that span the spectrum from headache to brain damage and can also lead to alterations in acute and chronic cognitive function [9]. It has long been known that heading of the soccer ball could produce "footballer's migraine" [34]. There are few biomechanical studies on subconcussive head trauma and implementing such studies requires highly technical and intricate technology and knowledge. Furthermore, biomechanical studies of full blown concussive episodes have gone to great lengths to quantify and identify a threshold of concussion to no avail [35], as this is very difficult given the fact that each concussion is different [36].

Cognitive Assessment of Subconcussive Head Trauma

These subconcussive impacts that are below the threshold of concussion and do not result in any clinically identifiable signs or symptoms are a controversial topic as researchers and clinicians are divided on their true effect. Some research has shown that subconcussive head trauma may have minimal impact on cognitive functions [37] although there is mounting evidence that subconcussive blows have detrimental effects on cognitive and cerebral functions [5, 14]. It has been hypothesized that exposure to repeated and multiple subconcussive blows throughout an athlete's career may compromise cognitive function [38]. It is becoming ever more apparent that brain injury does not only come from concussive episodes, but that the accumulation of these subconcussive blows may be detrimental [13]. A history of multiple concussions and subconcussive blows is known to result in depression, cognitive deficits, and progressive neuropathologies that include neurofibrillary tangles and deposits of amyloid plaques seen in Alzheimer's disease [39].

A majority of the literature that exists on acute and chronic sports-related subconcussive head trauma has been focused on soccer as purposeful heading represents a form of repetitive subthreshold mild brain injury [29]. In a preliminary study, it was found that out of 77 retired Norwegian professional soccer players, 50 % reported symptoms linked to heading, and 75 % suffered from disorientation, headache, and nausea [40]. Further studies by Tysvaer et al. used electroencephalograph (EEG) to evaluate professional soccer players. They found that 35 % of the participants had abnormal EEGs and 70 % displayed some form of neurological impairment [41, 42]. In addition to these findings, neuropsychological testing (Wechsler Adult Intelligence Scale) of the same soccer players revealed significant differences compared to controls with one-third of participants' scores low enough to suggest evidence of organic brain damage [43]. Matser et al. [44] reported significant deficits in neuropsychological assessment of amateur soccer players associated with heading. Specifically, they reported impaired performance in memory, planning, and visual perception processing that was exacerbated by the number of previous concussions a player had sustained. Downs and Abwender [45] reported that subjects with a long history of soccer heading demonstrated slower patterns of motor speed and reaction time. Another study looking at purposeful heading by Witol and Webbe [7] revealed that players with the most reported number of headers had the lowest attention, concentration, and IQ scores. Decreased reaction time and reduced speed performing a motor task have been documented when assessing the effects of subconcussive head trauma in soccer [45], as well as in athletes following a concussion [46], suggesting that reaction time is impaired following repeated subconcussive and concussive head trauma [38]. Although there is evidence that a long career which accounts to many instances of heading the soccer ball can lead to impaired brain function, it is not clear whether or not this increased likelihood is caused by numerous subconcussive blows or from full blown concussive episodes [33]. Jordan et al. [47] found that there was a correlation between a history of concussion with increased symptoms in the United Stated national soccer team players and may suggest that full blown concussions as compared to repetitive subconcussive impacts may be the cause of encephalopathic changes. But it seems evident in the literature that a long soccer career, which amounts to a higher frequency of heading and accumulation of subconcussive blows, contributes to impairments in cognitive function [33, 48]. Whereas, in a review by Rutherford et al. [15] on neuropsychological testing and purposeful heading in soccer literature, they raise certain methodological concerns with a majority of the studies. They conclude that there is preliminary evidence that full blown concussive episodes can have deleterious effects based upon neuropsychological examination, whereas the effects of subconcussive impacts on neuropsychological tests awaits more supporting evidence. Not all studies on heading in soccer have reported neuropsychological deficits [34]. In a recent study, Kontos and colleagues [49] used computerized testing in the form of Immediate Post-Concussion Assessment and Cognitive Testing (ImPACT) to test 63 adolescent soccer players. All subjects under study had no current (less than 3 months) history of concussion and were placed into one of the three groups based upon the number of documented headers as observed by the researchers over the course of two practices and games. Their results showed no significant differences between the low, moderate, and high frequency heading groups on computerized neuropsychological assessment. However, the authors did note that the males showed lower scores on verbal memory, visual memory, and motor processing compared to female participants. This decreased performance was attributed to differences based upon sex despite the fact that males headed the ball more often than females.

Similar to the studies looking at the chronic effects of repetitive subconcussive head trauma, initial research looking at the acute effects has reported mixed results. Schmitt et al. [33] tested postural control and recorded subjects' self-reported symptoms immediately and at 24 h following a controlled session of intentional soccer ball heading. They found that prior to, immediately following, and at 24 h after the 40 min session of heading, there were no differences in postural control as assessed by center of pressure (COP) area and velocity between the heading group and a control kicking group. In spite of not finding any significant difference in postural control after an acute bout of heading, an increase in concussion-related symptoms were found immediately following the heading session, but not at 24 h after in the heading cohort. The main complaints were headache, dizziness, and feeling lethargic. This reported finding was similar to Tysvaer [50] who found that 10 min following a session of purposeful heading, all subjects reported suffering from a headache. Consistent with these findings, Mangus et al. [51] also reported no differences in balance following an acute bout of soccer ball heading. Additionally, Broglio et al. [52] found no significant acute changes in postural control following a study that looked at the effects that purposeful heading in soccer can have on balance. In a recent study by Rieder and Jansen [53], they took subjects and divided them into three groups to investigate the effects that a bout of acute heading would have on neuropsychological exam. The three groups consisted of subjects exposed to aerobic training and purposeful heading drills, the second group consisted of subjects only doing the aerobic training, and the third group did not exert themselves physically before neuropsychological testing. Neuropsychological testing was performed 1 week prior to training session and immediately after. The results showed no differences between groups and or any deficits caused by heading drills. However, there was a higher incidence of headache during and after in the heading cohort which the authors attributed to the most minor form of head trauma, cranial contusion, which is associated with local or diffuse transient headache. However, Putukian et al. [54] did not report any differences in self-reported symptoms and cognitive function in a pilot study after a soccer training session that included heading. Therefore, symptoms from subconcussive blows may be shorter lived and only detectable immediately after insult as the training session was substantially longer and less focused on heading than the Schmitt et al. [33] study. Employing the use of a computerized tablet, Zhang et al. [55] devised a variant of common eye tracking research, prosaccade, and antisaccade by having participants point towards a target (Pro-Point) or point to the opposite target (Anti-Point). Eye tracking research has been shown to be more sensitive in picking up cognitive and functional deficits compared to standard neuropsychological testing [56–58]. In their study, Zhang et al. [55] tested 12 female high school soccer players following practice that included heading of the soccer ball. No difference was seen between the soccer group compared to sex and age matched control group on the Pro-Point task. Although the Anti-Point task, similar to the antisaccade task used in eye tracking studies, showed that subjects in the soccer group that were exposed to heading demonstrated significantly slower response times compared to the control group.

In an early study of boxers, Heilbronner and colleagues [59] were the first to demonstrate changes in cognitive function immediately following a fight when compared to a prefight assessment. Specifically they noted a decline in verbal and incidental memory, and noted that numerous subconcussive blows may be more deleterious than less frequent full blown concussions as the number of rounds a boxer fights better predicts the development of encephalopathy compared to the number of knockouts. In a study by Ravdin et al. [60] investigating the effects of subconcussive blows, boxers were administered neuropsychological examinations before a fight, after the fight, and at a 1-month follow-up session.

Their results were interesting and questioned the validity of a return-to-baseline as an appropriate criterion for return-to-play decisions. They noted that at 1-month post-fight, neuropsychological performance had increased beyond baseline assessment taken prior to the fight and was believed to be caused by the repeated subconcussive blows the boxers received while training for the fight. Repetitive subconcussive head trauma has been hypothesized to be the main cause of neurocognitive dysfunction in boxers and that the accumulation of subconcussive blows may lead to cognitive deterioration of brain function [61].

Shuttleworth-Edwards and Radloff [62] investigated the differences between rugby players and athletes involved in non-contact sports and found that rugby players had a poorer performance on visuomotor processing speed. Additionally, they subdivided the rugby players into two groups based upon the frequency of the positions to be exposed to subconcussive head trauma. This within group analysis revealed that the group that regularly receives more subconcussive impacts displayed lower scores on the digit symbol substitution visuomotor task. Interestingly enough, it has been reported that despite a five times greater frequency of head injuries, rugby players out perform soccer players on neuropsychological testing [63]. Additionally, Parker et al. [38] found that subjects exposed to repeated subconcussive blows in football, rugby, and lacrosse showed increased medial–lateral sway in their gaits. In a study by Killam et al. [64] examining athletes with and without a history of concussion and athletes recovering from concussion to a control group without any history of head trauma, researchers concluded that subconcussive head trauma seen in contact sports produces subclinical cognitive impairments. Similarly, Stephens et al. [65] performed neuropsychological testing on adolescent soccer and rugby players in addition to a group of noncontact athletes. They reported no evidence of neurological dysfunction in both the soccer and rugby players when compared to their noncontact counterparts. Although no individual has suffered a recent (within the past 3 years) head injury, those with a previous concussion showed poorer performance on attention measures.

In a recent study by Miller et al. [37], neuropsychological assessment of collegiate football players in the form of the Standardized Assessment of Concussion (SAC) and the ImPACT were performed at three time intervals: preseason, midseason, and postseason. No subjects under study received a clinically diagnosable concussion, yet were exposed to numerous subconcussive blows throughout the season. There were no significant decreases in overall SAC and ImPACT scores reported, yet significant improvements in visual memory and reaction time were noted. Additionally, improvement in verbal memory and processing speed were close to reaching the limits of significance at a p-value of 0.06 and 0.05, respectively. Recently, Talavage et al. [14] reported changes in cerebral functions attributed to multiple subconcussive impacts as evidenced by declines in the visual working memory in high school football players in the absence of clinical signs of concussion. Although it is common for football players to report headaches following practice, it is not yet known whether this is a posttraumatic phenomenon or caused from subconcussive impacts [66].

Neuroimaging of Subconcussive Head Trauma

Few reports in the literature have found any gross structural differences in the brain following a concussive or subconcussive head trauma as evaluated by computed tomography (CT) and standard magnetic resonance imaging (MRI). CT and MRI for the most part are usually found to be normal following concussion, as it is more of a metabolic reaction to trauma than a structural injury [67]. Although, their use can be invaluable in ruling out more serious injuries like skull fractures and hemorrhages. However, one study that looked at boxers longitudinally saw evidence in 13 % of the boxers of progressive brain injury, as well as several boxers presenting with cortical atrophy and *cavum septum pellucidum* [68]. Another CT study evaluating soccer players saw an increase in cerebral atrophy and ventriculomegaly in 27 % and 18 % of the professional soccer players, respectively [41, 42]. This shortcoming highlights the importance in using more sensitive and specific testing measures in concussion and subconcussive research such as advanced neuroimaging techniques. These newer advanced MRI techniques, like functional magnetic resonance imaging (fMRI), magnetic resonance spectroscopy (MRS), diffusion tensor imaging (DTI), and susceptibility weighted imaging (SWI) may offer promise in providing some insight on the injured brain due to concussion and subconcussive head trauma [2].

Experiments utilizing fMRI into the effects of subconcussive repetitive head trauma is scarce, and no studies have specifically used advanced neuroimaging techniques to investigate the acute effects of subconcussive blows. Talavage et al. [14] took 11 high school football players and performed an fMRI visual working memory paradigm and baseline neuropsychological testing. They found that the number of collisions was significantly correlated to changes in the subject's fMRI activation. Specifically, subjects that showed no clinical symptoms of concussion, yet showed poorer neuropsychological tests, exhibited a significant reduction of fMRI activation in the dorsolateral prefrontal cortex, middle and superior frontal gyri, and cerebellum. In an extension of this study, Breedlove et al. [69] reported that despite not sustaining a concussion, a large portion of their cohort under study showed significant neuropsychological changes as assessed by fMRI due to repetitive subconcussive head trauma. Additionally, they found a significant relationship between the number of blows and the documented changes in the neuropsychological testing, which reinforced their hypothesis that repetitive subconcussive head trauma may be connected to pathologically altered neurophysiology. Bazarian et al. [70] took a cohort of nine high school student athletes and performed DTI pre- and postseason at an interval of 3 months apart and subjects sustained between 26 and 399 subconcussive blows. One subject received a concussion during the season and demonstrated the highest number of voxels in the white matter with a significant change in fractional anisotropy (FA) and mean diffusivity (MD) values from pre- to postseason. The subconcussive group showed the next highest number of voxels with a significant FA and MD change with most subjects displaying an increase in FA and a decrease in MD. In contrast, Chappell et al. [71] reported an increase in ADC and a decrease in FA in the deep white matter of 81 professional boxers. They inferred that these abnormalities reported may reflect the cumulative effects of repetitive subconcussive head trauma. Similarly, using DTI, Koerte et al. [72] reported widespread differences in white matter integrity between a small cohort of soccer players with no previous concussive episode compared to swimmers. Specifically, they observed significantly increased radial diffusivity in a number of major white matter tracts including the corpus callosum, suggestive of compromised myelin integrity. An MRS pilot study of retired professional athletes with a known exposure to concussions and subconcussive head trauma revealed a significant increase in choline (Cho) and glutamate/glutamine (Glx) concentrations [73].

Looking at CTBI in boxers, Bailey and colleagues [74] used transcranial Doppler ultrasound to assess cerebral hemodynamic function. Specifically, the authors looked at dynamic cerebral autoregulation, cerebrovascular reactivity to changes in carbon dioxide (CVR CO_2), orthostatic tolerance, in addition to the neurocognitive examination of 12 current professional male boxers compared to 12 male non-boxers matched for age and physical fitness levels. Results of this study revealed neurocognitive dysfunction and impaired cerebral hemodynamic function compared to the control group. The CVR CO_2 metric was also correlated with the amount of sparring training the boxers had undergone, not the number of competitive bouts. This study was the first to demonstrate that cerebral hemodynamic function is compromised in CTBI. The authors contributed this hemodynamic and neurocognitive impairment to the mechanical trauma, mostly in the form of subconcussive impacts, experienced from sparring during a career in boxing. These advanced neuroimaging techniques, especially when combined in a multi-modal approach have the potential to obtain additional and specialized information about the neuropathology of subconcussive head trauma and offer researchers and medical practioners valuable insight.

Conclusion

Impacts to the head in collision sports are unavoidable, and as serious as concussion is, subconcussive impacts happen much more often and are now being implicated as a source for the deterioration of cerebral structures and function later in life [10]. Despite being labeled as subconcussive, subthreshold, or subclinical, it is apparent that athletes in contact sports are subjected to a staggering number of these impacts. Contradictory to what the "subconcussive" moniker may imply, subconcussive impacts can cause brain injury [9]. However, the effect of subconcussive blows has not been fully addressed although there is now a focus surrounding the immediate and long-term effects they may have [13]. It is important for future research to focus not only on concussive blows, but on varying degrees of head trauma that include subconcussive impacts, as well as time intervals between repetitive sports-related head trauma [2]. Furthermore, empirical evidence suggests that a history of concussion leads to an increased susceptibility to sustain recurrent concussions [75, 76] and further study is needed to explore the effects that subconcussive head trauma may have on those with a history or prior concussion and those without [77]. It appears that in subconcussive head trauma research, much in the fashion of concussion research, the only consistency is inconsistency. However, it is not hard to believe despite the overall lack of agreement based on neuropsychological measures, subconcussive impacts can cause microstructural and biochemical changes in the brain [30]. Whether or not subconcussive impacts not only have acute effects on the brain which need to be taken seriously and managed correctly or are amassed over time and manifest clinically later in life remains to be seen.

References

1. McKee AC, Cantu RC, Nowinski CJ, Hedley-Whyte ET, Gavett BE, Budson AE, et al. Chronic traumatic encephalopathy in athletes: progressive tauopathy after repetitive head injury. J Neuropathol Exp Neurol. 2009;68(7):709–35.
2. Dashnaw ML, Petraglia AL, Bailes JE. An overview of the basic science of concussion and subconcussion: where we are and where we are going. Neurosurg Focus. 2012;33(6):1–9.
3. Langlois JA, Rutland-Brown W, Wald MM. The epidemiology and impact of traumatic brain injury—a brief overview. J Head Trauma Rehabil. 2006;21(5):375–8.
4. Signoretti S, Vagnozzi R, Tavazzi B, Lazzarino G. Biochemical and neurochemical sequelae following mild traumatic brain injury: summary of experimental data and clinical implications. Neurosurg Focus. 2010;29(5):E1.
5. Gavett BE, Stern RA, McKee AC. Chronic traumatic encephalopathy: a potential late effect of sport-related concussive and subconcussive head trauma. Clin Sports Med. 2011; 30(1):179–88.
6. Martini DN, Sabin MJ, DePesa SA, Leal EW, Negrete TN, Sosnoff JJ, et al. The chronic effects of concussion on gait. Arch Phys Med Rehabil. 2011;92(4):585–9.
7. Witol AD, Webbe FM. Soccer heading frequency predicts neuropsychological deficits. Arch Clin Neuropsychol. 2003;18(4):397–417.
8. Shultz SR, MacFabe DF, Foley KA, Taylor R, Cain DP. Sub-concussive brain injury in the Long-Evans rat induces acute neuroinflammation in the absence of behavioral impairments. Behav Brain Res. 2012;229(1):145–52.
9. Bauer JA, Thomas TS, Cauraugh JH, Kaminski TW, Hass CJ. Impact forces and neck muscle activity in heading by collegiate female soccer players. J Sports Sci. 2001;19(3):171–9.
10. Broglio SP, Eckner JT, Martini D, Sosnoff JJ, Kutcher JS, Randolph C. Cumulative head impact burden in high school football. J Neurotrauma. 2011;28(10):2069–78.
11. Baugh CM, Stamm JM, Riley DO, Gavett BE, Shenton ME, Lin A, et al. Chronic traumatic encephalopathy: neurodegeneration following repetitive concussive and subconcussive brain trauma. Brain Imaging Behav. 2012;6(2):244–54.
12. Broglio SP, Eckner JT, Paulson HL, Kutcher JS. Cognitive decline and aging: the role of concussive and subconcussive impacts. Exerc Sport Sci Rev. 2012;40(3):138–44.
13. Spiotta AM, Shin JH, Bartsch AJ, Benzel EC. Subconcussive impact in sports: a new era of awareness. World Neurosurg. 2011;75(2):175–8.
14. Talavage TM, Nauman E, Breedlove EL, Yoruk U, Dye AE, Morigaki K, et al. Functionally-detected cognitive impairment in high school football players without clinically-diagnosed concussion. J Neurotrauma. 2013. epub ahead of print.

15. Rutherford A, Stephens R, Potter D. The neuropsychology of heading and head trauma in association football (soccer): a review. Neuropsychol Rev. 2003;13(3):153–79.
16. Tedeschi CG. Cerebral injury by blunt mechanical trauma—special reference to the effects of repeated impacts of minimal intensity—observations on experimental animals. AMA Arch Neurol Psychiatry. 1945;53(5):333–54.
17. Iverson GL, Gaetz M, Lovell MR, Collins MW. Cumulative effects of concussion in amateur athletes. Brain Inj. 2004;18(5):433–43.
18. Govons SR, Govons RB, Heusner WW, Vanhuss WD. Brain concussion in the rat. Exp Neurol. 1972;34(1):121–8.
19. Spiegel EA, Henny GC, Wycis HT, Spiegeladolf M. Effect of concussion upon the polarizability of the brain. Am J Physiol. 1946;146(1):12–26.
20. Barkhoudarian G, Hovda DA, Giza CC. The molecular pathophysiology of concussive brain injury. Clin Sports Med. 2011;30(1):33–48.
21. Ramlackhansingh AF, Brooks DJ, Greenwood RJ, Bose SK, Turkheimer FE, Kinnunen KM, et al. Inflammation after trauma: microglial activation and traumatic brain injury. Ann Neurol. 2011;70(3):374–83.
22. Schmidt OI, Heyde CE, Ertel W, Stahel PF. Closed head injury—an inflammatory disease? Brain Res Rev. 2005;48(2):388–99.
23. Allen GV, Gerami D, Esser MJ. Conditioning effects of repetitive mild neurotrauma on motor function in an animal model of focal brain injury. Neuroscience. 2000;99(1):93–105.
24. Noble RL, Collip JB. A quantitative method for the production of experimental traumatic shock without haemorrhage in unanaesthetized animals. Q J Exp Physiol Cogn Med Sci. 1942;31:187–99.
25. Slemmer JE, Weber JT. The extent of damage following repeated injury to cultured hippocampal cells is dependent on the severity of insult and inter-injury interval. Neurobiol Dis. 2005;18(3):421–31.
26. Fujita M, Wei EP, Povlishock JT. Intensity- and interval-specific repetitive traumatic brain injury can evoke both axonal and microvascular damage. J Neurotrauma. 2012;29(12):2172–80.
27. Bamac B, Tamer GS, Colak T, Colak E, Seyrek E, Duman C, et al. Effects of repeatedly heading a soccer ball on serum levels of two neurotrophic factors of brain tissue, BDNF and NGF in professional soccer players. Biol Sports. 2011;28(3):177–81.
28. Pellman EJ, Viano DC, Tucker AM, Casson IR. Concussion in professional football: location and direction of helmet impacts—part 2. Neurosurgery. 2003;53(6):1328–40.
29. Spiotta AM, Bartsch AJ, Benzel EC. Heading in soccer: dangerous play? Neurosurgery. 2012;70(1):1–11.
30. Khurana VG, Kaye AH. An overview of concussion in sport. J Clin Neurosci. 2012;19(1):1–11.
31. Bartsch A, Benzel E, Miele V, Prakash V. Impact test comparisons of 20th and 21st century American football helmets. J Neurosurg. 2012;116(1):222–33.
32. Rabadi MH, Jordan BD. The cumulative effect of repetitive concussion in sports. Clin J Sport Med. 2001;11(3):194–8.
33. Schmitt DM, Hertel J, Evans TA, Olmsted LC, Putukian M. Effect of an acute bout of soccer heading on postural control and self-reported concussion symptoms. Int J Sports Med. 2004;25(5):326–31.
34. Kirkendall DT, Jordan SE, Garrett WE. Heading and head injuries in soccer. Sports Med. 2001;31(5):369–86.
35. Duma SM, Rowson S. Past, present, and future of head injury research. Exerc Sport Sci Rev. 2011;39(1):2–3.
36. Cantu RC. Athletic concussion current understanding as of 2007. Neurosurgery. 2007;60(6):963–4.
37. Miller JR, Adamson GJ, Pink MM, Sweet JC. Comparison of preseason, midseason, and postseason neurocognitive scores in uninjured collegiate football players. Am J Sports Med. 2007;35(8):1284–8.

38. Parker TM, Osternig LR, van Donkelaar P, Chou LS. Balance control during gait in athletes and non-athletes following concussion. Med Eng Phys. 2008;30(8):959–67.

39. Packard RC. Chronic post-traumatic headache: associations with mild traumatic brain injury, concussion, and post-concussive disorder. Curr Pain Headache Rep. 2008;12(1):67–73.

40. Tysvaer A, Storli O. Association football injuries to the brain. A preliminary report. Br J Sports Med. 1981;15(3):163–6.

41. Sortland O, Tysvaer AT. Brain-damage in former association football players—an evaluation by cerebral computed-tomography. Neuroradiology. 1989;31(1):44–8.

42. Tysvaer AT, Storli OV, Bachen NI. Soccer injuries to the brain—a neurologic and electroencephalographic study of former players. Acta Neurol Scand. 1989;80(2):151–6.

43. Tysvaer AT, Lochen EA. Soccer injuries to the brain—a neuropsychological study of former soccer players. Am J Sports Med. 1991;19(1):56–60.

44. Matser EJT, Kessels AG, Lezak MD, Jordan BD, Troost J. Neuropsychological impairment in amateur soccer players. JAMA. 1999;282(10):971–3.

45. Downs DS, Abwender D. Neuropsychological impairment in soccer athletes. J Sports Med Phys Fitness. 2002;42(1):103–7.

46. Bleiberg J, Cernich AN, Cameron K, Sun WY, Peck K, Ecklund J, et al. Duration of cognitive impairment after sports concussion. Neurosurgery. 2004;54(5):1073–8.

47. Jordan SE, Green GA, Galanty HL, Mandelbaum BR, Jabour BA. Acute and chronic brain injury in United States National Team soccer players. Am J Sports Med. 1996;24(2):205–10.

48. Matser JT, Kessels AGH, Lezak MD, Troost J. A dose-response relation of headers and concussions with cognitive impairment in professional soccer players. J Clin Exp Neuropsychol. 2001;23(6):770–4.

49. Kontos AP, Dolese A, Elbin RJ, Covassin T, Warren BL. Relationship of soccer heading to computerized neurocognitive performance and symptoms among female and male youth soccer players. Brain Inj. 2011;25(12):1234–41.

50. Tysvaer AT. Head and neck injuries in soccer—impact of minor trauma. Sports Med. 1992;14(3):200–13.

51. Mangus BC, Wallmann HW, Ledford M. Analysis of postural stability in collegiate soccer players before and after an acute bout of heading multiple soccer balls. Sports Biomech. 2004;3(2):209–20.

52. Broglio SP, Guskiewicz KM, Sell TC, Lephart SM. No acute changes in postural control after soccer heading. Br J Sports Med. 2004;38(5):561–7.

53. Rieder C, Jansen P. No neuropsychological consequence in male and female soccer players after a short heading training. Arch Clin Neuropsychol. 2011;26(7):583–91.

54. Putukian M, Echemendia RJ, Mackin S. The acute neuropsychological effects of heading in soccer: a pilot study. Clin J Sport Med. 2000;10(2):104–9.

55. Zhang MR, Red SD, Lin AH, Patel SS, Sereno AB. Evidence of cognitive dysfunction after soccer playing with ball heading using a novel tablet-based approach. PLoS One. 2013;8(2):e57364.

56. Heitger MH, Anderson TJ, Jones RD, Dalrymple-Alford JC, Frampton CM, Ardagh MW. Eye movement and visuomotor arm movement deficits following mild closed head injury. Brain. 2004;127:575–90.

57. Heitger MH, Anderson TJ, Jones RD. Saccade sequences as markers for cerebral dysfunction following mild closed head injury. Prog Brain Res. 2002;140:433–48.

58. Capo-Aponte JE, Urosevich TG, Temme LA, Tarbett AK, Sanghera NK. Visual dysfunctions and symptoms during the subacute stage of blast-induced mild traumatic brain injury. Mil Med. 2012;177(7):804–13.

59. Heilbronner RL, Henry GK, Carson-Brewer M. Neuropsychologic test performance in amateur boxers. Am J Sports Med. 1991;19(4):376–80.

60. Ravdin LD, Barr WB, Jordan B, Lathan WE, Relkin NR. Assessment of cognitive head recovery following sports related trauma in boxers. Clin J Sport Med. 2003;13(1):21–7.

61. Jordan BD, Matser EJT, Zimmerman RD, Zazula T. Scarring and cognitive function in professional boxers. Phys Sportsmed. 1996;24(5):87–98.

62. Shuttleworth-Edwards AB, Radloff SE. Compromised visuomotor processing speed in players of Rugby Union from school through to the national adult level. Arch Clin Neuropsychol. 2008;23(5):511–20.
63. Rutherford A, Stephens R, Potter D, Fernie G. Neuropsychological impairment as a consequence of football (soccer) play and football heading: preliminary analyses and report on university footballers. J Clin Exp Neuropsychol. 2005;27(3):299–319.
64. Killam C, Cautin RL, Santucci AC. Assessing the enduring residual neuropsychological effects of head trauma in college athletes who participate in contact sports. Arch Clin Neuropsychol. 2005;20(5):599–611.
65. Stephens R, Rutherford A, Potter D, Fernie G. Neuropsychological consequence of soccer play in adolescent UK school team soccer players. J Neuropsychiatry Clin Neurosci. 2010;22(3):295–303.
66. Terrell TR. Concussion in athletes. South Med J. 2004;97(9):837–42.
67. Lovell M, Collins M, Bradley J. Return to play following sports-related concussion. Clin Sports Med. 2004;23(3):421–41.
68. McCrory P. Sports concussion and the risk of chronic neurological impairment. Clin J Sport Med. 2011;21(1):6–12.
69. Breedlove EL, Robinson M, Talavage TM, Morigaki KE, Yoruk U, O'Keefe K, et al. Biomechanical correlates of symptomatic and asymptomatic neurophysiological impairment in high school football. J Biomech. 2012;45(7):1265–72.
70. Bazarian JJ, Zhu T, Blyth B, Borrino A, Zhong J. Subject-specific changes in brain white matter on diffusion tensor imaging after sports-related concussion. Magn Reson Imaging. 2012;30(2):171–80.
71. Chappell MH, Ulu AM, Zhang L, Heitger MH, Jordan BD, Zimmerman RD, et al. Distribution of microstructural damage in the brains of professional boxers: a diffusion MRI study. J Magn Reson Imaging. 2006;24(3):537–42.
72. Koerte IK, Ertl-Wagner B, Reiser M, Zafonte R, Shenton ME. White matter integrity in the brains of professional soccer players without a symptomatic concussion. JAMA. 2012;308(18):1859–61.
73. Lin A, Ramadan S, Box H, et al. Neurochemical changes in athletes with chronic traumatic encephalopathy. Chicago: Radiological Society of North America; 2010.
74. Bailey DM, Jones DW, Sinnott A, Brugniaux JV, New KJ, Hodson D, et al. Impaired cerebral haemodynamic function associated with chronic traumatic brain injury in professional boxers. Clin Sci. 2013;124(3–4):177–89.
75. Giza CC, Hovda DA. The neurometabolic cascade of concussion. J Athl Train. 2001;36(3):228–35.
76. Guskiewicz KM. Cumulative effects associated with recurrent concussion in collegiate football players: the NCAA concussion study. JAMA. 2003;290(19):2549–55.
77. Kaminski TW, Cousino ES, Glutting JJ. Examining the relationship between purposeful heading in soccer and computerized neuropsychological test performance. Res Q Exerc Sport. 2008;79(2):235–44.

Chapter 20
The Role of the Quantitative EEG in the Diagnosis and Rehabilitation of the Traumatic Brain Injured Patients

Kirtley E. Thornton

Abstract The quantitative EEG (QEEG) has proven to be useful in the diagnosis and rehabilitation of the cognitive problems of the traumatic brain injured (TBI) subject. This chapter reviews the evidence on the use of the QEEG in discriminant analysis of TBI vs. normal individuals and the cognitive rehabilitation of the cognitive problems of the TBI patient. The research documents two cognitive activation approaches to QEEG analysis which have obtained 100 % accuracy in their diagnostic decision. Previous cognitive rehabilitation efforts have not been particularly effective in improving cognitive performance. The coordinated allocation of resource model of brain functioning was proposed as a conceptual framework to understand the brain's electrophysiological functioning. The model employs a cognitive activation evaluation and comparison to a normative activation database approach to determine the EEG biofeedback protocols. The approach has produced an average of 2.31 standard deviation improvements in auditory and reading memory in the TBI patient. Thus, the evidence supports the use of the activation database-guided QEEG in the diagnosis and rehabilitation of the TBI patient.

Keywords Quantitative EEG • Traumatic brain injury • Discriminant analysis • Cognitive rehabilitation • EEG biofeedback • Coordinated allocation of resource model of brain functioning • Memory improvement

K.E. Thornton, Ph.D. (✉)
The Brain Foundation, Lake Wylie, SC, USA
e-mail: ket@chp-neurotherapy.com

S.M. Slobounov and W.J. Sebastianelli (eds.), *Concussions in Athletics: From Brain to Behavior*, DOI 10.1007/978-1-4939-0295-8_20,
© Springer Science+Business Media New York 2014

Introduction

This chapter will examine how the quantitative EEG (QEEG) has been employed in the diagnosis of a TBI and rehabilitation efforts. The initial section will: (1) address the extent, focus, and costs of the TBI problem; (2) biological/neuroanatomical effects; (3) prognostic issues; (4) the spontaneous cure myth; (5) diagnostic issues with respect to the electrophysiological deficit pattern; (6) previous discriminant analysis attempts to distinguish between the TBI and normal population; (7) two proposed multiple cognitive discriminant methodologies which obtain 100 % accuracy in identification and discrimination of the TBI patient from the normal population.

The second section will address: (1) research results in the area of traditional cognitive rehabilitation intervention models; (2) the results obtained with the coordinated allocation of resource (CAR) model when employing EEG biofeedback as the intervention model; (3) the CAR model of brain functioning; and (4) a specific case example demonstrating the specificity and sensitivity of the approach.

The TBI Problem

Concussions are a major concern in three areas: (1) professional, college, high school, and elementary school athletic events; (2) returning soldiers from the Iraq and Afghanistan conflicts; and (3) Emergency Department patients.

Sports

There are 32 NFL teams that average of 0.62 concussions (2010) recorded per game [1]. It has been estimated that there is a 72 % chance of a concussion injury occurring during every NFL game [2]. There were 128 concussions in the NHL during the 2011–2012 seasons [3]. There is an estimated 650 college football teams in the USA [4]. There are about 67,000 players diagnosed with TBIs during HS football games each year and minimally 50 young football players have died or sustained serious head injuries during football games since 1997 [5]. Estimates of TBI in high school sports are probably on the low side. A survey of high school football players found that 47 % of the athletes reported a concussion at the time of injury [6]. The reasons provided by the students for not reporting were the belief that the injury was not serious enough to need medical attention (66 %), wanting to stay in the game (41 %), not recognizing the occurrence of a concussion (36 %), and not wanting to disappoint their teammates (22 %). An additional problematic research finding in this area was reported by Talavage et al. [7]. High school football players without a history of concussion were assessed with the ImPACT, fMRI, and longitudinal measures of head collision events (HIT system). They found players (about 50 %)

who exhibited no clinically observed symptoms associated with concussion demonstrated measurable neurocognitive (primarily visual working memory) and neurophysiologic (decreased activation in dorsolateral prefrontal cortex, dorsal lateral prefrontal cortex [DLPFC]) impairments.

Additional sports areas include rugby, boxing, soccer, basketball, hockey, and any sport that involves physical contact between the athletes or athletic situations where the athlete could fall (skiing, karate, etc.). There is an estimated 3.8 million sports-related concussion yearly in the USA [8]. Asken and Schwartz [9] provided an estimate that during a 300 game typical soccer career the player experiences some 2,000 head impacts.

Emergency Departments

Traumatic brain injury (TBI) incidence has been reported to result in more than 1,250,000 Emergency Department (ED) visits a year [10] in the USA with an estimated cost of 1.5 billion dollars a year. It has also been estimated that 56 % of mild TBI (mTBI) is not diagnosed in the ED [11]. As a comparison, each year, about 1.1 million Americans suffer a heart attack. The CDC estimates 1.7 million TBIs are experienced yearly. Thus, during the past 12 years roughly 20 million TBIs have been added to the TBI population. The CDC indicates, "direct medical costs and indirect costs such as lost productivity of TBI totaled an estimated $76.5 billion in the USA in 2000 [12]. Thus, over a similar 12 year period, the cost of TBI injuries could be estimated at $918 billion dollars. TBIs have been shown to be related to an increased risk of Alzheimer's (in NFL players) and increases the risk of the disease four times that of the general population [13]. Other NFL research has confirmed this general finding with results indicating, "retired players aged 30–49 receive a dementia-related diagnosis at a rate of 1.9 % or 20 times the rate of age-matched populations, while 6.1 % of players over the age of 50 receive a dementia-related diagnosis representing five times the national average of 1.2 % [14]. Thus, from any point of view TBI is a significant problem from a national health perspective as well as to the individual victim.

The Biological Effects of a TBI

There are a myriad of biological reactions to a TBI which underlie the electrophysiological effects, but the relation between biology and electrophysiology are not well understood at the present time.

The main biological mechanical effect of a TBI is diffuse axonal injury (DAI) [15]. Holbourn's focus was on non-brainstem effects which address the impact between the brain's surface and the skull, resulting in the shearing or tearing of the neurons. He conceptualized that shear injury is caused by rotational forces and not by linear or translational forces, which denote all of an object moving in a straight line in unison. Acceleration–deceleration forces can produce rotational movements. Two-thirds of DAI lesions (damaged tissue) occur at the gray-white matter junction (where the density differences are the greatest). The research in this area has supported the following: (1) magnitude and direction (vector) concepts: (2) "centripetal" force vector, where the pressure is highest at the outer cortex with a gradient to the subcortex and the brain stem [16]; (3) a rotational vector [15, 17]; and a (4) shear vector [18, 19]. Most TBI injuries affect the gray matter of the frontal and temporal lobes, which are independent of the direction of impact to the skull [20, 21] and reflect the effect of the brain impacting on the jagged sphenoid and ethmoid bones. The second non-brainstem effect involves a depressed skull bone which causes deformation. This effect has not received much attention in the literature. The third non brainstem effect is the percussion shock wave that moves from the impact point and makes contact with the opposite side of the skull in less than 200 ms. This shock wave can result in a "coup contra-coup" injury [20, 21].

A neurochemical cascade develops immediately following the biomechanical trauma to the brain and involves a multitude of cellular changes. The biomechanical effects are the stretching and tearing of the axons. Edema (fluid) and leakage occur in the axon as a result of the physical trauma. This effect is most intense during the first 2 weeks following injury. The resulting lesions (damage) involve small areas (0.04–0.60 in. diameter). The neuronal membranes are negatively affected. The axonal stretching leads to an increase in extracellular potassium, which is then followed by subsequent depolarization and then a release of excitatory neurotransmitters. This has been termed "neurotransmitter storm" [22]. This sequence includes a loss of ionic gradients, apoptosis (cell death), cell depolarization, cytotoxic edema (swelling of the cell elements), glutamate release, and many other biochemical effects. Due to these events the neuron breaks down, the axon splits into two sections, a retraction ball (collection of cytoplasm) is formed at the end of the axon, and Wallerian degeneration occurs which result in axonal collapse and resultant disconnection effects [23].

Non-brainstem Neuroanatomical Effects in TBI

When the brain moves enough to have an impact with the bone, a contusion (bruising) can occur. The bruising usually affects the superficial gray matter of the inferior, lateral, and anterior aspects of the frontal and temporal lobes. The occipital poles and the cerebellum are less involved. A subdural hemorrhage can occur when the movements of the brain are sufficient to tear the bridging veins on the surface, which bridge the brain surface to the dural venous sinus. These subdural hemorrhages are found in parietal and frontal locations. In the whiplash type injury, a sudden acceleration and no direct impact occurs (the brain's movement lags behind that of the skull). The forces affect the connections between the brain and the bridging veins and the brain tissue. The resultant ruptures of the bridging veins can result in axonal damage, subdural hematomas, and bleeding. When the skull stops moving, the brain is thrown against the skull and simultaneously pulls away from the posterior skull. Opposite the internal contact a contrecoup can result from the negative pressure which can possibly cause the formation of cavitation bubbles. The brain is then thrown backwards (deceleration) and a similar dynamic occurs. The reader is referred to Taber et al. [24] who presented figures representing nonpenetrating TBI injury locations for DAI, contusion, and subdural hemorrhages. The figures indicate that DAI affects the following locations: the gray matter—white matter (corticomedullary) junction (particularly frontal–temporal), deep gray matter, internal capsule, upper brainstem, and corpus callosum (CC).

Prognostic Issues for the TBI Patient

Initial studies on the long-term cognitive issues in the TBI patient have underestimated the effect of a TBI. Initially, it was thought that 50 % of MTBI cases experience recovery by 3 months post-injury, albeit incomplete in some cases [25]. Other research supports this general time frame in that post-concussive symptoms persisting between 3 and 6 months post injury occur in about 40 % of persons with mild TBI [26, 27] with 60 % showing no symptoms. However, more recent research [28] have documented information processing speed (Paced Visual Serial Addition Task) and working memory problems 1 year post-injury in a group of mTBI patients who were reporting post-concussion symptoms. The 6–12 months estimate has been challenged by Thornton and Carmody [29] who reported that long term effects have been documented in the protein S-100B serum. The serum S-100B is a peripheral biochemical marker of neural injury, including reactive gliosis, astrocytic death, and/or the blood–brain barrier dysfunction [30].

There have been associations found between MTBI and S-100B [31]. Neuropsychological deficits were evident in 74 % ($N = 36$) of MTBI cases (a 2-week testing point) and 67 % ($N = 29$) (a 6-month testing point). All of the patients were fully functional on the functional independence measure (FIM) in terms of activities of daily living. At the 6-month time period since the incident, the mild TBI (MTBI) group showed no signs of intracranial pathology or EEG abnormality (not QEEG data). The MTBI group did show significant neuropsychological deficits in the individuals with raised S-100B serum concentrations (about 50 % of sample of 79 patients) at the 6-month time since accident period. Patients with increased S-100B levels showed a twofold increase in severity of dizziness, memory problems, and headaches. The patients with normal S-100B levels 6 h after the injury and who did not report dizziness, nausea, or headaches were fully recovered at the 6-month time period. Thus, employing the S-100b level would indicate that about 50 % of the MTBI patients were still experiencing problems 6 months following the accident.

While it is no doubt the case that many mild TBI do not suffer long-term consequences, either because the initial injury was very mild or the brain effectively compensated, the initial picture being presented in the literature regarding no or minimal long-term effects is clearly in error.

Spontaneous Cure Myth vs. Compensation

Thornton [32] noted that the QEEG spectral correlation coefficient (SCC) deficits in the TBI population did not improve with greater time since the accident, resulting in the hypothesis that "time does not heal" the underlying physical damage to the brain. There was a significant positive correlation between the Shipley verbal IQ measure (eyes closed) and time since accident (+0.32) indicating some resolution over time of verbal abilities. The Thatcher et al. [33] article reported a similar finding in that the relations between T2 relaxation times and EEG amplitudes of the delta (0.5–3.5 Hz—positive relations) and alpha and beta (7–22 Hz—negative relations) were not affected by the time period since accident (eyes closed data). Additionally, longer reaction times were exhibited by symptomatic TBI athletes compared to asymptomatic athletes [34]. This effect was not influenced by the length of time since injury. Rutgers et al. [35], reported no significant relations between the time interval after injury and the DTI fiber tracking findings in TBI patients. Another study reported improvement in neuropsychological functioning with significantly greater gray and white matter change (2 vs. 12.7 months post-accident) in the TBI group compared to the control group [36]. If the brain hasn't spontaneously "cured" itself over time, then the appropriate interpretation of neuro-psychological improvements is that the brain has compensated for the deficits with a different response pattern. This was shown in the Thornton [37] article which showed a shift to the right hemisphere temporal lobe and higher frequencies to accomplish an auditory memory task.

In conclusion, the TBI patient experiences a 56 % probability that they will not be diagnosed in the ED, 50 % probability (if mTBI) that they still be experiencing cognitive issues 6 months following the accident, 53 % chance that they will not report the concussion symptoms if they occurred in a high school athletic event, and a 50 % chance that they will experience cognitive deficits and decreased DLPFC activation levels due to the accumulation of sub-concussive events, and increased risk of Alzheimer's. Thus, an accurate and immediate diagnostic method would appear to be very desirable with this problem.

Diagnostic Issues

Electrophysiological Effects

The electrophysiological effects of a TBI have been particularly informative. Lew et al. [38] reported on the differences between 11 TBI and 11 control participants. The results showed that the TBI patients (1) had significantly lower P300 amplitude in both auditory (11.2 vs. 22.7 μV) and visual (11.6 vs. 20.9 μV) domains, (2) had significantly longer P300 latency in both auditory (355 vs. 294 ms) and visual

(376 vs. 341 ms) modalities, and (3) although there was no significant difference in response accuracy between the two groups (97.7 % vs. 100 %), the reaction time for both auditory and visual tasks were significantly longer in TBI patients (auditory, 404 vs. 277 ms; visual, 397 vs. 346 ms). The P300 is an event-related potential (ERP) which occurs in the process of stimulus evaluation and categorization. There have been numerous research studies in the ERP and TBI area.

Leon-Carrion et al. [39] employed the QEEG to differentiate TBI ($N=81$) and cerebral vascular accident (CVA) ($N=41$) patients. They employed the FIM and the functional assessment measure (FAM) scales to group the participants according to their functional levels. The FIM and FAM scales are composed of 30 items (such as grooming, swallowing, memory, etc.) which are rated on an ordinal scale by evaluators and has been used to evaluate outcomes in rehabilitation settings. The QEEG discriminant showed an accuracy rate of 100 %, in discriminating low and high FIM and FAM scores, in the training set and a 75 % cross validation sample. The QEEG coherence measures were the most dominant measure employed by the discriminant.

There have been multiple studies addressing the use of the QEEG and discriminant analysis to differentiate the TBI patient from a normal population, with most of the results ranging between 82 and 100 % specificity [40–42]. There have been some confirmatory findings across research. However, methodological problems and differing TBI severity levels have contributed to the lack of consistency of results. Thatcher et al. [40] conducted the original discriminant analysis with 608 MTBI adult patients and 108 age-matched controls and obtained an accuracy rate of 90 %. Moderate to severe cases were not included in the analysis. The discriminating QEEG measures included, in the TBI patient, increased frontal theta coherence (Fp1-F3), decreased frontal beta (13–22 Hz) phase (Fp2-F4, F3-F4), increased coherence beta (T3-T5, C3-P3), and reduced posterior relative power alpha (P3, P4, T5, T6, O1, O2, T4). Three independent cross validations resulted in accuracy rates of 84, 93, and 90 %.

Thornton [32] focused on the damage to the Spectral Coherence Correlation Coefficients (SCC—based upon the Lexicor algorithms) and phase values in the beta2 (32–64 Hz) range when comparing the patients with TBI to the normal group during eyes closed condition and different cognitive activation tasks. The SCC algorithms employed in the Thornton studies were not the same as employed in the Barr et al. [42] study or Thatcher et al. [40] study. There are several hardware and software mathematical definitions of the coherence and phase concepts, which involve the similarity of the wave forms between different locations within a frequency range and within a time range. The Thornton results are opposite those of Thatcher et al. [40] study where higher (than normal) microvolt values of delta were found in the TBI group and related to white matter damage and lower values of beta microvolts related to gray matter damage. However, the correlation between microvolts and relative power values of a frequency range between 0.21 and 0.75 [32] and were nonsignificant in the delta frequency in the eyes closed condition and 0.53 for the beta1 frequency (13–32 Hz). Thatcher examined microvolts while Thornton examined the relative power values.

More recently, Zhou et al. [43] investigated the default-mode network (DMN) soon after a mTBI incident and correlated the DMN connectivity changes with neurocognitive measures and clinical symptoms. The TBI subject showed reduced connectivity in the posterior cingulate cortex and parietal regions and increased frontal connectivity around the medial prefrontal cortex in the MTBI group. These fronto-posterior opposing changes within the DMN were significantly correlated ($r=-0.44$, $P=0.03$). The reduced posterior connectivity correlated positively with neurocognitive dysfunction (e.g., cognitive flexibility), while the increased frontal connectivity correlated negatively with posttraumatic symptoms (i.e., depression, anxiety, fatigue, and post-concussion syndrome).

Although these reports present some overlapping patterns, there are several problems with some of the research in this area, which include: (1) use of a low frequency range (32 Hz and below); (2) use of eyes closed data; (3) lack of activation procedures; (4) empirically understanding exactly what QEEG variables relate directly to the poor cognitive performance of a TBI patient; (5) differences in coherence algorithms; and (6) differences in the severity of TBI which could be contributing to the different effects. Overall, the articles generally report increased levels of the lower frequency (delta, theta), decreased beta levels and connectivity issues.

The Multiple Cognitive Discriminant Approach

To address the problems raised in the preceding analysis, the author reanalyzed the data he has collected during the past 15 years with a different discriminant method. Rather than employ a single discriminant, the author decided to combine the different discriminant results across the different cognitive tasks.

Participants

The participants were 93 MTBI individuals and 50 normal subjects. The MTBI participants had obtained their head injury during auto accidents, sports events, slips and falls, or assaults. Neuropsychological evaluation and description of the event provided the basis of the diagnosis. Glasgow Coma Scale value was frequently unavailable and GCS was a screening instrument for triage purposes, thus unacceptable for diagnostic confirmation. The age range was between 15.08 and 72.42 years. The mean age was 41 for the mTBI group and 37.9 for the normal group. There were 53 males and 40 females in the EC TBI sample. The time between the date of the head injury and evaluation ranged from 12 days to 30 years. None of the patients were involved in long-term care facilities, thus ruling out a severe TBI, resulting in the major classification as being in the mild to moderate range.

EEG Recording

The brain activity was recorded using a 19-channel QEEG hardware device (Lexicor Medical Technology, Inc.). Bandpass filters were set between 0.0 and 64 Hz (3 dB points). The signals that passed were analyzed with a fast Fourier transform (FFT), which uses cosine-tapered windows and provides spectral magnitude in microvolts as a function of frequency. The sampling rate was set to 256 to allow for examination up to 64 Hz. An Electro-Cap was fitted to the participant. The electrodes were positioned at 19 scalp locations according to the standard 10–20 system [44] with ear-linked references. Impedances were maintained below 10 KΩ at all locations. Gain was set to 32,000 and the high pass filter was set to off. Only the six indicated frontal locations were examined. The algorithms available through the software provided by Lexicor Medical Inc. provided the numeric values of the QEEG variables. The data were examined for artifact (eye movements and EMG activity) as well as other possible sources of contamination. The bandwidths were grouped according to the following divisions: Delta: 0.00–4 Hz, Theta: 4–8 Hz, Alpha: 8–13 Hz, Beta1: 13–32 Hz, Beta2: 32–64 Hz.

Measures

Relative power. The microvolts of the particular band divided by the total microvolts generated by all bands at a location, averaged over the epoch time period. This measure is insensitive to the skull thickness as it measures the total microvolts at a location and determines the percentage of the total microvolts that are within a particular frequency range.

Spectral correlation coefficient. The average amplitude similarity between the waveforms of a particular band in two locations over an epoch. This variable is defined within a particular frequency range.

Phase. The time lag between two locations (A and B), in the 10–20 system, of a particular band as defined by how soon after the beginning of an epoch a particular waveform at location A is matched in amplitude at location B. The measurement time period for this variable is considerably less than for the SCC variable and can occur over a period of milliseconds.

Tasks

The cognitive tasks employed were part of the standard cognitive activation QEEG evaluation. The first task employed was a standard EC condition (300 s). Due to the high misclassification rate in the data, this task was not employed in the subsequent analyses.

Table 20.1 Individual misclassifications across tasks

AA data case #	MC as TBI	MC as N	VA data case #	MC as TBI	MC as N	L data case #	MC as TBI	MC as N	RS data case #	MC as TBI	MC as N
1		X	8	X		16		X	24		X
2		X	9	X		17		X	25		X
3		X	10	X		18		X	26	X	
4		X	11	X		19		X	27	X	
5		X	12	X		20		X	28	X	
6		X	13	X		21	X		29	X	
7	X		14	X		22	X		30	X	
			15	X		23	X				
	1	6		6	2		3	5		5	2
TBI-84[a]			TBI-91[a]			TBI-88[a]			TBI-76[a]		
N-57[a]			N-45[a]			N-55[a]			N-43[a]		

MC misclassified, *TBI* traumatic brain injured, *N* normal, *AA* auditory attention data, *VA* visual attention data, *L* listen to paragraphs, *RS* reading silently
[a]Sample size number in the groups

In the second task (auditory attention—AA) the participants were asked (while their eyes were closed) to raise their right index finger whenever they heard the sound of a pen tapping on the table (200 s). In the third task (visual attention—VA) the subjects were asked to raise their right index finger whenever a laser light was shown on the back of a laminated sheet of upside Spanish text (200 s—eyes open). In the fourth task (L-listening) the subjects listened to four stories (approximately 40–50 s in length—with their eyes closed) and were then asked to silently recall the story to themselves (eyes closed). In the fifth task (reading—RS) the participants were asked to read a story for 100 s that was presented on a laminated sheet and then recall the story to themselves (eyes closed). The total time required to collect this data was 11.6 min. These variables focused on six frontal locations with five of the seven involving SCC and phase relations.

Results

Table 20.1 presents the analysis which combines the different discriminant analysis to determine if the employment of the different activation approaches can improve the accuracy of the decision. The individual subjects are indicated by numbers. As the table indicates the subjects who were misclassified (as either normal or TBI patient) in the AA data were not subsequently misclassified in the VA, L, or RS conditions. Similarly, the subjects misclassified with the VA (visual attention) task were not misclassified in the subsequent listen (L) or RS tasks. No subject was misclassified twice across the four tasks.

There was a range of 119–143 subjects involved in the different conditions. If the decision regarding a TBI or normal requires that the classification (normal or TBI

Table 20.2 Individual SCC analysis of TBI vs. normal discriminant analysis across four different activation conditions

AA data case #	MC as TBI	MC as N	VA data case #	MC as TBI	MC as N	Listen data case #	MC as TBI	MC as N	RS data case #	MC as TBI	MC as N
1 R		X	**38**		X	44		X	55		X
31		X	39		X	45		X	**56**		X
2 R		X	**8 R**		X	16 R		X			
8 R		X	40		X	17 R		X			
32		X	41		X	46		X			
6 R		X	9 R		X	18 R		X			
33 R		X	**42**		X	47		X			
						20 R		X			
						48		X			
34	X		**10 R**	X		49	X		**28 R**	X	
28 R	X		43	X		50	X		57	X	
10 R	X		21 R	X		7 R	X		**58**	X	
11 R	X		**11 R**	X		51	X		59	X	
35	X		21 R	X		52	X		**60**	X	
36	X		**22 R**	X		53	X				
37	X		12 R	X		23 R	X				
15 R	X		13 R	X		**54**	X				
			14 R	X							
Total misclassifications	8	7		9	7		8	9		5	2
TBI-89[a]			TBI-89[a]			TBI-89[a]			TBI-73[a]		
Normal-52[a]			N-48[a]			N-54[a]			N-48[a]		

R—indicates that the subject had also been misclassified elsewhere
Cases in bold indicate misclassifications across different conditions
MC misclassified, *TBI* traumatic brain injured, *N* normal, *AA* auditory attention data, *VA* visual attention data, *Listen* listening to stories, *RS* reading silently
[a]Sample size number in the group

patient) be obtained in two of the three tasks, then the combined discriminant does not make any misclassifications. This result indicates a correct TBI and normal hit rate of 100 %, thus no false positives and no false negatives. This approach was developed on individuals who had experienced a TBI some 12 days to 30 years prior to the evaluation and is thus useful in determining if someone had a TBI within this time frame.

The second discriminant function method undertaken was to discern if the SCC data by itself is sufficient to result in 100 % accuracy. The data presently available to the author was examined with this problem in mind. The following summary Table 20.2 presents the results for the discriminant function analysis employing only the frontal SCC and phase values employed in the previously presented analysis. The EC data showed the highest error rates with 21 misclassifications and thus was not included in this analysis.

The critical question, however, is whether the combination of the SCC discriminants will result in 100 % accuracy. Table 20.2 presents the individual subject results of the cross activation task discriminant results, similar to Table 20.1. The case identification information is presented as numbers. The R label indicates that the subject had also been misclassified in Table 20.1. The bolded letters indicate that individual subjects were misclassified in two to three conditions (six in two conditions, one in three conditions) of the four employed. As the table indicates with the bolded letters, this problem occurred in eight subjects (of 143). There was no instance of consistent misclassifications in four of the four conditions. If diagnostic agreement across four conditions is set as the criterion, then the approach is 100 % accurate. The time required for the employed tasks was 700 s or 11.6 min.

QEEG and Rehabilitation

Thornton and Carmody [45] analyzed the effect sizes of different intervention models (computer, strategies, medications, QEEG biofeedback) on the cognitive problems in the TBI patient. The authors examined both the control group (CG) and pre–post comparison (PP) research. For auditory memory, the strategy approach (CG) showed a standard deviation (SD) improvement of 0.32 while the PP comparison showed a 0.21 SD improvement, neither of which was significant. Computer interventions showed a 0.44 SD (CG) effect size and medications showed (PP) a 0.52 SD effect size. The activation database-guided EEG biofeedback approach obtained a 2.61 SD improvement in auditory memory. The only intervention which was significant, employing confidence intervals, sample sizes, and effect size in the calculation was the activation database-guided EEG biofeedback approach.

Since that report Lundqvist et al. [46] reported on the use of computer interventions which results in significant improvement on working memory tasks at 4 and 20 weeks after training compared to baseline. The average effect size on the five measures employed (PASAT, Picture Span, Block Span, and a modified Stroop test) was 0.75 SD at 20 weeks. The subject pool of 21 patients had only one TBI patient in the sample.

Additionally, Rohling et al. [47] reviewed the two Cicerone's summaries of research on cognitive rehabilitation. Their analysis indicated a small treatment effect size (ES = 0.30) due to cognitive rehabilitation. They did report a larger treatment effect (ES = 0.71) for a single-group pretest to posttest outcomes. However, the no treatment control group demonstrated an ES of 0.41. Correcting for this effect resulted in a small, significant, overall estimate. Their conclusion was that the meta-analysis revealed sufficient evidence for the effectiveness of attention training after TBI and of language and visuospatial training for aphasia and neglect syndromes after stroke.

Maas et al. [48] reported, "Research in basic science has disclosed that multiple mechanisms are involved in the pathophysiology of TBI. This has led to the development of many neuroprotective agents with promising potential, but none have yielded benefits in clinical testing" [48, p. 2]. They also noted, "Recent findings

Table 20.3 TBI memory changes as a result of treatment

	Initial scores (SD)	Reevaluation (SD)	Effect size	% Change	Comparison to control group (SD/%)
Auditory (N = 14)	11.7 (7.7)	24 (5.8)	1.75	105	1.52 (53 %)
Reading (N = 13)	2.23 (1.38)	5.41 (1.9)	1.85	143	1.06 (50 %)

from the IMPACT studies have shown that the risk of poor outcomes could differ between centers, and is up to three times higher than would be expected by chance after adjustment for baseline prognostic risk [49]. The Institute of Medicine report to the Department of Defense on the effectiveness of cognitive rehabilitation therapy (CRT) concluded that there was "limited support for the efficacy of CRT interventions" [50, p. 2]. In conclusion, the research to date is not as encouraging as desired for efficacy statements regarding CRT.

The author recently analyzed his clinical files from the last 5 years to add to the analysis. Several groups (normal, learning disability, TBI) were examined. Table 20.3 presents the cognitive changes for the TBI patient as a result of the interventions. The initial scores were obtained from the original evaluation. For the auditory memory, the four stories of the original evaluation were averaged and, generally, the last two stories during the reevaluation were employed for the reevaluation results. The comparison to the control group values column represents the group's values greater (SD/%) than the control group.

Combining the TBI subjects available from previous research (45) results in an overall TBI sample size of 36. A weighted average of the auditory memory improvements across these three studies indicated an average SD improvement of 2.31.

Other Reported Relations Between QEEG Measures and Rehabilitation Outcomes

A new area of research focusing on the changes on QEEG measures as a result of rehabilitation attempts has begun to appear, with interesting but non-definitive results to date. Leon-Carrion et al. [51] reported on the relation between recovery at 6 months and delta–alpha ratios (eyes closed data). A higher delta–alpha initial value was associated with poorer recovery. Stathopoulou and Lubar [52] reported that the most systemic change on the EEG data (eyes closed, eyes open conditions) in the TBI patients following 22 sessions of a cognitive rehabilitation program (Captain's Log) was a decrease in alpha, contrary to the expectation of decreased delta, theta, and alpha (microvolts and relative power) and increases in beta. Vespa et al. [53] examined the daily percent alpha variability (PAV) variable on continuous EEG monitoring with moderate to severe TBI (GCS scores 2–12) 0–10 days after injury. The lower the alpha variability, the poorer was the clinical outcome. In patients with a GCS score of 8 or lower, a PAV value of 0.1 or lower was highly predictive of a poor outcome or death.

The Coordinated Allocation of Resource
Model of Brain Functioning

The treatment protocols employed the coordinated allocation of resource (CAR) model of brain functioning [54]. The model states that specific cognitive functions are a function of different, albeit overlapping in some situations, electrophysiological resources. Thus, a cognitive skill, such as auditory memory, requires high SCC alpha values in the left hemisphere [55] in the normal adult, while reading memory is dependent upon the F7 SCC beta1 and beta2 and T5 SCC alpha flashlights. The flashlight metaphor states that each location in the 10–20 system sends out a signal to all other locations (within a specific frequency) [55]. The metaphor is employed due to a need to reduce the number of variables being examined as well as based upon support in the literature for the concept of cortical/subcortical generators [56]. Normative values were obtained for the individual relations within a frequency and between locations. The rehabilitation model is to conduct an activation cognitive QEEG evaluation which involves ten tasks. The evaluation is a mini-neuropsychological evaluation which reports on the subject's critical (and all values) QEEG values during the task. The subject's QEEG values are compared to the QEEG values in the normative database on the critical variables which have been shown to be relevant to effective cognition (as well as all variables). The deficient values become the focus on the interventions. The treatment seeks to raise the subject's values to above the normal values. While the model provides a good structure to the interventions, other factors can influence the treatment protocol decisions. These factors could involve excessive theta or delta activity as well as decreased SCC beta2 values which are not involved as predictive variables in the normative sample but which are contributing to the subject's problems. It is a systems model which strives to improve the overall system while addressing specific problems on specific cognitive tasks.

Conclusion

TBI has presented a difficult problem in diagnosis with presently available medical diagnostic technologies. This chapter presents a methodology which offers a significant advance in the diagnostic problem of the TBI and has obtained a 100 % accuracy in the diagnostic problem. The field of cognitive rehabilitation has not realized what was the implicit original goal of the intervention methodology—a complete remediation of the cognitive problems in TBI patients. An alternative approach (CAR directed EEG biofeedback approach) may be a viable alternative in this situation.

References

1. Hagen B. Attorney at law. NFL concussions in 2010. http://www.hagen-law.com/nfl-concussion-statistics/. Accessed 6 Jan 2013.
2. Hagen B. Attorney at law. NFL concussions in 2011. http://www.hagen-law.com/nfl-concussion-statistics/. Accessed 6 Jan 2013.
3. USA Today Sports. Concussion policies by league. 2012. http://www.usatoday.com/story/sports/2012/10/11/concussions-nascar-nfl-mlb-nhl-nba/1628129/. Accessed 6 Jan 2013.
4. NCAA Football Teams. By Howie Long and John Czarnecki from football for dummies. 4th US ed. http://www.dummies.com/how-to/content/ncaa-football-teams.html. Accessed 6 Jan 2013.
5. Miller JR. Football continues to dominate high school sports despite concussion risk. 2012. http://www.foxnews.com/sports/2012/09/08/football-continues-to-dominate-high-school-sports-despite-concussion-risk/#ixzz2f3otab70. Accessed 6 Jan 2013.
6. McCrea M, Hammeke T, Olsen G, Leo P, Guskiewicz K. Unreported concussion in high school football players: implications for prevention. Clin J Sport Med. 2004;14(1):13–7.
7. Talavage TM, Nauman E, Breedlove EL, et al. Functionally-detected cognitive impairment in high school football players without clinically-diagnosed concussion. J Neurotrauma. 2010;765:1–46. doi:10.1089/neu.2010.1512.
8. Langlois JA, Rutland-Brown W, Wald MM. The epidemiology and impact of traumatic brain injury: a brief overview. J Head Trauma Rehabil. 2006;21(5):375–8.
9. Asken MJ, Schwartz RC. Heading the ball in soccer: what's the risk of brain injury? Phys Sportsmed. 1998;26(11):11.
10. Brewer TL, Metzger BL, Therrien B. Trajectories of cognitive recovery following a minor brain injury. Res Nurs Health. 2002;25:269–81.
11. Powell JM, Ferraro JV, Dikmen SS, Temkin NR, Bell KR. Accuracy of mild traumatic brain injury diagnosis. Arch Phys Med Rehabil. 2008;89(8):1550–5.
12. Injury Prevention & Control: Traumatic Brain Injury. http://www.cdc.gov/traumaticbraininjury/statistics.html. Accessed 6 Jan 2013.
13. Burleigh N. Would football without concussions still be football? 2012. http://observer.com/2012/11/would-football-without-concussions-still-be-football/. Accessed 6 Jan 2013.
14. Amen D. J Neuropsychiatry Clin Neurosci. 2011. http://www.dignityafterfootball.org/Families.htm. Accessed 6 Jan 2013.
15. Holbourn AHS. The mechanics of head injuries. Lancet. 1943;2:438–41.
16. Ommaya AK, Goldsmith W, Thibault L. Biomechanics and neuropathology of adult and paediatric head injury. Br J Neurosurg. 2002;16(3):220–42.
17. Holbourn AHS. The mechanics of brain injuries. Br Med Bull. 1945;622:147–9.
18. Advani SH, Ommaya AK, Yang WJ. Head injury mechanisms, characteristics and clinical evaluation. In: Chista D, editor. Human body dynamics. Oxford: Clarendon; 1982. p. 3–37.
19. Ommaya AK, Thibault LE, Bandak FA. Mechanisms of impact head injury. Int J Impact Eng. 1994;15(4):535–60.
20. Ommaya AK. Head injury mechanisms and the concept of preventive management: a review and critical synthesis. J Neurotrauma. 1995;12(4):527–46.
21. Sano K, Nakamura N, Hirakaws K. Mechanism of and dynamics of closed head injuries. Neurol Med Chir. 1967;9:21–3.
22. Mendez DR, Corbett R, Macias C, Laptook A. Total and ionized plasma magnesium concentrations in children after traumatic brain injury. Pediatr Res. 2005;57(3):347–52.
23. Povlishock JT, Katz DI. Update of neuropathology and neurological recovery after traumatic brain injury. J Head Trauma Rehabil. 2005;20(1):76–94.
24. Taber KH, Warden DL, Hurley RA. Blast-related traumatic brain injury: what is known? J Neuropsychiatry Clin Neurosci. 2006;18(2):141–5.
25. Dikmen S, McLean Jr A, Temkin NR, Wyler AR. Neuropsychologic outcome at one-month postinjury. Arch Phys Med Rehabil. 1986;67(8):507–613.

26. Ingebrigtsen T, Waterloo K, Marup-Jensen S, Attner E, Romner B. Quantification of post-concussion symptoms 3 months after minor head injury in 100 consecutive patients. J Neurol. 1998;245(9):609–12.

27. McCullagh S, Oucherlony D, Protzner A, Blair N, Feinstein A. Prediction of neuropsychiatric outcome following mild trauma brain injury: an examination of the Glasgow Coma Scale. Brain Inj. 2001;15(6):489–97.

28. Dean PJA, Sterr A. Long-term effects of mild traumatic brain injury on cognitive performance. Front Hum Neurosci. 2013;7:30.

29. Thornton K, Carmody D. Traumatic brain injury and the role of the quantitative EEG in the assessment and remediation of cognitive sequelae. In: Carlstedt RA, editor. Integrative clinical psychology, psychiatry and behavioral medicine: perspectives, practices and research. New York, NY: Springer; 2009. p. 463–508.

30. Wong CH, Rooney SJ, Bonser RS. S-100beta release in hypothermic circulatory arrest and coronary artery surgery. Ann Thorac Surg. 1999;67(6):1911–4.

31. De Kruijk JR, Leffers P, Menheere PP, Meerhoff S, Rutten J, Twijnstra A. Prediction of post-traumatic complaints after mild traumatic brain injury: early symptoms and biochemical markers. J Neurol Neurosurg Psychiatry. 2002;73(6):727–32.

32. Thornton K. Exploratory analysis: mild head injury, discriminant analysis with high frequency bands (32–64 Hz) under attentional activation conditions & does time heal? J Neurother. 2002;3(3/4):1–10.

33. Thatcher RW, Biver C, McAlaster R, Salazar A. Biophysical linkage between MRI and EEG coherence in closed head injury. Neuroimage. 1998;8(4):307–26.

34. Lavoie ME, Dupuis F, Johnston KM, Leclerc S, Lassonde M. Visual p300 effects beyond symptoms in concussed college athletes. J Clin Exp Neuropsychol. 2004;26(1):55–73.

35. Rutgers DR, Toulgoat F, Cazejust J, Fillard P, Lasjaunias P, Ducreux D. White matter abnormalities in mild traumatic brain injury: a diffusion tensor imaging study. Am J Neuroradiol. 2008;29(3):514–9.

36. Bendlin BB, Ries ML, Lazar M, et al. Longitudinal changes in patients with traumatic brain injury assessed with diffusion-tensor and volumetric imaging. Neuroimage. 2008;2(2):503–14.

37. Thornton K. Electrophysiology of the reasons the brain damaged subject can't recall what they hear. Arch Clin Neuropsychol. 2003;17:1–17.

38. Lew HL, Lee EH, Pan SS, Elaine S. Electrophysiologic abnormalities of auditory and visual information processing in patients with traumatic brain injury. Am J Phys Med Rehabil. 2004;83(6):428–33.

39. Leon-Carrion J, Martin-Rodriguez JF, Damas-Lopez J, Martin JM, Dominguez-Morales Mdel R. A QEEG index of level of functional dependence for people sustaining acquired brain injury: the Seville Independence Index (SINDI). Brain Inj. 2008;22(1):61–74.

40. Thatcher RW, Walker RA, Gerson I, Geisler FH. EEG discriminant analyses of mild head trauma. Electroencephalogr Clin Neurophysiol. 1998;73(2):94–106.

41. Hughes JR, John ER. Conventional and quantitative electroencephalography in psychiatry. J Neuropsychiatry Clin Neurosci. 1999;11(2):190–208.

42. Barr WB, Prichep LS, Chabot R, Powell MR, McCrea M. Measuring brain electrical activity to track recovery from sport-related concussion. Brain Inj. 2012;26(1):58–66.

43. Zhou Y, Milham MP, Lui YW, et al. Default-mode network disruption in mild traumatic brain injury. Radiology. 2012;265:882–92.

44. Jasper HH. Report of the committee on methods of clinical examination in electroencephalography. Electroencephalogr Clin Neurophysiol. 1958;10:370–1.

45. Thornton K, Carmody D. Efficacy of traumatic brain injury rehabilitation: interventions of QEEG-guided biofeedback, computers, strategies, and medications. Appl Psychophysiol Biofeedback. 2008;33(2):101–24.

46. Lundqvist A, Grundström K, Samuelsson K, Rönnberg J. Computerized training of working memory in a group of patients suffering from acquired brain injury. Brain Inj. 2010;24(10):1173–83.

47. Rohling ML, Faust ME, Beverly B, Demakis G. Effectiveness of cognitive rehabilitation following acquired brain injury: a meta-analytic re-examination of Cicerone et al.'s (2000, 2005) systematic reviews. Neuropsychology. 2009;23(1):20–39.
48. Maas AIR, Menon DK, Lingsma HF, Pineda JAM, Sandel E, Manley GT. Re-orientation of clinical research in traumatic brain injury: report of an international workshop on comparative effectiveness research. J Neurotrauma. 2012;29:32–46.
49. Lingsma HF, Roozenbeek B, Li B, Marmarou A, Murray GD, Maas AI, Steyerberg EW. Large between center differences in outcome after moderate and severe traumatic brain injury in the IMPACT study. Neurosurgery. 2011;68:601–7.
50. Shoulson I, et al. Cognitive rehabilitation therapy for traumatic brain injury. Evaluating the evidence. Institute of Medicine of the National Academies. 2011. http://www.iom.edu/CRTforTBI
51. Leon-Carrion J, Martin-Rodriguez JF, Damas-Lopez J, Barroso y Martin JM, Dominguez-Morales MR. Delta-alpha ratio correlates with level of recovery after neurorehabilitation in patients with acquired brain injury. Clin Neurophysiol. 2009;120(6):1039–45.
52. Stathopoulou S, Lubar JF. EEG changes in traumatic brain injured patients after cognitive rehabilitation. J Neurother. 2004;2:21–51.
53. Vespa PM, Boscardin WJ, Hovda DA, et al. Early and persistent impaired percent alpha variability on continuous electroencephalography monitoring as predictive of poor outcome after traumatic brain injury. J Neurosurg. 2002;97(1):84–92.
54. Thornton K, Carmody D. Eyes-closed and activation QEEG databases in predicting cognitive effectiveness and the inefficiency hypothesis. J Neurother. 2009;13(1):1–22.
55. Thornton K. NCLB goals (and more) are attainable with neurocognitive interventions, vol. 1. Charleston, SC: BookSurge Press; 2006.
56. Schreckenberger M, Lange-Asschenfeldt C, Lochmann M, et al. The thalamus as the generator and modulator of EEG alpha rhythm: a combined PET/EEG study with lorazepam challenge in humans. Neuroimage. 2004;22(2):637–44.

Chapter 21
Current Understanding of Concussion: Treatment Perspectives

Michael R. Gay and Scott L. Rosenthal

Abstract Concussion or mild traumatic brain injury (mTBI) represents a significant portion of sport-related traumatic brain injury. Much research in the past decade has provided the medical community with an increased knowledge base focused on the biological pathophysiology surrounding trauma to the brain. Given this increased knowledge however current clinical standards of care remain unchanged. As a result many groups studying mTBI have called for increased research in the area of treatment for concussion or mTBI. Treatment strategies in mTBI have been researched across many disciplines of brain science. Treatments can be characterized by their pharmaceutical, nutriceutical, and psychological approach to therapeutic intervention. Each intervention should be examined for the treatment it provides and how it relates to structural and functional healing concepts in the acute, subacute, and chronic stages of healing. Using this knowledge, clinicians should be able to determine how these interventions may benefit the individual recovering from concussion. In addition, it may provide a platform for making critical "Return to Play" activity recommendations so the athlete can return safely to sports participation. The purpose of this chapter on treatment perspectives in the field of sports-related concussion is to provide clinicians and researchers with a summary of interventions across disciplines.

M.R. Gay, Ph.D., A.T.C. (✉)
Penn State Center for Sports Concussion Research and Services, University Park, PA, USA

Pennsylvania State Intercollegiate Athletics, Pennsylvania State University,
19 Recreation Hall, University Park, PA 16802, USA
e-mail: mrg201@psu.edu

S.L. Rosenthal, B.S.
Department of Kinesiology, Pennsylvania State University,
201 Old Main, University Park, PA 16802, USA
e-mail: slr5284@psu.edu

S.M. Slobounov and W.J. Sebastianelli (eds.), *Concussions in Athletics:*
From Brain to Behavior, DOI 10.1007/978-1-4939-0295-8_21,
© Springer Science+Business Media New York 2014

Keywords Concussion • Mild traumatic brain injury • Post-concussion syndrome • Treatment • Therapy • Neuroinflammation • Metabolic dysregulation • Antioxidants

Introduction

Sports-related concussion or mild traumatic brain injury (mTBI) is a growing public health concern with increased attention being focused on treatment and management strategies aimed at reducing the impact on patients and athletes. The complexities of the pathophysiologic sequelae in the brain combined with the clinical manifestation of behavioral signs and symptoms are what can make the treatment of concussion challenging. Combine the difficulties in diagnosing and treating an athlete with concussion with the pressure surrounding an athletic sports culture and you create a potentially dangerous environment for the concussed athlete.

Research in mTBI has increased significantly within the past decade and has furthered our understanding of the complexities involved. Awareness, education, and attention have come on the heels of injuries to high profile athletes on professional sports teams like those in the NFL or NHL which are constantly in the media spotlight. In addition, there are alarming numbers of military personnel returning from multiple battle fronts overseas that have suffered traumatic brain injury (TBI) and are in need of treatment. With some researchers reporting 1.6–3.8 million concussions occurring in sports each year [1], mTBI accounts for 80 % of all reported TBIs [2]. Recent research into high school sports injury rates has revealed an alarming increase in the number of diagnosed concussions each year [3]. This staggering increase in the number of reported concussions has focused the research community's efforts into further understanding the pathophysiological response to injury as well as short- and long-term clinical manifestations. These investigations develop a platform by which we understand the injury and then develop strategies to treat individuals and athletes with concussion to improve their quality of life.

Definition of Concussion

Reviewing the literature surrounding the treatment for concussion or mTBI requires that we examine the definition and events surrounding concussive injury. There is disparity among researchers on the issue of a unified definition of the term "concussion." The current accepted definition of concussion was re-tasked by the Concussion in Sport Group (CISG) during the first International Conference on Concussion in Sport in Vienna 2001 and has remained unchanged in subsequent examinations by the CISG. This group comprised researchers and clinicians from the fields of neuropsychology, sports medical physicians, neurologists, and neurosurgeons among other allied health professionals. These experts were highly involved in research as well as with the diagnosis, treatment, and management of sports-related concussion in patients. The CISG definition is as follows [4].

"Concussion is defined as a complex pathophysiological process affecting the brain, induced by traumatic biomechanical forces. Several common features that incorporate clinical, pathological, and biomechanical injury constructs that may be used in defining the nature of a concussive head injury include:

1. Concussion may be caused by a direct blow to the head, face, neck, or elsewhere on the body with an 'impulsive' force transmitted to the head.
2. Concussion typically results in the rapid onset of short lived impairment of neurological function that resolves spontaneously.
3. Concussion may result in neuropathological changes but the acute clinical symptoms largely reflect a functional disturbance rather than structural injury.
4. Concussion results in a graded set of clinical syndromes that may or may not involve loss of consciousness. Resolution of the clinical and cognitive symptoms typically follows a sequential course.
5. Concussion is typically associated with grossly normal structural neuroimaging studies."

Although some medical experts and researchers vary in their approach to the term, in the research literature and in clinical terminology concussion is often considered to be interchangeable with mTBI. In contrast to the CISG-based definition of concussion in 1993 the American Congress of Rehabilitative Medicine defined mTBI as a traumatically induced physiological disruption of brain function, as manifested by focal neurologic deficit(s) that may or may not be transient [5]. This contrasting definition is inclusive in that mTBI involves some level of both functional and structural disruption to normal brain tissue that may or may not be permanent. The scope of this debate is beyond the intention of this chapter but considering the lack of a true clinical- or research-based distinction between concussion and mTBI, the terms will be used interchangeably throughout the text of this chapter.

Definition of Post-concussion Syndrome

Patients that suffer from concussion experience a variety of symptoms caused by minor damage and transient neurologic dysfunction at the cellular level in the brain. A majority of these individuals experience a clinical recovery from symptoms within 7–10 days post-injury. Approximately 10 % of mTBI patients experience symptoms lasting longer than 3 months [6]. At this point a diagnosis of post-concussion syndrome (PCS) based on clinical symptoms can be made. PCS is defined by the fifth edition of the *Diagnostic and Statistics Manual* (*DSM-IV*) as (1) cognitive deficits in attention or memory and (2) at least three or more of the following symptoms: fatigue, sleep disturbance, headache, dizziness, irritability, affective disturbance, apathy, or personality change [7].

Biomechanics of Concussion

Acute concussion or mTBI is characterized by the disruption of neuronal homeostasis through physical forces transferred to the neuron through direct or indirect mechanical forces. The biomechanics of mTBI are important to understand when looking at the associated physiological damage that is created. These damaging forces include acceleration/deceleration, compression, and distraction or shear forces. Each of these forces creates a different signature within the brain and can have slight differing affects across the relatively isomeric characteristic of brain tissue. Each of these forces should be explored and defined as concussion injury to the brain represents some level of combination of these forces. Rarely is brain trauma isotopic in nature (i.e., just stretch or just compression).

The acceleration force injury occurs when the head is fixed and is accelerated rapidly by an external force of an object colliding into it. These acceleration forces drive the inner cranium to collide with the fixed brain within the cranial cavity. In athletics an example of an acceleration injury would be like the forces absorbed through punches being taken by a boxer or when a football player is "blind sided" by an opposing athlete and the head becomes violently accelerated. In contrast, the deceleration force is created when the head is already in motion and it is rapidly decelerated by a fixed object. A player's head coming into contact with the playing surface or with a fixed object on the playing field like a goal post would be an example of a deceleration force.

Acceleration and deceleration forces of a linear nature produce contusion type injuries to the brain due to the absorption of compressive forces. A contusion located on the same side relative to the location of the applied external force is labeled a "coup" type injury. A contusion received by the brain on a side opposite the side of the acceleration/deceleration forces is commonly referred to a counter coup injury. The degree and depth of penetration for linear forces are modified by their intensity [8]. Mild acceleration/deceleration forces affect namely superficial layers in the brain. In addition moderate to severe compressive forces affect deeper structures within the brain. Thus cell viability and structural and functional disturbance of neurons can involve both cortical (superficial) and subcortical (deep) structures in the brain.

In addition to the damaging nature of linear acceleration/deceleration compressive forces, angular acceleration/deceleration stretch or shear forces can generate significant trauma in the brain and are often considered more damaging [9]. These may be considered more damaging as the viscoelastic and gelatinous properties of the brain, with its subsequent high water content, are highly resistant to compression and less resistant to distraction or shear tensile forces. These acceleration/deceleration forces contribute to the destructive shear forces or "stretch" on the white and grey matter of the brain. In addition, regardless of etiology focal injury has a tendency to accumulate at the site of a transition in density as in the transition zones of grey matter (neuronal cell bodies) to white matter (neuronal axons) as well as along areas where vessels penetrate the gelatinous matrix of the brain [10]. Angular acceleration/deceleration shear forces can create stretch injuries to the white matter or axons [11, 12].

Neurophysiologic Cascade of Injury

Seminal papers on the pathophysiology of concussion have been developed which have been foundational to our understanding of the traumatic sequelae resulting from the adverse biomechanical forces absorbed in the brain [13–16]. Researchers exploring treatment strategies base their interventions on the ensuing cascade of cellular events within the injured tissue in order to influence adverse effects downstream and ultimately limit the amount of damage to the brain. A brief overview of the different affective pathophysiologies of concussion will be helpful as we describe the different treatment strategies outlined in this chapter and give context to the intervention.

Metabolic Dysregulation

Of the most damaging forces, stretch and shear strain forces applied to the neuronal cell body and axon can cause significant membrane disruption with a cascade of neurometabolic events [17]. Disrupted membranes and altered membrane potentials result in a massive efflux of intracellular excitatory amino acids (EAA) and potassium (K^+) [18]. Additionally, mechanically induced depolarization contributes to the release of EAA like glutamate. Once glutamate is released and subsequently bound more intracellular K^+ is released compounding the distressed environment. In an effort to restore intracellular homeostasis, the Na^+/K^+ ATP-dependent pumps work in excess. This excess function demands increased amounts of ATP. However, the immediate ATP stores become quickly depleted as normal oxidative metabolism of ATP is diminished and less effective glycolysis begins. This depletion of ATP available for the cell has been linked to mitochondrial dysregulation in the cell after mTBI [19].

Metabolic dysregulation mediated by compromised mitochondrial function also leads to a decreased glucose metabolic rate and depressed oxidative metabolism [20, 21]. This was primarily due to mitochondrial dysfunction and decreased respiration that is well documented in the literature after concussive injury to the neuron [19, 22]. Di Pietro et al. developed a broader theory that the proteins associated with ATP-dependent processes within the cell and associated with the mitochondrial electron transport chain were down-regulated at the time of injury as a form of "hibernation" state. It's theorized that this hibernation and hypometabolic state may be neuroprotective in nature and spare the cell from secondary metabolic cell death [23]. However a prolonged state of metabolic dysregulation and hypometabolism may contribute to the deleterious long-lasting cognitive or behavioral symptoms often experienced in patients with prolonged symptoms or PCS [24].

Oxidative Damage and Apoptosis

The unregulated release of EAA contributes to an increased cellular concentration of calcium. Increased amounts of intracellular Ca^{2+} have direct and indirect consequences in the cell. A direct consequence of the cytosolic presence of Ca^{2+} is the altered membrane potentials across the mitochondrial membrane [25]. Moreover if not corrected the increasing presence of Ca^{2+} within the cell and within the mitochondria can stimulate the release of apoptotic precursor proteins (Caspase 3). The indirect consequence of Ca^{2+} accumulation in the cell is on the ATP-dependent voltage-gated Ca^{2+} channels. This becomes another ATP-dependent process in the cell which requires energy. In the axon, Ca^{2+}-mediated activation of catabolic enzymes will affect the cytoarchitecture in the effected microtubule causing compaction [26]. In addition, Ca^{2+}-mediated release of phospholipases works to disrupt cellular membranes of both the neuron and mitochondria as they both have phospholipid bilayers regulating and protecting intracellular processes. Indirectly glutamate induces neuronal cell death via stimulation of the N-methyl-D-aspartate (NMDA) receptor site. Through this action extracellular Ca^{2+} continues to enter the cell and activates Ca^{2+}-dependent nitric oxide (NO) synthase, resulting in excessive nitric oxide formation. Production of free radicals combined with mitochondrial dysfunction, and the resultant up-regulation of apoptotic precursor signaling proteins can ultimately contribute to cell death [21, 25, 27, 28].

Among cells which remain viable there has been some evidence of differential recovery of function between the soma (cell body) and axons of the groups of neurons exposed to injury [29]. The cell body has the density in organelles with the capability of earlier restoration of cell body homeostasis. This is in stark contrast to the axon which has microtubule structures that are more vulnerable to the stretch and shear forces seen in mTBI. Through the stretch biomechanical forces absorbed, intracellular Ca^{2+} stores are released resulting in increased intra-axonal concentrations [30]. Dysregulation of resting membrane potentials across the axonal cellular membrane contributes to sustained heightened Ca^{2+} concentrations which contribute to secondary axonotomy in some stretched axons [30, 31]. This acute and sustained increase in Ca^{2+} concentration leads to a cleaving of neurofilament side arms (leading to compaction) and microtubule disassembly [32]. The healing rates for axonal or white matter tracks can take days, months, or years according to diffuse tensor imaging research and delays in FA value recovery [29].

Inflammation and Concussion

Neuroinflammation plays a role in neuronal cell death and regeneration and can be activated in mild TBI or concussion [33]. There are many effects contributing to neuronal injury in TBI. Physical disruption of cellular membranes, subsequent excitotoxicity, altered cerebrovascular response, and mitochondrial dysfunction all contribute to the neurochemical milieu surrounding affected tissues and can contribute to neuronal injury and cell death. Each of these cellular responses contributes to the activation of inflammatory process within the brain. Activation of the complement cascade and up-regulation in the production of proinflammatory cytokines and chemokines are responsible for both a neuronal inflammatory response and neuronal regenerative response in the brain [34]. Up-regulation of proinflammatory cytokines like tumor necrosis factor-alpha (TNF-α[alpha][alpha]) and a subgroup of interleukins (IL-1, IL-6, IL-18) can facilitate the inflammatory response through activation of local microglial cells as well as stimulating the expression of various endothelial cellular adhesion molecules (CAM) [35–39]. CAM are then responsible for local infiltration of neutrophils, leukocytes, and other inflammatory cells [40].

Cerebrovascular Response to Concussive Injury

In addition to the other cellular responses to injury, cerebral blood flow can also be compromised from TBI. Cerebral blood flow can remain compromised in the acute and chronic stages of recovery from mTBI [14, 41]. This is possible through uncoupling of the autonomic nervous system's ability to regulate heart rate based on vascular feedback loops from the sympathetic and parasympathetic nervous system [42, 43]. Local release of cytokines leads to perturbations in local perfusion rates within vascular beds surrounding lesion sites [44]. Alterations in cerebral blood flow can last longer than 1 week in patients recovering from mTBI and can be significantly altered in patients suffering from chronic PCS [45].

Ultimately, correction of these cellular dysfunctions lies in the brain's ability to restore adequate blood flow to the site of injury, restore/preserve cellular membranes, restore/preserve mitochondrial function, increase substrate availability, and limit the inflammatory response to cellular injury. As the brain restores homeostasis, the normal physiologic function of largely intact neuronal cells can remain disrupted. Proposed treatment interventions for concussion or mTBI should attempt to address some of the deleterious pathophysiologic effects outlined above and investigated in the literature. The remainder of this chapter will provide a summary of interventions currently being researched in the area of TBI.

Animal Studies: Acute/Subacute Injury

Hypothermia Treatment (Posttraumatic Cooling)

Hypothermia is well researched in the TBI literature. Although there is some debate on the guidelines for proper clinical use of posttraumatic hypothermia treatment, it is generally accepted that hypothermic intervention has some benefit to TBI patients. Some of the reported benefits of hypothermia intervention in TBI include reduced lesion volume, decreased neuroinflammatory response, decreased total number of damaged axons, and increased post-injury cognitive and behavioral measures in animal models [46–51]. Hypothermia treatment in animal models of TBI ranges between 30 °C (mild) and 33 °C (moderate) to elicit a therapeutic dose to the patient. Treatment doses in the literature range from 60 min to several hours of sustained cranial temperatures within therapeutic ranges [46, 47, 50, 52]. There are currently no studies to date which use hypothermia and mTBI models. However, there is research which demonstrates that post-injury hyperthermia in a rat model of mTBI resulted in significantly larger contusion sizes and volumes than under normothermic conditions [53]. This parallels what is seen in the moderate to severe TBI injury model research. We can thus make an educated assumption that we may see the opposite effect under post-injury hypothermic conditions; however, animal model and clinical research still remain to be performed.

Donepezil

Donepezil is a selective acetylcholinesterase inhibitor that up-regulates nicotinic acetylcholine receptor (nAChR) activity. When taken immediately post-injury, 12 mg/kg Donepezil was effective in preventing apoptotic neuronal death at 9 days post-trauma in rats [54]. Donepezil also significantly reduced cognitive impairment on the Morris water maze test [54]. The mechanism of neuronal attenuation of apoptosis is unknown; however, it is thought that Donepezil prevents neuronal death by enhancing phosphorylation of the threonine kinase protein called Akt as well as glycogen synthase kinase-3 beta (GSK-3β[beta]) which inhibits glycogen synthase kinase 3 (GSK-3), a proapoptotic regulator. Donepezil also up-regulates expression of α7 nicotinic acetylcholine receptors (α7-nAChRs) which protects against glutamate toxicity through restoration of calcium membrane permeability via the Ca^{2+}-dependent phosphatidylinositol 3-kinase (PI3K) pathway. Both PI3K and Akt have been shown to be crucial for neuronal survival [55].

Donepezil was most effective when administered immediately following injury; however, it still showed significant attenuation of neuronal death when administered up to an hour following mTBI [54]. Although this is a rather short period of time, it does provide a feasible time frame for administration in human settings as immediate diagnosis is difficult in some cases and consequently delayed. Future studies should investigate the efficacy of Donepezil in clinical treatments of mTBI in addition to identifying the downstream cellular processes affected by administration of the drug.

Dehydroepiandrosterone Sulfate

Dehydroepiandrosterone sulfate (DHEAS) is a naturally occurring steroid found in the brain and is an allosteric weak inhibitor of GABA type A receptors. DHEAS has been shown to alter neuronal excitability and cognitive processes [56]. DHEAS also has antioxidant characteristics, can inhibit glial cell proliferation, and has demonstrated general protection against glutamate neurotoxicity [56].

In an animal model of mTBI, post-injury weekly administration of 20 mg/kg DHEAS, started at 7 days post-injury, was found to normalize cognition at 60 days post-injury and depressive behavior at 90 days post-injury [56]. While the exact mechanism of DHEAS within this clinical study is unknown, it is hypothesized that it inhibits calcium entry into cells, thus maintaining intracellular calcium concentrations and preventing excitotoxicity [57]. In addition it has been demonstrated previously that cognition or memory can be enhanced through DHEAS administration [58]. Specifically, DHEAS enhances expression of NMDA receptors which have a significant role in neural plasticity or memory [59].

Given the uncertainty of DHEAS' efficacy in the treatment of mTBI, future preclinical studies should include in-depth histological investigation. While DHEAS was effective in normalizing cognition and behavior, initial injections caused increased cognitive dysfunction in both control and injured mice. This cognitive dysfunction may possibly have been due to the early expression of NMDA receptors in the acutely injured brain. Early expression of these receptor sites can contribute to Ca^{2+} influx during a period of intracellular Ca^{2+} dysregulation. Further investigation is needed to determine the full effects and tolerance of this adverse initial response.

MK-801 and Scopolamine

MK-801, a noncompetitive NMDA antagonist, was found to significantly reduce neuronal death when combined with scopolamine, a muscarinic antagonist. Acetylcholine is liberated following TBI and appears in large quantities in cerebrospinal fluid. Muscarinic antagonists block acetylcholine receptors which reduces the behavioral deficits induced by the excess liberated acetylcholine [60]. At 7 days post-injury, combined MK-801 (0.3 mg/kg) and scopolamine (1 mg/kg) significantly reduced neuronal death in rats more than either treatment alone and was effective regardless of administered before or 45 min after mTBI. At 15 days post-injury, spatial memory deficits were significantly reduced when MK-801 and scopolamine were administered before injury but not after [61]. The combined treatment most likely increased neuronal survival via reduction of glutamate-induced excitotoxicity and mitigation of acetylcholine-induced deficits. However, the combined treatment did also produce unexpected motor deficits during initial administration. Further preclinical research is needed to investigate the extent of the induced motor deficits; however, given the demonstrated success of this study, investigation of additional combined treatment studies should be considered.

Excitotoxicity and Antioxidant Mechanism (Bacalein and Bacalin)

One of the major contributors to neuronal cell death in mTBI is the dysregulated release of EAA like glutamate. Excessive release of glutamate can lead to excitotoxicity and the production of nitric oxide and free radicals. *Scutellaria baicalensis*

Georgi is a very important traditional Chinese medicine comprising three polyphenols: wogin, bacalein, and bacalin. These three polyphenols are known to have antioxidant properties as free radical scavengers. An in vitro study examined the protective capacity of these free radical scavengers against glutamate toxicity [62]. In this study wogin was found to increase necrotic cell death in rat neuron cultures, but both bacalin and bacalein increased neuronal survival. Bacalein and bacalin decreased NMDA-mediated intracellular calcium and helped reduce neuronal death. While both bacalin and bacalein reduced intracellular calcium, bacalein appears to be more potent due to its greater membrane permeability and antioxidant strength. Bacalein reduced nitric oxide (NO), an indicator of NMDA activation but bacalin did not [62].

Bacalein is believed to prevent glutamate excitotoxicity through disruption of NO production rather than scavenging free radicals. NO combines with a superoxide anion to form glutamate; thus, a reduction of NO reduces glutamate levels. Bacalin is hypothesized to exert its effects through reduction of free radicals [62]. The current evidence surrounding bacalein and bacalin is limited to in vitro examination and future in vivo studies are needed to understand their effect on the body.

Cytokine Intervention (Proinflammatory Inhibitors: Minocycline)

Minocycline is a semisynthetic tetracycline drug that has strong anti-inflammatory capabilities. It has been demonstrated that administration of minocycline reduces the expression of proinflammatory cytokines IL-1β[beta] and TNF-α[alpha][alpha] [63]. In stroke research, therapeutic administration of minocycline significantly reduces the size of infarction and decreases neuronal apoptosis through these augmented anti-inflammatory mechanisms [64]. In an mTBI model, 50 mg/kg minocycline, injected for 4 days following injury, normalized rat behavior compared to controls and significantly reduced serum markers of inflammation [65]. In this investigation the authors monitored the presence of C-reactive protein (CRP), a complement system activator, and monocyte chemotactic protein-1 (MCP-1) which recruits monocytes to the site of injury. Therefore, CRP and MCP-1 can be considered clinical markers of inflammation. CRP expression is stimulated by proinflammatory cytokines and elevated MCP-1 indicates axonal damage. Minocycline normalized MCP-1, CRP, and TLR9, a regulator of the inflammatory response, indicating a reduction in neuronal damage and inflammation [65]. The presence of corticosterone (CORT), an indicator of stress levels, was also significantly reduced by minocycline. The normalization of CORT and the reduction in inflammation and neuronal damage were demonstrated in both the subacute and chronic phases of mTBI. This suggests that minocycline may be effective in reducing both the acute and long-term consequences of mTBI [65].

Although minocycline was effective in both the subacute and chronic phases of injury, it caused significant weight loss as a result of gastrointestinal problems.

Further preclinical investigation is necessary to determine the extent of minocycline's side effects before it can be considered for clinical trials.

Cytokine Intervention (TNF-alpha)

The inflammatory response elicited by mTBI is a potential target for therapeutic intervention. Administration of 3,6'-dithiothalidomide, which, like minocycline, is a potent anti-inflammatory drug, normalized behavior in rats and mice [65]. 3,6'-Dithiothalidomide, also known as tumor necrosis factor-alpha synthesis inhibitor (TNF-α[alpha][alpha] inhibitor), is a lipophilic analog of thalidomide (N-phthaloylglutamimide) that inhibits the cytokine TNF-α[alpha].

TNF-α[alpha] is a proinflammatory cytokine that is central in initiating and regulating the cytokine cascade during the inflammatory response. TNF-α[alpha] inhibitor appears to reduce TNF-α[alpha] by reducing mRNA translation of TNF-α[alpha] and decreasing its half-life. TNF-α[alpha] inhibitor was effective in normalizing mouse and rat behavior following mTBI when administered either pre- or post-injury [66]. Both low (28 mg/kg) and high (56 mg/kg) doses were safe and effective in normalizing animal behavior, regardless of injection 1 h before, 1 h after, or 12 h after injury [66]. A dose-dependent reduction in TNF-α[alpha] was demonstrated in cell cultivations, indicating that TNF-α[alpha] inhibitor is effective in reducing TNF-α[alpha] levels [66].

The strong success of TNF-α[alpha] inhibitor warrants further investigation. While no research has investigated TNF-α[alpha] inhibitor in humans, the effects of administration 12 h post-injury provides a feasible timeline for treatment in human settings that could potentially mitigate the inflammatory cascade following injury.

Cytokine Intervention (GSK-3)

Inhibitors of GSK-3, like TNF-α[alpha] inhibitor, target a specific molecule of the neurometabolic cascade following injury. Lithium, L803-mts, and GSK-3β[beta] inhibit GSK-3 which has been shown to provoke proapoptotic signals, has been linked directly to cell death, and is associated with depressive behavior following mTBI [67]. GSK-3β[beta] inhibits GSK-3 via phosphorylation of serine 9 which inactivates the kinase. In an animal model of injury, mice injected with GSK-3 inhibitors (1 μL of 50 mM lithium or L803mts at 1 μL of 25 mM in DMSO) 30 min before injury had no evidence of apoptotic cell death and significantly reduced depressive behavior at 24 h post-injury [67]. More preclinical research is needed before human trials can be recommended. Future research should focus on the duration of the antiapoptotic effects and the results of administration post-injury.

Antioxidant and Neurometabolic Intervention

Curcumin is a naturally occurring phenol that gives the Indian spice turmeric its yellow color. It has a strong history of use in oriental and Ayurvedic medicine and is known to have antioxidant, anti-inflammatory, and cytoprotective capabilities that can potentially offset the neuroinflammatory and metabolic disturbances observed following a concussion [68, 69].

In one study, researchers examined the effects of curcumin on acute to subacute mild fluid percussion injury in rats [70]. They randomly assigned rats to a regular diet or a diet supplemented with 500 ppm curcumin and then induced a mild fluid percussion injury on the brain. This investigation found that supplementation significantly lowered levels of oxidized proteins, normalized brain-derived neurotrophic factor (BDNF) levels and all BDNF downstream-dependent molecules, and restored cognition [70].

This treatment effect is important as BDNF facilitates synaptic transmission, promotes neuronal excitability, and is crucial for maintaining the molecular processes underlying cognition [71–73]. In addition, BDNF is crucial for the synthesis of synapsin I, a modulator of neurotransmitter release, axonal elongation and maintenance of synaptic connections, and cyclic AMP-response element-binding protein (CREB) [74, 75]. As important, CREB is a transcription factor involved in spatial learning and cellular processes underlying long-term memory [74]. Following a concussion, oxidative stress decreases BDNF levels and its subsequent downstream effects. This may be one factor which contributes to the post-injury decrease in cognition and neuronal synaptic plasticity seen in mTBI models of injury which was then modulated through dietary consumption of curcumin in the above study.

In another nutritional study, the investigators analyzed curcumin's protective effect on energy homeostasis following mild fluid percussion injury on rats [76]. The results demonstrated that curcumin supplementation had significant neurometabolic preservation effects following fluid percussion injury. Investigators observed these effects by monitoring mitochondrial proteins responsible for metabolic processes in the neuron. Cytochrome c oxidase II (Cox-II) is a mitochondrial enzyme partly responsible for oxidative metabolism. Ubiquitous mitochondrial creatine kinase (uMtCK) is namely responsible for synthesizing PCr from ATP in the intermembranous space within the neuron; this is one of the mechanisms for ATP maintenance in the cell. Mitochondrial uncoupling protein 2 (UCP2) is an additional regulator of metabolic function in the mitochondrial electron transport chain. Researchers demonstrated in this model of mild fluid percussion injury Cox-II, uMtCK, and UCP2 were decreased following a concussion, resulting in a depletion of available ATP. Nutritional intervention with curcumin significantly increased Cox-II, uMtCK, and UCP2 thus counteracting the disruptive effects of mTBI on metabolic homeostasis [76].

These investigations provide evidence to suggest that dietary supplementation with curcumin may augment the deleterious effects of concussion by supporting neurometabolic homeostasis and early restoration of pre-injury levels of cognition.

While curcumin appears effective when supplied before injury, it is still unknown whether supplementation begun after injury is beneficial, and if these effects can be replicated in human subjects. Further research is needed to fully investigate the benefits of curcumin as a post-injury treatment intervention in sports-related concussion.

Antioxidant and Anti-inflammatory Intervention

Omega-3 Fatty Acids

Omega-3 fatty acids, specifically docosahexaenoic acid (DHA) and eicosapentaenoic acid (EPA), have demonstrated anti-inflammatory and antioxidant properties in the mTBI research [69]. DHA is an abundant polyunsaturated fatty acid in neuronal phospholipids that has a high turnover rate in the brain and has been shown to stimulate neurite outgrowth in animal models of neural plasticity, as well as support overall neuronal membrane functional homeostasis [77, 78].

A few studies have investigated the efficacy of therapeutic DHA supplementation in a concussion injury model with rats. Two studies found that a diet containing 8 % fish oil (12.4 % DHA and 13.5 % EPA), administered for 4 weeks prior to mTBI, normalized BDNF, BDNF-associated downstream substances, cognition, and Sir2 1 week post-injury [79, 80]. A third study looked at the effects of 10 and 40 mg/kg/day of DHA supplementation for 30 days post-fluid percussion injury [81]. Oral supplementation of DHA significantly reduced the number of injured axons and the levels of amyloid precursor protein (APP)-positive axons, a marker of axonal injury. Additionally, the researchers reported the AA:EPA ratio, a marker of inflammation, decreased 72–109 % in supplemented rats and increased 65 % in unsupplemented rats. In this investigation the researchers summarized that DHA reduced inflammation by inhibiting the formation of proinflammatory eicosanoids and cytokines such as tumor necrosis factor, interleukin 1 (IL-1), and interleukin 6 (IL-6) [81].

The collective results from these investigations provide strong evidence for future research into the clinical application of omega-3 fatty acids in the pretreatment and treatment strategy for sports-related concussion.

Vitamin E

Alpha-tocopherol is a major component of vitamin E and is another antioxidant that has neuroprotective properties demonstrated in cultured cells in vitro [82, 83]. In vivo animal studies using supplemental dietary intake of 500 IU/kg of vitamin E, for 4 weeks prior to mild fluid percussion injury, also demonstrated various neuroprotective effects [84]. Researchers in this study demonstrated that vitamin E is effective in reducing oxidative damage, maintaining energy homeostasis, cognition, and synaptic plasticity [84]. These results indicated normalization of BDNF, calcium/calmodulin-dependent protein kinase II (CaMKII), cognition via Morris water maze performance, Sir2, and superoxide dismutase (SOD). Vitamin E also significantly reduced the level of oxidized proteins. CaMKII is a signaling system required for learning and memory that is modulated by BDNF. SOD is regulated by Sir2 and is an endogenous reactive oxidant species scavenger that helps to buffer oxidation. Both CaMKII and SOD are typically reduced following concussion [84].

An additional in vivo study involving vitamin E administration in guinea pigs found a significant decrease in the amount of lipid peroxidation following mTBI [85]. In this experiment vitamin E attenuates lipid peroxidation by donating a hydrogen to free radicals thus forming a stable radical that doesn't attack the cell membranes. SOD and vitamin E administration prevent oxidation of the phospholipid bilayers of the neuron and mitochondria which minimizes the accumulation of cerebral edema and ionic gradient shifts that can result in excitotoxicity and neuronal death [85].

Vitamin E is a well-researched nutriceutical with neuroprotective capabilities. These in vivo studies of vitamin E supplementation demonstrate neuroprotective results when administered before concussion; however, it remains to be determined if post-injury administration is beneficial. Questions about dosage and time-dependent administration remain largely unanswered in the mTBI injury model. Additionally, no studies have examined the efficacy of vitamin E in clinical settings with the specific treatment of mTBI. More research is needed to validate these findings however progress is being made.

Hydrogen-Rich Saline

As can be seen in this review the role of oxidative stress is a specific therapeutic target for the treatment of mTBI. The use of hydrogen-rich saline as a potent antioxidant has demonstrated beneficial effects in treating neuronal death from acute carbon monoxide poisoning [86, 87], spinal cord injury [88], cerebral ischemia [89], and TBI [72, 90] through antioxidant pathways. Hydrogen-rich saline is made by dissolving hydrogen gas in saline under high pressure (0.4 MPa) until supersaturated. In previous research it has been demonstrated that hydrogen gas can enter the cell through the cytoplasm and into the mitochondria and nucleus of neurons [91]. It offsets oxidative stress and lipid peroxidation by scavenging free hydroxyl radicals with minimal side effects [91]. In a recent investigation of mTBI the researchers demonstrated beneficial effects of hydrogen-rich saline administration [72]. These results were consistent with the antioxidative effects seen in other neuronal injury models and suggest that cognition, synaptic plasticity, and energy homeostasis are normalized by administration of hydrogen-rich saline for 7 days following mild fluid percussion injury in rats [72]. Given the proven benefits of hydrogen gas and early researched benefits of hydrogen-rich saline across neuronal injury mechanisms additional research is needed to fully understand the best treatment dose, time-dependent administration, and efficacy in human clinical trials of concussion.

N-Acetylcysteine

N-Acetylcysteine (NAC) is the N-acetyl derivative of naturally occurring cysteine. It is an antioxidant and anti-inflammatory drug that is capable of passing the blood–brain barrier. NAC directly scavenges hydroxyl and hypochlorous radicals as well as inhibits free radical formation. It inhibits radical formation by promoting the formation of glutathione (GSH). GSH enhances the activity of glutathione peroxidase, an inhibitor of hydroxyl radical formation, via inactivation of endogenous hydrogen peroxide.

Post-injury administration of NAC has been shown to reduce free radical activity in animal mTBI models [92] and has been found beneficial in a clinical trial of servicemen exposed to blast-induced mTBI [93]. The clinical study on servicemen was a randomized, double-blind, placebo-controlled study. Subjects were administered a dosage of 500 mg NAC given ranging from 0 to 72 h post-injury in an active combat zone. The NAC-administered group reported an 86 % resolution of mTBI symptoms after 7 days of treatment and were significantly more likely to experience symptom resolution than the placebo group [93]. The treatment group also demonstrated significantly improved and normalized performance on neuropsychological tests at 7 days post-injury [93]. The results of this clinical study are promising; however, there are a few limitations to this study. While the study was somewhat large ($n = 81$), approximately 99 % of the subjects were male, most of the subjects came from the same combat units, resulting in similar environmental exposure histories, and there was no follow-up past 7 days post-injury. Finally, it is not clear if treatments that are effective in blast-induced mTBI have the same efficacy in sport-related mTBI injury models. These limitations make it difficult to generalize these results to a normal population suffering from concussion but they are encouraging and warrant further investigation.

Antioxidant Intervention (PEG-HCC: Nanoparticles)

A rapidly developing area of medical intervention for oxidative stress is the engineering of nanoparticles. Poly(ethylene glycol)-functionalized hydrophilic carbon clusters (PEG-HCCs) are carbon-based nanovectors that have antioxidant characteristics. This new class of nanoparticles as antioxidants can be functionalized with antibodies to target specific molecules. These inorganic antioxidants combat the biologically damaging effects of oxidative stress by disrupting and/or halting the production of reactive oxygen species (ROS) or reactive nitrogen species (RNS).

An in vitro study of cultured brain endothelial cells found that PEG-HCCs were able to sufficiently protect against oxidative death to be considered biologically relevant [94]. They were also successfully functionalized to target and reduce P-selectin which is involved in the recruitment of leukocytes to sites of inflammation and injury [94]. Additional in vitro examination of PEG-HCCs demonstrated greater reduction of oxidative stress than traditional antioxidants such SOD and phenyl-α-*tert*-butyl nitrone (PBN). In vivo administration of PEG-HCCs at 2 mg/kg restored cerebral perfusion and normalized the radical profile when administered post-injury in a rat model of mTBI complicated with hemorrhagic hypotension [95]. While the results of this study are very promising it is uncertain whether PEG-HCCs are effective in normalizing cerebral blood flow in uncomplicated mTBI and it is uncertain if PEG-HCC is an effective in vivo antioxidant. Future studies are needed to address these questions.

Apoptotic Inhibition (pHBSP)

Much research has been done on the therapeutic effects of erythropoietin (EPO) in the treatment of severe anemia associated with renal failure and certain forms of cancer. To date little has been done to investigate the potential benefits of EPO and EPO-like medical delivery systems for treatment other than red blood cell production. Recently, therapeutic benefits of EPO-mimetic peptides have been explored for their healing capabilities and decreased numbers of side effects. Pyroglutamate helix B surface peptide (pHBSP), an EPO-mimetic peptide, demonstrates similar anti-inflammatory activity to EPO without increasing the risk of thrombotic adverse events and has been used in TBI injury models. Two recent investigations by Robertson et al. found that a 30 µg/kg dose of pHBSP administered every 12 h for 3 days significantly reduced cellular inflammation and significantly improved cognition, reduced contusion volume, and improved neurobehavioral impairment in a rodent model of mTBI [96, 97]. Additionally, pHBSP administration resulted in inflammatory and cognitive improvements whether administered 1 or 24 h post-injury. pHBSP is thought to activate Akt which inhibits a proapoptotic regulator and is crucial for neuronal survival [97]. Given pHBSP's reduced risk for thrombotic adverse events and its efficacy when administered within 24 h post-injury, future studies should investigate its effects in clinical settings.

PCS/Chronic mTBI

Exercise: Benefits and Neuroprotection

Exercise has been demonstrated in the literature to have neuroprotective or beneficial effects on neuronal conditions like stroke [98–101], stress-induced oxidative damage [102, 103], Parkinson's disease [104], Alzheimer's disease [105], and TBI [106, 107]. Exercise is capable of counteracting the deleterious effects of concussion through restoration of cerebral blow flow [108, 109], increasing mitochondrial biogenesis and function [110], increased up-regulation of BDNF [109, 111], and a mediated neuroinflammatory response and inhibition of neuronal apoptosis [109, 112]. These effects have been demonstrated using exercise as a preconditioning intervention as well as a post-injury treatment strategy. In concussion management exercise prescription isn't indicated until the patient has had at least a 24 h symptom-free waiting period *and* has been cleared for exercise by a supervising physician [4]. For those with persistent symptoms that have been diagnosed with PCS exercise can be administered to counteract the chronic deleterious effects of mTBI. In recent publications sub-symptom threshold exercise was prescribed in patient populations suffering from PCS [113]. The investigators demonstrated a significant reduction in subjects' post-concussion symptom score and cognitive improvement in both cohorts studied [113]. Interestingly the authors also found that athletes using the exercise protocol with PCS recovered at a quicker rate than sedentary PCS patients. The investigators postulated that preconditioning with regular exercise may be beneficial in the restoration of premorbid symptoms and levels of cognition in patients recovering from PCS [113].

Hyperbaric Oxygen

Hyperbaric oxygen therapy involves breathing 100 % pure oxygen in a pressurized room or compartment. During hyperbaric oxygen treatment, the air pressure is raised up to three times higher than normal atmospheric pressure. Increased atmospheric pressure increases oxygen saturation by dissolving oxygen in to the blood plasma. This increased oxidative capacity then delivers more oxygen to tissue recovering from injury. In animal models of TBI hyperbaric oxygen treatment ameliorated the effects of TBI through decreasing neuronal cell loss and cellular apoptosis [114], and restoring aerobic metabolic function in the injured neuron [115]. In clinical case studies using hyperbaric oxygen therapy, patients diagnosed with PCS or posttraumatic stress disorder demonstrated improvements in post-concussion symptoms scores, computer-based neuropsychological testing, cerebral blood flow, sleep disturbance, and quality of life measurements [116–119]. However, in one clinical trial, medical researchers examined the effects of hyperbaric oxygen on servicemen with reported symptoms stemming from a combat related-mTBI. This investigation was a double-blind, randomized, sham-controlled study which administered a treatment dose of oxygen at 2.4 ATA for 90 min/day for 30 days. In this investigation it was found that hyperbaric oxygen had no effect on cognitive measures and reported symptoms following mTBI [120].

Although this clinical trial was contrary to other demonstrated improvements in the literature, it is generally accepted that hyperbaric oxygen therapy improves symptoms of PCS in servicemen suffering a mild to moderate TBI.

Symptom Management: Naltrexone

Naltrexone, a congener of naloxone, is an opioid antagonist that is commonly used to treat alcoholism [121]. There is limited evidence suggesting that endogenous opioids may be elevated following TBI and their presence may complicate cognitive function [60, 122, 123]. Two case studies have demonstrated successful management of PCS symptoms through the use of naltrexone at 100 or 50 mg/day; however, the subjects' symptoms reappeared whenever an identical looking placebo was administered [123, 124]. The patients' symptoms remained in remission only via continued naltrexone utilization, indicating only treatment of the symptoms [124]. The results of this study are quite limited by its case study design; however, it seems that naltrexone is not an effective means of addressing the underlying etiology of PCS.

Symptom Management: Dihydroergotamine and Metoclopramide

Dihydroergotamine (DHE) is an ergotamine derivative that has a strong attraction to serotonin receptor subtypes and is commonly used in the treatment of migraines. Metoclopramide is an anti-nauseate; however, it is also effective in treating migraine pain via intrathecal administration. Metoclopramide acts as a dopamine inhibitor through its binding action as a dopamine receptor antagonist. 0.5 mg DHE and 10 mg metoclopramide were combined to treat individuals suffering from subacute mTBI and PCS [125]. The combined treatment was administered intravenously every 8 h for 24–48 h, followed by maintenance on tricyclic antidepressants (beta-blocker or calcium-channel blocker) after discharge. All patients had chronic headache as well as at least three other concussive symptoms. Eighty-five percent of patients treated self-reported improvements in headache, 91 % had improvements in memory, 94 % reported reduced sleep problems, and 88 % reported reduced dizziness. Upon cessation of the maintenance medication, the symptoms reappeared but were quickly resolved again upon re-administration of DHE [125]. This resurgence of symptoms following treatment cessation suggests that combined DHE and metoclopramide does not effectively treat the underlying cause of concussive symptoms. Confident interpretation of these results is limited by the lack of a control group, randomization, a small sample size, and the subjective nature of measures used.

Cognitive Treatment (Postsynaptic Enhancement)

Guanfacine is a selective alpha-2-adrenergic (A2A) agonist that has been shown to improve working memory. Guanfacine is a catecholamine agonist and is thought to improve working memory by stimulating postsynaptic α[alpha]2A-adrenoceptors in the prefrontal cortex, a crucial component of working memory circuitry [126].

The effect of 2 mg oral guanfacine on working memory 1 month post-mTBI was examined in a placebo-controlled, double-blind study [127]. A statistically significant improvement was demonstrated by the guanfacine mTBI group on an N-back working memory task. Additionally, fMRI analysis of the mTBI subjects' N-back performance under the guanfacine condition demonstrated similar activation patterns to that of healthy controls in the placebo condition [127]. This suggests that guanfacine enhances the circuitry through postsynaptic stimulation of the brain areas involved in working memory, but the small sample size and the failure to examine the long-term effects of guanfacine limit the interpretation of this particular mTBI study.

PCS: Posttraumatic Headaches

Divalproex

Divalproex sodium is a GABA activator that has been found to be useful for the treatment of migraine and chronic daily headache. GABA is an inhibitory neurotransmitter naturally found in the brain. Synaptic binding of GABA decreases neuronal excitability and firing rate through a change in resting membrane potential. It is hypothesized that patients with chronic, posttraumatic headaches (PTHA) suffer from hyperexcitability of central neurons in response to increased levels of EAA [128]. The increased or dysregulated release of EAA is a pathophysiological consequence of mTBI.

Investigators in one study looked to determine the effect of pharmaceutical administration of divalproex sodium on a cohort of mild traumatic brain-injured patients suffering from PTHA. A retrospective chart review of 100 patients with chronic daily PTHA resulting from mTBI was conducted [129]. Patients included had PTHA for at least 2 months and were administered divalproex for at least 1 month. Doses ranged from 250 to 1,500 mg administered daily. Sixty percent of the patients self-reported at least 25 % improvement in headaches, but only 6 % of the subjects reported complete amelioration of headaches [129]. This study lacked randomization, blinding, control groups, statistical analysis, and standardized treatment procedures. Furthermore, the retrospective and subjective nature of this study greatly limits the interpretation of the results. Future studies should address these limitations to provide a more complete analysis of divalproex's efficacy in mTBI-induced PTHA.

PCS: Depression Management

Sertraline

Sertraline is a selective serotonin reuptake inhibitor (SSRI) and has been used in the treatment of depression and anxiety disorder [130, 131]. Serotonin and dopamine cerebrospinal fluid levels have been shown to decrease following experimental concussion [132]. SSRIs increase serotonin availability by blocking reabsorption of serotonin.

A nonrandomized, single blind, placebo-controlled trial design analyzed sertraline's effects on measures of depression symptoms in subjects diagnosed with PCS [133]. All subjects were treated with a placebo for the first week, followed by 7 weeks of sertraline at doses of 25–200 mg/day. After completing the study, two thirds of the subjects had complete remission of their depression and statistically significant improvements in psychological distress, anger, aggression, PCS symptoms, and general functioning. While the measures employed in this study are subjective, the reduction in PCS symptoms suggests that treating depression could reduce the subjective level of other symptoms. This study had a small sample size, lacked randomization, and had negative side effects. Approximately 20 % of the participants in this study experienced nausea, diarrhea, abdominal cramps, and/or headaches [133].

An additional study compared sertraline to methylphenidate and a placebo; however, this study included individuals who had suffered mild to moderate TBI [134]. Methylphenidate blocks the reuptake of dopamine and noradrenaline which are catecholamines or neuromodulators of synaptic function. This study using methylphenidate lasted 4 weeks and utilized a double-blind, placebo-controlled, parallel group trial design. Sertraline started at a dose of 25 mg/day and was increased 25 mg every 2 days until reaching 100 mg/day. Methylphenidate started at 5 mg/day and was increased daily by 2.5 mg/day until reaching 20 mg/day. Researchers found that sertraline significantly improved depression but diminished cognitive performance compared to placebo and methylphenidate [134]. Methylphenidate was found to significantly reduce depression without negatively impacting cognitive performance. While this study replicated the aforementioned study's reduction in measures of symptoms related to depression, sertraline had less effect on PCS symptoms than placebo [134].

PCS: Psychological/Psychosocial

Education

There is some evidence to support the use of early education about expected symptoms and recovery of concussion. Several studies providing early reassurance regarding expected recovery, guidance about managing symptoms, and guidance in resuming pre-injury roles in the acute phase of injury found a significant effect of reported symptoms 3 months later [135]. Minderhoud, Boelens, Huizenga, and Saan provided patients with a manual on the nature and recovery of symptoms seen in PCS, and found significantly reduced reports of PCS symptoms 6 months post-injury [136]. In two different studies where patients were issued a manual or pamphlet specifying what symptoms to expect and how to manage symptoms and stress, the patients claimed that the information helped or reported fewer symptoms [135, 136]. This trend of reduced symptom reporting has shown up in several other studies involving early education as well. This would indicate that early education does not prevent the development of symptoms but rather facilitates better coping strategies and symptom management. This is exactly what Wade and colleagues concluded in their 1997 study [137]. They provided patients with an informational sheet about potential symptoms and additional clinical support as needed but found no objective difference in symptom severity at 6 months post-injury. They did, however, find significant improvement in daily functioning and activity [137]. In 2002, Ponsford and her coworkers provided patients with a pamphlet on potential symptoms and coping strategies [138]. They found almost identical results to Wade with no significant improvements on neuropsychological assessments but significantly fewer symptoms reported by the treatment group when compared to controls [138]. This is not to say that early education does not have a place in treatment of concussion. It has long been established that patients' appraisal of recovery can have a strong effect on their rate of recovery and overall perceived quality of life. Furthermore, it has been shown that stress can exacerbate concussion symptoms and slow recovery; therefore, early education may be beneficial simply by helping to foster management of symptoms and stress [139]. The inclusion of early education practices in managing patients recovering from concussion is indicated to manage injury-related stress.

Cognitive Behavioral Therapy

Cognitive behavioral therapy (CBT) takes the results of early education and improved symptom coping and management, and attempts to apply them to individuals suffering from PCS. CBT targets individuals' maladaptive beliefs, emotions, and cognitive processes [140]. It seeks to improve emotional appraisal of symptoms, coping, and stress management. In studies of individuals with head injuries subjects often underestimate the frequency and severity of PCS-like symptoms pre-injury. Also, healthy controls were better able to predict or anticipate potential symptoms of PCS. This difference in perception and expectation of injury can lead to cognitive bias and result in focusing on and exacerbation of symptoms. It has also been found that negative causal attributions and expectation predict persistent symptoms 3 months post-injury [140]. Whittaker et al. found patients that expected serious negative consequences were more likely to have persistent symptoms [141]. They also found that severity of injury and symptoms did not better predict persistent symptoms than negative expectations [141].

Although there are limited studies on maladaptive behaviors and coping in concussed individuals, some studies of more severe TBI have shown that poor coping and maladaptive behaviors such as self-blame and symptom focusing have been associated with poorer outcome. It is believed that maladaptive behaviors and perceptions may contribute to the maintenance of PCS and PCS-like symptoms.

Given an incomplete knowledge of how cognitive appraisal, strategies, and emotions contribute to the development and maintenance of PCS, and the lack of randomized control trials of CBT, more research is needed before CBT can be recommended as an appropriate method for treating patients recovering from concussions or that have been diagnosed with PCS.

Mindfulness-Based Stress Reduction

Mindfulness-based stress reduction (MBSR) is another psychological treatment that focuses on the management of negative thoughts, emotions, and behaviors. It involves mind–body-focused practices such as yoga and meditation that are intended to make one more aware of one's internal state and resources. MBSR like other psychological intervention platforms aims to combat the effects of stress, anxiety, and depression that sometimes accompany mTBI or TBI patients post-injury.

Unfortunately, an intervention strategy using MBSR has resulted in inconclusive results with regard to objective improvements in traumatic brain-injured individuals. Two studies using an MBSR intervention on TBI patients produced rather differing results [142, 143]. McMillan and colleagues found no significant effects on objective or subjective measures of cognition, mood, or symptom reporting in a cohort of TBI patients [142]. In contrast, Bédard and colleagues used MBSR interventions at a frequency of one session per week for 8 weeks and demonstrated statistically significant improvements in depression symptoms, reduced pain intensity, and increased energy levels [143]. However, it should be noted that Bédard had a small sample size and the MBSR intervention was used as a supplement to another group-based treatment plan; therefore, its result cannot solely be attributed to MBSR intervention. In a pilot study of MBSR in treating PCS, patients were led by neuropsychological experts trained in MBSR for a 2 h session once a week for 10 weeks [144]. The study found significant changes in perceived quality of life and self-efficacy but no significant improvements in symptoms [144].

It would appear that MBSR helps patients cope better but does not provide objective improvement with regard to recovery. At this time it cannot be recommended that MBSR be used as a means to treat concussions or PCS; however, it may be of some use in conjunction with a treatment plan that provides objective improvement based on reported improvements in depressive symptoms that sometimes follow mTBI.

Cognitive Rehabilitation

A final area of interest in the domain of psychological treatment is cognitive rehabilitation/remediation. Studies involving cognitive rehabilitation have found improvement in patients' performance on neuropsychological measures of executive function, cognition, and attention as well as self-reported PCS symptoms [145]. A study by Cicerone found significant improvement in neuropsychological measures of working memory and attention in addition to an improvement of overall PCS symptoms in subjects after applying a cognitive rehabilitation program [146]. However, this study had large bias in assignment to treatment groups and small sample sizes ($n=4$). In one study by Ho and Bennet, the researchers carried out a two-component cognitive rehabilitation program focused on improving daily independence in mTBI individuals [147]. These components consisted of activities designed to regain previous function and strategies to compensate for cognitive deficits. The authors summarized that the cognitive compensatory training makes the results of this study difficult to analyze as any improvement in neuropsychological testing may be a result of compensatory tactics given to the subjects and not from objective improvements. As a result of cognitive training intervention, subjects had significant improvement on most outcomes measured, including behavioral performance and cognitive neuropsychological tests measures [147]. The authors go on to conclude because each subject in this study had a customized rehabilitation plan and the length of each plan varied by subject's need, this makes it difficult to generalize these results and methods to larger populations.

These limitations outlined by these particular studies make it difficult to make a sound and objective report on the validity of cognitive rehabilitation for concussed individuals. While the results of these studies themselves are quite promising, cognitive rehabilitation cannot be recommended as an effective means of treatment until more research is done using tools which can objectively discriminate for true cognitive improvement.

References

1. Langlois J, Rutland-Brown W, Wald M. The epidemiology and impact of traumatic brain injury: a brief overview. J Head Trauma Rehabil. 2006;21(5):375–8.
2. Ruff R. Mild traumatic brain injury and neural recovery: rethinking the debate. NeuroRehabilitation. 2011;28:167–80.
3. Lincoln A, Caswell S, Almquist J, Dunn R, Norris J, Hinton R. Trends in concussion incidence in high school sports: a prospective 11-year study. Am J Sports Med. 2011; 30(10):958–63.
4. McCrory P, Johnston K, Meeuwisse W, Aubry M, Cantu R, Dvorak J, et al. Summary and agreement statement of the 2nd international conference on concussion in sport, Prague 2004. Br J Sports Med. 2005;39:196–204.
5. American Congress of Rehabilitation Medicine, Mild Traumatic Brain Injury Committee. Definition of mild traumatic brain injury. J Head Trauma Rehabil. 1993;8(3):86–7.
6. Willer B, Leddy J. Management of concussion and post-concussion syndrome. Curr Treat Options Neurol. 2006;8(5):415–26.
7. American Psychiatric Association. Diagnostic and statistical manual of mental disorders. Washington, DC: American Psychiatric Association; 1994.
8. Ommaya AK, Gennarelli TA. Cerebral concussion and traumatic unconsciousness. Correlation of experimental and clinical observations of blunt head injuries. Brain. 1974;97(4):633–54.
9. Holbourn A. Mechanics of head injuries. Lancet. 1943;242(6267):438–41.
10. Bigler ED, Maxwell WL. Neuropathology of mild traumatic brain injury: relationship to neuroimaging findings. Brain Imaging Behav. 2012;6(2):108–36.

11. Strich S. Shearing of nerve fibers as a cause of brain damage due to head injury. Lancet. 1961;2:443–8.
12. Povlishock J, Becket D, Cheng C, Vaughan G. Axonal change in minor head injury. J Neuropathol Exp Neurol. 1983;42:225–42.
13. Denny-Brown D, Russell W. Experimental cerebral concussion. Brain. 1941; 64(2–3):93–164.
14. Giza CC, Hovda DA. The neurometabolic cascade of concussion. J Athl Train. 2001;36(3):228–35.
15. Signoretti S, Vagnozzi R, Tavazzi B, Lazzarino G. Biochemical and neurochemical sequelae following mild traumatic brain injury: summary of experimental data and clinical implications. Neurosurg Focus. 2010;29(5):E1–12.
16. Barkhoudarian G, Hovda D, Giza C. The molecular pathophysiology of concussive brain injury. Clin Sports Med. 2010;30:33–48.
17. Farkas O, Lifshitz J, Povlishock JT. Mechanoporation induced by diffuse traumatic brain injury: an irreversible or reversible response to injury? J Neurosci. 2006;26(12):3130–40.
18. Katayama Y, Becker DP, Tamura T, Hovda DA. Massive increases in extracellular potassium and the indiscriminate release of glutamate following concussive brain injury. J Neurosurg. 1990;73:889–900.
19. Gilmer L, Roberts K, Joy K, Sullivan P, Scheff S. Early mitochondrial dysfunction after cortical contusion injury. J Neurotrauma. 2009;26:1271–80.
20. Hovda D, Yoshino A, Kawamata T, Katayama Y, Becker D. Diffuse prolonged depression of cerebral oxidative metabolism following concussive brain injury in the rat: a cytochrome oxidase histochemistry study. Brain Res. 1991;567:1–10.
21. Vagnozzi R, Marmarou A, Tavazzi B, Signoretti S, Di Pietro D, et al. Changes of cerebral energy metabolism and lipid peroxidation in rats leading to mitochondrial dysfunction after diffuse brain injury. J Neurotrauma. 1999;16(10):903–13.
22. Singh IN, Sullivan PG, Deng Y, Mbye LH, Hall ED. Time course of post-traumatic mitochondrial oxidative damage and dysfunction in a mouse model of focal traumatic brain injury: implications for neuroprotective therapy. J Cereb Blood Flow Metab. 2006;26:1407–18.
23. Di Pietro V, Amorini A, Tavazzi B, Hovda D, Signoretti S, Giza C, et al. Potentially neuroprotective gene modulation in an in vitro model of mild traumatic brain injury. Mol Cell Biochem. 2013;375:185–98.
24. Peskind E, Petrie E, Cross D, Pagulayan K, McCraw K, et al. Cerebrocerebellar hypometabolism associated with repetitive blast exposure mild traumatic brain injury in 12 Iraq war veterans with persistent post-concussive symptoms. Neuroimage. 2011;54 Suppl 1:S76–82.
25. Lifshitz J, Sullivan P, Hovda D. Mitochondrial damage and dysfunction in traumatic brain injury. Mitochondrion. 2004;4(5–6):705–13.
26. Povlishock J, Pettus E. Traumatically induced axonal damage: evidence for enduring changes in axolemmal permeability with associated cytoskeletal change. Acta Neurochir Suppl. 1996;66:81–6.
27. Dawson VL, Dawson TM, London ED, Bredt DS, Snyder SH. Nitric oxide mediates glutamate neurotoxicity in primary cortical cultures. Proc Natl Acad Sci U S A. 1991;88: 6368–71.
28. Tamura Y, Sato Y, Akaike A, Shiomi H. Mechanisms of cholecystokinin-induced protection of cultured cortical neurons against N-methyl-D-aspartate receptor-mediated glutamate cytotoxicity. Brain Res. 1992;592:317–25.
29. Vagnozzi R, Signoretti S, Cristofori L, Alessandrini F, Floris R, et al. Assessment of metabolic brain damage and recovery following mild traumatic brain injury: a multicentre, proton magnetic resonance spectroscopic study in concussed patients. Brain. 2010;133:3232–42.
30. Staal JA, Dickson TC, Gasperini R, Liu Y, Foa L, Vickers JC. Initial calcium release from intracellular stores followed by calcium dysregulation is linked to secondary axotomy following transient axonal stretch injury. J Neurochem. 2010;112(5):1147–55.
31. Chung RS, Staal JA, McCormack GH, Dickson TC, Cozens MA, Chuckowree JA, et al. Mild axonal stretch injury in vitro induces a progressive series of neurofilament alterations ultimately leading to delayed axotomy. J Neurotrauma. 2005;22(10):1081–91.

32. Okonkwo DO, Pettus EH, Moroi J, Povlishock JT. Alteration of the neurofilament sidearm and its relation to neurofilament compaction occurring with traumatic axonal injury. Brain Res. 1998;784(1–2):1–6.

33. Holmin S, Soderlund J, Biberfeld P, Mathiesen T. Intracerebral inflammation after human brain contusion. Neurosurgery. 1998;42:291–9.

34. Schmidt O, Heyde C, Ertel W, Stahel P. Closed head injury—an inflammatory disease? Brain Res Brain Res Rev. 2005;48:388–99.

35. Hurwitz A, Lyman W, Guida M, Calderon T, Berman J. Tumor necrosis factor alpha induces adhesion molecule expression on human fetal astrocytes. J Exp Med. 1992;176:1631–6.

36. Otto V, Heinzel-Pleines U, Gloor S, Trentz O, Kossmann T, Morganti-Kossmann M. sICAM-1 and TNF-alpha induce MIP-2 with distinct kinetics in astrocytes and brain microvascular endothelial cells. J Neurosci Res. 2000;60:733–42.

37. Stoll G, Jander S, Schroeter M. Detrimental and beneficial effects of injury-induced inflammation and cytokine expression in the nervous system. Adv Exp Med Biol. 2002;513:87–113.

38. Barksby HE, Lea SR, Preshaw PM, Taylor JJ. The expanding family of interleukin-1 cytokines and their role in destructive inflammatory disorders. Clin Exp Immunol. 2007;149(2):217–25.

39. Helmy A, Carpenter KL, Menon DK, Pickard JD, Hutchinson PJ. The cytokine response to human traumatic brain injury: temporal profiles and evidence for cerebral parenchymal production. J Cereb Blood Flow Metab. 2011 Feb;31(2):658–70.

40. Casarsa C, De Luigi A, Pausa M, De Simoni M, Tedesco F. Intracerebroventricular injection of terminal complement complex causes inflammatory reaction in the rat brain. Eur J Immunol. 2003;33:1260–70.

41. Bonne O, Gilboa A, Louzounb Y, Kempf-Sherfc O, Katza M, et al. Cerebral blood flow in chronic symptomatic mild traumatic brain Injury. Psychiatry Res. 2003;124:141–52.

42. Lewelt W, Jenkins LW, Miller JD. Autoregulation of cerebral blood flow after experimental fluid percussion injury of the brain. J Neurosurg. 1980;53:500–11.

43. La Fountaine MF, Gossett JD, De Meersman RE, Bauman WA. Increased QT interval variability in 3 recently concussed athletes: an exploratory observation. J Athl Train. 2011;46(3):230–3.

44. Philip S, Udomphorn Y, Kirkham FJ, Vavilala MS. Cerebrovascular pathophysiology in pediatric traumatic brain injury. J Trauma. 2009;67(2 Suppl):S128–34.

45. Amen DG, Wu JC, Taylor D, Willeumier K. Reversing brain damage in former NFL players: implications for traumatic brain injury and substance abuse rehabilitation. J Psychoactive Drugs. 2011;43(1):1–5.

46. Lyeth BG, Jiang JY, Liu S. Behavioral protection by moderate hypothermia initiated after experimental traumatic brain injury. J Neurotrauma. 1993;10:57–64.

47. Dietrich D, Alonso O, Busto R, Globus MY, Ginsberg M. Post-traumatic brain hypothermia reduces histopathological damage following concussive brain injury in the rat. Acta Neuropathol. 1994;87:250–8.

48. Bramlett HM, Green EJ, Dietrich WD, Busto R, Globus MY, Ginsberg MD. Posttraumatic brain hypothermia provides protection from sensorimotor and cognitive behavioral deficits. J Neurotrauma. 1995;12:289–98.

49. Büki A, Koizumi H, Povlishock JT. Moderate posttraumatic hypothermia decreases early calpain-mediated proteolysis and concomitant cytoskeletal compromise in traumatic axonal injury. Exp Neurol. 1999;159(1):319–28.

50. Chatzipanteli K, Alonso O, Kraydieh S, Dietrich WD. Importance of posttraumatic hypothermia and hyperthermia on the inflammatory response after fluid percussion brain injury: biochemical and immunocytochemical studies. J Cereb Blood Flow Metab. 2000;20:531–42.

51. Seo JW, Kim JH, Kim JH, Seo M, Han HS, et al. Time-dependent effects of hypothermia on microglial activation and migration. J Neuroinflammation. 2012;9:164.

52. Bramlett HM, Dietrich WD. The effects of posttraumatic hypothermia on diffuse axonal injury following parasagittal fluid percussion brain injury in rats. Ther Hypothermia Temp Manag. 2012;2(1):14–23.

53. Sakurai A, Atkins C, Alonso O, Bramlett H, Dietrich WD. Mild hyperthermia worsens the neuropathological damage associated with mild traumatic brain injury in rats. J Neurotrauma. 2012;29(2):313–21.

54. Fujiki M, Kubo T, Kamida T, Sugita K, Hikawa T, et al. Neuroprotective and antiamnesic effect of donepezil, a nicotinic acetylcholine-receptor activator, on rats with concussive mild traumatic brain injury. J Clin Neurosci. 2008;15:791–6.

55. Noh M, Koh S, Kim Y, Kim HY, Cho GW, Kim SH. Neuroprotective effects of donepezil through inhibition of GSK-3 activity in amyloid-β[beta]-induced neuronal cell death. J Neurochem. 2009;108:1116–25.

56. Milman A, Zohar O, Maayan R, Weizman R, Pick C. DHEAS repeated treatment improves cognitive and behavioral deficits after mild traumatic brain injury. Eur Neuropsychopharmacol. 2008;18:181–7.

57. Kimonides V, Khatibi N, Sendsen C, Sofroniew M, Herbert J. Dehydroepiandrosterone (DHEA) and DHEA-sulfate (DHEAS) protect hippocampal neurons against excitatory amino acid-induced neurotoxicity. Proc Natl Acad Sci U S A. 1998;95:1852–7.

58. Flood J, Roberts E. Dehydroepiandrosterone sulfate improves memory in aging mice. Brain Res. 1988;448(1):178–81.

59. Wen S, Dong K, Onolfo JP, Vincens M. Treatment with dehydroepiandrosterone sulfate increases NMDA receptors in hippocampus and cortex. Eur J Pharmacol. 2001;430(2–3):373–4.

60. Lyeth B, Hyes R. Cholinergic and opioid mediation of traumatic brain injury. J Neurotrauma. 1992;9:S463–70.

61. Jenkins L, Lu Y, Johnston W, Lyeth B, Prough D. Combined therapy affects outcomes differentially after mild traumatic brain injury and secondary forebrain ischemia in rats. Brain Res. 1999;817:132–44.

62. Lee H, Yang L, Wang C, Hu SY, Chang SF, Lee YH. Differential effects of natural polyphenols on neuronal survival in primary cultured central neurons against glutamate and glucose deprivation-induced neuronal death. Brain Res. 2003;986:103–13.

63. Pabreja K, Dua K, Sharma S, Padi SS, Kulkarni SK. Minocycline attenuates the development of diabetic neuropathic pain: possible anti-inflammatory and anti-oxidant mechanisms. Eur J Pharmacol. 2011;661(1–3):15–21.

64. Tang XN, Wang Q, Koike MA, Cheng D, Goris ML, Blankenberg FG, Yenari MA. Monitoring the protective effects of minocycline treatment with radiolabeled annexin V in an experimental model of focal cerebral ischemia. J Nucl Med. 2007;48(11):1822–8.

65. Kovesdi E, Kamnaksh A, Wingo D, Ahmed F, Grunberg NE, et al. Acute minocycline treatment mitigates the symptoms of mild blast-induced traumatic brain injury. Front Neurol. 2012;3:111.

66. Baratz R, Tweedie D, Rubovitch V, Luo W, Yoon JS, et al. Tumor necrosis factor-α[alpha] synthesis inhibitor, 3,6′-dithiothalidomide, reverses behavioral impairments induced by minimal traumatic brain injury in mice. J Neurochem. 2011;118(6):1032–42.

67. Shapira M, Licht A, Milman A, Pick CG, Shohami E, Eldar-Finkelman H. Role of glycogen synthase kinase-3β[beta] in early depressive behavior induced by mild traumatic brain injury. Mol Cell Neurosci. 2007;34:571–7.

68. Bisht K, Wagner KH, Bulmer AC. Curcumin, resveratrol and flavonoids as anti-inflammatory, cyto- and DNA-protective dietary compounds. Toxicology. 2010;278(1):88–100.

69. Petraglia A, Winkler E, Bailes J. Stuck at the bench: potential natural neuroprotective compounds for concussion. Surg Neurol Int. 2011;2:146.

70. Wu A, Ying Z, Gomez-Pinilla F. Dietary curcumin counteracts the outcome of traumatic brain injury on oxidative stress, synaptic plasticity, and cognition. Exp Neurol. 2006;197:309–17.

71. Vaz SH, Jørgensen TN, Cristóvão-Ferreira S, Duflot S, Ribeiro JA, et al. Brain-derived neurotrophic factor (BDNF) enhances GABA transport by modulating the trafficking of GABA transporter-1 (GAT-1) from the plasma membrane of rat cortical astrocytes. J Biol Chem. 2011;286(47):40464–76.

72. Hou Z, Luo W, Sun X, Hao S, Zhang Y, et al. Hydrogen-rich saline protects against oxidative damage and cognitive deficits after mild traumatic brain injury. Brain Res Bull. 2012;88(6):560–5.
73. Leal G, Comprido D, Duarte CB. BDNF-induced local protein synthesis and synaptic plasticity. Neuropharmacology. 2013. pii: S0028-3908(13):00142-1.
74. Silva A, Kogan J, Frankland P, Kid S. Creb and memory. Annu Rev Neurosci. 1998;21:127–48.
75. Valente P, Casagrande S, Nieus T, Verstegen AM, Valtorta F, et al. Site-specific synapsin I phosphorylation participates in the expression of post-tetanic potentiation and its enhancement by BDNF. J Neurosci. 2012;32(17):5868–79.
76. Sharma S, Zhuang Y, Ying Z, Wu A, Gomez-Pinilla F. Dietary curcumin supplementation counteracts reduction in levels of molecules involved in energy homeostasis after brain trauma. Neuroscience. 2009;161:1037–44.
77. He C, Qu X, Cui L, Wang J, Kang J. Improved spatial learning performance of fat-1 mice is associated with enhanced neurogenesis and neuritogenesis by docosahexaenoic acid. Proc Natl Acad Sci U S A. 2009;106(27):11370–5.
78. Walczewska A, Stępień T, Bewicz-Binkowska D, Zgórzyńska E. The role of docosahexaenoic acid in neuronal function. Postepy Hig Med Dosw (Online). 2011;65:314–27.
79. Wu A, Ying Z, Gomez-Pinilla F. Dietary omega-3 fatty acids normalize BDNF levels, reduce oxidative damage, and counteract learning disability after traumatic brain injury in rats. J Neurotrauma. 2004;21:1457–67.
80. Wu A, Ying Z, Gomez-Pinilla F. Omega-3 fatty acids supplementation restores mechanisms that maintain brain homeostasis in traumatic brain injury. J Neurotrauma. 2007;24(10):1587–95.
81. Bailes J, Mills J. Docosahexaenoic acid (DHA) reduces traumatic axonal injury in a rodent head injury model. J Neurotrauma. 2010;27(9):1617–24.
82. Crouzin N, de Jesus Ferreira MC, Cohen-Solal C, Aimar RF, Vignes M, Guiramand J. Alpha-tocopherol-mediated long-lasting protection against oxidative damage involves an attenuation of calcium entry through TRP-like channels in cultured hippocampal neurons. Free Radic Biol Med. 2007;42(9):1326–37.
83. Crouzin N, Ferreira MC, Cohen-Solal C, Barbanel G, Guiramand J, et al. Neuroprotection induced by vitamin E against oxidative stress in hippocampal neurons: involvement of TRPV1 channels. Mol Nutr Food Res. 2010;54(4):496–505.
84. Wu A, Ying Z, Gomez-Pinilla F. Vitamin E protects against oxidative damage and learning disability after mild traumatic brain injury in rats. Neurorehabil Neural Repair. 2010;24:290–8.
85. Inci S, Ozcan OE, Kilinc K. Time-level relationship for lipid peroxidation and the protective effect of alpha-tocopherol in experimental mild and severe brain injury. Neurosurgery. 1998;43(2):330–6.
86. Wang W, Li Y, Ren J, Xia F, Li J, Zhang Z. Hydrogen rich saline reduces immune-mediated brain injury in rats with acute carbon monoxide poisoning. Neurol Res. 2012;34(10):1007–15.
87. Shen MH, Cai JM, Sun Q, Zhang DW, Huo ZL, He J, Sun XJ. Neuroprotective effect of hydrogen-rich saline in acute carbon monoxide poisoning. CNS Neurosci Ther. 2013;19(5):361–3.
88. Zhou L, Wang X, Xue W, Xie K, Huang Y, et al. Beneficial effects of hydrogen-rich saline against spinal cord ischemia-reperfusion injury in rabbits. Brain Res. 2013;1517:150–60.
89. Li J, Dong Y, Chen H, Han H, Yu Y, Wang G, Zeng Y, Xie K. Protective effects of hydrogen-rich saline in a rat model of permanent focal cerebral ischemia via reducing oxidative stress and inflammatory cytokines. Brain Res. 2012;1486:103–11.
90. Ji X, Tian Y, Xie K, Liu W, Qu Y, Fei Z. Protective effects of hydrogen-rich saline in a rat model of traumatic brain injury via reducing oxidative stress. J Surg Res. 2012;178(1):e9–16.
91. Ohsawa I, Ishikawa M, Takahashi K, Watanabe M, Nishimaki K, Yamagata K, et al. Hydrogen acts as a therapeutic antioxidant by selectively reducing cytotoxic oxygen radicals. Nat Med. 2007;13:688–94.

92. Ellis E, Dodson L, Police J. Restoration of cerebrovascular responsiveness to hyperventilation by the oxygen radical scavenger N-acetylcysteine following experimental traumatic brain injury. J Neurosurg. 1991;75:774–9.

93. Hoffer M, Balaban C, Slade M, Tsao J, Hoffer B. Amelioration of acute sequelae of blast induced mild traumatic brain injury by N-acetyl cysteine: a double-blind, placebo controlled study. PLoS One. 2013;8(1):e54163.

94. Marcano DC, Bitner BR, Berlin JM, Jarjour J, Lee JM, et al. Design of poly(ethylene glycol)-functionalized hydrophilic carbon clusters for targeted therapy of cerebrovascular dysfunction in mild traumatic brain injury. J Neurotrauma. 2012;29:1–8.

95. Bitner BR, Marcano DC, Berlin JM, Fabian RH, Cherian L, et al. Antioxidant carbon particles improve cerebrovascular dysfunction following traumatic brain injury. ACS Nano. 2012;6(9):8007–14.

96. Robertson CS, Cherian L, Shah M, Garcia R, Navarro JC, et al. Neuroprotection with an erythropoietin mimetic peptide (pHBSP) in a model of mild traumatic brain injury complicated by hemorrhagic shock. J Neurotrauma. 2012;29:1156–66.

97. Robertson CS, Garcia R, Gaddam SS, Grill RJ, Cerami Hand C, et al. Treatment of mild traumatic brain injury with an erythropoietin-mimetic peptide. J Neurotrauma. 2012;29:1–10.

98. Hayes K, Sprague S, Guo M, Davis W, Friedman A, et al. Forced, not voluntary, exercise effectively induces neuroprotection in stroke. Acta Neuropathol. 2008;115(3):289–96.

99. Zhang P, Zhang Q, Pu H, Wu Y, Bai Y, et al. Very early-initiated physical rehabilitation protects against ischemic brain injury. Front Biosci. 2012;4:2476–89.

100. Zhang P, Zhang Y, Zhang J, Wu Y, Jia J, et al. Early exercise protects against cerebral ischemic injury through inhibiting neuron apoptosis in cortex in rats. Int J Mol Sci. 2013;14(3):6074–89.

101. Zhang Q, Wu Y, Sha H, Zhang P, Jia J, et al. Early exercise affects mitochondrial transcription factors expression after cerebral ischemia in rats. Int J Mol Sci. 2012;13(2):1670–9.

102. Leite HR, Mourão FA, Drumond LE, Ferreira-Vieira TH, Bernardes D, et al. Swim training attenuates oxidative damage and promotes neuroprotection in cerebral cortical slices submitted to oxygen glucose deprivation. J Neurochem. 2012;123(2):317–24.

103. Gerecke KM, Kolobova A, Allen S, Fawer JL. Exercise protects against chronic restraint stress-induced oxidative stress in the cortex and hippocampus. Brain Res. 2013; 1509:66–78.

104. Alonso-Frech F, Sanahuja JJ, Rodriguez AM. Exercise and physical therapy in early management of Parkinson disease. Neurologist. 2011;17(1):S47–53.

105. García-Mesa Y, López-Ramos JC, Giménez-Llort L, Revilla S, Guerra R, et al. Physical exercise protects against Alzheimer's disease in 3xTg-AD mice. J Alzheimers Dis. 2011; 24(3):421–54.

106. Lima FD, Oliveira MS, Furian AF, Souza MA, Rambo LM, et al. Adaptation to oxidative challenge induced by chronic physical exercise prevents Na+, K+-ATPase activity inhibition after traumatic brain injury. Brain Res. 2009;1279:147–55.

107. Piao CS, Stoica BA, Wu J, Sabirzhanov B, Zhao Z, et al. Late exercise reduces neuroinflammation and cognitive dysfunction after traumatic brain injury. Neurobiol Dis. 2013;54:252–63.

108. Archer T, Svensson K, Alricsson M. Physical exercise ameliorates deficits induced by traumatic brain injury. Acta Neurol Scand. 2012;125(5):293–302.

109. Zhang P, Yu H, Zhou N, Zhang J, Wu Y, et al. Early exercise improves cerebral blood flow through increased angiogenesis in experimental stroke rat model. J Neuroeng Rehabil. 2013;10(1):43.

110. Steiner JL, Murphy A, McClellan JL, Carmichael MD, Davis JM. Exercise training increases mitochondrial biogenesis in the brain. J Appl Physiol. 2011;111:1066–71.

111. Baker L, Frank L, Foster-Schubert K, Green P, Wilkinson C, et al. Effects of aerobic exercise on mild cognitive impairment: a controlled trial. Arch Neurol. 2010;67(1):71–9.

112. Zhang F, Wu Y, Jia J. Exercise preconditioning and brain ischemic tolerance. Neuroscience. 2011;177:170–6.
113. Leddy J, Kozlowski K, Donnelly J, Pendergast D, Epstein L, et al. A preliminary study of subsymptom threshold exercise training for refractory post-concussion syndrome. Clin Sports Med. 2010;20:21–7.
114. Wang G, Zhang XG, Jiang Z, Li X, Peng L, et al. Neuroprotective effects of hyperbaric oxygen treatment on traumatic brain injury in the rat. J Neurotrauma. 2010;27:1733–43.
115. Daugherty W, Levasseur J, Sun D, Rockswold G, Bullock MR. Effects of hyperbaric oxygen therapy on cerebral oxygenation and mitochondrial function following moderate lateral fluid-percussion injury in rats. J Neurosurg. 2004;101:499–504.
116. Wright JK, Zant E, Groom K, Schlegel RE, Gilliland K. Case report: treatment of mild traumatic brain injury with hyperbaric oxygen. Undersea Hyperb Med. 2009;36(6):391–9.
117. Harch PG, Fogarty EF, Staab PK, Van Meter K. Low pressure hyperbaric oxygen therapy and SPECT brain imaging in the treatment of blast-induced chronic traumatic brain injury (post-concussion syndrome) and post-traumatic stress disorder: a case report. Cases J. 2009;2:6538.
118. Harch PG, Andrews SR, Fogarty EF, Amen D, Pezzullo JC, et al. A phase I study of low-pressure hyperbaric oxygen therapy for blast-induced post-concussion syndrome and post-traumatic stress disorder. J Neurotrauma. 2012;29(1):168–85.
119. Weaver LK, Cifu D, Hart B, Wolf G, Miller S. Hyperbaric oxygen for post-concussion syndrome: design of Department of Defense clinical trials. Undersea Hyperb Med. 2012;39(4):807–14.
120. Wolf G, Cifu D, Baugh L, Carne W, Profenna L. The effect of hyperbaric oxygen on symptoms after mild traumatic brain injury. J Neurotrauma. 2012;29:1–7.
121. Mitchell J, Tavares V, Fields H, D'Esposito M, Boettiger C. Endogenous opioid blockade and impulsive responding in alcoholics and healthy controls. Neuropsychopharmacology. 2007;32:439–49.
122. Hayes R, Galinat B, Kulkarne P, Becker D. Effects of naloxone on systemic and cerebral responses to experimental concussive brain injury in cats. J Neurosurg. 1983;58:720–8.
123. Messing R, Jensen R, Martinez J. Naloxone enhancement of memory. Behav Neural Biol. 1979;27:266–75.
124. Tennant F, Wild J. Naltrexone treatment for postconcussional syndrome. Am J Psychiatry. 1987;144:813–4.
125. McBeath J, Nanda A. Use of dihydroergotamine in patients with postconcussion syndrome. Headache. 1994;34:148–51.
126. Wang M, Ramos BP, Paspalas CD, Shu Y, Simen A, et al. Alpha2A-adrenoceptors strengthen working memory networks by inhibiting cAMP-HCN channel signaling in prefrontal cortex. Cell. 2007;129(2):397–410.
127. McAllister TW, McDonald BC, Flashman LA, Ferrell RB, Tosteson TD, et al. Alpha-2 adrenergic challenge with guanfacine one month after mild traumatic brain injury; altered working memory and BOLD response. Int J Psychophysiol. 2011;82(1):107–14.
128. Welch KM, D'Andrea G, Tepley N, Barkley G, Ramadan NM. The concept of migraine as a state of central neuronal hyperexcitability. Neurol Clin. 1990;8:817–28.
129. Packard R. Treatment of chronic daily posttraumatic headache with divalproex sodium. Headache. 2000;40:736–9.
130. Khanzode SD, Dakhale GN, Khanzode SS, Saoji A, Palasodkar R. Oxidative damage and major depression: the potential antioxidant action of selective serotonin re-uptake inhibitors. Redox Rep. 2003;8(6):365–70.
131. Kennard B. Twelve weeks' sertraline and CBT in young people with anxiety disorders increases likelihood of no longer having the diagnosis compared with placebo or monotherapy, but residual symptoms remain. Evid Based Ment Health. 2012;15(3):71.
132. Kmieciak-Kolada K, Felinska W, Stachura Z, Majchrzak H, Herman Z. Concentration of biogenic amines and their metabolites in different parts of brain after experimental cerebral concussion. Pol J Pharmacol. 1987;39(1):47–53.

133. Fann J, Uomoto J, Katon W. Sertraline in the treatment of major depression following mild traumatic brain injury. J Neuropsychiatry Clin Neurosci. 2000;12(2):226–32.

134. Lee H, Kim SW, Kim JM, Shin IS, Yang SJ, et al. Comparing effects of methylphenidate, sertraline and placebo on neuropsychiatric sequelae in patients with traumatic brain injury. Hum Psychopharmacol. 2005;20:97–104.

135. Snell DL, Surgenor LJ, Hay-Smith EJ, Siegert RJ. A systematic review of psychological treatments for mild traumatic brain injury: an update on the evidence. J Clin Exp Neuropsychol. 2009;31(1):20–38.

136. Miller LJ, Mittenberg W. Brief cognitive behavioral intervention in mild traumatic brain injury. Appl Neuropsychol. 1998;5(4):172–83.

137. Wade DT, Crawford S, Wenden FJ, King NS, Moss NE. Does routine follow up after head injury help? A randomized controlled trial. J Neurol Neurosurg Psychiatry. 1997;62(5):478–84.

138. Ponsford J, Willmott C, Rothwell A, Cameron P, Kelly AM, et al. Impact of early intervention on outcome following mild head injury in adults. J Neurol Neurosurg Psychiatry. 2002;73:330–2.

139. King NS. Post-concussion syndrome: clarity amid the controversy? Br J Psychiatry. 2003;183:276–8.

140. Potter S, Brown RG. Cognitive behavioural therapy and persistent post-concussional symptoms: integrating conceptual issues and practical aspects in treatment. Neuropsychol Rehabil. 2012;22(1):1–25.

141. Whittaker R, Kemp S, House A. Illness perceptions and outcome in mild head injury: a longitudinal study. J Neurol Neurosurg Psychiatry. 2007;78(6):644–6.

142. McMillan T, Robertson I, Brock D, Chorlton L. Brief mindfulness training for attentional problems after traumatic brain injury: a randomized control treatment trial. Neuropsychol Rehabil. 2002;12(2):117–25.

143. Bédard M, Felteau M, Marshall S, Dubois S, Gibbons C, et al. Mindfulness-based cognitive therapy: benefits in reducing depression following a traumatic brain injury. Adv Mind Body Med. 2012;26(1):14–20.

144. Azulay J, Smart CM, Mott T, Cicerone KD. A pilot study examining the effect of mindfulness-based stress reduction on symptoms of chronic mild traumatic brain injury/postconcussive syndrome. J Head Trauma Rehabil. 2012;8:1–9.

145. Comper P, Bisschop SM, Carnide N, Tricco A. A systematic review of treatments for mild traumatic brain injury. Brain Inj. 2005;19(11):863–80.

146. Cicerone K. Remediation of 'working attention' in mild traumatic brain injury. Brain Inj. 2002;16(3):185–95.

147. Ho MR, Bennett TL. Efficacy of neuropsychological rehabilitation for mild-moderate traumatic brain injury. Arch Clin Neuropsychol. 1997;12(1):1–11.

Chapter 22
Post-concussion Syndrome, Persistent Symptomatic Concussion, Related Sequelae, and Treatment of Mild Closed Head Injury

Jonathon Cooke and J. Christopher Zacko

Abstract Concussion, particularly sport-related concussion, has recently seen a revival of academic and clinical interest. While most concussions are self-limited and resolve over 7–10 days, there is a small subset of patients who experience prolonged symptoms. These prolonged symptoms are often refractory to treatment. Once the symptoms of a concussion become protracted they can prove to be very difficult to treat. This constellation of symptoms is most commonly referred to as post-concussive syndrome (PCS) but several synonymous terms exist in the literature, most notably post-concussive disorder, persistently symptomatic concussion, and difficult concussion.

While there has been an explosion of research regarding *acute* concussion, more chronic injuries are just now being investigated as a distinct entity. To be frank, we simply do not know enough about the PCS to accurately describe the risk factors, common features, or ideal treatment for PCS. At this time, *treatment is largely anecdotal* and derived from a combination of successful treatment paradigms used in acute concussion and more severe traumatic brain injuries. Fortunately PCS is beginning to also see an upsurge in attention that will hopefully provide valuable insight into the pathophysiology needed to treat it more effectively. For now, an active and comprehensive rehabilitation program focusing on the persistent symptoms and managed from an experienced concussion clinic is the best course of action.

Keywords Post-concussive syndrome • Post-concussive disorder • Persistently symptomatic concussion • Difficult concussion

J. Cooke, M.D.
Department of Neurological Surgery, Penn State Hershey
Medical Center, Hershey, PA, USA

J.C. Zacko, M.S., M.D. (✉)
Penn State Hershey Medical Center, 30 Hope Drive—EC110,
Hershey, PA 17033, USA
e-mail: jzacko@hmc.psu.edu

S.M. Slobounov and W.J. Sebastianelli (eds.), *Concussions in Athletics:*
From Brain to Behavior, DOI 10.1007/978-1-4939-0295-8_22,
© Springer Science+Business Media New York 2014

Introduction

The first decade of the twenty-first century has seen a resurgence of interest in concussion (particularly sports-related concussion) and mild traumatic brain injury (mTBI). The global war on terror has produced a patient population with a high incidence of symptomatic closed head injury that will sadly require healthcare services for many years to come. However, it is the efforts of the National Football League (NFL) that have fueled a lot of the change in domestic concussion practices. We are seeing athletes being taken out of games after on-field collisions and rules being amended to protect players and make the game safer. Similar changes are now being adopted in the National Hockey League (NHL), Major League Baseball (MLB), and the National Basketball Association (NBA). Additionally, mainstream media coverage and public relations efforts have raised awareness of concussion in amateur athletics from the collegiate level all the way to junior athletic leagues. This has carried over into clinical practices across the country as practitioners have increased vigilance towards non-sports-related concussions. These developments have dramatically changed the public's view on the consequences of concussion and have led to a favorable impact on the historical paradigm that concussions are a universally benign and self-limited condition. The culture that a concussion, or even sub-concussive blows, is something one should "just shake off" is rapidly vanishing. From a clinician's perspective, this resurgence of interest has resulted in increased funding for concussion research causing the body of information on concussion and related disorders to grow exponentially.

Despite this, there is still a large amount of frustration surrounding our understanding of concussion and how to treat it. This is especially true for the persistently symptomatic concussion patient (>10 days). This small subset of all concussion patients (~10–15 %) [1] has been called several things in the past, most commonly the post-concussion syndrome (PCS) and post-concussion disorder (PCD). To further blur the literature, the term "difficult concussion" has been used with increasing frequency to describe the same patients. Though PCS has been recognized for over a century, much of our methodology remains unsettled. Questions remain regarding definition, diagnostic criteria, identification of high-risk patients, and treatments. This chapter will review the last decade of advances in the understanding of PCS, persistently symptomatic concussions, and their related sequelae.

The field of concussion is increasingly more complex and dynamic. As our understanding of concussion evolves, so does the nomenclature used to describe it. Additionally, as of this writing, there is no universally accepted term to describe persistently symptomatic concussions and many object to the use of the word syndrome. This objection stems from two main points: (1) many of the symptoms recognized in these patients are indistinct and can be associated with concurrent conditions and comorbidities; (2) a "syndrome" implies that if any number of predetermined symptoms is present the diagnosis of PCS can definitively be made. This traditional view of making a diagnosis does not work well with post-concussive patients leading to the adoption of the term post-concussion disorder.

Until our understanding of this condition improves, some will argue to simplify matters and use the term persistently symptomatic concussion or "difficult concussion" (although it is acknowledged that PCS is the most common and familiar term used to identify these patients). Throughout this chapter you will see several of these terms used interchangeably as attempts were made to adhere to the nomenclature used by the primary reference being reviewed.

Historical Perspective

While descriptions of concussion and persistent symptoms go back hundreds of years, the first attempt to quantify this constellation was put forth by Erichsen in the nineteenth century [2]. The increased use of rail travel led to a high incidence of railroad-associated injury caused by sudden stops and train collisions. In his 1866 text, On Railway and Other Injuries of the Nervous System, Erichsen described patients who had neurological symptoms without identifiable injury. This became known as Erichsen's disease or "railway spine" in the vernacular. He also described a subset of patients with nonspecific, prolonged neurological symptoms some of which were cerebral in nature. Erichsen's theories were supported by other prominent physicians of the time including Leydon, Erb, and Lidell [3]. The result of this was increased concern by the public over railway travel and litigation against the railroad companies for damages [3]. In the 1880s Page and Charcot each published challenges to Erichsen and proposed a psychological etiology [3, 4]. The symptoms were thought to be the result of hysteria and predilection towards neurological injury and not an organic injury. This theory would be challenged by survivors of The Great War who were subjected to high energy injuries and did not appear to have this component of hysteria. It was not until the 1930s that we saw the term PCS appear, cited in a historical article by Strauss and Savitsky [5].

Debate raged over the twentieth century as to whether PCS was of an organic nature or an overriding posttraumatic neurosis. Each side had its supporters with British neurologists Symonds and Miller championing each viewpoint, respectively [6]. The next major contribution was made by Lishman [7] who combined the two theories. He proposed that organic pathology was prominent in the early stages of the disease while neurotic decompensation occurred late. However, this did not seem to settle the debate as many attempted to link posttraumatic stress disorder, depression, mTBI, trauma without mTBI, and several other factors with PCS symptoms.

Definition

Perhaps the biggest challenge of PCS is defining it. Post-concussion syndrome/post-concussive disorder (PCS/PCD) is a constellation of clinical symptoms persisting for a prolonged period of time that interferes with the patient's ability to carry

Table 22.1 ICD-10 criteria for post-concussion syndrome

- Head injury usually severe enough to cause loss of consciousness within 4 weeks of symptom onset
- Preoccupation with symptoms and fear of brain damage with hypochondrial concern and adaptation of sick role
- Three of eight from below
  - Headache, dizziness, malaise, fatigue, noise intolerance
  - Irritability, depression, anxiety, emotional lability
  - Concentration, memory, or intellectual deficit without neuropsychological evidence of deficit
  - Insomnia
  - Reduced alcohol intolerance

Table 22.2 DSM-4 criteria for post-concussion syndrome

- History of severe concussion
- Neuropsychological evidence of attention or memory impairment
- At least three of the following occurring shortly after injury lasting for 3 months
  - Fatigue
  - Sleep impairment
  - Irritability or aggression
  - Anxiety, depression, or labile affect
  - Headache
  - Dizziness
  - Personality change
  - Apathy

out his or her chosen lifestyle. Howe organized these symptoms into three categories: *somatic* (headache, dizziness, fatigue, noise/light sensitivity, and sleep disturbance), *cognitive* (confusion, attention problems, reduced processing speed, memory difficulties, and executive dysfunction), and *emotional/behavioral* (depression, anxiety, irritability, apathy, and mood changes) [8]. The most common symptoms experienced in these patients include headache, difficulty concentrating, a feeling of imbalance, depression, decreased energy, sleeping difficulties, and "not feeling quite right, in a fog" [9]. Currently, there are two accepted definitions for PCS: the International Classification for Diseases 10th Revision (ICD-10) [10] and the Diagnostic and Statistical Manual of Mental Disorders 4th Edition (DSM-4) [11]. Criteria for each are found in Table 22.1 [10] and Table 22.2 [11], respectively. Each of these diagnostic references incorporates organic and neuropsychiatric properties in diagnosing PCS. Because of this the incidence of PCS is difficult to quantify with ranges being between 15 and 47 % of concussed patients [12].

As each of these resources enters its second decade of service, questions arise as to the efficacy and accuracy of these definitions. Boake et al. followed a cohort of patients 3 months after injury and evaluated them using the DSM-4 and ICD-10 criteria [13]. They found that the prevalence of PCS at that time was significantly higher using the ICD-10 (64 % met criteria) versus the DSM-4 (11 % met criteria).

Furthermore both of these definitions require the presence of a head injury. However, mounting evidence in the literature suggests that the symptoms of PCS are not specific for mTBI and can be applied to patients with many conditions including depression, extracranial trauma, pain, and posttraumatic stress disorder [8, 14–18]. Mickeviciene et al. suggest that even expectation of symptoms can contribute to over-reporting of PCS [19]. Garden and Sullivan recently looked at a cohort of healthy participants. Almost half the cohort met the criteria for PCS and showed significant elevations in many psychiatric scales, including depression, anxiety, and borderline personality disorder [20]. Culture may also play a role in PCS symptoms. Zakzanis examined a multicultural cohort of healthy volunteers and found that certain cultures endorsed many of the symptoms of PCS and that culture could contribute to a false-positive diagnosis [21]. Conversely, Spinos et al. looked at a cohort of mTBI patients in Greece and noted there to be a markedly lower incidence of PCS than is quoted in the literature [22]. Covassin et al. suggest that female gender and younger age may contribute to PCS [23]. Another possible confounder to diagnosing PCS is the idea of the "Good Old Day" Bias. Lange et al. were able to show that patients with PCS falsely elevated their pre-injury level of functioning thereby inflating their functional decline post-injury [24]. As we develop a better understanding of the organic and psychological properties of PCS we may need to update our diagnostic resources to appropriately identify patients.

Pathophysiology

While there is growing understanding of the pathophysiology of mTBI and acute concussion, the investigation into the pathophysiology of PCS/PCD is truly in its infancy. It is generally presumed that many of the secondary injury mechanisms involved in more severe TBIs may also contribute, in varying degrees, to the deleterious effects seen after mTBI and concussion. The magnitude, time scale, and interrelationship of these injurious cascades in mTBI are being investigated. A detailed overview of the pathophysiology is beyond the scope of this chapter and premature in its applicability to PCS/PCD. Secondary injury mechanisms recognized in TBI include [25]:

- Excitotoxicity
- Calcium dysregulation
- Cytoskeletal proteolysis/diffuse axonal injury
- Cerebral edema
- Alterations in cerebral blood flow
- Metabolic and mitochondrial dysfunction
- Oxidative stress/free radical formation
- Neuroinflammation/immunoexcitotoxicity

At this time it is unclear if any of these secondary injury mechanisms predominates in the development of PCS/PCD. It is also unclear if there may be a novel secondary injury mechanism of concussion not appreciated in more severe TBIs.

As of today, a concussion is felt to be a functional or biochemical disturbance rather than a structural injury. However, it may be that our current imaging techniques are not advanced enough to pick up the exact structural damage occurring with concussion. It follows that PCS may be the result of persistent similar biochemical (and possibly structural) processes. Lastly, the contribution of psychogenic factors in the development of PCS engenders much debate and is currently unknown.

Predictor of Disease

Accurate diagnosis of PCS is essential because these patients are severely disabled and use a disproportionate amount of healthcare. Therefore, it would be advantageous to be able to assess and identify early those patients who are likely to progress to PCS/PCD. Several methods have been explored including clinical symptoms, serum markers, and radiological studies.

The most cost-effective method of predicting PCS/PCD would be to determine which clinical signs and symptoms patients have at presentation of their initial injury that makes them high risk to progress to PCS/PCD. Lau looked at a cohort of high school football players and determined that out of many on-field signs and symptoms, only dizziness was significantly prognostic of prolonged recovery from concussion [26]. Sheedy et al. looked at a cohort of mTBI patients in the ED and at 1 month post injury. They found neurocognitive impairment, pain, and balance deficits were significantly associated with post-concussive symptoms [27]. Dischinger et al. looked at a similar cohort at 3-month follow-up and found anxiety and noise sensitivity were significantly associated with PCS [28]. Savola found skull fracture, headache, and dizziness as being significantly associated with the development of PCS [29]. Recently, Heitger et al. looked at impairment of eye movements and found that the duration of this impairment overlapped cerebral impairment in PCS/PCD [30]. Despite much effort there does not seem to be agreement in the literature about hallmark signs or symptoms that can select patients at high risk for PCS. More work is needed on the subject.

Of the many serum markers possibly linked to PCS three have received the most study: S100 protein, neuron-specific enolase, and cleaved tau protein. There are reports throughout the literature finding significance and no significance with each of these markers. However, a meta-analysis by Begaz et al. in 2006 incorporating 11 studies found that none of the above was significantly associated with development of PCS/PCD [31]. They proposed that while serum markers alone were inaccurate, perhaps a combination of serum markers and clinical signs and symptoms would be and suggested further exploration. Many imaging and monitoring techniques have been explored in an attempt to visualize structural changes in PCS patients. From electroencephalography (EEG) to positron emission tomography (PET) and most recently magnetic resonance (MR) technology, more research is being done exploring quantifiable physical changes in the parenchyma of PCS patients.

Korn et al. found higher power in the delta band and lower power in the alpha band on quantitative EEG and focal reduction in perfusion and blood–brain barrier breakdown on single photon emission computed tomography (SPECT) in PCS/PCD patients versus healthy controls [32]. However, other studies found no benefit to EEG [33]. Peskind et al. looked at a cohort of 12 Iraq War Veterans with blast injuries and mTBI with fluorodeoxyglucose-PET [34]. They found hypometabolism in the cerebellar hemispheres, vermis, pons, and medial temporal lobe. They also found impairments in verbal fluency, cognitive processing speed, attention, and working memory similar to patients with non-traumatic cerebellar lesions. Though this was a small cohort, this line of research is encouraging and further investigation is warranted. Several different studies have looked at magnetic resonanace imaging (MRI) in PCS/PCD [35]. Smits et al. correlated diffusion-weighted imaging (DWI) and gradient echo images with Rivermead Postconcussion Symptoms Questionnaire. They found reduction of white matter correlated with severity of post-concussion symptoms. Though this study was limited by the small number of patients ($n = 12$). Messe et al. also used DWI to look at mTBI patients with PCS/PCD symptoms [36]. They found a loss of structural integrity at the subacute phase that resolved over time. Those PCS/PCD patients had larger deficits and longer duration of symptoms than controls. These studies strengthened the evidence of a structural derangement in PCS. Smits et al. looked at patients with PCS/PCD with functional MRI (fMRI) [37]. They found increased activation in the posterior parietal area, parahippocampal gyrus, and posterior cingulate gyrus. This was also proportional to severity of PCS/PCD symptoms. Though much encouraging work has been done there is a lack of consensus over imaging findings in patients with PCS. Though results are promising more work needs to be done.

Treatment

As discussed above, defining, diagnosing, and predicting persistently symptomatic concussions can be a challenging endeavor. That said, treating PCS and these "difficult concussions" is often even more problematic. At this point, *there are no evidence-based guidelines addressing the optimum management of persistently symptomatic concussions*. This distinct clinical challenge is only recently getting the specific attention required to advance our approach to treatment. Our current treatment strategy remains largely anecdotal and incorporates many tenets from the management of acute concussions as well as more serious (and often structural) head injuries. This is obviously a suboptimal approach as these are broadly considered to be different categories of head injury. One could argue that concussion and some mTBIs fall along the same injury spectrum but it is certainly not established that these more "minor" head injuries are similar enough to severe brain injuries to justify comparable treatment paradigms. However, with our current knowledge, sharing some treatment strategies is an understandable and sensible approach while the medical community awaits more clarity on best practice strategies specifically for PCS/PCD. Lastly, severity of concussion and PCS/PCD has been notoriously hard to predict and classify. In this "new era" of concussion research most agree that there is no accurate grading scale to measure concussion severity. Most recommend against using concussion grading scales until a greater understanding of the condition is achieved. Once a grading scale can be developed that actually affords a clinician the ability to prognosticate a time frame for recovery and outcome it would be appropriate to reintroduce grading scales into the assessment of concussion. For now, it is best felt to simply gauge if a person "did" or "did not" have a concussion. The severity of a given concussion is then determined during the subsequent treatment period and stratified by the number, severity, persistence, and refractoriness of symptoms.

A treatment program for a patient with PCS/PCD should be multidisciplinary in nature and comprehensive in its scope. It is crucial to be conscious of, and treat, potential co-existing medical conditions that may be clouding the clinical picture and hampering the recovery process. During the initial evaluation of a patient with potential PCS/PCD, the fundamental tenet used in the treatment of acute concussion may still apply (depending on the symptoms and how long they have been present). This consists of physical and cognitive rest until asymptomatic with graded return to functional activity. However, continued and prolonged rest is not always a practical option, nor has it been shown to be beneficial in cases of PCS/PCD. Furthermore, prolonged rest (particularly with an ambiguous endpoint) is not feasible for many patients as socioeconomic concerns such as maintaining employment, planning for adequate short-term disability, or scheduling a substitute for a team or work environment become very genuine concerns.

As aforementioned, management of persistent (or "difficult") concussions differs from acute concussions in that continued rest is not necessary or recommended. In contrast, the initiation of an active multidisciplinary rehabilitation and recovery program is advocated—even in the face of symptoms [38–40]. An approach to treating the persistently symptomatic concussion patient is outlined below.

Overall Strategy

1. *Multidisciplinary approach*: A physician experienced in evaluating a concussion should oversee the entire process to ensure all problems are adequately addressed. Involved disciplines include but are not limited to sports medicine physician/neurologist/neurosurgeon, neuropsychologists, speech therapists, physical therapists, occupational therapists, otolaryngologists, psychiatrist, social worker, behavioral therapists, and ophthalmologists. See non-pharmacologic treatment below for more details.

2. *Detailed H + P*: Gathering pertinent information when evaluating a concussion should be an obvious first step. It is crucial to understand the circumstances of the concussion, identify the new symptoms (and how they may have evolved since the time of injury), and be careful to identify co-existing pathologies that

have a tendency to be lumped into "post-concussive" sequelae. Adequately addressing these co-existing pathologies (e.g., depression, anxiety, musculoskeletal injuries, and socioeconomic stressors) can result in dramatic improvements for the patient before the concussion-specific symptoms have even been addressed. Lastly, understanding what treatments, if any, have already been attempted to date is also vital.

3. *Prioritize symptom management*: Many times a patient suffering from difficult concussion has multiple vague or generalized symptoms. Trying to treat all the symptoms at once can be a daunting task. Furthermore, if pharmacotherapy is initiated, the side effects from a given medication can confound future clinical assessment for resolution of symptoms. In other words, the "solution" may become confused with the problem. For this reason, we recommend carefully explaining to patients that *while you want to treat all their symptoms, it is best to focus on the 1–2 most bothersome symptoms initially with full intention to fold in treatments for any remaining symptoms during future visits*.

4. *Non-pharmacological treatment*:

   (a) Initiate a multidisciplinary and active rehabilitation program: some common symptoms and treatment options to address them are listed below.

   (b) *Vertigo/imbalance/dizziness*: PT evaluation for vestibular rehabilitation has been shown to benefit patients [9, 41, 42]. If symptoms remain refractory consider a consultation with ENT to rule out inner ear disorders such as posttraumatic Meniere's disease or benign positional vertigo.

   (c) *Blurry vision/diplopia/visual field deficits*: May benefit from referral to an ophthalmologist for visual rehabilitation or occupational therapy for light therapy, convergence therapy, etc.

   (d) *Headaches*: Consider ophthalmologic exam to ensure disorders of visual acuity are not contributing to headaches. Cervicogenic headaches from nuchal musculature strain are also common and important to consider as the source of headache (refractory headaches are one of the most common symptoms treated in PCS and are most commonly treated medically).

   (e) *Myofascial pain/cervicogenic headaches*: Consider physical therapy (PT) and/or deep tissue massage.

   (f) *Insomnia*: Sleep hygiene should be discussed, including eliminating distractions and avoiding caffeine, alcohol, and nicotine. Obstructive sleep apnea may not be a result of concussion, but if this is an untreated preexisting condition it can interfere with efficient recovery.

   (g) *Short-term memory loss or word-finding difficulties*: Both formal neuropsychological assessment and speech therapy for cognitive rehabilitation are pillars of PCS/PCD treatment.

   (h) *Anxiety/depression/panic attacks/posttraumatic stress disorder*: These can all be seen after TBI and referral to a mental health specialist trained in treating these disorders is important. Treatment options include cognitive behavioral therapy, biofeedback, meditation, and psychological counseling [43, 44].

5. *Pharmacologic treatment*:

   (a) The senior author prefers to limit us pharmacotherapy after the first visit until other assessments can be made and assimilated. There are obviously exceptions to this practice but the thought is to reduce the risk of introducing medication side effects into the constellation of symptoms while initial assessments are ongoing. That said, it is often quite reasonable to prescribe homeopathic medications such as antioxidants and natural supplements at the first visit as treatment options are being initiated. If symptoms continue to persist there are several pharmacologic options for specific symptoms after head injury but most lack true scientific rigor when considered for the treatment of PCS. For an excellent review, see an article by *Petralgia, Marron, and Bailes*: *From the Field of Play to the Field of Combat: A Review of the Pharmacological Management of Concussion* [45]. Some agents will be briefly discussed below.

   (b) *Headaches*: A short trial with over-the-counter analgesics and/or NSAIDS is worthwhile (Tylenol, Excedrin, Excedrin Migraine). Other medications to consider are Fioricet, Indomethacin (if headaches are consistent with hemicrania continua), antidepressants (Amitriptyline), anticonvulsants (Valproate) [46], beta-blockers (Propranolol) [47], antimigrainous triptans (Imitrex), and Ergot preparations [48].

   (c) *Depression*: Amitriptyline is a common first choice as it has also been shown to help with headache control.

   (d) *Cognitive dysfunction*: There has been recent interest in using amantadine for TBI, including a clinical trial involving severe TBI [49]. Reddy et al. recently published a paper showing symptoms improvement in subjects with PCS >21 days who were prescribed amantadine 100 mg BID [9, 50].

   (e) *Dizziness*: Aside from vestibular rehab, agents such as meclizine, scopolamine, and Dramamine have been used for dizziness.

   (f) *Fatigue*: Commonly attempted medications include methylphenidate, modanafil, and amantadine.

   (g) *Nausea*: Zofran is a typical choice.

   (h) *Sleep aid*: Melatonin is felt to be a good first choice.

   (i) *Antioxidants/supplements*: Multivitamins with vitamin E, vitamin C, and fish oil are worth considering as initial treatments.

6. *Role of testing*:

   (a) *Neuropsychological testing*: This can be achieved both with computer-based programs and formal testing. Both of these are important for detecting more subtle alterations in cognition and can guide treating physicians in gauging severity of concussion.

   (b) *Imaging*: At this point in time, the role of imaging (CT or MRI) is to rule out the presence of anatomical injury. If revealed, consultation with a neurologist and/or neurosurgeon is strongly recommended. There are more advanced imaging techniques being investigated and remain an important source of optimism for future breakthroughs in our understanding and recognition of mTBI and concussion. Examples include MRI, DWI, fMRI, MR spectroscopy (MRS), diffusion tensor imaging (DTI), and diffusion kurtosis imaging (DKI). White-matter integrity is estimated with advanced imaging modalities such as DTI and DWI. Studies have been performed which seem to show a relationship between PCS and reduced white-matter integrity [35, 36].

(c) *Genetic testing*: This is another area of interesting research but has not reached the point where usage in the clinical realm is practical or recommended. Again, extrapolating from the severe TBI literature, apolipoprotein E is an active area of investigation. The presence of the APOE4 genotype has been linked to worse outcomes in TBI. For now, the scientific foundation for such a relationship is still being explored. Suffice it to say that there is some preliminary evidence to support a complex interrelationship between head injury, genetics, and the risk of worse outcome.

7. *Future directions*:

(a) *Hyperbaric oxygen therapy* (*HBOT*): HBOT has long been explored as a medical treatment for a variety of conditions—including chronic neurological disorder such as stroke and brain injury. Typically HBOT is applied at 2.0–3.0 atmospheres absolute (ATA) for selected approved conditions (TBI is not one of them at this time). Harch et al. completed a Phase I trial demonstrating significant improvement in symptoms of patients suffering from PCS and/or PTSD who underwent low-pressure HBOT (1.5 ATA) for 40 sessions [51].

Summary

PCS remains an ill-defined and much debated constellation of symptoms used to describe the persistent symptoms experienced by a patient after a head injury. While a head injury of any severity can lead to the symptoms described in PCS, it is a term most commonly used in the setting of concussion and sports-related concussion. PCS continues to be a challenging, and at times frustrating, clinical condition to manage. It is hoped that this new age of interest in concussion research will bring to light the answers we seek regarding the risk factors, pathophysiology, and treatment of PCS. The fact that the terms post-concussive syndrome, post-concussive disorder, persistently symptomatic concussion, and difficult concussion are all terms used to describe essentially the same condition only speaks to the uncertainty surrounding this extremely common problem.

It is important to distinguish PCS from acute concussion. At this time, PCS is considered to be present when symptoms are present longer than 10 days. The optimum treatment of acute concussion is widely promoted as physical and cognitive rest until asymptomatic and then graded return to activity. In contrast, PCS responds to a more active and multidisciplinary rehabilitation program.

While the prognosis for PCS remains good, some patients remain symptomatic for a prolonged period of time. At 1 month most cases have resolved [52] and at 3 months almost all have recovered [53]. Incidence of persistent symptoms at 1 year remains controversial, but is commonly estimated 10 %. However, many feel this may be confounded by bias, over-reporting, and in some cases malingering.

This is an exciting time to be involved in concussion research. As recently as the last 5 years the diagnosis and management of concussion were seemingly taken for granted. Now public awareness and medical research on this topic have grown exponentially. With the development of new imaging and diagnostic technologies there is true optimism that our understanding of PCS will continue to grow and our treatments will become even more effective.

Corresponding Author's Disclaimer

The views expressed in this presentation are those of the author and do not necessarily reflect the official policy or position of the Department of the Navy, Department of Defense, or the US Government. I am a military service member (or employee of the US Government). This work was prepared as part of my official duties. Title 17, USC, §105 provides that "Copyright protection under this title is not available for any work of the U.S. Government." Title 17, USC, §101 defines a US Government work as a work prepared by a military service member or employee of the US Government as part of that person's official duties.

References

1. Mccrory P, Meeuwisse WH, Aubry M, Cantu B, Dvořák J, Echemendia RJ, et al. Consensus statement on concussion in sport: the 4th international conference on concussion in sport held in Zurich, November 2012. Br J Sports Med. 2013;47(5):250–8.
2. Erichsen JE. On railway and other injuries of the nervous system. Philadelphia, PA: Henry C. Lea; 1867. p. 91–103.
3. Keller T. The rise and fall of Erichsen's disease. Spine. 1996;21(13):1597–601.
4. Macleod AD. Post-concussion syndrome: the attraction of the psychological by the organic. Med Hypotheses. 2010;74:1033–5.
5. Strauss I, Savitsky N. Head injury neurologic and psychiatric aspects. Arch Neurol Psychiatr. 1934;31(5):893–955.
6. Evans RW. Persistent post traumatic headache, postconcussion syndrome, and whiplash injuries: the evidence for a non-traumatic basis with historical review. Headache. 2010;50(4):716–24.
7. Lishman WA. Physiogenesis and psychogenesis in the post concessional syndrome. Br J Psychiatry. 1988;153:460–9.
8. Howe LL. Giving context to post deployment post concussive like symptoms: blast related potential mild traumatic brain injury and comorbidities. Clin Neurophysiol. 2009;23:1315–37.
9. Makdissi M, Cantu RC, Johnston KM, McCrory P, Meeuwisse WH. The difficult concussion patient: what is the best approach to investigation and management of persistent (>10 days) postconcussive symptoms? Br J Sports Med. 2013;47(5):308–13.

10. World Health Organization. International statistical classification of diseases and related health problems. 10th ed. Geneva, Switzerland: World Health Organization; 1992.
11. American Psychiatric Association. Diagnostic and statistical manual of mental disorders. 4th ed. Washington, DC: American Psychiatric Association; 1994.
12. Williams WH, Potter S, Ryland H. Mild traumatic brain injury and postconcussion syndrome: a neuropsychological perspective. J Neurol Neurosurg Psychiatry. 2010;81:1116–22.
13. Boake C, McCauley SR, Levin HS, Pedroza C, Contant CF, Song JX, et al. Diagnostic criteria for postconcussional syndrome after mild to moderate traumatic brain injury. J Neuropsychiatry Clin Neurosci. 2005;17(3):350–6.
14. Iverson GL. Misdiagnosis of persistent post-concussion syndrome in patients with depression. Arch Clin Neuropsychol. 2006;21:303–10.
15. Meares S, Shores EA, Taylor AJ, Batchelor J, Bryant RA, Baguley IJ, Chapman J, et al. Mild traumatic brain injury does not predict acute post-concussion syndrome. J Neurol Neurosurg Psychiatry. 2008;79:300–6.
16. Meares S, Shores EA, Taylor AJ, Batchelor RA, Baguley IJ, Chapman J, Gurka J, Marosszeky JE. The prospective course of postconcussion syndrome: the role of mild traumatic brain injury. Neuropsychology. 2011;25(4):454–65.
17. Tsai J, Whealin JM, Cobb Scoff J, Harpaz-Rotem I, Pietzak R. Examining the relation between combat related concussion, a novel 5 factor model of posttraumatic stress symptoms and health related quality of life in Iraq and Afghanistan veterans. J Clin Psychiatry. 2012;73(8): 1110–8.
18. Schneiderman AI, Braver ER, Kang HK. Understanding the sequelae of injury mechanisms and mTBI incurred during conflicts in Iraq and Afghanistan: persistent postconcussive symptoms and post traumatic stress disorder. Am J Epidemiol. 2008;167(12):1446–52.
19. Mickeviciene D, Schrader H, Obelieniene D, Surkiene D, Kunickas R, Stovner LJ, et al. A controlled prospective inception cohort study on the post-concussion syndrome outside the medicolegal context. Eur J Neurol. 2004;11:411–9.
20. Garden N, Sullivan KA. The relationship between personality characteristics and postconcussion symptoms in a nonclinical sample. Neuropsychology. 2009;24(2):168–75.
21. Zakzanis KK, Yeung E. Base rates of post-concussive symptoms in a nonconcussed multicultural sample. Arch Clin Neuropsychol. 2011;26:461–5.
22. Spinos P, Sakellaropoulos G, Georgiopoulos M, Stavridi K, Apostolopoulou K, Ellul J, et al. Postconcussion syndrome after MTBI in Western Greece. J Trauma. 2010;69(4):789–94.
23. Covassin T, Elbin RJ, Harris W, Parker T, Kontos A. The role of age and sex in symptoms, neurocognitive performance, and postural stability in athletes after concussion. Am J Sports Med. 2012;40(6):1303–12.
24. Lange RT, Iverson GL, Rose A. Post-concussion symptom reporting and the "good old days" bias following mTBI. Arch Clin Neuropsychol. 2010;25:442–50.
25. Winn HR. Youman's neurological surgery. In: Zacko JC, Hawryluk GWJ, Bullock R, editors. Neurochemical pathomechanisms in traumatic brain injury. 6th ed. Elsevier; 2011.
26. Lau BC. Which on field signs/symptoms predict protracted recovery from sport related concussion among high school football players? Am J Sports Med. 2011;39:2311–8.
27. Sheedy J, Geffen G, Donnelly J, Faux S. Emergency department assessment of mTBI and prediction of post-concussion symptoms at one month post injury. J Clin Exp Neuropsychol. 2006;28:755–72.
28. Dischinger PC, Ryb GE, Kufera JA, Auman KM. Early predictors of postconcussive syndrome in a population of trauma patients with mild traumatic brain injury. J Trauma. 2008;66(2):289–97.
29. Savola O, Hillborn M. Early predictors of post-concussion symptoms in patients with mild head injury. Eur J Neurol. 2003;10:175–81.
30. Heitger MH, Jones RD, Macleod AD, Snell DL, Frampton CM, Anderson TJ. Impaired eye movements in post-concussion syndrome indicate suboptimal brain function beyond the influence of depression, malingering or intellectual ability. Brain. 2009;132:2850–70.
31. Begaz T, Kyriacou DN, Segal J, Bazarian JJ. Serum biochemical markers for post-concussion syndrome in patients with mTBI. J Neurotrauma. 2006;23(8):1201–10.

32. Korn A, Golan H, Melamed I, Pascual-Marqui R, Friedman A. Focal cortical dysfunction and blood brain barrier disruption in patients with postconcussion syndrome. J Clin Neurophysiol. 2005;22:1–9.

33. Korinthenberg R, Schreck J, Weser J, Lehmkuhl G. Post-traumatic syndrome after minor head injury cannot be predicted by neurological investigations. Brain Dev. 2004;26:113–7.

34. Peskind ER, Petrie EC, Cross DJ, Pagulayan K, McCraw K, Hoff D, et al. Cerebrocerebellar hypometabolism associated with repetitive blast exposure mild traumatic brain injury in 12 Iraq war veterans with persistent post concussive symptoms. Neuroimage. 2011;54(1):576–82.

35. Smits M, Houston GC, Dippel DW, Wielopolski PA, Vernooij MW, Koudstaal PJ, et al. Microstructural brain injury in post-concussion syndrome after minor head injury. Neuroradiology. 2011;53:553–63.

36. Messe A, Caplain S, Pelegrini-Issac M, Blancho S, Montreuil M, Levy R, Benali H. Structural integrity and post-concussion syndrome in mTBI patients. Brain Imaging Behav. 2012; 6:283–92.

37. Smits M, Dippel DW, Houston GC, Wielopolski PA, Koudstaal PJ, Hunink MG, et al. Postconcussion syndrome after minor head injury: brain activation of working memory and attention. Hum Brain Mapp. 2009;30:2789–803.

38. Gagnon I, Galli C, Friedman D, et al. Active rehabilitation for children who are slow to recover following sport-related concussion. Brain Inj. 2009;23:956–64.

39. Leddy JJ, Kozlowski K, Donnelly JP, et al. A preliminary study of subsymptom threshold exercise training for refractory post-concussion syndrome. Clin J Sport Med. 2010;20:21–7.

40. Baker JG, Freitas MS, Leddy JJ, et al. Return to full functioning after graded exercise assessment and progressive exercise treatment of postconcussion syndrome. Rehabil Res Pract. 2012;2012:705309.

41. Leddy JJ, Baker JG, Kozlowski K, et al. Reliability of a graded exercise test for assessing recovery from concussion. Clin J Sport Med. 2011;21:89–94.

42. Gottshall K. Vestibular rehabilitation after mild traumatic brain injury with vestibular pathology. NeuroRehabilitation. 2011;29:167–71.

43. Sayegh AA, Sandford D, Carson AJ. Psychological approaches to treatment of postconcussion syndrome: a systematic review. J Neurol Neurosurg Psychiatry. 2010;81:1128–34.

44. Potter S, Brown RG. Cognitive behavioural therapy and persistent post-concussional symptoms: integrating conceptual issues and practical aspects of treatment. Neuropsychol Rehabil. 2012;22(1):1–25.

45. Petraglia AL, Maroon JC, Bailes JE. From the field of play to the field of combat: a review of the pharmacological management of concussion. Neurosurgery. 2012;70:1520–33.

46. Packard RC. Treatment of chronic daily posttraumatic headache with divalproex sodium. Headache. 2000;40:736–9.

47. Weiss HD, Stern BJ, Goldberg J. Post-traumatic migraine: chronic migraine precipitated by minor head or neck trauma. Headache. 1991;31:451–6.

48. McBeath JG, Nanda A. Use of dihydroergotamine in patients with postconcussion syndrome. Headache. 1994;34:148–51.

49. Giacino JT, Whyte J, Bagiella E, Kalmar K, Childs N, Khademi A, et al. Placebo-controlled trial of amantadine for severe traumatic brain injury. N Engl J Med. 2012;366(9):819–26.

50. Reddy CC, Collins M, Lovell M, et al. Efficacy of amantadine treatment on symptoms and neurocognitive performance among adolescents following sports-related concussion. J Head Trauma Rehabil. 2013;28(4):260–5.

51. Harch PG, Andrews SR, Fogarty EF, Amen D, Pezzullo JC, Lucarini J, et al. A phase I study of low-pressure hyperbaric oxygen therapy for blast-induced post-concussion syndrome and post-traumatic stress disorder. J Neurotrauma. 2012;29(1):168–85.

52. Triebel KL, Martin KC, Novack TA, et al. Treatment consent capacity in patients with traumatic brain injury across a range of injury severity. Neurology. 2012;78(19):1472–8.

53. Kashluba S, Paniak C, Blake T, et al. A longitudinal, controlled study of patient complaints following treated mild traumatic brain injury. Arch Clin Neuropsychol. 2004;19(6):805–16.

Index

S.M. Slobounov and W.J Sebastianelli (eds.), *Concussions in Athletics:*
From Brain to Behavior, DOI 10.1007/978-1-4939-0295-8,
© Springer Science+Business Media New York 2014

Printed by Publishers' Graphics LLC
JCIMO140222.15.16.1